Amebiasis: Diagnosis, Prevention and Treatment

Amebiasis: Diagnosis, Prevention and Treatment

Editor: Kiara Hurst

AMERICAN
MEDICAL PUBLISHERS
www.americanmedicalpublishers.com

AMERICAN
MEDICAL PUBLISHERS
www.americanmedicalpublishers.com

Cataloging-in-Publication Data

Amebiasis : diagnosis, prevention and treatment / edited by Kiara Hurst.
p. cm.
Includes bibliographical references and index.
ISBN 978-1-63927-867-1
1. Amebiasis. 2. Amebiasis--Diagnosis. 3. Amebiasis--Prevention.
4. Amebiasis--Treatment. 5. Protozoan diseases. I. Hurst, Kiara.
RC121.A5 A443 2023
616.9--dc23

American Medical Publishers,
41 Flatbush Avenue,
1st Floor, New York,
NY 11217, USA

ISBN 978-1-63927-867-1 (Hardback)

Contents

Preface

In my initial years as a student, I used to run to the library at every possible instance to grab a book and learn something new. Books were my primary source of knowledge and I would not have come such a long way without all that I learnt from them. Thus, when I was approached to edit this book; I became understandably nostalgic. It was an absolute honor to be considered worthy of guiding the current generation as well as those to come. I put all my knowledge and hard work into making this book most beneficial for its readers.

Amebiasis refers to an infection caused by entamoeba histolytica. There can be several symptoms of amebiasis such as abdominal pain, lethargy, diarrhea, colonic ulcerations, loss of weight, etc. Complications related with amebiasis may involve inflammation and ulceration of the colon with tissue death or perforation that can cause peritonitis. Amebiasis is most commonly transmitted through the fecal-oral route. The disease can also transmit via touching with dirty hands or objects and through anal-oral contact. Preventive measures to avoid amebiasis may include frequently washing hands with soap, improving sanitation, avoiding unhealthy foods, drinking boiled water, avoiding the sharing of towels, etc. There are several ways to treat amebiasis infected tissues, such as nitazoxanide, dehydroemetine and tinidazole. Luminal infection is treatable with iodoquinoline or diloxanide furoate. Efficient treatment to tackle this disease at all stages requires a combination of various medications. The aim of this book is to present researches that have transformed the study of amebiasis, as well as its diagnosis, prevention and treatment. Those in search of information to further their knowledge will be greatly assisted by it.

I wish to thank my publisher for supporting me at every step. I would also like to thank all the authors who have contributed their researches in this book. I hope this book will be a valuable contribution to the progress of the field.

Editor

1

Non-Vesicular Lipid Transport Machinery in *Entamoeba histolytica*

*Koushik Das and Tomoyoshi Nozaki**

Graduate School of Medicine, The University of Tokyo, Bunkyō, Japan

***Correspondence:**
Tomoyoshi Nozaki
nozaki@m.u-tokyo.ac.jp

Eukaryotic cells are organized into separate membrane-bound compartments that have specialized biochemical signature and function. Maintenance and regulation of distinct identity of each compartment is governed by the uneven distribution and intra-cellular movement of two essential biomolecules, lipids, and proteins. Non-vesicular lipid transport mediated by lipid transfer proteins plays a pivotal role in intra-cellular lipid trafficking and homeostasis whereas vesicular transport plays a central role in protein trafficking. Comparative study of lipid transport machinery in protist helps to better understand the pathogenesis and parasitism, and provides insight into eukaryotic evolution. Amebiasis, which is caused by *Entamoeba histolytica,* is one of the major enteric infections in humans, resulting in 40–100 thousand deaths annually. This protist has undergone remarkable alterations in the content and function of its sub-cellular compartments as well represented by its unique diversification of mitochondrion-related organelle, mitosome. We conducted domain-based search on AmoebaDB coupled with bioinformatics analyses and identified 22 potential lipid transfer protein homologs in *E. histolytica*, which are grouped into several sub-classes. Such *in silico* analyses have demonstrated the existence of well-organized lipid transport machinery in this parasite. We summarized and discussed the conservation and unique features of the whole repertoire of lipid transport proteins in *E. histolytica*.

Keywords: lipid, *E. histolytica*, signaling, protozoan parasites, pathogenesis

INTRODUCTION

Eukaryotic cells are organized into distinct membrane-enclosed organelles or compartments. Each organelle has distinctive lipid and protein signature and dedicated function (Holthuis et al., 2003; Lev, 2010). Each cell organelle also assures proper segregation of complex cellular processes catalyzed by metabolic enzymes, structural and regulatory proteins (Lev, 2010). Proteins are precisely distributed to different cell organelles either by their intrinsic signal peptides or through post-translational modifications (Lev, 2010). In contrast, lipids do not have any such signal sequence that determine their accurate intracellular distribution (Lev, 2010). Nevertheless, each organelle differs in its lipid composition (Voelker, 1991; Sprong et al., 2001; Lev, 2010). In general, ER is the main site for lipid synthesis (Blom et al., 2011) and lipids are then transported from ER to site of function. Previous studies suggest that both vesicular and non-vesicular transport machinery are responsible for the delivery of lipids to their final destinations (Lev, 2010). Vesicular transport has an important role in protein trafficking, endocytic and exocytic (secretory) pathways

(Lev, 2010). It is an energy dependent process and involves cytoskeletal reorganization (Lev, 2010). However, significant amount of lipids can be transferred by vesicular transport as lipids are the major component of transport vesicles (Lev, 2010). Nonetheless, lipid transport was still identified when vesicular transport was impaired by either depletion of ATP, reduced temperature, or treatment with pharmacological inhibitors (such as brefeldin A and colchicine) (Kaplan and Simoni, 1985; Vance et al., 1991; Li et al., 2014). Lipid transportation was also detected among cell organelles, those are not linked by vesicular transport machinery (e.g., ER/mitochondria and ER/peroxisomes) (Levine, 2004; Holthuis and Levine, 2005). These observations suggest that non-vesicular transport mechanisms have a significant role in intracellular lipid trafficking. Non-vesicular lipid transport in and between organellar membranes is mostly facilitated by three possible methods: lateral diffusion, trans-bilayer flip-flop, and monomeric lipid exchange (Sleight, 1987; Van Meer, 1989; Lev, 2010). Lateral diffusion is responsible for the lateral movement of lipid in a membrane bilayer (Lev, 2010). Although lateral diffusion mostly transport lipid within membranes, this process was also identified between membranes which are linked via membrane bridges (Lev, 2010). Lipids are moved between two layers of the membrane bilayer by the process called trans-bilayer flip-flop (Lev, 2010). This type of movement takes place either spontaneously or mediates by flippases and translocases (Sprong et al., 2001; Lev, 2010). Trans-bilayer flip-flop do not participate directly in inter-organelle lipid transport (Lev, 2010). It can either encourage non-vesicular lipid transport by monomeric lipid exchange or influence vesicular transport through the alteration of membrane curvature, vesicle budding and fusion (Sprong et al., 2001; Lev, 2006, 2010). Monomeric lipid exchange, the primary mechanism of intra-cellular lipid transport is an energy-independent process (Lev, 2010). In this process, lipid monomer is transported from a donor membrane to an acceptor membrane through the cytosol either spontaneously or facilitated by lipid transfer proteins (LTPs) (Lev, 2010). Spontaneous transport of lipid molecule from donor to the acceptor membrane through cytosol is a time- consuming process and insufficient for substantial transport of major lipids (Jones and Thompson, 1989; Mesmin and Maxfield, 2009; Lev, 2010, 2012).

Non-vesicular lipid transport between cellular membranes are greatly facilitated by LTPs, which are the key contributor of organelle-specific lipid distribution and cellular lipid homeostasis (Helle et al., 2013). LTP-mediated lipid transport locally modulates the lipid composition of membranes and consequently regulates various cellular processes including vesicular trafficking, lipid metabolism, and signal transduction (Ohashi et al., 1995; Kim et al., 2015). Furthermore, LTPs can also act as membrane contact sites (MCSs) between the endoplasmic reticulum (ER) and virtually all other organelles, and are involved in the transport of Ca^{2+}, metabolites, and lipids (Lev, 2010; Helle et al., 2013).

Amebiasis is caused by a protozoan parasite *Entamoeba histolytica* and one of the major enteric infections in humans. An estimated 50 million people are infected with *E. histolytica* worldwide, resulting in 40–100 thousand human deaths annually (Haque et al., 2003; Stanley, 2003; Hung et al., 2012). *In-vivo* growth and survival of *E. histolytica* as an enteric parasite depends on its efficient cellular processes to thrive in adverse host environment (Mittal et al., 2008; Nakada-Tsukui et al., 2009; Vicente et al., 2009). The parasite has two inter-changeable stages consisting of the infective dormant cyst and the proliferative motile trophozoite stages in the life cycle. Inter-conversion between cysts and trophozoites involves complex cellular metabolic processes and essential for transmission of the disease. Lipid and its metabolism apparently play important roles in stage conversion (De Cádiz et al., 2013). Furthermore, this anaerobic or microaerophilic parasite has to overcome a wide variety of environmental and host-derived oxidative and nitrosative stresses during its life cycle (Vicente et al., 2009; Baumel-Alterzon and Ankri, 2014; Pineda and Perdomo, 2017). The pathogenic behavior of this parasite depends on their ability to uptake host nutrients through ingestion and degradation of mammalian cells and tissues. *E. histolytica* trophozoites engulf live and dead host cells through trogocytosis and phagocytosis, respectively (Nakada-Tsukui et al., 2009; Ralston et al., 2014). Contact dependent cytolysis of host cells depends on the secretion of cytolytic proteins, including cysteine proteases (CP) (Que and Reed, 2000) and pore forming peptides (Zhang et al., 2004). Such contact dependent killing and uptake of host cells are likely primed with a receptor-ligand interaction on the surface, which leads to activation of lipid signaling cascades to downstream effectors (Nakada-Tsukui et al., 2009; Somlata et al., 2017).

Lipids can either directly affect the membrane charge and the curvature by their altered local distribution or act as precursors to accelerate the local lipid synthesis by lipid metabolizing enzymes. Furthermore, it has also been established that in the nucleus, distribution and metabolism of lipids and lipid-mediated signaling play essential roles in cell proliferation, differentiation, and stress adaptation in higher eukaryotes (Shah et al., 2013). By analogy, non-vesicular lipid transport mediated by LTPs are likely indispensable for *E. histolytica*. As *E. histolytica* resides in the anaerobic or microaerophilic environment, its mitochondrial functions have highly diverged, resulting in the atypical mitochondrion-related organelles (MROs), called mitosomes, which have drastically modified morphological, structural, and functional features compared to those of the aerobic mitochondria (Makiuchi and Nozaki, 2014). Likewise, *E. histolytica* also lacks well-defined morphologically discernible ER and Golgi apparatus (Perdomo et al., 2016). Lipid transport machinery between such highly divergent organelles in *E. histolytica* could be significantly different from those in the well characterized higher eukaryotes. Thus, investigation on the LTP-mediated lipid transfer in *E. histolytica* should certainly help us to better understand conservation and diversity of this important biological process. Here, we conducted an InterPro domain search (PFAM) analysis on AmoebaDB in order to identify the potential LTP candidates in *E. histolytica.* We also discussed the conservation and unique features of LTPs, and their possible mechanisms and roles in biology and pathophysiology of amebiasis.

GENERAL BACKGROUND OF LIPID TRANSPORT BY LIPID TRANSFER PROTEINS (LTPs)

Domains of LTPs

Non-vesicular lipid transport is catalyzed by LTPs. LTPs can extract lipids from the donor membrane and deliver them to the acceptor membrane. This type of transfer involves a special lipid-transfer domain (LTD) that can form a lipid binding cavity, which binds and accommodate the hydrophobic moieties of lipid molecules from the aqueous environment (Helle et al., 2013). A combination of hydrogen bonds and hydrophobic interactions secure the lipid binding and influence the binding affinity (Lev, 2010). In addition to LTDs, LTPs often possess different combinations of membrane/organelle targeting domains, which direct them to special cellular compartments (Helle et al., 2013), such as pleckstrin homology (PH), protein kinase C (PKC) conserved 1 (C1) and PKC conserved 2 (C2) domains. C1 domain (~50 amino acids, a cysteine-rich compact structure) was first identified in protein kinase C (PKC) as the binding site for di-acyl-glycerol (DAG) and phorbol ester (Cho, 2001). The binding site has cationic residues, which accelerate the Ca^{+2} dependent recruitment and adsorption of the C1 domain to the anionic membrane surfaces (Cho, 2001), while the hydrophobic tip of the domain penetrates the membrane to bind with DAG that is partially buried in the membrane (Cho, 2001). C2 domain (~130 amino acids, Ca^{+2} binding site) was found in PKC, cytosolic phospholipase A_2 (PLA_2), phospholipase C (PLC), phospholipase D (PLD) and phosphoinositide (PtdIns phosphate, PI) 3-Kinase (Cho, 2001). Ca^{+2} ions assist the membrane targeting of C2 domain either through providing a bridge between the C2 domain and anionic phospholipids or induce intra-domain conformational change which in turn triggers membrane protein interactions (Cho, 2001). Sub-cellular localization of C2 domain depends on its phospholipid specificities. C2 domain of PKC prefers anionic phospholipids rapidly translocate to PM, while the C2 domain of PLA_2 is selective to phosphatidylcholine (PC) localized to the perinuclear region in response to Ca^{+2} import (Cho, 2001). LTPs are broadly classified into two major classes based on their domain architecture: (i) cytosolic LTPs, which lack any membrane binding domain, and (ii) membrane anchored LTPs, which contain some membrane binding domain(s) and function to form a MCS. Cytosolic LTPs could possibly facilitate intra-cellular transport of lipid through a sequential process involving interaction of the LTP with donor membrane (Lev, 2012) followed by the opening of hydrophobic cavity, lipid extraction and dissociation of LTP from donor membrane, movement through cytosol in a "closed" transport competent conformation (Kasper and Helmkamp, 1981; Helmkamp, 1986; Nichols, 1988; Rueckert and Schmidt, 1990; Wirtz, 1991; Gadella and Wirtz, 1994; Wirtz et al., 2005; Lev, 2012). The transport is completed by the interaction of LTP with an acceptor membrane, opening of the lipid binding cavity, and desorption of lipid molecule (Lev, 2012) **(Figure 1A)**. In contrast to cytosolic LTPs, LTPs with two targeting domains/motifs for two different organelle membranes are naturally directed to membrane contact sites (MCSs) between these two cellular compartments (Lev, 2010; Helle et al., 2013). Such MCSs bring two membranes from different organelles in a close vicinity (at 10-20 nm), which favor lipid exchange between such closely apposed membranes **(Figure 1B)** and also regulate intra-cellular Ca^{+2} and signaling processes (Levine, 2004; Voelker, 2005; Levine and Loewen, 2006; Giorgi et al., 2009; Lebiedzinska et al., 2009; Lev, 2010).

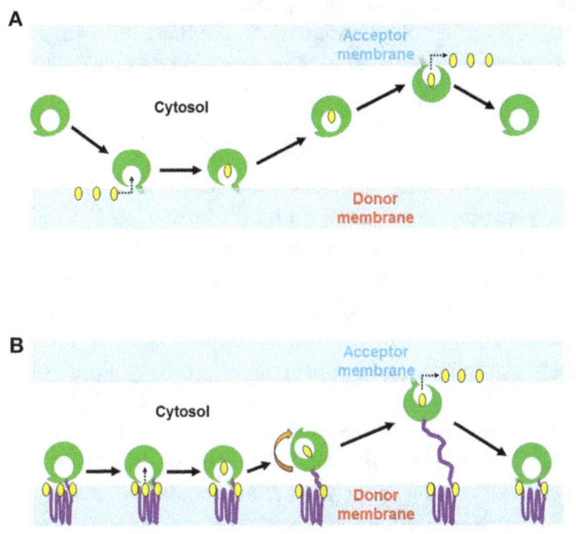

FIGURE 1 | Two proposed mechanisms of lipid transport by lipid transfer proteins (LTPs). **(A)** Lipid conveyance across the cytoplasm by cytosolic LTP. Cytosolic LTP (e.g., STARD containing proteins 1-7) contains only lipid-transfer domain (LTD) (green) but lacks any membrane binding domain. A ligand-free form of LTP interacts with the donor membrane to acquire a lipid molecule (yellow). This interaction induces a conformational change of LTP and opens its lipid binding pocket. Once the lipid molecule (yellow) has occupied the pocket, the protein conformational change occurs again, leading to a lid closure. The ligand-bound form of LTP is targeted to the acceptor membrane to deliver the lipid. **(B)** Lipid transport at MCSs by membrane anchored LTP (e.g., ceramide transfer protein, CERT; oxysterol-binding protein, ORP3). LTP anchors with the donor membrane via its membrane binding domain (purple) and exposes its LTD (green) to the cytoplasm. LTD can extract the lipid molecule (yellow) from the donor membrane and deliver it to a closely positioned acceptor membrane.

Biological Roles of LTPs

LTPs have different modes of action: First, LTPs can facilitate vectorial and often bidirectional lipid transfer as shown in intact living cells and *in vitro* (Helle et al., 2013). Second, LTPs have been recognized as lipid presenting proteins for lipid metabolizing enzymes (Kular et al., 1997, 2002; Cockcroft and Garner, 2013). It can transiently modulates the intracellular lipid metabolism by providing lipid substrates to lipid metabolizing enzymes during signal transduction pathways under various physiological and cellular conditions (Cockcroft and Garner, 2013; Fayngerts et al., 2014). Third, LTPs can act as lipid sensors by altering their affinity to other associated proteins in response to the binding to lipids or bio-membranes (Lev, 2010). Fourth, LTPs can facilitate transient alterations in lipid distribution of a bio-membrane by extracting or delivering of lipid molecules to a certain region of the membrane, or through changing the lipid phase in a particular membrane portion to which it is bound (Lev, 2010). LTP can employ more than one of these mechanisms and regulates the following cellular process (Ohashi et al., 1995; Kim et al., 2015).

Intra-Cellular Lipid Trafficking

Inter-organelle lipid transport facilitated by steroidogenic acute regulatory protein-related lipid transfer (START) domain containing proteins is mostly studied. Mammalian START domain containing proteins are sub-divided into broad sub-families based on their domain organization (membrane targeted and soluble START) and lipid specificities (cholesterol/oxysterol binding proteins and phospholipid/ sphingolipid binding proteins). STARD1 sub-family (contain of STARD1 and STARD3/MLN64) and STARD4 sub-family (comprised of STARD4, STARD5, and STARD6) transport cholesterol to various cell organelles (Alpy and Tomasetto, 2005; Clark, 2012). STARD2 sub-family is composed of STARD2, STARD7, STARD10, and STARD11/CERT (Alpy and Tomasetto, 2005; Clark, 2012). STARD2, 7 and 10 transport PC/PE (Alpy and Tomasetto, 2005; Clark, 2012), while STARD11/CERT transport ceramide from ER to Golgi complex (Alpy and Tomasetto, 2005; Clark, 2012; Kumagai et al., 2014). Among the above mentioned START proteins, STARD3/MLN64 and STARD11/CERT have additional membrane targeted domain, rest possess only STARD domain and are cytosolic (Alpy and Tomasetto, 2005; Clark, 2012).

Lipid Supply for Metabolism and Signal Transduction

The receptor-ligand mediated signaling processes such as trogocytosis, phagocytosis, pinocytosis and exocytosis involves an array of PIs and their metabolizing enzymes (PI 4-kinases, PtdIns4P 5-kinases, PI 3-phosphatases, PI 5-phosphatases, and non-specific phosphatases), residing in various cell organelles (Kölsch et al., 2008; Thomas, 2012; Haastert et al., 2013; Levin et al., 2015). However, PtdIns, the main precursor of PIs is synthesized in the ER and needs to be transported by LTPs (also known as PtdIns transfer proteins, PITPs) to cell organelles for the generation of PIs pools during these cellular processes. PA is produced from diacylglycerol (DAG) by DAG kinases at the plasma membrane (PM), also transported back to the ER by PITPs for replenishment of PtdIns at the ER (Cockcroft and Garner, 2013). This example illustrates that LTPs can function as lipid presenting proteins for lipid metabolizing enzymes and subsequently modulates the lipid metabolism associated with signal transduction pathways under various physiological and cellular conditions.

Lipid Sensing, and Regulation of Vesicular Trafficking

LTPs can function as lipid sensors and regulate Golgi-mediated vesicular trafficking, exocytosis (Litvak et al., 2005; Peretti et al., 2008; Mattjus, 2009), as well explained for Sec14 in *S. cerevisiae* (Curwin et al., 2009). Sec14 involved in intra-cellular transport of either phosphatidylcholine (PC) or phosphatidylinositol (PtdIns) between the ER and the Golgi complex (Bankaitis et al., 1990; Lev, 2010). However, the PtdIns–PC exchange activity of Sec14 is not involved in the Golgi secretory function. Instead, Sec14 functions as PC sensor, can sense the PC level in Golgi and respond to increased PC level by inhibiting its production from diacylglycerol (DAG) through cytidine diphosphate (CDP)-choline pathway (McGee et al., 1994; Skinner et al., 1995; Lev, 2010). In this way, Sec14 regulates a critical level of DAG and PC in Golgi, which is crucial for Golgi mediated vesicular trafficking, exocytosis and viability of *S. cerevisiae* (Bankaitis et al., 1989; Lev, 2010). Sec14 can function as both as a PC sensor and as a PtdIns-presenting protein, which transmits PC metabolic information to PI synthesis (Schaaf et al., 2008; Lev, 2010). Oxysterol-binding-protein-related proteins (ORPs) interact with Rab GTPases and control intra-cellular movement of transport vesicles as described for ORP1L from higher eukaryotes (Johansson et al., 2007; Rocha et al., 2009; Lev, 2010). ORP1L can induce the formation of the membrane contact site (MCS) between the ER and late endosomes, by undergoing conformational changes in response to lower cholesterol content in late endosomes (Johansson et al., 2007; Rocha et al., 2009; Lev, 2010). Priming and docking of the exocytic vesicle complex with the PM also requires an PITP mediated transient alteration in lipid [e.g., PtdIns(4,5)P2] distribution at the site of exocytosis (Lev, 2010; Thomas, 2012).

Modulation of Nuclear Lipid Signaling and Associated Nuclear Functions

A repertoire of lipid (PI, PA, and DAG) metabolizing enzymes, their lipid substrates, byproducts and downstream effectors, involved in various aspects of transcription, chromatin remodeling, mRNA maturation, cell proliferation, differentiation, and stress management (Tanaka et al., 1999; Martelli et al., 2002; Audhya and Scott, 2003; Irvine, 2003; Balla and Balla, 2006; Matsubara et al., 2006; Carman and Henry, 2007; Demmel et al., 2008; Mishkind et al., 2009; Ren et al., 2010; Jang and Min, 2011; Shah et al., 2013; Symeon, 2013; Jülke and Ludwig-Müller, 2015; Karlsson et al., 2016), have been identified in eukaryotic nucleus. In order to maintain the critical level of lipid in the nucleus, the precursor for lipid biosynthetic enzymes needs to be transported to the nucleus by LTPs. Other than function as a lipid exchanger, LTP can interacts with other nuclear associated proteins and regulates the nuclear functions as described for microsomal triglyceride transfer protein, which regulate lipid homeostasis and interacts with RNA helicase DDX3, hepatocyte nuclear factor 4 (HNF4) and small heterodimer partner (SHP) (Tsai et al., 2017). An LTP can also modify nuclear transport via its interaction with a nuclear pore component (Nup62) as described for sterol transporter, ORP8 (Zhou et al., 2011; Béaslas et al., 2012).

Cytoskeleton Organization, Adhesion, and Motility

Several LTP homologs in higher eukaryotes were reported to be associated with cytoskeleton organization, cell adhesion, and motility. For instances, ORP3 and its close relative ORP7 interacts with R-Ras and regulates cytoskeleton organization, cell adhesion, migration (Goldfinger et al., 2007; Weber-Boyvat et al., 2013), while STARD8/12/13 (START proteins with Rho GTPase activating protein (Rho-GAP) domain) are also involved in cytoskeleton organization and migration of a cancer cell line (Alpy and Tomasetto, 2005).

IDENTIFICATION OF LIPID TRANSFER PROTEIN (LTP) HOMOLOGS IN *E. histolytica*

Identification, Domain Organization of *E. histolytica* LTP Homologs

We conducted an InterPro domain search (PFAM) analysis on AmoebaDB version 38 (released 5th July, 2018) in order to identify the potential LTP candidates in *E. histolytica* HM-1:IMSS. The *E. histolytica* HM-1:IMSS genome encodes a diverse repertoire of 22 potential lipid transfer protein (LTP) homologs [four oxysterol-binding-protein-related (ORP) proteins, 15 steroidogenic acute regulatory protein-related lipid transfer (START) proteins, two Sec14 like proteins, and one protein of relevant evolutionary and lymphoid interest (PRELI) domain containing protein] (**Figure 2**) with different E-value (as E-value provided by AmoebaDB). We further verify each of these twenty two potential LTP homologs for possessing of the indicated lipid transfer domain (LTD) [for instances, STARD, ORD, Sec14 and PRELI domains] by NCBI conserved domain search analysis and position of individual domain in each homolog were defined. Twenty two potential LTP homologs were then compared with LTP homologs previously studied in other eukaryotes, in particular, human and *Saccharomyces sp.*, and grouped based on their domain organization (**Figure 2**). Note that information on non-vesicular lipid transport are mostly available in human (Curwin and McMaster, 2008), yeast (Bankaitis et al., 1989, 1990; Im et al., 2005), plant (Li et al., 2016) and little in *Plasmodium sp.* (Van Ooij et al., 2013; Hill et al., 2016)]. Mutual amino acid identities among LTP homologs from *E. histolytica* and their counterparts in human and yeast (as per the classification in **Figure 2**), calculated with ClustalW, revealed that *E. histolytica* LTPs are significantly divergent from those of human and other eukaryotes (Data not shown in this review). A summary table indicates the repertoire of LTP homologs will be analyzed in *E. histolytica* (**Table 1**).

ORPs

E. histolytica possess four ORP homologs (EHI_086250, EHI_050360, EHI_023470, and EHI_074110), which could mediate sterol transport between the ER and other organelles (**Figure 2**). Among four ORP homologs, two of them (EHI_023470 and EHI_074110) contain only ORP-related domain (ORD) and lacks any potential membrane anchoring domain, which indicates that they are likely localized in the cytosol. The two other ORP homologs (EHI_086250 and EHI_050360) possess the PH domain and the diphenylalanine-in-an-acidic-tract (FFAT) motif in the amino terminus and a single TM domain in the carboxyl terminus (**Figure 2**). PH domain is known to interact with specific PIs such as PtdIns4P found on the Golgi membrane and the PM (Helle et al., 2013), while FFAT is known to bind to ER proteins (Helle et al., 2013). Thus, these two TM domain-containing ORP candidates likely act to form a potential MCS between the ER and the Golgi and/or the ER and the PM. They potentially bring these two organelle membranes close enough to facilitate lipid transport as observed in OSBP-mediated sterol transport (Raychaudhuri et al., 2006; Schulz and Prinz, 2007; Raychaudhuri and Prinz, 2010; Olkkonen, 2015) and CERT-mediated ceramide transport at the ER–Golgi MCSs in mammals (Hanada, 2010; Lev, 2010; Kumagai et al., 2014).

START Domain Containing Proteins

Among 15 START domain containing proteins, most of them (except EHI_155260) contain only START domain, which likely indicate their cytosolic localization (**Figure 2**). Only one protein (EHI_155260) has an additional BUD13 domain (**Figure 2**), which was previously reported to have a role in mRNA splicing and retention in higher eukaryotes (Scherrer and Spingola, 2006). EHI_155260 also has the potential NLS and NES, which indicates that it can potentially relocate between the nucleus and the cytoplasm, depending upon physiological and environmental conditions. This domain organization of EHI_155260 is unique to *E. histolytica*. Low mutual similarity among *E. histolytica* START protein homologs (Data not shown in this review) indicate their diverse ligand specificities and functions, as observed in higher eukaryotes (Alpy and Tomasetto, 2005).

Sec14s

E. histolytica has two potential Sec14 homologs (EHI_146930 and EHI_158090), which also possess Ras GTPase activating protein (Ras-GAP) or Rho-GAP, respectively (**Figure 2**). Sec14 protein was first identified in budding yeast, essential for the transport of secretory proteins from the Golgi complex (Mousley et al., 2006; Sirokmány et al., 2006; Curwin et al., 2009). Sec14 homologs possessing Ras- GAP or Rho-GAP domain has also been identified in human (Curwin and McMaster, 2008). p50Rho-GAP/ARH-GAP1 (Sec14 homolog with Rho-GAP domain) (**Figure 2**) is present on the endosomal membrane, where it co-localizes with internalized transferrin receptor (Sirokmány et al., 2006). The Sec14 domain of p50Rho-GAP is essential for its endosomal targeting. p50Rho-GAP forms *in vivo* a complex with Rab5 and Rab11 on endosomal membranes through its Sec14 domain. Thus, Sec14 domain, which was previously known as a phospholipid binding module, mediates protein-protein interactions with Rab and Rho-GTPases and regulates receptor-mediated endocytosis (Sirokmány et al., 2006). *E. histolytica* Sec14 homolog with Rho-GAP domain (EHI_158090) could potentially play a similar function in endocytic and trogo/phagocytic processes.

PRELI Domain Containing Proteins

The *E. histolytica* genome contains a single PRELI-like domain containing protein (EHI_143630) (**Figure 2**), which may be involved in lipid homeostasis of its highly divergent mitochondrion-related organelle, as previously described for aerobic mitochondria from higher eukaryotes (Miliara et al., 2015; Tatsuta and Langer, 2016). *E. histolytica* possesses a highly divergent form of the mitochondrion called mitosome, which is unique in its content and function to *Entamoeba* (Makiuchi and Nozaki, 2014). It is mainly involved in sulfate activation, and important for parasite growth and differentiation (Mi-ichi et al., 2009, 2015). Since, *E. histolytica* do not possess any canonical

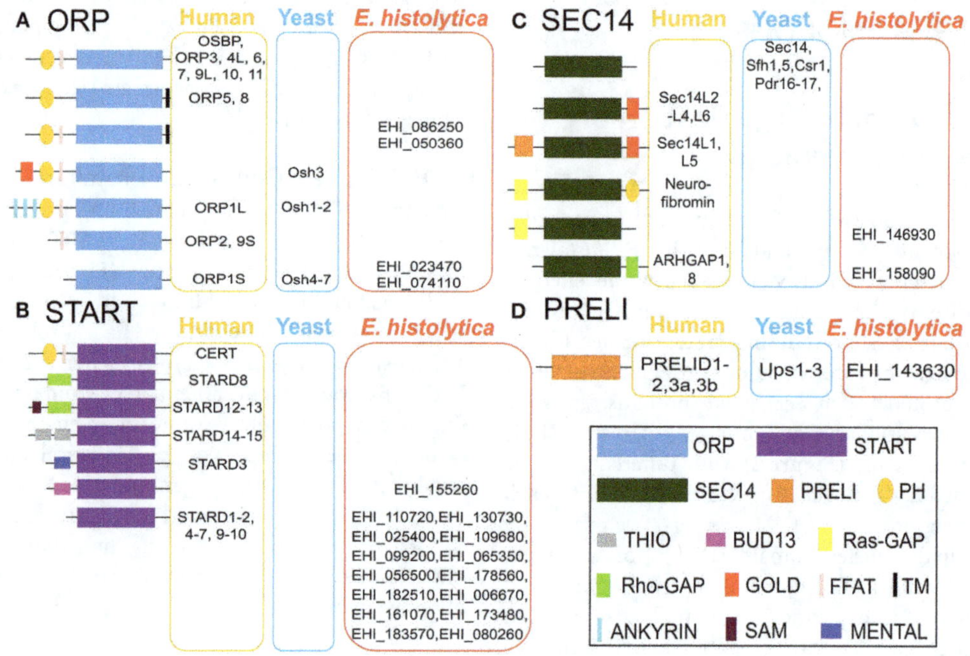

FIGURE 2 | Classification and domain organization of lipid transfer proteins (LTPs) from human, yeast, and *E. histolytica*. Based on domain organization and cellular localization, LTPs are classified into cytosolic and membrane-bound LTPs. Cytosolic LTPs possess only lipid transfer domains (LTDs) such as oxysterol-binding protein (OSBP)-related domain (ORD, bind to sterols and to PtdIns4P), steroidogenic acute regulatory protein (StAR)-related lipid transfer (START) domain (bind to either sterols, phospholipids, or ceramides), Sec14 domain (bind to PC and PtdIns), and protein of relevant evolutionary and lymphoid interest (PRELI domain, binds to PA), all of which can shelter the hydrophobic moieties of various lipid ligands from the aqueous environment. Membrane bound LTPs have various combinations of LTDs with other additional membrane-anchored domains/motifs such as pleckstrin-homology (PH) domain, diphenylalanine-in-an-acidic-tract (FFAT) motif, Golgi dynamics (GOLD) domain, function as membrane contact sites (MCSs). *E. histolytica* genome has 22 potential LTP homologs, **(A)** four OSBP-related protein (ORP), **(B)** 15 START, **(C)** two Sec14, and **(D)** single PRELI candidates. AmoebaDB ID of *E. histolytica* LTP homologs are shown.

mitochondria (Makiuchi and Nozaki, 2014), it will be interesting to study whether function of PRELI homolog in *E. histolytica* (EHI_143630) is evolutionary conserved or it has a distinct cellular function unique to this protozoan parasite.

Other Proteins Known to Be Involved in Lipid Transfer in Other Organisms, but Missing in *E. histolytica*

E. histolytica lacks some of LTP homologs known to be present and functional in other eukaryotes (**Figure 2**). *E. histolytica* has no homologs for human PITPs, similar as *Saccharomyces sp.* (Nile et al., 2010). The *Saccharomyces* genomes contain several Sec14 homologs that function as PITPs (Phillips et al., 2006). *E. histolytica* possesses a panel of START domain protein homologs, some of which could potentially function as PITP as reported in *Plasmodium falciparum* (Van Ooij et al., 2013; Hill et al., 2016). *E. histolytica* also lacks a homolog of eukaryotic synaptotagmin-like, mitochondrial and PH domain (SMP) containing proteins (Helle et al., 2013). In yeast SMP-containing homologs (Nvj2, Tcb1, Tcb2 and Tcb3) are localized at various MCSs, which indicates their common function at MCSs (Helle et al., 2013). Moreover, the ER–mitochondria encounter structure (ERMES) components (the ER protein, Mmm1, the cytosolic protein, Mdm12, and the OMM protein, Mdm34) also possess SMP domain (Helle et al., 2013). Since the *E. histolytica* genome encodes none of ERMES components and other SMP homologs (**Figure 2**), it is plausible that some LTP homologs could potentially function at the MCSs. It is known in other organisms that some LTP homologs with unique domain organization are unique to a particular organism. For instance, Osh3 (of ORP sub-class), Sec14, Pdr16, Pdr 17, Sfh1 and Sfh5 (of Sec14 sub-class) are unique to yeast (**Figure 2**). Similarly, EHI_155260 (of START sub-class), EHI_086250 and EHI_050360 (of ORP sub-class) are unique to *E. histolytica* (**Figure 2**).

mRNA Expression of LTP Homologs in *E. histolytica* HM-1:IMSS

Relative steady-state levels of mRNA expression of a panel of 22 potential LTP homologs from *E. histolytica* (15 START proteins, 4 ORPs, 2 Sec14s and 1 PRELI domain proteins) were investigated using data available at AmoebaDB (Hon et al., 2013). Three members of *E. histolytica* START protein homologs showed higher mRNA expression in HM-1:IMSS compared to other LTP candidates (in a descending order of EHI_080260, EHI_161070, and EHI_173480) (**Figure 3**). Three START protein homologs (EHI_182510, EHI_155260 and EHI_130730) showed very low levels of expression (**Figure 3**). Interestingly, the reptilian sibling *Entamoeba* species, *E. invadens*, has two EHI_155260 homologs (EIN_257190, EIN_107840). Similar patterns of upregulation of these two gene transcripts were observed during encystation

TABLE 1 | The repertoire of LTP homologs from *E. histolytica* identified and analyzed in this study.

LTP homolog[a]	Accession number[b]	Domain organization[c]
START	EHI_110720, EHI_130730, EHI_025400, EHI_109680, EHI_099200, EHI_065350, EHI_056500, EHI_178560, EHI_182510, EHI_006670, EHI_161070, EHI_173480, EHI_183570, EHI_080260	START[e]
	EHI_155260	BUD13[f], START
ORP	EHI_023470, EHI_074110	ORP[g]
	EHI_086250, EHI_050360	PH[h], FFAT[i], ORP, TM[j]
Sec14	EHI_146930	Ras-GAP[k], Sec14[l]
	EHI_158090	Sec14, Rho-GAP[m]
PRELI	EHI_143630	PRELI[n]

Twenty two potential LTP homologs of E. histolytica, their accession numbers and domain structure. Refer to ***Figure 2*** *for classification and domain organization.*
[a]*LTP homolog in E. histolytica as per AmoebaDB database.*
[b]*AmoebaDB ID.*
[c]*Domain organization based on NCBI conserved domain search analysis.*
[e]*steroidogenic acute regulatory protein-related lipid transfer (START) domain.*
[f]*BUD (BurrH domain) 13 domain.*
[g]*oxysterol-binding-protein-related (ORP) domain.*
[h]*pleckstrin-homology (PH) domain.*
[i]*diphenylalanine-in-an-acidic-tract (FFAT) motif.*
[j]*Transmembrane (TM) domain.*
[k]*Ras-GAP domain.*
[l]*Sec14 domain.*
[m]*Rho-GAP domain.*
[n]*protein of relevant evolutionary and lymphoid interest (PRELI) domain.*

(data not shown) (De Cádiz et al., 2013), which indicates their potential roles in cell differentiation, as previously shown for LTP during somatic embryogenesis in *Arabidopsis thaliana* (Potocka et al., 2012). Among 4 ORP candidates, EHI_023470 and EHI_074110 are more highly expressed than EHI_086250 and EHI_050360 (**Figure 3**). Two Sec14 homologs (EHI_146930 and EHI_158090) showed relatively low expression levels among all identified LTP candidates (**Figure 3**).

BIOLOGICAL SIGNIFICANCE OF LIPID TRANSFER IN *E. histolytica*

Previous Reports on Lipids and Their Trafficking in *E. histolytica*

The structure and PM components of *E. histolytica* were studied previously (Espinosa-Cantellano and Martínez-Palomo, 1991), which has identified several surface antigens, adherence proteins, amoebic enzymes (for instances, collagenase, phospholipase A, neuraminidase, cysteine proteases) and fibronectin receptor. PM of *E. histolytica*, enriched in cholesterol, phosphatidylethanolamine (PE), ceramide aminoethyl phosphonate (CAEP) was also reported (Espinosa-Cantellano and Martínez-Palomo, 1991). Previous studies on lipids in *E. histolytica* mostly suggested their roles in parasite growth, proliferation, differentiation, and virulence. It was shown that PC-cholesterol liposomes enabled *in vitro* cultured trophozoites to retain their virulence-associated biological functions such as endocytosis, erythrophagocytosis, expression of surface molecules, protease activity, and liver abscess formation in hamsters. This indicates the contribution of lipids to parasite virulence (Serrano-Luna et al., 2010). Both the unique phospholipid compositions and the high cholesterol content in the amoebic membranes were shown to protect the parasite from self-destruction by its own pore-forming toxins (Andrä et al., 2004). Castellanos-Castro et al. has recently shown that lysobisphosphatidic acid is generally involved in endocytosis (i.e., pinocytosis and erythrophagocytosis). Lysobisphosphatidic acid was demonstrated to be localized in Rab7A positive vesicles in quiescent (non-phagoctytic) conditions and during a late phase of erythrophagocytosis (Castellanos-Castro et al., 2015). It was shown that lipopeptidophosphoglycan (EhLPPG) is also involved in adherence of *E. histolytica* trophozoites to intestinal epithelial cells, similar to other adhesive molecules like, Gal/GalNAc lectin, serine rich *E. histolytica* proteins (SREHP), and lysine glutamic acid rich protein 1 (KERP1) (Stanley et al., 1990; Dodson et al., 1999; Lauwaet et al., 2004; Seigneur et al., 2005). EhLPPG is also recognized by both the innate and the adaptive immune systems and stimulates cytokine production from human monocytes, macrophages, and dendritic cells (Wong-Baeza et al., 2010). EhLPPG induces *in vitro* formation of human neutrophil extracellular traps (NETs) (Ávila et al., 2016). Sulfolipids are one of the terminally synthesized bio-molecules of sulfur metabolism, shown to play an important role in trophozoites proliferation and differentiation processes (Mi-Ichi et al., 2017). For instance, fatty alcohol disulfates plays a crucial role in trophozoites proliferation (Mi-Ichi et al., 2017). Cholesteryl sulfate, another sulfolipid plays a central role in encystation, a differentiation process from the motile trophozoites to the dormant cysts (Mi-Ichi et al., 2017). Furthermore, sulfur metabolism, in which sulfolipids are generated, is not conserved in other free-living amoebae, indicating a causal relationship of sulfur metabolism with parasitism (Mi-Ichi et al., 2017). Lysophosphatidylinositol was shown to stimulate natural killer T (NKT) cells and to induce selective production of IFN-γ but not IL-4 in a CD1-d restricted manner in murine systems (Aiba et al., 2016).The

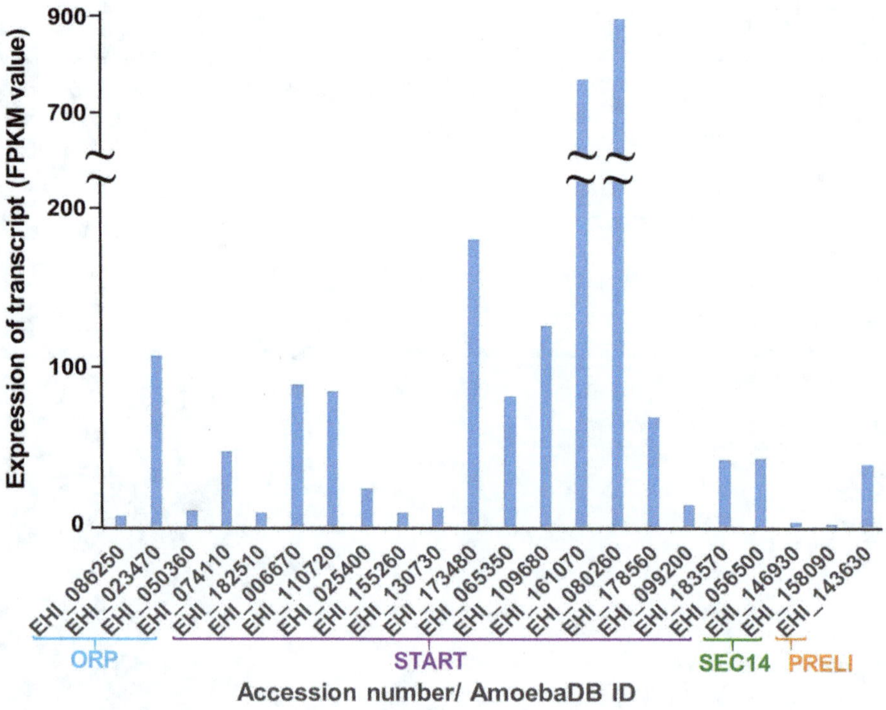

FIGURE 3 | Relative mRNA expression of LTP homologs in *E. histolytica* HM-1:IMSS. Survey of the *E. histolytica* genome has identified a total of 22 LTP homologs. The levels of mRNA expression are shown with FPKM (fragments per kilobase of exon per million fragments mapped) value as per AmoebaDB. Three members of *E. histolytica* START protein homologs (EHI_080260 followed by EHI_161070 and EHI_173480) show the highest mRNA expression in HM-1:IMSS strain among all LTP candidates. Among 4 ORP candidates, EHI_023470, and EHI_074110, both of which contain only ORD and are possibly cytosolic (see **Figure 2** for their classification and domain organization), show higher levels of expression compared to the two remaining membrane-bound LTP homologs (EHI_086250 and EHI_050360). Sec14 homologs (EHI_146930 and EHI_158090) show low expression levels among all identified LTP candidates.

localization of PI (3,4,5)-trisphosphate [PI(3,4,5)P3 or PIP(3)] in *E. histolytica* during various endocytic processes was studied using glutathione S-transferase (GST)- and green fluorescent protein (GFP)-labeled PH domains as lipid biosensors (Byekova et al., 2010). PIP(3) specific biosensor was accumulated at extending pseudopods and also localized in the phagocytic cup during erythrophagocytosis. However, no such localization of the biosensor was observed in pinocytic compartment during pinocytosis. *E. histolytica* maintains a high steady state level of PIP(3) in its PM irrespective of serum concentration (Byekova et al., 2010).

However, non-vesicular lipid transport machinery and the function of LTPs remained largely unexplored in *E. histolytica*. There are two previous reports where the lipid trafficking in *E. histolytica* was described (Pina-Vázquez et al., 2014; Bolaños et al., 2016). Piña- Vázquez et al. identified a START domain containing protein in *E. histolytica* (EHI_110720, also present in our list of *E. histolytica* LTP homologs) and named it as *E. histolytica* phosphatidylcholine transfer protein-like (EhPCTP-L). They identified EhPCTP-L by virtue of interaction with anti-chicken embryo caveolin-1 monoclonal antibody, which indicates their potential role in caveola-mediated endocytosis. EhPCTP-L mainly binds to anionic phospholipids phosphatidylserine (PS) and PA, and is localized to the PM and the cytosol (Pina-Vázquez et al., 2014). However, the essential biochemical characteristics as LTPs, i.e., lipid transport activity, was not reported in this study. START protein homolog (EHI_178560) of *E. histolytica* is essential for parasite growth as observed in the previous study by Solis et al. Double stranded RNA (dsRNA) mediated silencing of EHI_178560 causes growth retardation of *E. histolytica* trophozoites (Solis et al., 2009). Mfotie et al. also reported that plant derivatives that showed anti-amoebic activity also caused the repression of gene expression of another START homolog (EHI_161070) of *E. histolytica* (Mfotie Njoya et al., 2014). Bolaños et al. recently reported that *E. histolytica* NPC1 (EhNPC1) and EhNPC2 proteins responsible for the trafficking of exogenous cholesterol in *E. histolytica* trophozoites and also influence the phagocytosis process (Bolaños et al., 2016). However, these previous studies only partially characterized the roles of LTPs in the trafficking of ingested lipids in *Entamoeba*. The complex network of intra-cellular lipid transport machinery mediated by diverse LTP homologs in *E. histolytica* remains elusive.

Predicted Roles of LTPs in *E. histolytica*

Role of *E. histolytica* LTPs in Phagocytosis, Trogocytosis, Endocytosis, Signal Transduction, and Lipid Presentation

E. histolytica is highly capable of engulfment of the host cells and microorganisms by two distinct processes. In phagocytosis, the parasite engulfs the dead host cells and bacteria as whole, while in trogocytosis the parasite nibbles parts of the live host cells (Nakada-Tsukui et al., 2009; Ralston et al., 2014; Somlata et al., 2017). These two distinct cellular processes are initiated by being triggered by different ligands (on dead/live host cells and microorganisms), and likely activate similar but different cascades of events (Somlata et al., 2017). It is possible that different LTPs may be selectively involved in phagocytosis and trogocytosis. Similarly, *Entamoeba* also depends on receptor-mediated endocytosis/pinocytosis for the transport of nutrients from the extracellular environment (Avalos-Padilla et al., 2015). Such receptor-ligand mediated signaling process is often initiated by PIs (Nakada-Tsukui et al., 2009; Somlata et al., 2017).

E. histolytica possess several classes of PI metabolizing enzymes such as: PtdIns 4-kinase (EHI_148700) and PtdIns4P 5-kinases (EHI_153770, EHI_049480), and a panel of PI phosphatases (14 isotypes of PI 3-phosphatase, 6 isotypes of PI 5- phosphatase, and 3 isotypes of non-specific PI phosphatase). Identification of a repertoire of PI kinases and phosphatases enforces the notion that *E. histolytica* LTPs also participate in the constant replenishment of PIs at all cellular compartments at various physiological conditions. *E. histolytica* also possesses 5 putative DAG kinases (data not shown), thus is able to produce PA from DAG. This is consistent with the hypothesis that the reciprocal transport of PtdIns and PA between the ER and the PM (Cockcroft and Garner, 2013) occurs and is mediated by some members of LTPs as lipid presenting proteins.

Role of *E. histolytica* LTPs in the Secretion of Hydrolytic Enzymes and Regulation of Vesicular Trafficking

Trafficking and secretion of lysosomal hydrolases such as CPs contributes to both cytolysis of host tissues and degradation of internalized host cells and microorganisms (Nakada-Tsukui et al., 2005; Mitra et al., 2007). Thus, vesicular trafficking that regulates intracellular CP transport plays a pivotal role in virulence and parasitism of *E. histolytica*. CP trafficking and secretion are regulated via cysteine protease binding family protein (CPBF) 1 (Furukawa et al., 2012; Nakada-Tsukui et al., 2012; Marumo et al., 2014), Rab GTPases (Saito-Nakano et al., 2004, 2005; Mitra et al., 2007; Hanadate et al., 2016), the retromer-like complex (Nakada-Tsukui et al., 2005), and intrinsic CP inhibitors (Sato et al., 2006), and also presumably by priming and docking of CP-containing vesicles with the exo-cyst complex that tethers at the site of exocytosis on the PM (Nakada-Tsukui et al., 2005). As LTPs can function as lipid sensors to regulate Golgi-mediated (or post-Golgi) vesicular trafficking, as above explained for Sec14, it is possible that two Sec14 homologs (EHI_146930 and EHI_158090) that also possess either Rho-GAP or Ras-GAP domain **(Figure 2)** can regulate the Golgi-mediated secretory function, in a similar mechanism as described previously (Curwin et al., 2009). The four ORP homologs **(Figure 2)** may interact with Rab GTPase and control trafficking of the transport vesicles as described for ORP1L in higher eukaryotes (Johansson et al., 2007).

Role of *E. histolytica* LTPs in Nuclear Lipid Transport and Signaling

The nucleus plays indispensable roles in cell proliferation, differentiation, and stress management (Shah et al., 2013). Stage conversion between the two forms in the life cycle requires remarkable alterations in cellular components, metabolism, transcriptional, and post- transcriptional/translational regulations of gene expression, and involves a complex and dynamic signaling events induced by extracellular stimuli (Mittal et al., 2008; Vicente et al., 2009; De Cádiz et al., 2013). Moreover, *E. histolytica* is also harassed by a wide variety of environmental and host-derived stresses, such as fluctuation in glucose concentrations, changes in pH, pO2, temperature, and attack by oxidative and nitrosative stresses from neutrophils and macrophages (Husain et al, 2010; Husain et al., 2012; Nagaraja and Ankri, 2018). *E. histolytica* senses extracellular stress and accordingly makes necessary amendment in its physiology and metabolism for survival and transmission.

Although the lipid transport, metabolism and signaling in the nucleus and the roles of LTPs in nuclear associated functions are largely unknown, it is conceivable that one START domain containing protein (EHI_155260), which possess BUD13 domain and potential NLS and NES, is involved in nuclear lipid transport, more specifically shuttling between the nucleus and the cytoplasm, and signaling, and thus may be important for growth, stage conversion, and/or evasion from various stresses. In addition, some of the PI and PA metabolizing enzymes in *E. histolytica* (data not shown here) contain putative NLS and NES, indicating their potential roles in nuclear lipid homeostasis by nuclear-cytoplasmic shuttling, as well described in higher eukaryotes (Davis et al., 2015). The *E. histolytica* genome encodes a few PI-binding downstream effectors including a plant homeodomain (PHD) finger-containing protein (EHI_138970), which also contains NLS. Thus, it is conceivable that a panel of these proteins coordinately function in the nucleus. As mentioned above (3.2), *E. invadens* apparently possesses two homologs (EIN_257190, EIN_107840) of the BUD13/NLS/NES-containing START domain containing protein (a single protein in *E. histolytica*, EHI_155260). These *E. invadens* genes showed upregulation of gene expression during encystation (De Cádiz et al., 2013), which indicates their potential role in the nucleus during differentiation, as observed in other eukaryotes (Potocka et al., 2012).

Role of *E. histolytica* LTPs in Motility, Adherence, and Cytoskeletal Reorganization

It is conceivable that two SEC14 homologs containing Rho-GAP and Ras-GAP (EHI_146930 and EHI_158090, respectively) are involved in cytoskeletal reorganization associated with cell motility and adherence to the host cells and microorganisms. The genome of *E. histolytica* also contains four ORP (EHI_086250, EHI_050360, EHI_023470, and EHI_074110), 15 START domain homologs other than Sec14 (**Figure 2**). ORP homologs might be associated with cytoskeleton organization, cell adhesion, and motility, as reported in higher eukaryotes (Goldfinger et al., 2007) and previously discussed in section Cytoskeleton organization, adhesion, and motility Other than ORP, a few

START domain homologs could also be associated with cytoskeletal reorganization and migration, as previously reported in a cancer cell line (Alpy and Tomasetto, 2005). Adhesion with the host gut epithelia and migration through the tight junction between host cells are two key pathogenic processes presented by *E. histolytica* trophozoites (Tavares et al., 2005; Franco-Barraza et al., 2006), which also involve the receptor-ligand mediated signaling cascades, in which PIs play indispensable roles.

CONCLUDING REMARKS

We have discovered a panel of conserved and lineage-specific LTPs in *E. histolytica* by domain-based survey of LTP homologs in AmoebaDB. The *E. histolytica* genome possess single PRELI domain containing protein (EHI_143630). It is worth investigating whether this PRELI domain containing protein is involved in mitosomal transport. *E. histolytica* possess a single START domain containing protein (EHI_155260) with potential NLS and NES, indicating its potential role as a nuclear lipid transporter and its ability of nucleocytoplasmic shuttling depending upon physiological conditions. Upregulation of gene expression of its two homologs (EIN_257190, EIN_107840) in *E. invadens* during encystation (De Cádiz et al., 2013), indicates its potential role in cell differentiation as well as disease transmission. The *E. histolytica* genome possess a repertoire of START domain containing proteins. Some of them can function as potential PITP similarly as in *Plasmodium* sp. (Van Ooij et al., 2013; Hill et al., 2016). This is also conceivable because phosphoinositides are the essential signaling phospholipids for *E. histolytica*, which depends greatly on receptor-ligand mediated signaling processes. On the other hand, *E. histolytica* lacks canonical PITP homologs from higher eukaryotes. Furthermore, *E. histolytica* lacks any homologs of SMP containing proteins, which are involved in the organization of various MCSs and ERMES complex (Helle et al., 2013). The absence of canonical mitochondria, ER, and Golgi apparatus, in the forms found in higher eukaryotes, could possibly justify this observation. The identified LTP repertoire encompassing ORP, START, SEC14, and PRELI present in *E. histolytica* ensures the complexity and biological significance of LTPs in a variety of cellular processes: lipid transport between cellular compartments, adherence, phagocytosis, trogocytosis, endocytosis, signal transduction, vesicular traffic, cytoskeletal reorganization, nuclear regulation, lipid presentation, and sensing. Further studies are needed to elucidate the role of individual LTPs on the biology and pathogenesis of this parasite. Once *E. histolytica*-specific LTPs and lipid transfer mechanisms are identified, they may potentially provide a novel drug target against this medically important parasite. Since most of existent chemical interventions against lipid signaling pathways target particular lipid metabolizing enzymes (Nile et al., 2014; Khan et al., 2016), such intervention often exerts specific and limited overall effects to the eukaryotic cells, e.g., cancer cells. In addition, parasitic organisms often have highly adaptable nature and a bypass mechanism to overcome the effects caused by various chemical insults, results in the generation of drug resistance. Thus, chemical inhibition of parasite-specific LTPs might be a reasonable solution to the problem because LTPs are involved in a wide range of multiple cellular processes described above.

AUTHOR CONTRIBUTIONS

All authors listed have made a substantial, direct and intellectual contribution to the work, and approved it for publication.

ACKNOWLEDGMENTS

We acknowledge The Tokyo Biochemical Research Foundation (TBRF) for providing TBRF postdoctoral fellowship for foreign researchers for KD (TBRF-RF17-105). This work was supported in part by Grants-in-Aid from TBRF (TBRF-RF17-105), Grant-in- Aid for Challenging Exploratory Research (17K19416) and Grant-in-Aid for Scientific Research (B) (18H02650) from the Japan Society for the Promotion of Science, and a grant for Research Program on Emerging and Re-emerging Infectious Diseases from the Japan Agency for Medical Research and Development (AMED) (JP17fk0108119) to TN.

REFERENCES

Aiba, T., Sato, M., Umegaki, D., Iwasaki, T., Kambe, N., Fukase, K., et al. (2016). Regioselective phosphorylation of myo-inositol with BINOL-derived phosphoramidites and its application for protozoan Lysophosphatidylinositol. *Org. Biomol. Chem.* 14:6672. doi: 10.1039/C6OB01062H

Alpy, F., and Tomasetto, C. (2005). Give lipids a START: the StAR-related lipid transfer (START) domain in mammals. *J. Cell Sci.* 118, 2791–2801. doi: 10.1242/jcs.02485

Andrä, J., Berninghausen, O., and Leippe, M. (2004). Membrane lipid composition protects *Entamoeba histolytica* from self-destruction by its pore-forming toxins. *FEBS Lett.* 564, 109–115. doi: 10.1016/S0014-5793(04)00324-2

Audhya, A., and Scott, D. (2003). Regulation of PI4,5P2 synthesis by nuclear-cytoplasmic shuttling of the Mss4 lipid kinase. *EMBO J.* 22, 4223–4236. doi: 10.1093/emboj/cdg397

Avalos-Padilla, Y., Betanzos, A., Javier-Reyna, R., García-Rivera, G., Chávez-Munguía, B., Lagunes-Guillén, A., et al. (2015). EhVps32 Is a vacuole-associated protein involved in pinocytosis and phagocytosis of *Entamoeaba histolytica*. *PLoS Pathog.* 11:e1005079. doi: 10.1371/journal.ppat.1005079

Ávila, E. E., Salaiza N, Pulido, J., Rodríguez, M. C., Díaz-Godínez, C., Laclette, J. P., et al. (2016).*Entamoeba histolytica* trophozoites and lipopeptidophosphoglycan trigger human neutrophil extracellular traps. *PLoS ONE* 11:e0158979. doi: 10.1371/journal.pone.0158979

Balla, A., and Balla, T. (2006). Phosphatidylinositol 4-kinases: old enzymes with emerging functions. *Trends Cell Biol.* 16, 351–361. doi: 10.1016/j.tcb.2006.05.003

Bankaitis, V. A., Aitken, J. R., Cleves, A. E., and Dowhan, W. (1990). An essential role for a phospholipid transfer protein in yeast Golgi function. *Nature* 347, 561–562. doi: 10.1038/347561a0

Bankaitis, V. A., Malehorn, D. E., Emr, S. D., and Greene, R. (1989). The Saccharomyces cerevisiae SEC14 gene encodes a cytosolic factor that is required for transport of secretory proteins from the yeast Golgi complex. *J. Cell Biol.* 108, 1271–1281. doi: 10.1083/jcb.108.4.1271

Baumel-Alterzon, S., and Ankri, S. (2014). *Entamoeba histolytica* adaptation to glucose starvation: a matter of life and death. *Curr. Opin. Microbiol.* 20, 139–145. doi: 10.1016/j.mib.2014.06.005

Béaslas, O., Vihervaara, T., Li, J., Laurila, P. P., Yan, D., and Olkkonen, V. M. (2012). Silencing of OSBP-related protein 8 (ORP8) modifies the macrophage transcriptome, nucleoporinp62 distribution, and migration capacity. *Exp. Cell Res.* 318, 1933–1945 doi: 10.1016/j.yexcr.2012.05.026

Blom, T., Somerharju, P., and Ikonen, E. (2011). Synthesis and biosynthetic trafficking of membrane lipids. *Cold Spring Harb. Perspect. Biol.* 8:a004713. doi: 10.1101/cshperspect.a004713

Bolaños, J., Betanzos, A., Javier-Reyna, R., García- Rivera, G., Huerta, M., Pais-Morales, J., et al. (2016). EhNPC1 and EhNPC2 proteins participate in trafficking of exogenous cholesterol in Entamoeba histolytica Trophozoites: relevance for phagocytosis. *PLoS Pathog.* 12:e1006089. doi: 10.1371/journal.ppat.1006089

Byekova, Y. A., Powell, R. R., Welter, B. H., and Temesvari, L. A. (2010). Localization of phosphatidylinositol (3,4,5) triphosphate to phagosome in *Entamoeba histolytica* achieved using glutathione S-transferase and green fluorescent protein tagged lipid biosensors. *Infect. Immun.* 78:125–137. doi: 10.1128/IAI.00719-09

Carman, M., and Henry, S. A. (2007). Phosphatidic acid plays a central role in the transcriptional regulation of glycerophospholipid synthesis in *Saccharomyces cerevisiae*. *J. Biol. Chem.* 282, 37293–37297. doi: 10.1074/jbc.R700038200

Castellanos-Castro, S., Cerda-García-Rojas, C. M., Javier-Reyna, R., Pais-Morales, J., Chávez-Munguía, B., and Orozco, E. (2015). Identification of the phospholipid lysobisphosphatidic acid in the protozoan Entamoeba histolytica: An active molecule in endocytosis. *Biochem. Biophys. Rep.* 5,224–236. doi: 10.1016/j.bbrep.2015.12.010

Cho, W. (2001). Membrane targeting by C1 and C2 domains. *J. Biol. Chem.* 276, 32407–32410. doi: 10.1074/jbc.R100007200

Clark, B. J. (2012). The mammalian START domain protein family in lipid transport in health and disease. *J. Endocrinol.* 212, 257–275. doi: 10.1530/JOE-11-0313

Cockcroft, S., and Garner, K. (2013). Potential role for phosphatidylinositol transfer protein (PITP) family in lipid transfer during phospholipase C signaling. *Adv. Biol. Regul.* 53, 280–291. doi: 10.1016/j.jbior.2013.07.007

Curwin, A., and McMaster, C. (2008). Structure and function of the enigmatic Sec14 domain-containing proteins and the etiology of human disease. *Future Lipidol.* 4, 399–410. doi: 10.2217/17460875.3.4.399

Curwin, A. J., Fairn, G. D., and McMaster, C. R. (2009). Phospholipid transfer protein sec14 is required for trafficking from endosomes and regulates distinct trans-golgi export pathways. *J. Biol. Chem.* 284, 7364–7375. doi: 10.1074/jbc.M808732200

Davis, W. J., Lehmann, P. Z., and Li, W. (2015). Nuclear PI3K signaling in cell growth and tumorigenesis. *Front. Cell Dev. Biol.* 3:24. doi: 10.3389/fcell.2015.00024

De Cádiz, A. E., Jeelani, G., Nakada-Tsukui, K., Caler, E., and Nozaki, T. (2013).Transcriptome analysis of encystation in Entamoeba invadens. *PLoS ONE* 8:e74840 doi: 10.1371/journal.pone.0074840

Demmel, L., Mike Beck, M., Christian Klose, C., Anne-Lore Schlaitz, A. L., Yvonne, G., and Peggy, P., et al (2008). Nucleocytoplasmic shuttling of the golgi phosphatidylinositol 4-kinase Pik1 is regulated by 14-3-3 proteins and coordinates golgi function with cell growth. *MBoC* 19, 1046–1061. doi: 10.1091/mbc.E07-02-0134

Dodson, J. M., Lenkowski, P. W. Jr, Eubanks, A. C., Jackson, T. F., Napodano, J., Lyerly, D. M., et al. (1999). Infection and immunity mediated by the carbohydrate recognition domain of the *Entamoeba histolytica* Gal/GalNAc lectin. *J. Infect. Dis.* 179, 460–466. doi: 10.1086/314610

Espinosa-Cantellano, M., and Martínez-Palomo, A. (1991). The plasma membrane of *Entamoeba histolytica:* structure and dynamics. *Biol Cell.* 72, 189–200. doi: 10.1111/j.1768-322X.1991.tb03015.x

Fayngerts, S. A., Wu, J., Oxley, C. L., Liu, X., Vourekas, A., Cathopoulis, T., et al. (2014). TIPE3 is the transfer protein of lipid second messengers that promote cancer. *Cancer Cell.* 26, 465–478. doi: 10.1016/j.ccr.2014.07.025

Franco-Barraza, J., Zamudio-Meza, H., Franco, E., del Carmen Domínguez-Robles, M., Villegas-Sepúlveda, N., and Meza, I. (2006). Rho signaling in Entamoeba histolytica modulates actomyosin-dependent activities stimulated during invasive behavior. *Cell Motil. Cytoskeleton* 63, 117–131. doi: 10.1002/cm.20105

Furukawa, A., Nakada-Tsukui, K., and Nozaki, T. (2012). Novel transmembrane receptor involved in phagosome transport of lysozymes and b-hexosaminidase in the enteric protozoan *Entamoeba histolytica*. *PLoS Pathog.* 8:e1002539. doi: 10.1371/journal.ppat.1002539

Gadella, T. W. Jr., and Wirtz, K. W. (1994). Phospholipid binding and transfer by the nonspecific lipid-transfer protein (sterol carrier protein 2). A kinetic model. *Eur. J. Biochem.* 220, 1019–1028. doi: 10.1111/j.1432-1033.1994.tb18707.x

Giorgi, C., De Stefani, D., Bononi, A., Rizzuto, R., and Pinton, P. (2009). Structural and functional link between the mitochondrial network and the endoplasmic reticulum. *Int. J. Biochem. Cell Biol.* 41, 1817–1827. doi: 10.1016/j.biocel.2009.04.010

Goldfinger, L. E., Ptak, C., Jeffery, E. D., Shabanowitz, J., Han, J., Haling, J. R., et al. (2007). An experimentally derived database of candidate Ras-interacting proteins. *J. Proteome Res.* 6, 1806–1811. doi: 10.1021/pr060630l

Haastert, B., Mellanby, R. J., Anderton, S. M., and O'Connor, R. A. (2013). T cells at the site of autoimmune inflammation show increased potential for trogocytosis. *PLoS ONE* 8:e81404. doi: 10.1371/journal.pone.0081404

Hanada, K. (2010). Intracellular trafficking of ceramide by ceramide transfer protein. *Proc. Jpn. Acad. Ser. B Phys. Biol. Sci.* 86, 426–437. doi: 10.2183/pjab.86.426

Hanadate, Y., Saito-Nakano, Y., Nakada-Tsukui, K., and Nozaki, T. (2016). Endoplasmic reticulum resident Rab8A GTPase is involved in phagocytosis in protozoan parasite *Entamoeba histolytica*. *Cell. Microbiol.* 10, 1358–1373. doi: 10.1111/cmi.12570

Haque, R., Hughes, M., Houpt, E., and Petri, W. A. (2003). Amebiasis. *N. Engl. J. Med.* 348, 1565–1573. doi: 10.1056/NEJMra022710

Helle, S. C., Kanfer, G., Kolar, K., Lang, A., Michel, A. H., and Kornmann, B. (2013). Organization and function of membrane contact sites. *Biochimica et Biophysica Acta* 1833, 2526–2541. doi: 10.1016/j.bbamcr.2013.01.028

Helmkamp, G. M. Jr. (1986). Phospholipid transfer proteins: mechanism of action. *J. Bioenerg. Biomembr.* 18, 71–91. doi: 10.1007/BF00743477

Hill, R. J., Ringel, A., Knuepfer, E., Moon, R. W., Blackman, M. J., and van Ooij, C. (2016). Regulation and essentiality of the StAR-related lipid transfer (START) domain-containing phospholipid transfer protein PFA0210c in malaria parasites. *J. Biol. Chem.* 291, 24280–24292. doi: 10.1074/jbc.M116.740506

Holthuis, J. C., and Levine, T. P. (2005). Lipid traffic: floppy drives and a superhighway. *Nat. Rev. Mol. Cell Biol.* 6, 209–220. doi: 10.1038/nrm1591

Holthuis, J. C., van Meer, G., and Huitema, K. (2003). Lipid microdomains, lipid translocation and the organization of intracellular membrane transport. *Mol. Membr. Biol.* 20, 231–241. doi: 10.1080/0988768031000100768

Hon, C. C., Weber, C., Sismeiro, O., Proux, C., Koutero, M., Deloger, M., et al. (2013). Quantification of stochastic noise of splicing and polyadenylation in Entamoeba histolytica. *Nucleic Acids Res.* 41, 1936–1952. doi: 10.1093/nar/gks1271

Hung, C. C., Chang, S. Y., and Ji, D. D. (2012). *Entamoeba histolytica* infection in men who have sex with men. *Lancet Infect. Dis.* 12, 729–736. doi: 10.1016/S1473-3099(12)70147-0

Husain, A., Sato, D., Jeelani, G., Mi-ichi, F., Ali, V., Suematsu, M., et al. (2010). Metabolome analysis revealed increase in S-methylcysteine and phosphatidylisopropanolamine synthesis upon L-cysteine deprivation in the anaerobic protozoan parasite *Entamoeba histolytica*. *J. Biol. Chem.* 285, 39160–39170. doi: 10.1074/jbc.M110.167304

Husain, A., Sato, D., Jeelani, G., Soga, T., and Nozaki, T. (2012). Dramatic increase in glycerol biosynthesis upon oxidative stress in the anaerobic protozoan parasite *Entamoeba histolytica*. *PLoS Negl. Trop. Dis.* 6:e1831. doi: 10.1371/journal.pntd.0001831

Im, Y. J., Raychaudhuri, S., Prinz, W. A., and Hurley, J. H. (2005). Structural mechanism for sterol sensing and transport by OSBP-related proteins. *Nature* 437, 154–158. doi: 10.1038/nature03923

Irvine, R. F. (2003). Nuclear lipid signaling. *Nat. Rev. Mol. Cell Biol.* 4, 349–361. doi: 10.1038/nrm1100

Jang, Y. H., and Min, do. S. (2011). Nuclear localization of phospholipase D1 mediates the activation of nuclear protein kinase Cα and extracellular signal-regulated kinase signaling pathways. *J. Biol. Chem.* 286, 4680–4689. doi: 10.1074/jbc.M110.162602

Johansson, M., Rocha, N., Zwart, W., Jordens, I., Janssen, L., Kuijl, C., et al. (2007). Activation of endosomal dynein motors by stepwise assembly of Rab7- RILP-p150Glued, ORP1L, and the receptor βIII spectrin. *J. Cell Biol.* 176, 459–471. doi: 10.1083/jcb.200606077

Jones, J. D., and Thompson, T. E. (1989). Spontaneous phosphatidylcholine transfer by collision between vesicles at high lipid concentration. *Biochem* 28, 129–134. doi: 10.1021/bi00427a019

Jülke, S., and Ludwig-Müller, J. (2015). Response of Arabidopsis thaliana roots with altered lipid transfer protein (LTP) gene expression to the club root diseases and salt stress. *Plants* 5:2. doi: 10.3390/plants5010002

Kaplan, M. R., and Simoni, R. D. (1985). Intracellular transport of phosphatidylcholine to the plasma membrane. *J. Cell Biol.* 101, 441–445. doi: 10.1083/jcb.101.2.441

Karlsson, T., Altankhuyag, A., Dobrovolska, O., Turcu, D. C., and Lewis, A. E. (2016). A polybasic motif in ErbB3-binding protein 1 (EBP1) has key functions in nucleolar localization and polyphosphoinositide interaction. *Biochem. J.* 473, 2033–2047. doi: 10.1042/BCJ20160274

Kasper, A. M., and Helmkamp, G. M. Jr. (1981). Intermembrane phospholipid fluxes catalyzed by bovine brain phospholipid exchange protein. *Biochim. Biophys. Acta* 664, 22–32. doi: 10.1016/0005-2760(81)90025-4

Khan, D., McGrath, K. R., O., Dorosheva, Bankaitis, V. A., and Tripathi, A. (2016). Structural elements that govern Sec14-like PITP sensitivities to potent small molecule inhibitors. *J. Lipid Res.* 57, 650–662. doi: 10.1194/jlr.M066381

Kim, Y. J., Guzman-Hernandez, M., Wisniewski, E., and Balla, T. (2015). Phosphatidylinositol-phosphatidic acid exchange by Nir2 at ER-PM contact sites maintains phosphoinositide signaling competence. *Dev Cell.* 33, 549–561. doi: 10.1016/j.devcel.2015.04.028

Kölsch, V., Charest, P. G., and Firtel, R. A. (2008). The regulation of cell motility and chemotaxis by phospholipid signaling. *J. Cell Sci.* 121, 551–559. doi: 10.1242/jcs.023333

Kular, G., Loubtchenkov, M., Swigart, P., Whatmore, J., Ball, A., Cockcroft, S., et al. (1997). Co-operation of phosphatidylinositol transfer protein with phosphoinositide 3-kinase gamma in the formylmethionyl-leucylphenylalanine-dependent production of phosphatidylinositol 3,4,5-trisphosphate in human neutrophils. *Biochem. J.* 325, 299–301. doi: 10.1042/bj3250299

Kular, G. S., Chaudhary, A., Prestwich, G., Swigart, P., Wetzker, R., and Cockcroft, S. (2002). Co-operation of phosphatidylinositol transfer protein with phosphoinositide 3-kinase gamma *in vitro*. *Adv. Enzyme Regul.* 42, 53–61. doi: 10.1016/S0065-2571(01)00023-1

Kumagai, K., Kawano-Kawada, M., and Hanada, K. (2014). Phosphoregulation of the ceramide transport protein CERT at serine 315 in the interaction with VAMP-associated protein (VAP) for inter-organelle trafficking of ceramide in mammalian cells. *J. Biol. Chem.* 289, 10748–10760. doi: 10.1074/jbc.M113.528380

Lauwaet, T., Oliveira, M. J., De Bruyne, G., Bruchhaus, I., Duchêne, M., and Mareel, M., et al (2004). *Entamoeba histolytica* trophozoites transfer lipophosphopeptidoglycans to enteric cell layers. *Int. J. Parasitol.* 34, 549–556. doi: 10.1016/j.ijpara.2003.11.013

Lebiedzinska, M., Szabadkai, G., Jones, A. W., Duszynski, J., and Wieckowski, M. R. (2009). Interactions between the endoplasmic reticulum, mitochondria plasma membrane and other subcellular organelles. *Int. J. Biochem. Cell Biol.* 41, 1805–1816. doi: 10.1016/j.biocel.2009.02.017

Lev, S. (2006). Lipid homoeostasis and Golgi secretory function. *Biochem. Soc. Trans.* 34, 363–366. doi: 10.1042/BST0340363

Lev, S. (2010). Non-vesicular lipid transport by lipid-transfer proteins and beyond. *Nature Rev. Mol. Cell Biol.* 11, 739–750. doi: 10.1038/nrm2971

Lev, S. (2012). Nonvesicular lipid transfer from the endoplasmic reticulum. *Cold Spring Harb. Perspect. Biol.* 4:a013300. doi: 10.1101/cshperspect.a013300

Levin, R., Grinstein, S., and Schlam, D. (2015). Phosphoinositides in phagocytosis and macropinocytosis. *Biochim. Biophys. Acta* 1851, 805–823. doi: 10.1016/j.bbalip.2014.09.005

Levine, T. (2004). Short-range intracellular trafficking of small molecules across endoplasmic reticulum junctions. *Trends Cell Biol.* 14, 483–490. doi: 10.1016/j.tcb.2004.07.017

Levine, T., and Loewen, C. (2006). Inter-organelle membrane contact sites: through a glass, darkly. *Curr. Opin. Cell Biol.* 18, 371–378. doi: 10.1016/j.ceb.2006.06.011

Li, J., Guizhen, G.ao, Kun, X.u, Biyun, C.hen, Guixin, Y.an, Feng, L.i, et al. (2014). Genome-wide survey and expression analysis of the putative non-specific lipid transfer proteins in *Brassica rapa* l. *PLoS ONE* 9:e84556. doi: 10.1371/journal.pone.0084556

Li, N., Xu, C., Li-Beisson, Y., and Philippar, K. (2016). Fatty acid and lipid transport in plant cells. *Trends Plant Sci.* 21, 145–158. doi: 10.1016/j.tplants.2015.10.011

Litvak, V., Dahan, N., Ramachandran, S., Sabanay H., and Lev S. (2005). Maintenance of the diacylglycerol level in the Golgi apparatus by the Nir2 protein is critical for Golgi secretory function. *Nat. Cell Biol.* 7, 225–234. doi: 10.1038/ncb1221

Makiuchi, T., and Nozaki, T. (2014). Highly divergent mitochondrion-related organelles in anaerobic parasitic protozoa. *Biochimie* 100, 3–17. doi: 10.1016/j.biochi.2013.11.018

Martelli, A. M., Bortul, R., Tabellini, G., Bareggi, R., Manzoli, L., Narducci, P., et al. (2002). Diacylglycerol kinases in nuclear lipid-dependent signal transduction pathways. *Cell. Mol. Life Sci.* 59, 1129–1137. doi: 10.1007/s00018-002-8492-9

Marumo, K., Nakada-Tsukui, K., Tomii, K., and Nozaki, T. (2014).Ligand heterogeneity of the cysteine protease binding protein family in the parasitic protist *Entamoeba histolytica*. *Int. J. Parasitol.* 44, 625–635. doi: 10.1016/j.ijpara.2014.04.008

Matsubara, T., Shirai, Y., Miyasaka, K., Murakami, T., Yamaguchi, Y., Ueyama, T., et al.,(2006). Nuclear transportation of diacylglycerol kinase and its possible function in the nucleus. *J. Biol. Chem.* 281, 6152–6164. doi: 10.1074/jbc.M509873200

Mattjus, P. (2009).Glycolipid transfer proteins and membrane interaction. *Biochim. Biophys. Acta* 1788, 267–272. doi: 10.1016/j.bbamem.2008.10.003

McGee, T. P., Skinner, H. B., Whitters, E. A., Henry, S. A., and Bankaitis, V. A. (1994). A phosphatidylinositol transfer protein controls the phosphatidylcholine content of yeast Golgi membranes. *J. Cell Biol.* 124, 273–287. doi: 10.1083/jcb.124.3.273

Mesmin, B., and Maxfield, F. R. (2009). Intracellular sterol dynamics. *Biochim. Biophys. Acta* 1791, 636–645. doi: 10.1016/j.bbalip.2009.03.002

Mfotie Njoya E., Weber, C., Hernandez-Cuevas, N. A., Hon, C. C., Janin, Y., Kamini, M. F., et al. (2014). Bioassay-guided fractionation of extracts from Codiaeum variegatum against *Entamoeba histolytica* discovers compounds that modify expression of ceramide biosynthesis related genes. *PLoS Negl. Trop. Dis.* 8:e2607. doi: 10.1371/journal.pntd.0002607

Mi-ichi, F., Miyamoto, T., Takao, S., Jeelani, G., Hashimoto, T., Hara, H., et al. (2015). Entamoeba mitosomes play an important role in encystation by association with cholesteryl sulfate synthesis. *Proc. Natl. Acad. Sci. U.S.A.* 112, 2884–2890. doi: 10.1073/pnas.1423718112

Mi-Ichi, F., Miyamoto, T., and Yoshida, H. (2017). Uniqueness of Entamoeba sulfur metabolism: sulfolipid metabolism that plays pleiotropic roles in the parasitic life cycle. *Mol. Microbiol.* 106, 479–491. doi: 10.1111/mmi.13827

Mi-ichi, F., Yousuf, M. A., Nakada-Tsukui, K., and Nozaki, T. (2009). Mitosomes in *Entamoeba histolytica* contain a sulfate activation pathway. *Proc. Natl. Acad. Sci. U.S.A.* 106, 21731–21736. doi: 10.1073/pnas.0907106106

Miliara, X., Garnett, J. A., Tatsuta, T., Ali, F. A., Baldie, H., Pérez-Dorado, I., et al. (2015). Structural insight into the TRIAP1/PRELI-like domain family of mitochondrial phospholipid transfer complexes. *EMBO Rep.* 16, 824–835. doi: 10.15252/embr.201540229

Mishkind, M., Vermeer, J. E. M., Darwish, E., and Munnik, T. (2009). Heat stress activates phospholipase D and triggers PIP2 accumulation at the plasma membrane and nucleus. *Plant J.* 60, 10–21. doi: 10.1111/j.1365-313X.2009.03933.x

Mitra, B. N., Saito-Nakano, Y., Nakada-Tsukui, K., Sato, D., and Nozaki, T. (2007). Rab11B small GTPase regulates secretion of cysteine proteases in the enteric protozoan parasite *Entamoeba histolytica*. *Cell Microbiol.* 9, 2112–2125. doi: 10.1111/j.1462-5822.2007.00941.x

Mittal, K., B. H., and Temesvari, L. A. (2008). *Entamoeba histolytica*: lipid rafts are involved in adhesion of trophozoites to host extracellular matrix components. *Exp. Parasitol.* 120, 127–134. doi: 10.1016/j.exppara.2008.06.003

Mousley, C. J., Tyeryar, K. R., Ryan, M. M., and Bankaitis, V. A. (2006). Sec14p-like proteins regulate phosphoinositide homoeostasis and intracellular protein and lipid trafficking in yeast. *Biochem. Soc. Transact.* 34, 346–350. doi: 10.1042/BST0340346

Nagaraja, S., and Ankri, S. (2018) Utilization of different omic approaches to unravel stress response mechanisms in the parasite *Entamoeba histolytica*. *Front. Cell. Infect. Microbiol.* 8:19. doi: 10.3389/fcimb.2018.00019

Nakada-Tsukui, K., Okada, H., Mitra, B. N., and Nozaki, T. (2009). Phosphatidylinositol-phosphates mediate cytoskeletal reorganization during phagocytosis via a unique modular protein consisting of RhoGEF/DH and FYVE domains in the parasitic protozoon *Entamoeba histolytica*. *Cell Microbiol.* 11, 1471–1491. doi: 10.1111/j.1462-5822.2009.01341.x

Nakada-Tsukui, K., Saito-Nakano, Y., Ali, V., and Nozaki, T. (2005). A retromerlike complex is a novel Rab7 effector that is involved in the transport of the virulence factor cysteine protease in the enteric protozoan parasite *Entamoeba histolytica*. *Mol. Biol. Cell.* 16, 5294–5303. doi: 10.1091/mbc.e05-04-0283

Nakada-Tsukui, K., Tsuboi, K., Furukawa, A., Yamada, Y., and Nozaki, T. (2012). A novel class of cysteine protease receptors that mediate lysosomal transport. *Cell Microbiol.* 8, 1299–1317. doi: 10.1111/j.1462-5822.2012.01800.x

Nichols, J. W. (1988). Kinetics of fluorescent-labeled phosphatidylcholine transfer between nonspecific lipid transfer protein and phospholipid vesicles. *Biochemistry* 27, 1889–1896 doi: 10.1021/bi00406a014

Nile, A. H., Bankaitis, V. A., and Grabon, A. (2010). Mammalian diseases of phosphatidylinositol transfer proteins and their homologs. *Clin Lipidol.* 5, 867–897. doi: 10.2217/clp.10.67

Nile, A. H., Tripathi, A., Yuan, P., Mousley, C. J., Suresh, S., and Wallace, I. M., et al (2014). PITPs as Targets for selectively interfering with phosphoinositide signaling in cells. *Nat. Chem. Biol.* 10, 76–84. doi: 10.1038/nchembio.1389

Ohashi, M., Jan de Vries, K., Frank, R., Snoek, G., Bankaitis, V., Wirtz, K., et al. (1995). A role for phosphatidylinositol transfer protein in secretory vesicle formation. *Nature* 377, 544–547. doi: 10.1038/377544a0

Olkkonen, V. M. (2015). OSBP-related protein family in lipid transport over membrane contact sites. *Lipid Insights* 8, 1–9. doi: 10.4137/LPI.S31726

Perdomo, D., Manich, M., Syan, S., Olivo-Marin, J., Dufour, A. C., and Guillén, N. (2016). Intracellular traffic of the lysine and glutamic acid rich protein KERP1 reveals features of endomembrane organization in *Entamoeba histolytica*. *Cell. Microbiol.* 18, 1134 –1152. doi: 10.1111/cmi.12576

Peretti, D., Dahan, N., Shimoni, E., Hirschberg, K., and Lev, S. (2008). Coordinated lipid transfer between the endoplasmic reticulum and the Golgi complex requires the VAP proteins and is essential for Golgi-mediated transport. *Mol. Biol. Cell* 19, 3871–3884. doi: 10.1091/mbc.e08-05-0498

Phillips, S. E., Vincent, P., Rizzieri, K. E., Schaaf, G., Bankaitis, V. A., and Gaucher, E. A. (2006). The diverse biological functions of phosphatidylinositol transfer proteins in eukaryotes. *Crit. Rev. Biochem. Mol. Biol.* 41, 21–49. doi: 10.1080/10409230500519573

Pina-Vázquez, C., Reyes-Lopez M,Mendoza-Hern!andez, G., María Bermúdez-Cruz, R., and de la Garza, M. (2014). Identification of phosphatidylcholine transfer protein-like in the parasite *Entamoeba histolytica*. *Biochimie* 107, 223–234. doi: 10.1016/j.biochi.2014.09.007

Pineda, E., and Perdomo, D. (2017). *Entamoeba histolytica* under oxidative stress: what countermeasure mechanism are in place?. *Cells* 6:4. doi: 10.3390/cells6040044

Potocka, I., Baldwin, T. C., and Kurczynska, E. U. (2012). Distribution of lipid transfer protein 1 (LTP1) epitopes associated with morphogenic events during somatic embryogenesis of Arabidopsis thaliana. *Plant Cell Rep.* 31, 2031–2045. doi: 10.1007/s00299-012-1314-0

Que, X., and Reed, S. L. (2000). Cysteine proteinases and the pathogenesis of amebiasis. *Clin. Microbiol. Rev.* 13, 196–206. doi: 10.1128/CMR.13.2.196-206.2000

Ralston, K. S., Solga, M. D., Mackey-Lawrence, N. M., Somlata, Bhattacharya A., and Petri W. A. Jr., (2014). Trogocytosis by *Entamoeba histolytica* contributes to cell killing and tissue invasion. *Nature* 508, 526–530. doi: 10.1038/nature13242

Raychaudhuri, S., Im, Y. J., Hurley, J. H., and Prinz, W. A. (2006). Nonvesicular sterol movement from plasma membrane to ER requires oxysterol-binding protein related proteins and phosphoinositides. *J. Cell Biol.* 173, 107–119. doi: 10.1083/jcb.200510084

Raychaudhuri, S., and Prinz W. A. (2010).The diverse functions of oxysterol-binding proteins. *Annu. Rev. Cell Dev. Biol.* 26, 157–177. doi: 10.1146/annurev.cellbio.042308.113334

Ren, H., Federico, L., Huang, H., Sunkara, M., Drennan, T., Frohman, M. A., et al. (2010). A phosphatidic acid binding/nuclear localization motif determines lipin1 function in lipid metabolism and adipogenesis. *MBoC* 21, 3171–3181. doi: 10.1091/mbc.E10-01-0073

Rocha, N., Kuijl, C., van der Kant, R., Janssen, L., Houben, D., Janssen, H., et al. (2009). Cholesterol sensor ORP1L contacts the ER protein VAP to control Rab7-RILP-p150Glued and late endosome positioning. *J. Cell Biol.* 185, 1209–1225. doi: 10.1083/jcb.200811005

Rueckert, D. G., and Schmidt, K. (1990). Lipid transfer proteins. *Chem. Phys. Lipids* 56, 1–20. doi: 10.1016/0009-3084(90)90083-4

Saito-Nakano, Y., Loftus, B. J., Hall, N., and Nozaki, T. (2005). The diversity of Rab GTPases in *Entamoeba histolytica*. *Exp. Parasitol.* 110, 244–252. doi: 10.1016/j.exppara.2005.02.021

Saito-Nakano, Y., Yasuda, T., Nakada-Tsukui, K., Leippe, M., and Nozaki, T. (2004). Rab5-associated vacuoles play a unique role in phagocytosis of the enteric protozoan parasite *Entamoeba histolytica*. *J. Biol. Chem.* 279, 49497–49507. doi: 10.1074/jbc.M403987200

Sato, D., Nakada-Tsukui, K., Okada, M., and Nozaki, T. (2006). Two cysteine protease inhibitors, EhICP1 and 2, localized in distinct compartments, negatively regulate secretion in *Entamoeba histolytica*. *FEBS Lett.* 22, 5306–5312. doi: 10.1016/j.febslet.2006.08.081

Schaaf, G., Ortlund, E. A., Tyeryar, K. R., Mousley, C. J., Ile, K. E., Garrett, T. A., et al. (2008). Functional anatomy of phospholipid binding and regulation of phosphoinositide homeostasis by proteins of the Sec14 superfamily. *Mol. Cell* 29, 191–206. doi: 10.1016/j.molcel.2007.11.026

Scherrer, F. W. Jr., and Spingola, M. (2006). A subset of Mer1p-dependent introns require Bud13p for splicing activation and nuclear retention. *RNA* 12, 1361–1372. doi: 10.1261/rna.2276806.

Schulz, T. A., and Prinz, W., A (2007). Sterol transport in yeast and the Oxysterol Binding Protein Homologue (OSH) family. *Biochim. Biophys. Acta* 1771, 769–780. doi: 10.1016/j.bbalip.2007.03.003

Seigneur, M., Mounier, J., Prevost, M. C., and Guillén, N. (2005). A lysine- and glutamic acid-rich protein, KERP1, from *Entamoeba histolytica* binds to human enterocytes. *Cell Microbiol.* 7, 569–579. doi: 10.1111/j.1462-5822.2005.00487.x

Serrano-Luna, J., Gutiérrez-Meza, M., Mejía-Zepeda, R., Galindo-Gómez, S., Tsutsumi, V., and Shibayama, M. (2010). Effect of phosphatidylcholine-cholesterol liposomes on *Entamoeba histolytica* virulence. *Can. J. Microbiol.* 56, 987–995. doi: 10.1139/W10-088

Shah, Z. H., Jones, D. R., Sommer, L., Foulger, R., Bultsma, Y., D'Santos, C., et al. (2013). Nuclear phosphoinositides and their impact on nuclear functions. *FEBS J.* 280, 6295–6310. doi: 10.1111/febs.12543

Sirokmány, G., Szidonya, L., Káldi, K., Gáborik, Z., Ligeti, E., and Geiszt, M. (2006). Sec14 homology domain targets p50RhoGAP to endosomes and provides a link between Rab and Rho GTPases. *J. Biol. Chem.* 281, 6096–6105. doi: 10.1074/jbc.M510619200

Skinner, H. B., McGee, T. P., McMaster, C. R., Fry, M. R., Bell, R. M., and Bankaitis, V. A. (1995). The Saccharomyces cerevisiae phosphatidylinositol-transfer protein effects a ligand-dependent inhibition of choline-phosphate cytidylyltransferase activity. *Proc. Natl Acad. Sci. U.S.A.* 92, 112–116. doi: 10.1073/pnas.92.1.112

Sleight, R. G. (1987). Intracellular lipid transport in eukaryotes. *Annu. Rev. Physiol.* 49, 193–208. doi: 10.1146/annurev.ph.49.030187.001205

Solis, C. F., Santi-Rocca, J., Perdomo, D., Weber, C., Guillén N. (2009). Use of bacterially expressed dsRNA to downregulate *Entamoeba histolytica* gene expression. *PLoS ONE* 4:e8424. doi: 10.1371/journal.pone.0008424

Somlata, Nakada-Tsukui, K., and Nozaki, T. (2017). AGC family kinase 1 participates in trogocytosis but not in phagocytosis in *Entamoeba histolytica*. *Nat. Commun.* 101, 1–12. doi: 10.1038/s41467-017-00199-y

Sprong, H., van der Sluijs, P., and van Meer, G. (2001). How proteins move lipids and lipids move proteins. *Nat. Rev. Mol. Cell Biol.* 2, 504–513. doi: 10.1038/35080071

Stanley, S. L. Jr, Becker, A., Kunz-Jenkins, C., Foster, L., and Li, E. (1990). Cloning and expression of a membrane antigen of *Entamoeba histolytica* possessing multiple tandem repeats. *Proc. Natl. Acad. Sci. U.S.A.* 87, 4976–4980. doi: 10.1073/pnas.87.13.4976

Stanley, S. L. Jr. (2003). Amoebiasis. *Lancet* 361, 1025–1034. doi: 10.1016/S0140-6736(03)12830-9

Symeon, S. (2013). Phospholipid metabolism and nuclear function: roles of the lipin family of phosphatidic acid phosphatase. *Biochim. Biophys. Acta* 1831, 575–581. doi: 10.1016/j.bbalip.2012.09.014

Tanaka, K., Horiguchi, K., Yoshida, T., Takeda, M., Fujisawa, H., Takeuchi, K., et al. (1999). Evidence that a phosphatidylinositol 3,4,5-triphosphate binding protein can function in nucleus. *J. Biol. Chem.* 274, 3919–3922. doi: 10.1074/jbc.274.7.3919

Tatsuta, T., and Langer, T. (2016). Intramitochondrial phospholipid trafficking. *Biochim. Biophys. Acta* 1862, 81–89. doi: 10.1016/j.bbalip.2016.08.006

Tavares, P., Rigothier, M., Khun, H., Roux, P., Huerre, M., and Guillén, N. (2005). Roles of cell adhesion and cytoskeleton activity in Entamoeba histolytica pathogenesis: a delicate balance. *Infect Immun.* 73, 1771–1778. doi: 10.1128/IAI.73.3.1771-1778.2005

Thomas, F. J. M. (2012). Role of PI(4,5)P2 in vesicle exocytosis and membrane fusion. *Subcell Biochem.* 59, 111–130. doi: 10.1007/978-94-007-3015-1_4

Tsai, T. Y., Wang, W. T., Li, H. K., Chen, W. J., Tsai, Y. H., Chao, C. H., et al. (2017). RNA helicase DDX3 maintains lipid homeostasis through upregulation of the microsomal triglyceride transfer protein by interacting with HNF4 and SHP. *Sci Rep.* 7, 41452–41469. doi: 10.1038/srep41452

Van Meer, G. (1989). Lipid traffic in animal cells. *Annu. Rev. Cell Biol.* 5, 247–275. doi: 10.1146/annurev.cb.05.110189.001335

Van Ooij, C., Withers-Martinez, C., Ringel, A., Cockcroft, S., Haldar, K., and Blackman, M. J. (2013). Identification of a *Plasmodium falciparum* phospholipid transfer protein *J. Biol. Chem.* 44, 31971–31983. doi: 10.1074/jbc.M113.474189

Vance, J. E., Aasman, E. J., and Szarka, R. (1991). Brefeldin A does not inhibit the movement of phosphatidylethanolamine from its sites for synthesis to the cell surface. *J. Biol. Chem.* 266, 8241–8247.

Vicente, J. B., Ehrenkaufer, G. M., Saraiva, L. M., Teixeira, M., and Singh, U. (2009). *Entamoeba histolytica* modulates a complex repertoire of novel genes in response to oxidative and nitrosative stress: implications for amebic pathogenesis. *Cell Microbiol.* 11, 51–69. doi: 10.1111/j.1462-5822.2008.01236.x

Voelker, D. R. (1991). Organelle biogenesis and intracellular lipid transport in eukaryotes. *Microbiol. Rev.* 55, 543–560.

Voelker, D. R. (2005). Bridging gaps in phospholipid transport. *Trends Biochem. Sci.* 30, 396–404. doi: 10.1016/j.tibs.2005.05.008

Weber-Boyvat, M., Zhong, W., Yan, D., and Olkkonen, V. M. (2013). Oxysterol-binding proteins: functions in cell regulation beyond lipid metabolism. *Biochem Pharmacol.* 86, 89–95. doi: 10.1016/j.bcp.2013.02.016

Wirtz, K. W. (1991). Phospholipid transfer proteins. *Annu. Rev. Biochem.* 60, 73–99. doi: 10.1146/annurev.bi.60.070191.000445

Wirtz, K. W., Schouten, A., and Gros, P. (2005). Phosphatidylinositol transfer proteins: from closed for transport to open for exchange. *Adv. Enzyme Regul.* 46, 301–311. doi: 10.1016/j.advenzreg.2006.01.020

Wong-Baeza, I., Alcántara-Hernández, M., Mancilla-Herrera, I., Ramírez-Saldívar, I., Arriaga-Pizano, L., Ferat-Osorio, E., et al. (2010). The role of lipopeptidophosphoglycan in the immune response to *Entamoeba histolytica. J. Biomed. Biotechnol.* 2010:254521. doi: 10.1155/2010/254521

Zhang, X., Zhang, Z., Alexander, D., Bracha, R., Mirelman, D., Stanley, S. L., et al. (2004). Expression of amoebapores is required for full expression of *Entamoeba histolytica* virulence in amebic liver abscess but is not necessary for the induction of inflammation or tissue damage in amebic colitis. *Infect. Immun.* 72, 678–683. doi: 10.1128/IAI.72.2.678-683.2004

Zhou, T., Li, S., Zhong, W., Vihervaara, T., Béaslas, O., Perttil,ä J., et al. (2011). OSBP related protein 8 (ORP8) regulates plasma and liver tissue lipid levels and interacts with nucleoporin Nup62. *PLoS ONE* 6:e21078. doi: 10.1371/journal.pone.0021078

2

Telomeric Repeat-Binding Factor Homologs in *Entamoeba histolytica*: New Clues for Telomeric Research

Francisco Javier Rendón-Gandarilla[1†], Víctor Álvarez-Hernández[1], Elizabeth J. Castañeda-Ortiz[1], Helios Cárdenas-Hernández[1], Rosa Elena Cárdenas-Guerra[1], Jesús Valdés[2], Abigail Betanzos[3,4], Bibiana Chávez-Munguía[4], Anel Lagunes-Guillen[4], Esther Orozco[4], Lilia López-Canovas[1] and Elisa Azuara-Liceaga[1]*

[1] Posgrado en Ciencias Genómicas, Universidad Autónoma de la Ciudad de Mexico, Mexico City, Mexico, [2] Departamento de Bioquímica, Centro de Investigación y de Estudios Avanzados del Instituto Politécnico Nacional, Mexico City, Mexico, [3] Consejo Nacional de Ciencia y Tecnología, Mexico City, Mexico, [4] Departamento de Infectómica y Patogénesis Molecular, Centro de Investigación y de Estudios Avanzados del Instituto Politécnico Nacional, Mexico City, Mexico

***Correspondence:**
Elisa Azuara-Liceaga
elisa.azuara@uacm.edu.mx

†Present Address:
Francisco Javier Rendón-Gandarilla, Centro Regional de Educación Superior, Campus Zona Norte, Universidad Autónoma de Guerrero, Taxco Guerrero, Mexico

Telomeric Repeat Binding Factors (TRFs) are architectural nuclear proteins with critical roles in telomere-length regulation, chromosome end protection and, fusion prevention, DNA damage detection, and senescence regulation. *Entamoeba histolytica*, the parasite responsible of human amoebiasis, harbors three homologs of human TRFs, based on sequence similarities to their Myb DNA binding domain. These proteins were dubbed EhTRF-like I, II and III. In this work, we revealed that EhTRF-like I and II share similarity with human TRF1, while EhTRF-like III shares similarity with human TRF2 by *in silico* approach. The analysis of *ehtrf-like* genes showed they are expressed differentially under basal culture conditions. We also studied the cellular localization of EhTRF-like I and III proteins using subcellular fractionation and western blot assays. EhTRF-like I and III proteins were enriched in the nuclear fraction, but they were also present in the cytoplasm. Indirect immunofluorescence showed that these proteins were located at the nuclear periphery co-localizing with Lamin B1 and trimethylated H4K20, which is a characteristic mark of heterochromatic regions and telomeres. We found by transmission electron microscopy that EhTRF-like III was located in regions of more condensed chromatin. Finally, EMSA assays showed that EhTRF-like III forms specific DNA-protein complexes with telomeric related sequences. Our data suggested that EhTRF-like proteins play a role in the maintenance of the chromosome ends in this parasite.

Keywords: TRF, Myb-like DNA binding domain, lamin B1, H4K20, chromosome, DNA sequence

INTRODUCTION

Telomeres are specialized protein-DNA complexes localized at the end of eukaryotic chromosomes (Blackburn and Gall, 1978; Meyne et al., 1989; Giraud-Panis et al., 2013). Telomeric DNA consists of tandem arrays of G + T-rich repetitive sequences ending in a single-stranded G-rich overhang which is added by the ribonucleoprotein enzyme telomerase (O'Sullivan and Karlseder, 2010; Giraud-Panis et al., 2013). The length of these arrays varies among species, ranking from few hundred base pairs disposed in irregular tandem repeats in *Saccharomyces cerevisiae* (Lue, 2010), to thousands of base pairs of a TTAGGG repeat in vertebrate telomeres (Moyzis et al., 1988; Giraud-Panis et al., 2013). Proteins that bind to telomeric DNA play critical roles in telomere length regulation and chromosomal end protection in eukaryotic organisms. They conform a machinery known as Telosome or Shelterin complex (Palm and de Lange, 2008). These protein complexes include members or functional homologs of the TTAGGG Repeat Binding Factors, Telomeric Repeat Binding Factors (TRF) and telobox family members (Chong et al., 1995; Broccoli et al., 1997b). TRF proteins are architectural nuclear proteins involved in diverse roles, such as telomere length regulation, chromosome end protection, prevention of chromosomes fusion, sense of DNA damage, and regulation of senescence (de Lange, 2005; Palm and de Lange, 2008). These proteins are conserved from lower eukaryotes, to plants and mammals (Horvath, 2000–2013). The genome *of H. sapiens* contains two genes coding for TRF proteins: TRF1 and TRF2, these proteins bind as homodimers to the double-stranded DNA telomeric sequence (Chong et al., 1995; Broccoli et al., 1997b). TRF1 controls the length of telomeric repeats, whereas TRF2 is involved in the assembly of the terminal t-loop, negative telomere length regulation and chromosomal end protection (Palm and de Lange, 2008). Proteins of the TRF family have similar architectures, defined by the presence of two domains: (i) the conserved single MYB-type helix-turn-helix (HTH) DNA-binding domain (MYB DBD; 55 amino acids) located in their C-terminal; this domain contains three evenly spaced tryptophan residues and in the third α-helix presents a telobox motif (VDLKDKWRT, consensus VxxKDxxR) (Bilaud et al., 1996). (ii) The TRF-homology domain (TRFH; 200 amino acids) situated in the N-terminal, which is unique for members of this family (Broccoli et al., 1997b); and its function is related to homodimerization and protein-protein interactions with other telomeric proteins (Fairall et al., 2001). Additionally, TRF1 and TRF2 proteins diverge in their N-terminal domain, which is rich in acidic or basic residues, respectively (Broccoli et al., 1997a; Palm and de Lange, 2008). Gene encoding homologs to TRF1 and TRF2 have been found in the genomes of *Trypanosoma brucei*, *Trypanosoma cruzi* and *Leishmania. major* based on similarities to the C-terminal MYB DBD (Li et al., 2005; da Silva et al., 2010). Besides TRF1 and TRF2, telomeric DNA also requires the binding of other specific proteins, such as Rap1 (replication protein A 1), POT1 (protection of telomeres 1), TIN2 (TRF1-interacting nuclear factor 2) and TPP which together conform the Shelterin complex in *H. sapiens* (Palm and de Lange, 2008). In Trypanosomes besides the TRF2, a homolog of Rpa-1 has also been identified, suggesting that the telomeric function is conserved and that the telomeric machinery evolved early in eukaryotes (Lira et al., 2007).

In *Entamoeba histolytica*, the causative protozoan of human amoebiasis, the MYB DBD is the most abundant domain related to transcriptional regulation (Clark et al., 2007). MYB DBD-containing proteins in this parasite are clustered into three monophyletic groups. Families I and III are related to transcriptional factors and were dubbed as EhMybR2R3 and EhMybSHAQKYF, respectively (Meneses et al., 2010). Family II includes single-repeat proteins related to human telomeric binding proteins (Meneses et al., 2010). In *E. histolytica* the identification of telomeric signatures has been a challenging task. Although the first draft of *E. histolytica* genome was published in 2005, it has not been possible to identify sequences that referenced the terminal ends of the chromosomes neither canonical telomeric sequences nor orthologs of telomerase genes have been identified (Loftus et al., 2005; Clark et al., 2007; Lorenzi et al., 2010). However, 10% of the *E. histolytica* genome corresponds to tRNA genes which are associated with short tandem repeats (Loftus et al., 2005). There are 25 different types of long tandem arrays that contain between 1 and 5 tRNA types per repeat unit and STRs which resembles microsatellites (Clark et al., 2006; Tawari et al., 2008). It has been proposed that these arrays could localize at the chromosome ends, acting as telomeric regions that fulfill a structural role in the genome (Clark et al., 2006; Tawari et al., 2008). In addition, *E. histolytica* chromosomes do not completely condense and there is a considerable variation in their chromosome size, maybe due to expansion and contraction of telomeric repeats, as in other protists (Patarapotikul and Langsley, 1988; Melville et al., 1999; Willhoeft and Tannich, 2000). Until now, no telomeric sequences or protein complexes implicated in telomere function have been described in this parasite. The study of TRF homologs will help to gain insight into telomere biology of *E. histolytica*. Thus, in this work, we identified and characterized the TRF-like proteins of *E. histolytica* as homologous to human TRF1 and TRF2. We observed their nuclear localization in condensed chromatin regions, their co-localization with Lamin B1 and trimethylated H4K20, and their binding capacity to form DNA-protein complexes with telomeric related sequences. Our results suggest that the TRF-like proteins of *E. histolytica* play similar function as in their human counterparts. However, further experiments are still needed to address their role in the maintenance of telomeres in this parasite.

MATERIALS AND METHODS

E. histolytica Cultures

E. histolytica trophozoites (strain HM1:IMSS) were axenically cultured at 37°C in TYI-S-33 medium, supplemented with 15% bovine serum (Microlab), 1% Diamond vitamin mixture (Sigma-Aldrich), 100 μg ml^{-1} streptomycin sulfate and 100 U ml^{-1} penicillin (Diamond et al., 1978). Trophozoites were harvested during logarithmic growth phase.

In silico Analysis of the EhTRF-Like Proteins of *E. Histolytica*

Amino acid sequences of proteins coded by genes from *locus* EHI_001090, EHI_148140 and EHI_001110, EHI_009820 and EHI_074810 were obtained from AmoebaDB database (http://amoebadb.org/amoeba/). Such sequences were used as a bait to perform queries using the DELTA-BLAST (Domain Enhanced Lookup Time Accelerated BLAST) algorithm to identify orthologs in other members of Entamoeba or other eukaryotes (https://blast.ncbi.nlm.nih.gov/Blast.cgi). The Percent of Identity (PID) was calculated using the amino acids sequences from *E. histolytica* proteins coded by the above-mentioned genes,

TRF1, TRF2, and proteins from organisms corresponding with the best hits, taking gaps into account using the following equation: PID = (identical positions/length of the alignment) × 100. The predicted secondary structure of complete TRF1 and EhTRF-like I, II and III (corresponding to AmoebaDB ID: EHI_001090, EHI_001110, and EHI_148140, respectively) proteins was determined using PSIPRED (http://bioinf.cs.ucl.ac.uk/psipred/) tool and aligned by ClustalW2 software (https://www.ebi.ac.uk/Tools/msa/clustalw2/). Molecular weight, pI and post-translational modifications were analyzed using the ExPaSy: Compute pI/Mw (https://web.expasy.org/compute_pi/), ProtPi (https://www.protpi.ch/) and Mod Pred tools (http://www.modpred.org/). Nuclear localization signals (NLS) were located through SeqNLS (http://mleg.cse.sc.edu/seqNLS/) and cNLS (http://nls-mapper.iab.keio.ac.jp/cgi-bin/NLS_Mapper_help.cgi) tools. The amino acid sequence of DBD MYB from TRF proteins was aligned using ClustalW2 and phylogenetic analysis was inferred using Neighbor-Joining method. The evolutionary distances were computed using the Poisson correction method. Evolutionary analyses were conducted using MEGA 7 (Kumar et al., 2016). Phylogenetic tree was constructed through a bootstrap of 1,000 replicates. To identify orthologous components of the Sheltering machinery in *E. histolytica* genome, the amino acid sequences of *Homo sapiens* Rap1 (Q9NYB0), TIN2 (Q9BSI4), TPP1 (Q96AP0), and POT1 (Q9NUX5) were obtained from the UniProt database (http://www.uniprot.org/) and used as a bait to make queries with Blast algorithm (http://blast.ncbi.nlm.nih.gov). The presence of conserved functional domains in the identified proteins was analyzed in the Pfam database (http://pfam.xfam.org/).

RT-PCR Assays

Total RNA from *E. histolytica* trophozoites was isolated following the Trizol® LS Reagent (Invitrogen) protocol and then semi-quantitative RT-PCR assays were performed with 100 ng of total RNA. Primers used to amplify the *ehtrf-like I*, *ehtrf-like II*, *ehtrf-like III* and *40s rps2* genes were designed using Primer-BLAST (https://www.ncbi.nlm.nih.gov/tools/primer-blast/) and manually corrected (**Table S1**). To validate the specificity of these primers, we amplified the specific sequence from 50 ng of genomic DNA, obtained with the Wizard Genomic purification kit (Promega). PCR products were separated by gel electrophoresis in 2% agarose gels, stained with RedGel™ Nucleic AcidGel Stain 10,000X (BIOTUM) and visualized in a standard UV transilluminator. Relative quantification by qRT-PCR was performed using the QuantiFast SYBR Green RT-PCR kit (Qiagen) and 50 ng of the total RNA, according to the manufacturer's instructions. Relative changes in gene expression were calculated using *40s rps2* as an internal gene calculated by $\Delta\Delta$CT method. Absolute quantitation was performed using a 10-fold serially diluted standard curve of each *ehtrf-like I, II, III* and *40s rps2* genes in parallel with qRT-PCR of RNA from trophozoites grown in basal conditions. Reaction volumes were set with 25 μl QuantiFast SYBR Green RT-PCR kit (Qiagen) and qRT-PCR was performed using 50 ng of the total RNA and 1 μM each primer, according to the manufacturer's instructions. Initial thermal cycling conditions were 1 cycle of 50°C for 10 mins for reverse transcription, followed by 1 cycle of 95°C for 5 min and 40 cycles of denaturation at 95°C for 10 s and annealing/extension temperature of 55°C for 30 s. Plotting Ct values vs. copy number of the different genes in a standard curve allowed to approximate copies *ehtrf-like* genes from Ct values. The data shown was displayed as mean with standard error in triplicate and repeated in independent experiments by duplicate. GraphPad Prism 6.0e software was used for student *t*-test by two-tailed analyses.

Production of Polyclonal Antibodies Against EhTRF-Like I and EhTRF-Like III

The complete amino acid sequences from EhTRF-like I and EhTRF-like III proteins were aligned using the ClustalW2 tool to identify unique regions of these proteins. Subsequently, to determine hydrophobic regions, EhTRF-like I and III amino acid sequences were analyzed using the Hopp-Woods program (Hopp and Woods, 1981). Finally, a prediction of B epitopes was made using the ABCpred server (http://crdd.osdd.net/raghava/abcpred/). Differential peptides, CTLPSVGNALIPPS and CNKQKVQPQVSQPH for EhTRF-like I and III, respectively, were synthesized, conjugated to Keyhole Limpet Hemocyanin (KLH) (GL Biochem, Shanghai) and used to immunize New Zealand male rabbits. Before immunization, the pre-immune serum (PS) was obtained and then rabbits were subcutaneously inoculated with 400 μg of each peptide diluted in TiterMax® Gold (Sigma-Aldrich). Four booster injections (500 μg each) at 15-days intervals, were given. After 1 week of the last immunization, rabbits were bled, and polyclonal antisera were obtained and tested by western blot assays against total extracts of *E. histolytica* trophozoites.

Subcellular Fractionation

E. histolytica trophozoites were recovered by centrifugation and lysed as follows to obtain subcellular fractions. Soluble nuclear extracts (Ns) were prepared as described by Schreiber et al. (1989). Briefly, 1 × 10^6 trophozoites were resuspended by gentle pipetting in 400 μl of cold buffer A (10 mM HEPES pH 7.9, 10 mM KCl, 0.1 mM EDTA, 0.1 mM EGTA, 1 mM DTT, 0.5 mM PMSF). Trophozoites were allowed to swell on ice for 15 min, after which 25 μl of 10% NP-40 solution (Sigma-Aldrich) was added and vigorously vortexed for 30 s. Homogenate was centrifuged for 10 min at 14,000 rpm, to separate the supernatant containing cytoplasmic extracts (C), and the pellet containing nuclei. Pellet was resuspended in 1 ml of buffer A and layered on 1 ml of buffer A containing 0.34 M sucrose (Sigma-Aldrich), then mixed and centrifuged for 10 min at 14,000 rpm. The nuclear pellet was resuspended in 150 μl ice-cold buffer C (20 mM HEPES pH 7.9; 0.4 M NaCl; 1 mM EDTA; 1 mM EGTA; 1 mM DTT; 1 mM PMSF) and vigorously rocked at 4°C for 15 min. Nuclear soluble extracts (Ns) were obtained after centrifugation for 10 min at 13,000 rpm at 4°C and frozen in aliquots at −70°C until used. The remaining pellet was lysed in RIPA buffer (50 mM Tris-Cl, pH 8, 150 mM NaCl, 2 mM EDTA, 1% Triton X-100, 0.1% SDS) and sonicated with three pulses of 30 s (30% power) and 2 min refractory period each on ice, to disrupt the chromatin. Later, samples were centrifuged at 14,000 rpm at 4°C for 10 min and supernatants were labeled as nuclear insoluble fractions (Ni). Total extracts (T) were obtained by freeze-thawing trophozoites in the presence of 100 mM Tris-HCl pH 7.9, 100 mM p-hydroxymercuribenzoate (PHMB) (Sigma-Aldrich), Complete™ protease inhibitor cocktail (Sigma-Aldrich), 10 μM E64 (Sigma-Aldrich) and 100 mM PMSF (Sigma-Aldrich). Protein concentration was determined by Bradford method (Bradford, 1976) using the Bio-Rad protein assay or the DC Protein Assay (BIO-RAD).

SDS-PAGE Gels and Western Blot Assays

Protein extracts obtained as previously indicated (T, Ns, Ni or C), were separated by sodium dodecyl sulfate polyacrylamide gel, electrophoresed by (SDS-PAGE). Briefly, 40 μg of each extract was loaded in a 12% SDS-PAGE and transferred to 0.45 μm nitrocellulose membranes (BIO-RAD). For western blot (WB) assays, membranes were stained with Ponceau S Red staining solution (Sigma-Aldrich) and incubated 1 h with 5% non-fat milk. Then were incubated overnight (ON) with α-TRF-like I (1:2,500), α-TRF-like III (1:1,000), α-EhKMT4 (1:1,000) (Borbolla-Vázquez et al., 2015); α-H3K27me3 (1:1,000, Cell Signaling Technology), α-H4K20me3 (1:1,000, Abcam), α-Lamin B1 (1:1,000, Abcam), α-actin (1:1,000, Sigma-Aldrich) or α-Myc (1:1,000, Cell Signaling Technology) antibodies and then, incubated for 2 h with the corresponding horseradish peroxidase (HRP) labeled secondary antibodies (1:8,000, Santa Cruz Biotechnology). Protein bands were detected and visualized by chemiluminescence on X-ray films. All experiments were repeated at least three times.

Subcellular Localization by Confocal Microscopy

Trophozoites cultured on cover slides were fixed with absolute ethanol for 20 min at −20°C and washed with PBS pH 6.8. Then, coverslips were incubated with 50 mM NH_4Cl for 30 min at 37°C and blocked with 1% bovine serum albumin for 30 min. For co-localization experiments, α-EhTRF-like I, α-Lamin B1, α-EhTRF-like III and α-H4K20me3 antibodies were labeled with Alexa Flour 647, 555, 488 and 488, respectively, using Molecular Probes® Antibody Labeling kit (ThermoFisher Scientific) and following the manufacturer's instructions. In other experiments, samples were incubated ON at 4°C with α-TRF-like III (1:200) and α-Myc (1:100, Cell Signaling) antibodies. Cells were washed and then, incubated with fluorescein labeled secondary antibody (1:200, Jackson Immuno Research). Slides were mounted with Vectashield containing DAPI (Vector Lab), visualized through a Nikon inverted microscope attached to a laser Confocal scanning system (Leica TCS SP2) and analyzed by Confocal Assistant software image.

Construction of *pehtrf-like Iox*, *pehtrf-like IIIox*, and *pCold-ehtrf-like I* Plasmids

The *ehtrf-like I* (1,210 pb) and *ehtrf-like III* (1,383 bp) complete open reading frames (ORF) were cloned in the *pKT-3M* (Saito-Nakano et al., 2004) plasmid to express the EhTRF-like I and III proteins tagged with Myc sequence at their N-terminal. The *ehtrf-like I* gene was amplified by PCR using the following oligonucleotides: sense 5′-TCCC<u>CCCGGG</u>ATGAATAACCCTCAGTTGC-3′ and antisense 5′- GCGCGC<u>CTCGAG</u>TTATTGAGAAAGATCCAATTGTTTAAAT-3′. The *ehtrf-like III* gene was amplified using the following oligonucleotides: sense 5′-TCCCC<u>CCCGGG</u>ATGGAGAAAAAACTAA-3′ and antisense 5′-GGGGC<u>CTCGAG</u>TTAAAATTATCAGAATTA-3′. Forward primers contained a *Sma*I site and the reverse primers contained a *Xho*I site (underlined). PCR was performed with 100 ng of *E. histolytica* genomic DNA, using the following conditions: 92°C for 5 min, 92°C for 1 min, 55°C for 1 min, and 70°C for 1 min (28 cycles). PCR products were digested with *Sma*I and *Xho*I and cloned into a previously digested *pKT-3M* vector. For the EhTRF-like I recombinant protein (rEhTRF-like I), the 1,210 pb entire ORF was amplified using the forward primer 5-CGC<u>GGATCC</u>TTATTGAGAAAGATCCAATTG-3 and reverse primer 5-GGAATTC<u>CATATG</u>AATAACCCTCAGTTTGC-3, which contained *Bam*HI and *Nde*I restriction sites, respectively. The 1,210 bp amplicon was digested and cloned into a previously linearized *pCold I* vector (Takara). All plasmids obtained were confirmed by sequencing using the BigDye Terminator v3.1 Cycle Sequencing Kit and the ABI Prism® 310 Genetic Analyzer (Applied Biosystems).

Transfection of Trophozoites

Trophozoites were transfected by lipofection as previously described (Olvera et al., 1997; Abhyankar et al., 2008). Briefly, 8×10^5 trophozoites were placed for adhesion in 6-well plates during 20 min, and then washed with M-199 medium (Invitrogen) supplemented with 5.7 mM cysteine, 1 mM ascorbic acid and 25 mM HEPES pH 6.8. Later, 20 μg of *pKT-3M or pehtrf-like Iox* or *pehtrf-like IIIox* plasmids were added to a tube containing 20 μl of Superfect (Qiagen), incubated at room temperature (RT) for 20 to 30 min, mixed with 0.8 ml of M199 supplemented medium plus 15% bovine serum and added to each well-plate. Trophozoites were incubated for 4 h at 37°C and then harvested and added to a 125 mm cell culture tube, containing pre-warmed TYI-S-33 medium. Transfected trophozoites were grown for 48 h and selected initially with 3 μg ml^{-1} G-418 (Thermofisher Scientific) and gradually increased to 20 μg ml^{-1}.

Immunoelectron Microscopy

Immunoelectron microscopy was performed as described (Segovia-Gamboa et al., 2011). Briefly, transfected trophozoites were washed twice with PBS, pH 7.4 and fixed in 4% paraformaldehyde and 0.1% glutaraldehyde in serum-free medium for 1 h at RT. Samples were embedded in LR White resin and polymerized under UV at 4°C ON. Sections were obtained and mounted on formvar-covered nickel grids. Then, they were incubated with α-EhTRF-like III (1:1,000) and α-Myc (1:1,000) antibodies, followed by incubation with 30 nm gold-conjugated particles (Ted Pella Inc.) secondary antibodies (1:60). Thin sections (60–90 nm) were observed in a transmission electron microscope (JEM 1011).

Expression and Purification of rEhtRF-Like I

Escherichia coli Rosetta (DE3) competent cells (Novagen) were transformed with the *pCold-ehtrf-like I* construct. The expression of rEhTRF-like I was induced with 1 mM isopropyl-1-thio-β-D-galactopyranoside (IPTG) at 16°C for 18 h and analyzed by SDS-PAGE and WB assays. The WB assays were performed by using an anti-histidine monoclonal antibody (α-His) (Santa Cruz Biotechnology, Inc) (1:1,000) as the primary antibody and a peroxidase-conjugated goat anti-mouse polyclonal secondary antibody (Invitrogen-Gibco) at a dilution of 1:3,000. The recombinant protein was obtained from the soluble fraction and purified using an affinity chromatography by Ni Sepharose High Performance agarose (GE Healthcare), following the manufacturer's instructions. The rEhTRF-like I was dialyzed with 25 mM Tris–HCl pH 7.5 and 300 mM NaCl. Protein was quantified and used as described below.

Electrophoresis Mobility Shift Assays (EMSA)

DNA-binding activity was tested with four different DNA probes: HsTEL [TTAGGG, human telomeric sequence (Hwang et al., 2001)], EhTEL (the STR sequence TTAGTATT derived from the NK2 unit from the tRNA arrays of *E. histolytica*; Clark et al., 2006; Tawari et al., 2008), a mut-TEL (mutated telomeric sequence) and non-Rel (non-related sequence) probe (**Table S2**). Double-stranded oligonucleotides were end-labeled with 10 μCi [α-^{32}P] dATP (Perkin Elmer) or 10 μCi [γ-^{32}P] dATP, using Klenow fragment or a polynucleotide kinase (New England Biolabs) and purified with the QIAquick nucleotide removal kit (Qiagen). Nuclear soluble extracts (10 μg) from wild type or transfected trophozoites or 106.86 μM rEhTRF-like I were incubated for 20 min at 4°C with 1 ng of labeled oligonucleotides in binding buffer (12 mM HEPES pH 7.9, 60 mM KCl, 5 mM $MgCl_2$, 1 mM EDTA, 4 mM Tris–HCl, 5 mM DTT, 10% glycerol, 4 mM Spermidine, 4 mM MgCl, 50 ng of poly dI·dC and protease inhibitors cocktail). Competitions were carried out in the presence of a 50, 100 and 200-fold molar excess of unlabeled specific HsTEL, EhTEL, mut-Tel and non-Rel probes. Supershifts were performed by pre-incubating nuclear extracts from transfected trophozoites with α-EhTRF-like III or PS (2–4 μg/reaction) for 30 min on ice, before adding the probe. DNA–protein complexes were resolved on a 6% non-denaturing PAGE gel by electrophoresis at 160 V for 2 h at RT in 0.5× TBE buffer (44.5 mM Tris-borate, 44.5 mM boric acid, 1 mM EDTA). Gels were vacuum-dried and radioactive complexes were detected in a Phosphor Imager apparatus (BIO-RAD) or revealed by autoradiography using Kodak X-omat film (Sigma) exposed at −70°C.

Ethic Statement

The Institutional Animal Care and Use Committee (Cinvestav IACUC/ethics committee) reviewed and approved our protocol for the animal care and use of rabbits employed to produce antibodies (Protocol Number 0313-06, CICUAL 001). All steps were taken to ameliorate the welfare and to avoid the animals suffering. Food and water were available *ad libitum*. Animals were monitored pre- and post-inoculation. All procedures were conducted by trained personnel under the supervision of veterinarians and, all invasive clinical procedures were performed while animals were anesthetized and when it was required, animals were humanely euthanized. The ethics committee verified that our Institute fulfills the NOM-062-ZOO-1999, regarding the Technical Specifications for Production, Care and Use of Laboratory Animals given by the General Direction of Animal Health of the Minister of Agriculture of Mexico (SAGARPA-Mexico). The technical specifications approved by SAGARPA-Mexico fulfill of the international regulations/guidelines for use and care of animals used in laboratory and were verified and approved by Cinvestav IACUC/ethics committee (Verification Approval Number: BOO.02.03.02.01.908).

RESULTS

In silico Characterization of *E. Histolytica* EhTRF-Like Proteins

In this work, we focus on the family II of the MYB DBD-containing proteins of *E. histolytica* (Meneses et al., 2010). This family comprises genes encoding hypothetical proteins with AmoebaDB accession numbers (AE): EHI_001090, EHI_001110, EHI_148140, EHI_009820, and EHI_074810, which were reported as single-repeat telomeric proteins related to human telomeric binding proteins (Meneses et al., 2010). On one hand, analysis of the amino acid sequences of the proteins coded by genes from *locus* EHI_009820 and EHI_074810 showed identities with the MYB DBD-containing proteins related to c-Myb, with narrowed identity to TRF-related proteins (**Table 1**). In contrast, the amino acid sequences of proteins coded by genes from *locus* EHI_001090, EHI_001110, and EHI_148140 present about 25.8 to 29% identity with TRF1 from *H. sapiens* (**Table 1**). Moreover, these proteins share 29.6 to 30.3% identity with TRF proteins from other organisms, such as *Pan troglodytes* or *Desmus rotundus* (**Table 1**). Therefore, we considered these *E. histolytica* hypothetical proteins as TRF-like proteins and from now we named them as EhTRF-like I (EHI_001090), II (EHI_001110), and III (EHI_148140). *E. histolytica* EhTRF-like proteins showed higher homology between each other than with human homologs. The sequence conservation between full length EhTRF-like proteins was 35.89 to 63.94% identity, in contrast to human TRF1 and TRF2 which had a 27.77% identity between them. Interestingly, the Myb DBD domain, which characterizes TRF proteins, showed 80.32 to 93.44% identity in EhTRF-like proteins, exhibiting a higher identity between EhTRF-like I and II (**Table S3**).

The alignment of the MYB DBD of the EhTRF-like proteins with TRF1 and TRF2 from *H. sapiens* showed that the sequences conserved the three α-helices characteristics of the MYB DBD, as well as the positions of the second and third tryptophan residues responsible of HTH conformation (**Figure 1A**; **Figure S1**). In addition, EhTRF-like I, II and III have a telebox motif (VxKDxxR) in the third α-helix, and a lysine and arginine

TABLE 1 | Comparison of MYB DBD-containing proteins of *E. histolytica* with other organisms.

Entamoeba histolytica		*Homo sapiens*				Other organisms				
Locus^	**Annotation***	**Protein**	**Accession**	***e*-value**	**PID&**	**Protein**	**Species**	**Accession**	***E*-value**	**PID**
EHI_009820	Myb-like	c-Myb	Q708E3	7e-13	24	TFIIIB	*Camponotus floridanus*	E2ACRO	4e-13	34.7
EHI_074810	HP#	c-Myb	Q708E3	2e-10	29	Myb-like	*Tetrahymena thermophila*	Q23Q10	9.1e-9	35.1
EHI_148140	HP#	TRF1	P54274	4.8e-7	29.7	TRF1	*Pan troglodytes*	H2R473	2.2e-8	30.3
EHI_001090	HP#	TRF1	P54274	4.8e-7	29.7	TRF1	*Pan troglodytes*	H2R473	2.2e-8	30.3
EHI_001110	HP#	TRF1	P54274	9.9e-7	25.8	TRF1	*Desmodus rotundus*	K9J0W4	6.6e-10	29.6

*^According to AmoebaDB data base. *According to Uniprot. &Percentage of identity in global alignment. #Hypothetical protein.*

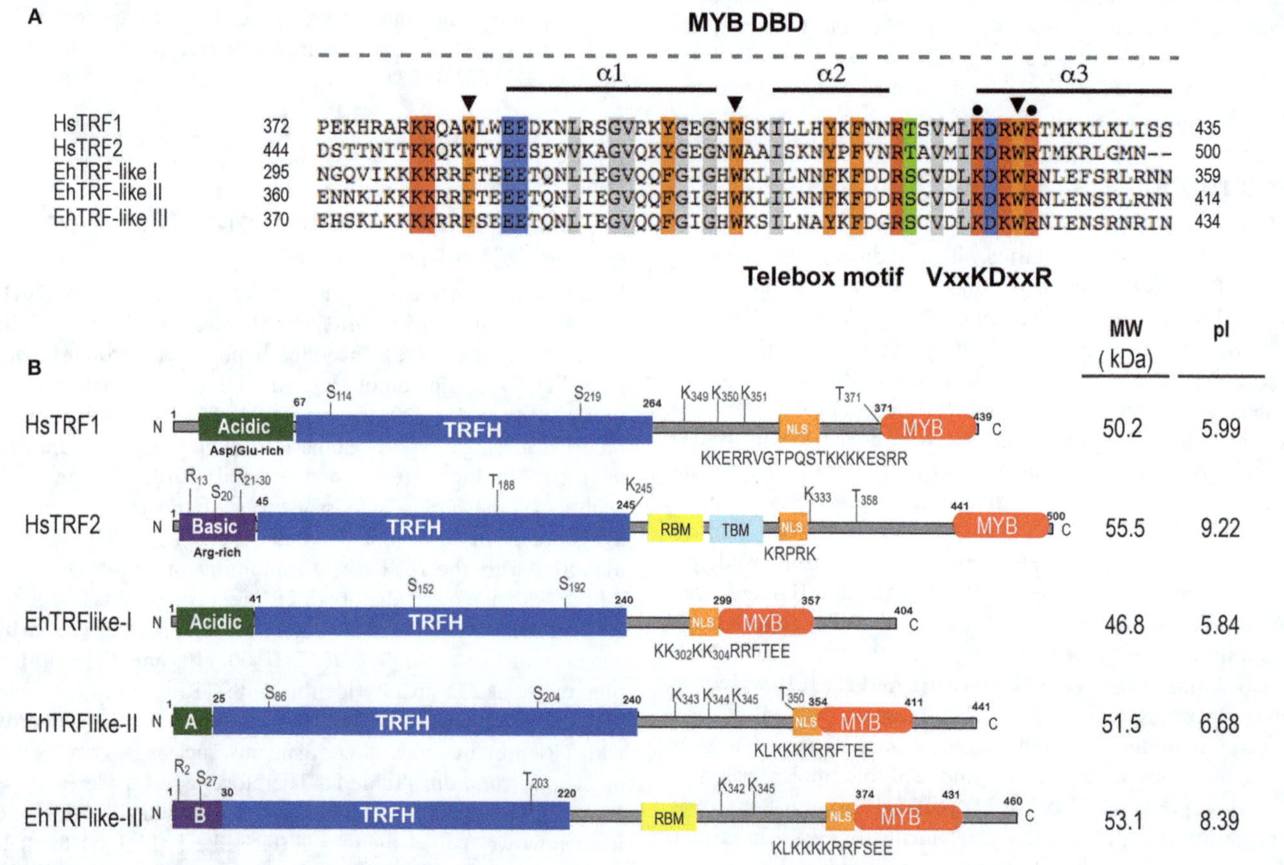

FIGURE 1 | EhTRF-like proteins in *E. histolytica*. **(A)** Multiple alignment of MYB DBD from *Homo sapiens* (HsTRF2 and HsTRF1) and *E. histolytica* (EhTRF-like I, II and III). Black bars illustrate the position of the three α-helices in MYB DBD. Conserved tryptophans or aromatic residues are marked with a black arrowhead. Telebox consensus is shown, conserved amino acids are marked with black dots and identical amino acids are highlighted in colors. **(B)** Schematic representation of major domains and post-translational modifications contained in TRF1 proteins. TRFH, dimerization domain; NLS, nuclear localization signal; MYB DBD, Myb-like DNA binding domain; A, acidic N-terminus; B, basic N-terminus; MW, molecular weight; and pI, isoelectric point.

residues involved in the DNA telomeric recognition in human TRF1 and TRF2 (**Figure 1A; Figure S1**).

Even though there was scarce amino acid identity among the TRFH domains from EhTRF-like proteins and human TRFs, several hydrophobic residues required for the dimer interface, such as leucines, isoleucines, and phenylalanines were conserved (**Figure S1**). In addition, we deduced the secondary structure of the complete amino acid sequences for EhTRF-like proteins and human TRF1 and we aligned them to have a structural comparison (**Figure S2**). Based on their secondary structure, we proposed the presence of a TRFH domain located in the N-terminal of EhTRF-like proteins, because we found at the same position, the nine α-helices essential for domain dimerization in human TRF1 (**Figure 1B; Figure S2**).

According to the ORFs size (1,215, 1,326, and 1,383 pb for *ehtrf-like I, II* and *III*, respectively), the predicted molecular

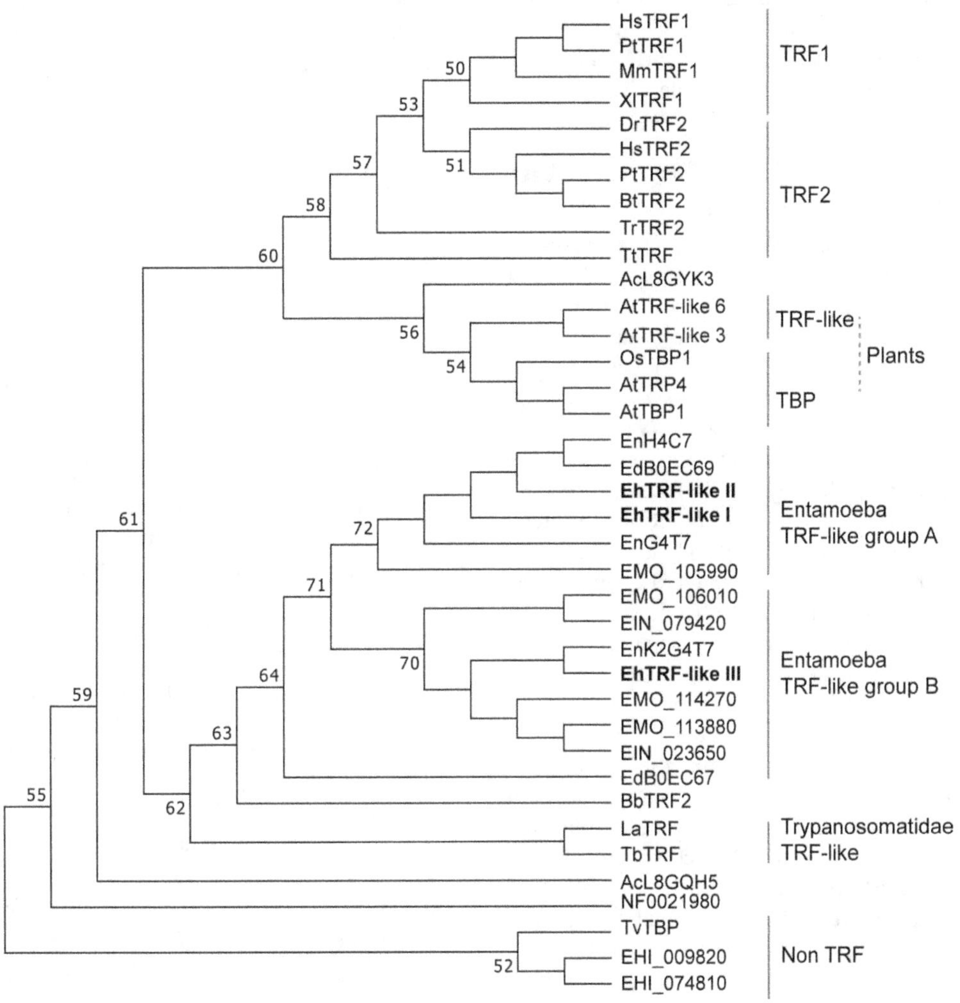

FIGURE 2 | Phylogenetic tree of TRF proteins. The amino acid sequence of DBD MYB from TRF proteins was aligned using ClustalW2 and phylogenetic analysis was inferred using Neighbor-Joining method. Evolutionary distances were computed by the Poisson correction method. Bootstrap values >50% (from 1,000 replicates) are shown near to the individual branches. Evolutionary analyses were conducted using MEGA 7 (Kumar et al., 2016). HsTRF1 (Homo sapiens, NP_059523.2), MmTRF1 (*Mus musculus,* NP_033378.1), PtTRF1 (*Pan troglodytes,* XP_016815057.1), XlTRF1 (*Xenopus laevis,* DQ146827.1), HsTRF2 (*H. sapiens*, NP_005643.2), PtTRF2 (*P. troglodytes,* XP_016785565.1), BtTRF2 (*Bos taurus,* NP_001341392.1), BbTRF2 (*Branchiostoma belcheri,* XP_019634930.1), DrTRF2 (*Danio rerio,* BC096857.1), TrTRF2 (*Thecamonas trahens*, XP_013759355.1), TtTRF (*Takifugu rubripes*, XP_011616883.1), AtTRF-like 3 (*A. thaliana*, NP_001185023.1), AtTRF-like 6 (*A. thaliana*, NP_974133.1), AtTBP1 (*A. thaliana*, XP_015625433.1), AtTRP4 (*A. thaliana*, NP_196886.1), OsTBP1 (*Oryza sativa*, XP_015625433.1), EhTRF-like I (*E. histolytica,* XP_649878.1), EhTRF-like II (*E. histolytica,* XP_649880.1), EhTRF-like III (*E. histolytica,* XP_657528.1), EdBOEC67 (*Entamoeba dispar*, XP_001735901.1), EdB0EC69 (*E. dispar*, XP_001735903.1), Ein079420 (*E. invadens*, XP_004184366.1), Ein023650 (*E. invadens*, XP_004257447.1), EnH4C7 (*E. nuttalli,* XP_008857362.1), EnK2H4C7 (*E. nuttalli,* XP_008860337.1), EnK2G4T7 (*E. nuttalli,* XP_008860339.1), NF0021980 (*Naegleria fowleri*), LaTRF2 (*Leishmania amazonensis*, ABU53006.1), TbTRF (*Trypanosoma brucei,* AAX86992.1), TvTBP (*Trichomonas vaginalis*, XP_001314728.1), EHI_009820 (*E. histolytica*, XP_001913661.1), and EHI_074810 (*E. histolytica,* XP_649576.1).

weight of EhTRF-like I, II and III is 46.8, 51. 5, and 53.1 kDa, respectively, showing similarity to their human counterparts (**Figure 1B**). TRF1 and TRF2 have isoelectric points (pI) of 5.99 and 9.22, respectively, which are related to their amino acids content in their N-terminal end. Theoretical pI of EhTRF-like I and II were predicted as 5.84 and 6.68, respectively, similar to that of TRF1, which is an acidic protein. On the contrary, EhTRF-like III presented a predicted pI of 8.39, alike to the basic protein TRF2. Consequently, the first 50 amino acids of EhTRF-like I and II were acidic residues, similar to those found at the same region of TRF1. On the other hand, the EhTRF-like III N-terminal was composed of basic residues as in TRF2 (**Figure 1B**). TRF2 also contains binding sites for the Shelterin proteins, Rap1 and TIN2 (de Lange, 2005). In concordance, in EhTRF-like III we identified the presence of two α-helices with conserved hydrophobic residues, corresponding to a Rap1-binding domain (RBM domain; **Figure 1B**). Likewise, all EhTRF-like proteins showed a nuclear localization signal (NLS) and susceptible sites of phosphorylation and SUMOylation, present in their human counterparts (**Figure 1B**). Altogether, we predict that EhTRF-like proteins from *E. histolytica* have a similar architecture to TRF1 and TRF2 from *H. sapiens* and are homologs to mammalian telomeric repeat-binding factors. In summary, EhTRF-like I and II share common properties with TRF1, while EhTRF-like III does with TRF2.

Phylogenetic Analysis of TRF Proteins With MYB DBD or Telebox Domain

In order to shed light into the evolutionary relationships of EhTRF-like proteins, we aligned the MYB DBD amino acid sequence of TRFs from *E. histolytica*, *H. sapiens*, representative vertebrates, plants and deep branching protozoa, including other members of Entamoeba genus and Trypanosomatids (**Figure S3**). Proteins coded by genes from *locus* EHI_009820 and EHI_074810 from *E. histolytica* and TvTBP protein from *Trichomonas vaginalis* served as outgroup for tree reconstruction. Interestingly, the alignment with the MYB DBD showed that the first tryptophan residue in TRF-like proteins from Entamoeba genus was replaced with the aromatic amino acid phenylalanine, and unlike to TRF1 and TRF2 they present serine or cysteine residues in the third α-helix of their MYB DBD. In addition, all Entamoeba TRF-like proteins conserved the Telebox signature in a greater extent than other unicellular organisms like Trypanosomatids, where homologs to TRF have been already characterized (Li et al., 2005; da Silva et al., 2010). The phylogenetic inference showed that the TRF proteins are separated into two branches, one of them included the vertebrate proteins related to TRF1 and TRF2 and the TRF-like proteins from plants, and in the other branch contained TRF-like proteins from protozoan parasites including members from the Entamoeba genus (**Figure 2**). It is important to highlight that all TRF-like proteins from Entamoeba genus were clustered into a unique clade and subdivided in two groups that separated members of the EhTRF-like I and II (group A) from members of the EhTRF-like III (group B). The topology observed in the phylogenetic analysis could be the result of a gene duplication event. Interestingly, genes that encoded EhTRF-like I and II proteins are contiguous located in the same genomic location (DS571146). These results suggest that TRF proteins evolved from a common ancestor before vertebrate TRFs diverged and that in the case of *E. histolytica*, a gene duplication events could occur and therefore increased the TRF gene number.

Shelterin Machinery Survey

To determine whether *E. histolytica* contains other components of Shelterin machinery besides TRFs, we searched for proteins homologous to Rap1, TIN2, TPP1 and POT1 in its genome. Through this analysis, we identified a hypothetical protein (AmoebaDB AN: EHI_064550, 156 residues) with 26% identity to *H. sapiens* Rap1 (399 amino acids; **Table 2**). Sequence analysis of this protein revealed the presence of a TRF2-interacting telomeric protein/Rap1 C-terminal domain (*e*-value of 2e-19), suggesting that in *E. histolytica* this hypothetical protein could bind to EhTRF-like III. For these reasons, we decided to name EHI_064550 as EhRap1-like protein. In *H. sapiens,* RAP1 binds to DNA through a MYB-type domain, which was absent in EhRap1-like protein, suggesting that its function is limited to telomeres protection. By using *H. sapiens* proteins as a bait, no other members of Shelterin machinery were identified in the *E. histolytica* genome. Nevertheless, the *E. histolytica* genome encodes a protein which is annotated in AmoebaDB database as the Replication Factor A1 (AN: EHI_062980), therefore this protein was dubbed EhRpa1-like. EhRpa1-like conserves an oligonucleotide/oligosaccharide (OB) domain (e-value of 9e-50 according to Pfam), which could be used for single-stranded telomeric DNA recognition in the absence of POT1 (**Table 2**). These findings, support the idea that *E. histolytica* exhibits a rudimentary Shelterin-like complex conformed by EhTRF-like I, II, III, and EhRap1-like. In addition, EhRpa1-like could have a possible role in telomere maintenance.

TABLE 2 | Candidate proteins to be part of the Shelterin-like complex of *E. histolytica*.

Entamoeba histolytica			*Homo sapiens*		
Locus^	**Annotation^**	**Amino acid size (aa)**	**% Identity**	**Score**	***E*-value**
EhRap1-like					
EHI_064550	UP#	156	26%	86.7	2e-19
EhRpa1-like					
EHI_062980	Replication factor A protein 1	310	17%	22%	9e-50

^According to Amoeba data base. #Putative uncharacterized protein.

Expression of the EhTRF-Like Proteins in Trophozoites of *E. Histolytica*

To determine whether all three *trf-like* genes were constitutively expressed by *E. histolytica,* the mRNA expression patterns were analyzed using qRT-PCR assays derived from trophozoites grown in basal culture conditions. Results showed that three *trf-like* genes had differential expression levels, being *ehtrf-like III* more apparently expressed than the other two (**Figure 3A**).

In order to analyse their protein expression, we produced polyclonal antibodies only against EhTRF-like I and III proteins, using synthetic peptides (N-term-CTLPSVGNALIPPS and N-term-CNKQKVQPQVSQPH, respectively) to immunize rabbits. In western blot analysis using trophozoites lysates, these antibodies revealed two bands of ~55 and 65 kDa, respectively (**Figure 3B**). Those bands are of higher molecular weight than the expected for EhTRF-like I (46 kDa) and III (53 kDa), respectively. Differences between theoretical and experimental molecular weights could be explained by post-translational modifications, such as phosphorylation, ubiquitination and SUMOylation of EhTRF-like I and III (**Figure 1B**). To determine the subcellular localization of both proteins, we carried out a cellular fractionation according to (Schreiber et al., 1989), in which cytoplasmic and soluble nuclear fractions were isolated. To extract the insoluble nuclear proteins, RIPA buffer was added to the remaining nuclei pellet. Results evidenced that EhTRF-like I was present in cytoplasmic and nuclear fractions; however, in cytoplasmic and soluble nuclear fractions the antibody

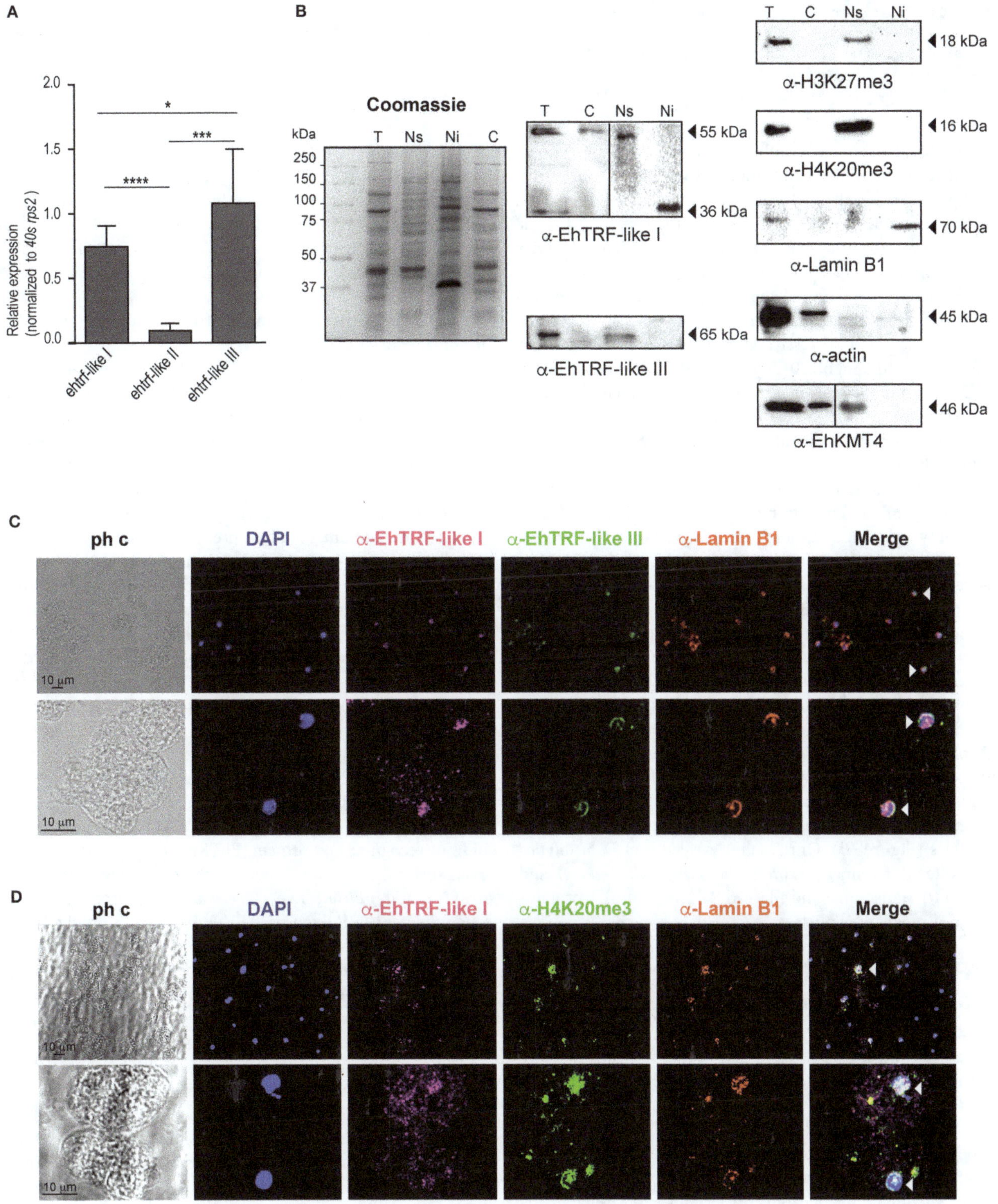

FIGURE 3 | Expression of the EhTRF-like proteins in *E. histolytica* trophozoites. **(A)** The *trf-like* genes have differential expression levels. Absolute RT-qPCR quantification of *ehtrf-like* genes in trophozoites grown in basal conditions. Ribosomal *40s rsp2* subunit gene was used as a control. **(B)** Detection of EhTRF-like I and EhTRF-like III proteins in different trophozoite fractions. Coomassie-blue stained SDS-PAGE of total protein (T), nuclear soluble (Ns), nuclear insoluble (Ni), and cytoplasmic **(C)** extracts. Replicates were transferred to nitrocellulose membranes to immunodetect EhTRF-like I and EhTRF-like III with the corresponding antibodies.

(Continued)

FIGURE 3 | WB were also performed using α-H3K27me3 (as a control for Ns fraction), α-H4K20me3 (as a telomeric label in Ns fraction), α-Lamin B1 (as a control for Ni fraction), α-EhKMT4 (as control for Ns and C fractions), and α-actin (as loading control). **(C,D)** Localization of EhTRF-like proteins in *E. histolytica*. Trophozoites were processed for immunofluorescence and incubated with α-EhTRF-like I (Alexa-647, magenta), α-EhTRF-like III (Alexa-488, green), α-Lamin B1 (Alexa-555, red) and α-H4K20me3 (Alexa-488, green) antibodies. Nuclei were counterstained with DAPI and preparations were analyzed by confocal microscopy. The white arrowheads indicate colocalization in the nuclear periphery. ph c, phase contrast. $^{*}p < 0.05$, $^{***}p < 0.0002$, $^{****}p < 0.0001$.

recognized a 55 kDa band, while in insoluble nuclear fractions, it only detected a 36 kDa band (**Figure 3B**). Otherwise, EhTRF-like III protein was only observed in the soluble nuclear fraction, with the same 65 kDa molecular weight than in total lysates. In these assays, to probe the fractions purity, different cellular fractionation markers were included. As a control of the soluble nuclear fraction, we detected the K27me3 modification of H3 in the total and soluble nuclear fractions previously identified in *E. histolytica* as a repressive epigenetic mark by Foda and Singh (Foda and Singh, 2015; **Figure 3B**). We also detected the K20me3 modification in the H4 histone, which is specific for heterochromatin and related to telomeric regions (Blasco, 2007) and was previously identified in *E. histolytica* by Borbolla-Vázquez (Borbolla-Vázquez et al., 2015). H4K20me3 was also present in the total soluble nuclear fractions. Then, we included the detection of the enzyme methyltransferase EhKMT4 as a control of cytoplasmic and soluble nuclear fractions. This protein was detected in total, cytoplasmic and soluble nuclear extracts (**Figure 3B**). For the insoluble nuclear fraction, we used Lamin B1, which has been reported at the nuclear periphery in contact with the inner side of nuclear envelope in this parasite (Lozano-Amado et al., 2016). This protein was only detected in the total and insoluble nuclear fractions (**Figure 3B**), as expected. Additionally, we used actin as loading control for all cellular fractionations; however, a lesser amount of protein was detected in insoluble and soluble nuclear fractions than in cytoplasm, maybe due to different polymerization state of the actin within the nucleus. Despite, gel stained with Coomassie blue of the fractions obtained, demonstrated a similar protein amount in all samples (**Figure 3B**). Our results revealed that *E. histolytica* trophozoites differentially express *ehtrf-like I, ehtrf-like II* and *ehtrf-like III* transcripts, and the EhTRF-like I and III proteins are concentrated at the nucleus.

EhTRF-Like I and III Are Nuclear Proteins That Co-localize With Lamin B1 and H4k20me3

In order to confirm the EhTRFs-like proteins localization, we performed immunofluorescence assays. Trophozoites cultured in basal conditions were processed for immunofluorescence using α-EhTRF-like I, α-EhTRF-like III, α-Lamin B1 and α-H4K20me3 antibodies coupled to Alexa-647,−488,−555 and−488, respectively. Confocal images evidenced EhTRF-like I and III mainly at trophozoite nuclei and EhTRF-like I was also localized at cytoplasm (**Figure 3C**). Staining of both proteins appeared at nuclear periphery, thus we employed Lamin B1 as a specific marker of this localization (Goldman et al., 2002; Lozano-Amado et al., 2016). Images revealed that EhTRF-like I and III co-localized with Lamin B1 at nuclear periphery, but EhTRF-like I presented a more diffused stain pattern inside nuclei. Therefore, we also investigated if EhTRF-like I was present in telomeric regions, employing H4K20me3 as a telomeric chromatin marker (Blasco, 2007). We found that EhTRF-like I colocalized with H4K20me3, showing sometimes diffused patterns or well-defined *foci* (**Figure 3D**). These results indicated that EhTRF-like I and III proteins are localized in specific nuclear regions as nuclear periphery or distributed in *foci*, co-localizing with Lamin B1 and H4K20me3. Considering the localization of EhTRF-like proteins they could be participating in the protection of the chromosome terminal ends of *E. histolytica.*

To validate the localization and to gain insight into the functional effect of EhTRF-like proteins, in *E. histolytica* trophozoites, we over-expressed the *ehtrf-like I and III* genes fused to the Myc tag and cloned in the *pKT-3M* vector to generate the *pTRF-like Iox and pTRF-like IIIox* overexpression vectors. Trophozoites were transfected with the *pTRF-like Iox, pTRF-like IIIox* or empty (*pKT-3M*) plasmid and stably selected in medium supplemented with 20 $\mu g\ ml^{-1}$ G-418. According to semi-quantitative and quantitative RT-PCR results, the expression of *ehtrf-like I and ehtrf-like III* was 10.2 and 8-fold higher, respectively compared to the expression in *pKT-3M* transfected trophozoites (**Figures 4A,B, 5A,B**). In agreement, WB experiments of lysates from *pEhTRF-like Iox* showed that EhTRF-like I was overexpressed (55 kDa band corresponding to EhTRF-like I), when they are compared with lysates derived from trophozoites transfected with the empty vector (**Figure 4B**). Similarly, WB experiments of lysates from *pEhTRF-like IIIox* transfected trophozoites and using α-Myc antibody, detected a 65 kDa band corresponding to EhTRF-like III (**Figure 5C**). As expected, in *pKT-3M* transfected trophozoites this antibody did not recognize any protein. EhTRF-like I and EhTRF-like III overexpression was confirmed in confocal images of *pEhTRF-like Iox* and *pEhTRF-like IIIox* transfected trophozoites and using the α-EhTRF-like I or α-EhTRF-like III antibody. In these parasites, proteins were more abundant at the nucleus, but they were also observed at cytoplasm (**Figures 4D, 5D**,j–l), in comparison to the lesser staining of trophozoites transfected with empty vector (**Figures 4D, 5D**,f–h). Similar nuclear and perinuclear staining were obtained using the α-Myc antibody, which detected only the heterologous proteins in trophozoites overexpressing EhTRF-like I and EhTRF-like III (**Figures 4D, 5D**,r–t). Comparison with trophozoites transfected with the empty vector no staining was detected (**Figures 4D, 5D**,n–p). No signal was obtained in trophozoites incubated with both pre-immune serums (**Figures 4, 5**,b–d). All of these data confirm the nuclear localization pattern of the EhTRF-like I and III proteins.

EhTRF-Like III Localizes at Nuclear Heterochromatin Regions

Results of EhTRF-like III localization at nuclear *foci* (**Figures 3–5**), suggested this protein could act in specific and functional regions of the nuclei. Thus, we analyzed the

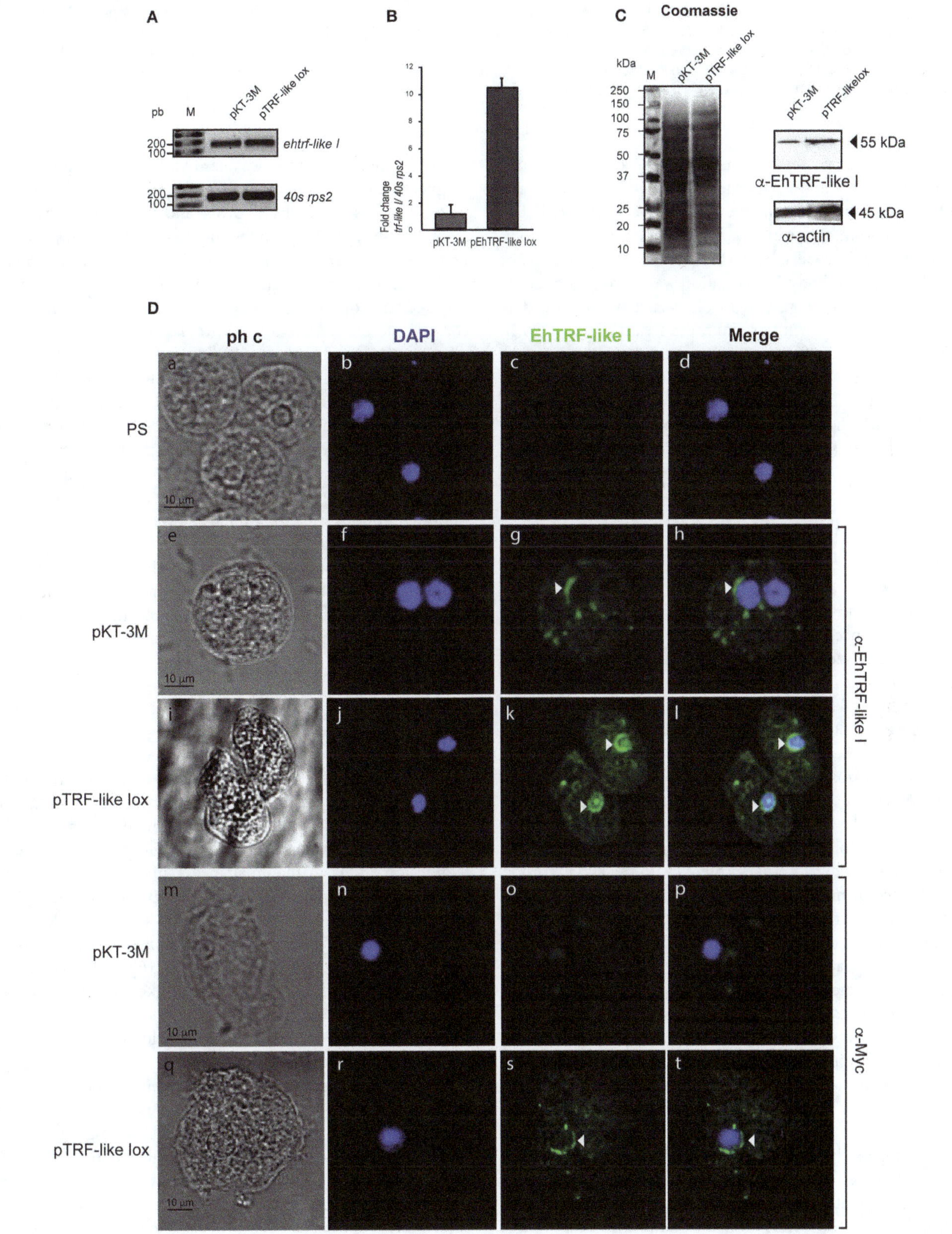

FIGURE 4 | Overexpression of EhTRF-like I in *E. histolytica* trophozoites. **(A)** RT-PCR analysis of the *ehtrf-like I* gene in stably transfected trophozoites with empty plasmid *pKT-3M* or *pEhTRF-like lox*. Ribosomal *40s rsp2* subunit gene was used as control. **(B)** Relative expression of *ehtrf-like I* gene was determined by qRT-PCR,

(Continued)

FIGURE 4 | using the *40s rsp2* gene as control. **(C)** Coomassie blue stained SDS-PAGE showing total extracts of transfected trophozoites (empty plasmid *pKT-3M* or *pEhTRF-like lox*). A duplicate gel was transferred to nitrocellulose membrane and submitted to WB using α-EhTRF-like I and α-actin antibodies. Anti-Actin antibody was used as loading control. **(D)** Transfected trophozoites were processed for immunofluorescence and incubated with pre-immune serum (PS), α-EhTRF-like I or α-Myc antibodies, followed by the α-rabbit FITC-coupled secondary antibody. Nuclei were stained with DAPI and preparations were visualized by confocal microscopy. Arrowheads: EhTRF-like I location at nuclei. ph c, phase contrast.

localization of this protein by transmission electron microscopy (TEM) in *pEhTRF-like IIIox* transfected trophozoites. We found EhTRF-like III abundantly in the trophozoite nuclei, enriched in the heterochromatin or highly condensed chromatin regions, close to the nuclear periphery (**Figures 6C,D**,g,h), using the α-EhTRF-like III antibody. This location was corroborated using the α-Myc antibody (**Figure 6F**,i). No signal was obtained in trophozoites incubated with pre-immune serum (**Figures 6A,B**) or in *pKT-3M* transfected trophozoites stained with the anti-Myc antibody (**Figure 6E**). These data showed that EhTRF-like III is found in chromatin regions with high degree of compaction, which is suggestive of telomeric areas, where EhTRF-like proteins could protect the chromosomes terminal ends.

EhTRF-Like III Forms DNA-Protein Complexes With Telomeres Related Sequences

TRF proteins bind as homodimers to double-stranded DNA telomeric sequences (Broccoli et al., 1997b; Blasco, 2007). Hence, we analyzed if in the nuclear extracts obtained from this parasite there were proteins that could recognize telomeric canonical sequences. We employed EMSA assays using nuclear extracts obtained from wild type trophozoites and the human telomeric sequence (HsTRF). The nuclear extracts from wild-type trophozoites formed three DNA-protein complexes (**Figure 7A**, lane 2). The presence of these three complexes is possibly due by the TRF homologs binding to the HsTEL DNA. Presumably, the formation of these complexes are due to the binding of the three EhTRF-like proteins with the HsTEL probe. In the absence of nuclear extract, no DNA-proteins complexes were formed (**Figure 7A**, lane 1). The HsTEL probe competed with the formation of the three complexes when it was added at increased concentrations (50, 100 and 200 molar). These results suggested that proteins forming these complexes are related to telomeric sequences (**Figure 7A**, lanes 3–5). Even more, when the competition was performed with an *E. histolytica* sequence, the EhTRF probe, it was more efficient (**Figure 7A**, lanes 6–8), showing a greater affinity for this sequence. Other mutated or non-related probes as mut-Tel or non-REL, did not competed with any of DNA-protein complexes (**Figure 7A**, lanes 9–14).

To investigate whether EhTRF-like proteins were able to bind to double-stranded telomeric DNA, we purified the EhTRF-like I recombinant protein (rEhTRF-like I) (**Figure S4**). As shown in **Figures 7B,C**, rEhTRF-like I bound specifically to the HsTEL and EhTEL probes. Competition assays showed that the formed complex by the recombinant protein was abolished in the presence of unlabeled HsTEL and EhTEL excess probes (**Figures 7B,C**, lanes 3–8). There was no competition for binding when the mut-TEL probe was used with the same molar excess (**Figures 7B,C**, lanes 9–11).

Next, we used the EhTEL probe and nuclear extracts derived from transfected trophozoites. In these EMSA assays, we also obtained three DNA-protein complexes, but the complex III was enriched when nuclear extracts from *pEhTRF-like IIIox* transfected trophozoites were used (**Figure 7D**, lane 3). To corroborate the identity of the proteins that formed the DNA-protein complex, a super-shift assay was performed using the oligonucleotide EhTEL, nuclear extracts from *pEhTRF-like IIIox* transfected trophozoites and the α-EhTRF-like III antibody. We observed a shifted complex in the presence of the α-EhTRF-like III antibody (**Figure 7E**, lane 3) and the pre-immune serum did not modify the formation of any DNA-protein complexes (**Figure 7E**, lane 4). We also included an anti-Myc antibody but in our conditions, we didn't obtain slower migration complexes, probably the Myc epitope become hidden upon binding to DNA (inducing a conformational change). This data indicated that pTRF-like III is able to form DNA-protein complexes with EhTEL sequences. Overall, these results indicated that in the nucleus of this parasite there are proteins interacting with telomeric sequences.

DISCUSSION

All eukaryotes protect their chromosome ends through telomere binding proteins, which are well-conserved among these organisms (Linger and Price, 2009). These proteins conform a protein complex dubbed Shelterin and bind specifically to telomeric regions in mammalian organisms (de Lange, 2005). However, less complex machineries are present in fission yeast, protozoan ciliates, and plants (Watson and Riha, 2010). The stable interaction of Shelterin with telomeres depends on the association of two proteins, TRF1 and TRF2 to double-stranded telomeric repeats. The presence of TRF-like proteins in primitive unicellular eukaryotes is outstanding and might represent the ancestral scenario during evolution of telomeres and its protein counterparts.

In silico analysis showed that *Entamoeba histolytica* has three genes coding for TRF-like proteins. These proteins conserve the Telobox motif in their MYB DBD, which is highly conserved as in higher eukaryotes, and showed high identity (25 to 35%) with the amino acid sequences of the human Sheltering proteins TRF1 and TRF2. It is very interesting that this parasite has three genes that encode for TRF proteins, which could be the result of a gene duplication event. It has been proposed that the selective pressure through mechanisms of recombination were involved during TRF paralog formation. Stress responses is a selection pressure which generate elevated paralog formation

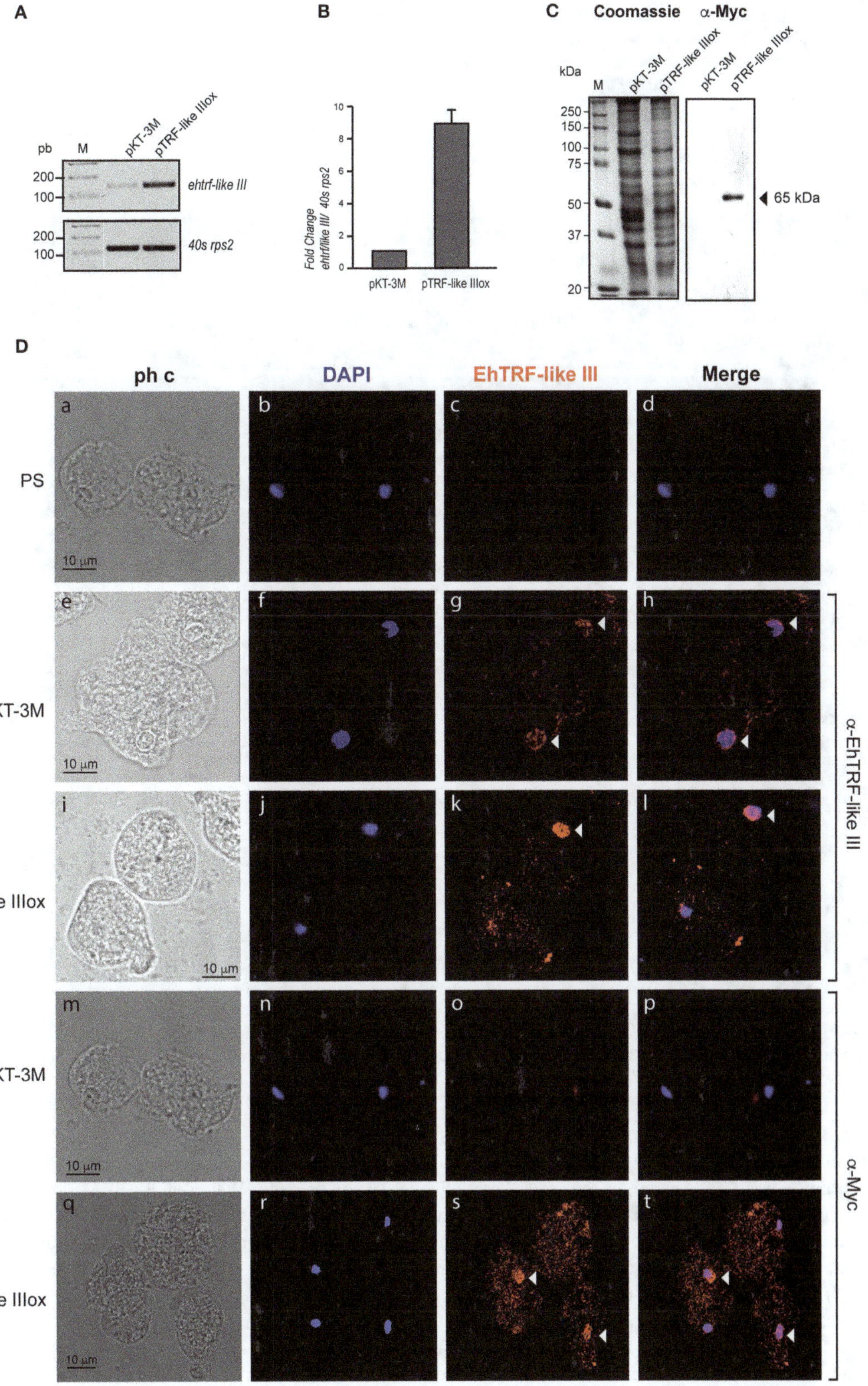

FIGURE 5 | Overexpression of EhTRF-like III in *E. histolytica* trophozoites. **(A)** RT-PCR analysis of the *ehtrf-like III* gene in stably transfected trophozoites with empty plasmid *pKT-3M* or *pEhTRF-like IIIox*. Ribosomal *40s rsp2* subunit gene was used as control. **(B)** Relative expression of *ehtrf-like III* gene was determined using

(Continued)

FIGURE 5 | qRT-PCR and the *40s rsp2* gene as control. **(C)** Coomassie-blue stained SDS-PAGE showing total extracts of transfected trophozoites (empty plasmid *pKT-3M* or *pEhTRF-like IIIox*). A duplicate gel was transferred to nitrocellulose membrane and submitted to WB using α-Myc antibody. **(D)** Transfected trophozoites were processed for immunofluorescence and incubated with pre-immune serum (PS), α-EhTRF-like III or α-Myc antibodies, followed by the α-rabbit TRITC-coupled secondary antibody. Nuclei were stained with DAPI and preparations were visualized by confocal microscopy. Arrowheads: EhTRF-like III location at nuclei. ph c, phase contrast.

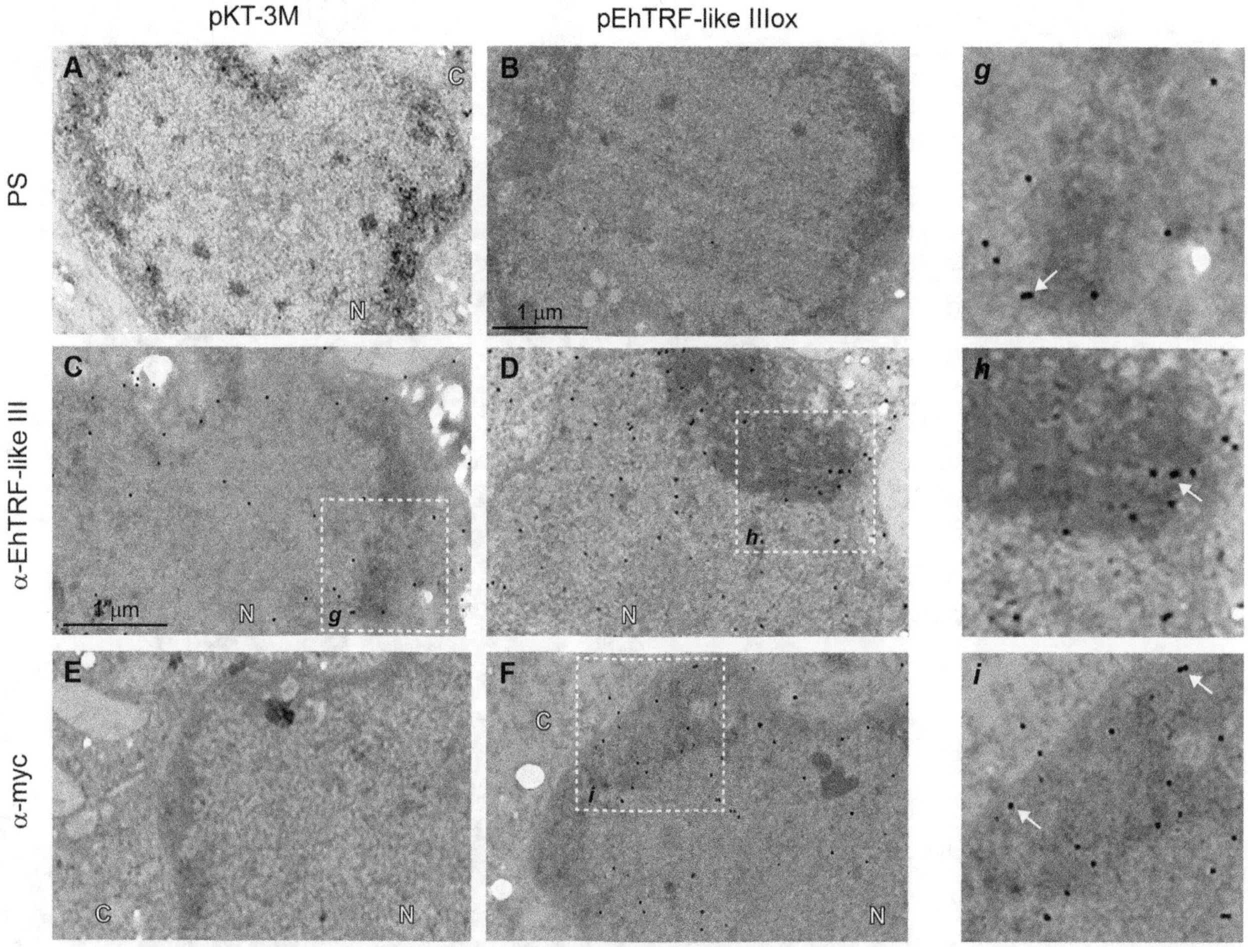

FIGURE 6 | Detection by TEM of EhTRF-like III at *E. histolytica* trophozoites nuclei. TEM of transfected trophozoites (*pKT-3M* and *pEhTRF-like IIIox*) incubated with pre-immune serum (PS; **A,B**), α-EhTRF-like III **(C,D)**, or α-Myc antibodies **(E,F)**, followed by the incubation with α-rabbit gold-labeled secondary antibody. Panels g–i: magnifications of squares on **(C,D,F)**, respectively. N, nuclei and C, cytoplasm. Arrows: gold particles.

and lead to an exceedingly high rate of Telomeric Binding Proteins evolution (Lustig, 2016). In the case of *E. histolytica,* the host's environment submits the parasite to a variety of stress conditions (oxidative stress derived from the immune response, tissue invasion, migration, or the simply need of persistence in the host). It has been proposed that gene duplication is the main process by which new genetic material is obtained by an organism. Our qRT-PCR results showed a differential expression pattern of *Ehtrf-like* genes. *ehtrf-like III* is more expressed in basal conditions while *ehtrf-like II* has the minor expression. These results suggest that the mechanisms that control gene expression could have changed depending on the environment conditions. This differential behavior of the trophozoite has been observed changing the growing conditions of the parasite (Weber et al., 2016). The presence of three *ehtrf-like* genes may result in a differential functionality of telomeric binding proteins improving the organisms' responses to the environmental challenges and protecting their chromosome ends.

Few telomeric binding proteins have been identified in protozoan parasites. Our analyses suggested that *E. histolytica* has a simpler machinery to protect their telomeric DNA. This machinery Shelterin-like could be similar to other unicellular parasites, such as *Trypanosoma* and *Leishmania*, were orthologs of TRF-2, Rpa-1 (replication protein A subunit 1) and RAP1 have been identified and characterized, suggesting that the telomeric

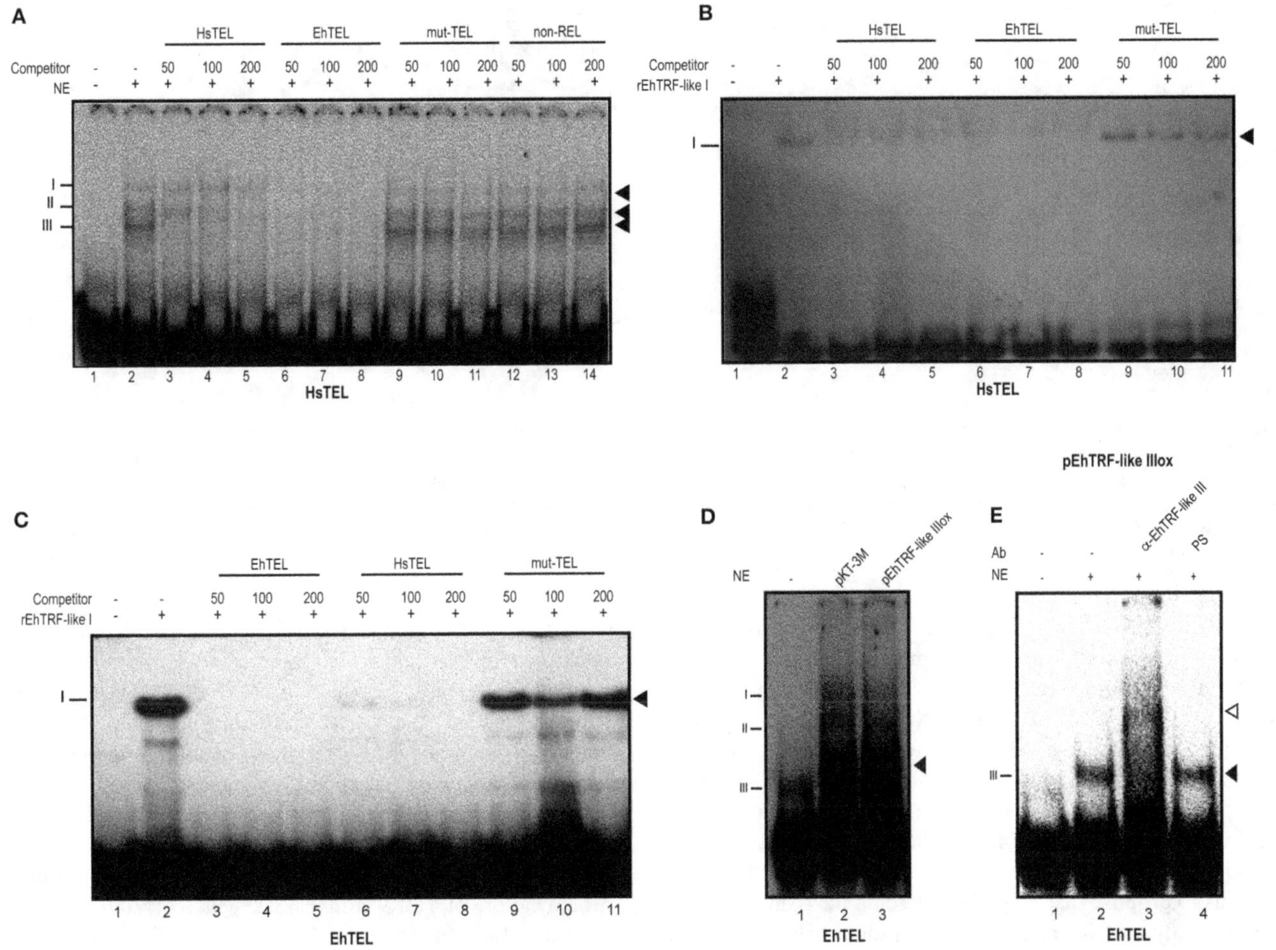

FIGURE 7 | TRF-like III forms DNA-protein complexes with telomeric sequences. **(A)** EMSA was done using radiolabeled double-stranded human canonical telomeric DNA (HsTEL) as probe and nuclear extracts obtained from *E. histolytica* trophozoites. Competition assays were done in the presence of 50, 100, and 200-fold excess of non-labeled sequences: HsTEL specific competitor, *E. histolytica* sequence (EhTEL), mutated telomeric sequence (mut-TEL) or non-related sequence (non-Rel). **(B)** EMSA assay using rEHTRF-like I recombinant protein and HsTEL probe competition assays were done in the presence of 50, 100, and 200-fold excess of non-labeled sequences (HsTEL, EhTEL and mut-TEL). **(C)** EMSA assay using rEHTRF-like I and EhTEL competition assays were done in the presence of 50, 100, and 200-fold excess of non-labeled sequences (HsTEL, EhTEL and mut-TEL). **(D)** EMSA assay using EhTEL sequence and nuclear extracts obtained from trophozoites transfected with the *pKT-3M* or *pEhTRF-like IIIox* plasmids. **(E)** Super-shift assay was done using radiolabeled double-stranded EhTEL sequence as probe, nuclear extracts obtained from transfected trophozoites and α-EhTRF-like III antibody or pre-immune serum (PS). Protein-DNA complexes were separated in a 6% PAGE. Black arrowheads: specific protein-DNA complexes. Open arrowhead: super shifted protein-DNA complex.

machinery evolved early in eukaryotes (Lira et al., 2007; Yang et al., 2009).

EhTRF-like I and III proteins span from 404 to 460 amino acids with theoretical molecular weight (MW) of 46.8 to 53.1 kDa, respectively; However, in our experiments, EhTRF-like I was recognized at a 55 or a 36 kDa band and EhTRFlike III was observed in all fractions at 60 kDa band. The MW increase observed in both proteins could be related to post-translational modifications (PTMs), such as phosphorylation, ubiquitinations and SUMOylations that change protein mobility (Audagnotto and Dal Peraro, 2017). This is relevant since the function of the TRF proteins, their ability to bind to the telomeric DNA, their dimerization and location as well as their degradation and interaction with other proteins (Walker and Zhu, 2012) is regulated through PTMs. Therefore, we performed an *in silico* analysis and found that EhTRF-like proteins can be modified by SUMOylations in different residues, some of them conserved with respect to TRF-1 and TRF-2. The K302 and K303 SUMOylation sites of EhTRF-like I were conserved with respect to TRF1 (K338 and K339), which explain the MW difference since it has been reported that SUMOylated proteins increase their MW from 8 to 17 kDa for each unit of the bound SUMO peptide (Hilgarth and Sarge, 2005). We propose similar scenario for EhTRF-like III. SUMOylation regulates proteins with nuclear function since it is related to nuclear transport, transcription, location in subnuclear compartments, chromatin organization, DNA damage repair of DNA and is linked to cell cycle regulation, growth and apoptosis (Flotho and Melchior, 2013). In TRF1,

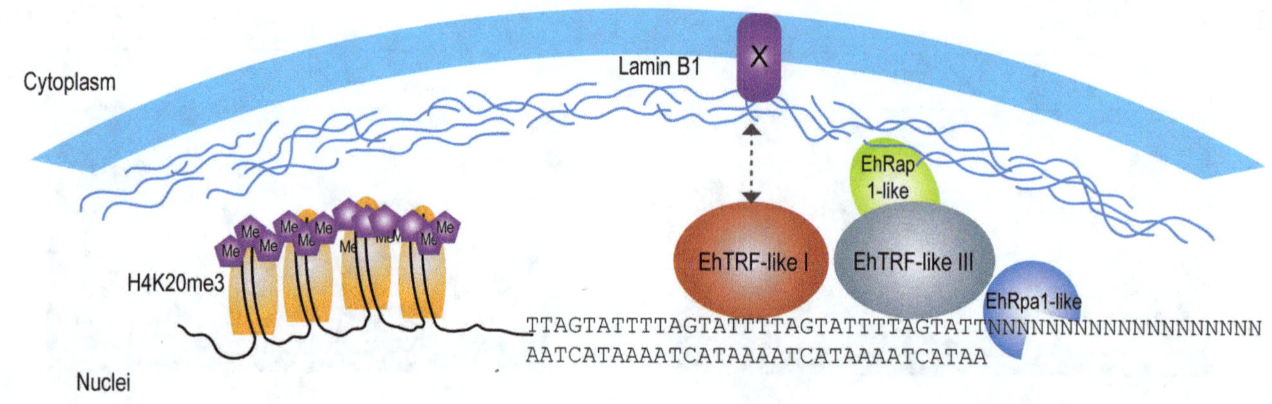

FIGURE 8 | Model of EhTRF-like participation in the protection of chromosome ends in *E. histolytica*. Scheme at the nuclear periphery location of EhTRF-like I and EhTRF-like III linked to the double-stranded DNA. These proteins are close to nuclear lamina, co-localizing with the telomeric heterochromatin label H4K20me3. EhTRF-like I and III could interact with lamin B1, probably through an unknown protein with a similar function to the Sun anchoring protein as in *H. sapiens* (Giraud-Panis et al., 2013). Additionally, some putative Shelterin proteins are shown: EhRap1-like (EHI_064550) and the single-stranded DNA-binding protein EhRpa1-like (EHI_062980).

SUMOylation is related to telomere maintenance through the ALT pathway (Alternative Lengthening of Telomeres), which occurs in the absence of telomerase. SUMOylated TRF-1 is recruited to the PML bodies where telomeric regions have been identified DNA (Yu et al., 2007; Royle et al., 2008). Therefore, the increase in the MW of the EhTRF-like I and III proteins could be explained by means of this PTM that suggest a similar role. Interestingly, all the enzymes involved in SUMOylation have been identified in *E. histolytica* (Bosch and Siderovski, 2013). This allows us to propose that EhTRF-like I could have similar PTMs as TRF-1 to modulate its activity and protect telomeric DNA. Detection of the EhTRF-like I protein in the insoluble nuclear fraction with a molecular weight of 36 kDa was also obtained. This molecular weight is lower than the predicted for EhTRF-like I. EhTRF-like I protein contains different residues susceptible to proteolytic cleavage, E352 was predicted as proteolytic cleavage site. If this site is functional, it would generate a peptide with a similar weight to that we found in the insoluble fraction. Interestingly, this residue is also conserved in *H. sapiens* TRF1. Finally, it has been reported that the presence of high content of acidic residues might affect the gel mobility shift of a protein and thereby explain the molecular weight variations found (Guan et al., 2015).

Human cells telomeres are tethered to the nuclear envelope during post-mitotic nuclear assembly. TRF proteins are associated with the nuclear membrane through Lamin B1. Binding of lamins to telomeres is partially mediated by TRF2, via its interaction with RAP1 which interacts with the nuclear envelope protein Sunl (Hediger et al., 2002; Crabbe et al., 2012; Gonzalo and Eissenberg, 2016). In agreement, we found that EhTRF-like I and III colocalized with Lamin B1 at the nuclear periphery suggesting that they occupy a similar position. In accordance with this localization, in EhTRF-like III over-expressing trophozoites, this protein was localized also in the nuclear periphery proximal to the nuclear membrane in condensed heterochromatin regions. Likewise, telomeres have been found located in interphase nuclei close to the nuclear envelope; However, not in all organisms telomeres occupy this position, for example in plants like *A. thaliana* they have been reported close to the nucleolus (Schrumpfová et al., 2014). Therefore, the subnuclear location of telomeres is species-, cell type- and cell-phase dependent (Giraud-Panis et al., 2013). Telomeres carry features of repressive chromatin associated with constitutive heterochromatin. Different histone signatures have recently been identified associated with mammalian telomeres: trimethylation of H3K9 and H4K20 (Blasco, 2007). Here we selected H4K20me3 because it was previously identified and described in this parasite (Borbolla-Vázquez et al., 2015) and could suggest its participation in the organization and regulation of telomeric DNA in the *E. histolytica* nuclear periphery. Consistent with this, we observed that EhTRF-like I colocalized with the H4K20me3 mark suggesting that EhTRF-like proteins occupy regions of silenced compacted chromatin, in consistence with the telomere compacted structure (Giraud-Panis et al., 2013). Given the position of EhTRF-like I and III at the nuclear periphery and their colocalization with Lamin B and the trimethylated H4K20, we propose that these proteins could participate in the protection of chromosome ends.

Finally, we explored whether nuclear proteins from *E. histolytica* recognized the human telomeric sequence (HuTRF). Interestingly, we found three DNA-protein specific complexes from nuclear extracts of trophozoites that were competed with the human canonical telomeric sequence and with the probe derived from the STR repeat of the NK2 array that could be related to telomeric DNA (EhTEL). These DNA-protein complexes were not competed with mutated telomeric sequence (mut-TEL) or non-related (non- REL), showing specificity for telomeric sequences. Moreover, in an attempt to evaluate the telomeric DNA binding properties of EhTRF-like proteins, we observed that rEhTRF-like I recognized both HuTRF and EhTEL sequences. Since *E. histolytica* has three genes that code for three proteins with telomeric MYB DBD it would be interesting to determine if DNA-protein complexes correspond to these three proteins. Using nuclear extracts from trophozoites overexpressing EhTRF-like III we found that this protein formed DNA protein complexes with the STR sequence of *E. histolytica*. In our conditions, only complex III was enriched when extracts from TRF-like III overexpressing clones were used with the EhTEL probe indicating that the TRF-like III protein interacts with the STR repeat of the tRNA genes. This is the first report were a sequence derived from the tRNA arrays ([NK2]) is used to determine its recognition by nuclear proteins and rTRF-like I in EMSA assays. Previously, the YE array was used in fluorescence *in situ* hybridization (FISH) analysis, detecting six distinct signals at the parasite nucleus (Willhoeft and Tannich, 2000). However, as the ploidy of *E. histolytica* remains to be determined the interpretation of this evidence was difficult. It will be interest to determine the *in vivo* association of EhTRF-like proteins with sequences derived from the tRNA arrays.

In conclusion, the protection of the chromosome ends is critical to the survival of any cell as their disruption can induce genomic instability and consequently compromise the viability of the organism. Although no canonical Shelterin proteins have been identified in this protozoan, TRF-like proteins might accomplish this role for their ability to recognize and interact with telomeric DNA through their MYB-DBD. Therefore, this work shows the first evidence of telomeric proteins in *E. histolytica* able to interact with the proposed *Entamoeba* telomeric DNA sequences conforming a simple Shelterin complex as in other protozoans (**Figure 8**). This work raises several interesting questions and further investigation will contribute to a better understanding of the role of EhTRF-like proteins in the telomeric function in *E. histolytica*.

AUTHOR CONTRIBUTIONS

All authors contributed equally to design and conception of this work. FR-G, VÁ-H, EC-O, and RC-G collected *E. histolytica* experimental data. HC-H performed the *in-silico* analysis; BC-M and AL-G performed MET analysis. AB contributes with confocal microscopy. FR-G, AB, JV, EO, LL-C, and EA-L contributed to experimental design, intellectual input, interpreting data and in writing the manuscript.

FUNDING

EA-L thanks CONACYT for a research grant to study proteins that preserve genome integrity in *Entamoeba histolytica* (Ciencia Básica # 222956).

ACKNOWLEDGMENTS

VÁ-H thanks fellowship 586852 from CONACYT. HC-H thanks fellowships BI 080530161142 and ICyTDF/179/2011. We thank Dr. Luis Brieba for reading the manuscript and providing constructive comments. The authors are grateful to Alfredo Barberi for graphical design and Brenda Herrera Villalobos for technical assistance.

REFERENCES

Abhyankar, M. M., Hochreiter, A. E., Hershey, J., Evans, C., Zhang, Y., Crasta, O., et al. (2008). Characterization of an *Entamoeba histolytica* high-mobility-group box protein induced during intestinal infection. *Eukaryot Cell* 7, 1565–1572. doi: 10.1128/EC.00123-08

Audagnotto, M., and Dal Peraro, M. (2017). Protein post-translational modifications: *in silico* prediction tools and molecular modeling. *Comput. Struct. Biotechnol. J.* 15, 307–319. doi: 10.1016/j.csbj.2017.03.004

Bilaud, T., Koering, C. E., Binet-Brasselet, E., Ancelin, K., Pollice, A., Gasser, S. M., et al. (1996). The telobox, a Myb-related telomeric DNA binding motif found in proteins from yeast, plants and human. *Nucleic Acids Res.* 24, 1294–1303. doi: 10.1093/nar/24.7.1294

Blackburn, E. H., and Gall, J. G. (1978). A tandemly repeated sequence at the termini of the extrachromosomal ribosomal RNA genes in *Tetrahymena*. *J. Mol. Biol.* 120, 33–53. doi: 10.1016/0022-2836(78)90294-2

Blasco, M. A. (2007). The epigenetic regulation of mammalian telomeres. *Nat. Rev. Genet.* 8, 299–309. doi: 10.1038/nrg2047

Borbolla-Vázquez, J., Orozco, E., Betanzos, A., and Rodríguez, M. A. (2015). Entamoeba histolytica: protein arginine transferase 1a methylates arginine residues and potentially modify the H4 histone. *Parasites Vectors* 8:219. doi: 10.1186/s13071-015-0820-7

Bosch, D. E., and Siderovski, D. P. (2013). Structural determinants of ubiquitin conjugation in *Entamoeba histolytica*. *J. Biol. Chem.* 288, 2290–2302. doi: 10.1074/jbc.M112.417337

Bradford, M. M. (1976). A rapid and sensitive method for the quantitation of microgram quantities of protein utilizing the principle of protein-dye binding. *Anal. Biochem.* 72, 248–254. doi: 10.1016/0003-2697(76)90527-3

Broccoli, D., Chong, L., Oelmann, S., Fernald, A. A., Marziliano, N., van Steensel, B., et al. (1997a). Comparison of the human and mouse genes encoding the telomeric protein, TRF1: chromosomal localization, expression and conserved protein domains. *Hum. Mol. Genet.* 6, 69–76.

Broccoli, D., Smogorzewska, A., Chong, L., and de Lange, T. (1997b). Human telomeres contain two distinct Myb-related proteins, TRF1 and TRF2. *Nat. Genet.* 17, 231–235.

Chong, L., van Steensel, B., Broccoli, D., Erdjument-Bromage, H., Hanish, J., Tempst, P., et al. (1995). A human telomeric protein. *Science* 270, 1663–1667.

Clark, C. G., Ali, I. K., Zaki, M., Loftus, B. J., and Hall, N. (2006). Unique organisation of tRNA genes in *Entamoeba histolytica*. *Mol Biochem Parasitol.* 146, 24–29. doi: 10.1016/j.molbiopara.2005.10.013

Clark, C. G., Alsmark, U. C., Tazreiter, M., Saito-Nakano, Y., Ali, V., Marion, S., et al. (2007). Structure and content of the Entamoeba histolytica genome. *Adv. Parasitol.* 65, 51–190. doi: 10.1016/S0065-308X(07)65002-7

Crabbe, L., Cesare, A. J., Kasuboski, J. M., Fitzpatrick, J. A., and Karlseder, J. (2012). Human telomeres are tethered to the nuclear envelope during postmitotic nuclear assembly. *Cell Rep.* 2, 1521–1529. doi: 10.1016/j.celrep.2012.11.019

da Silva, M. S., Perez, A. M., da Silveira Rde, C., de Moraes, C. E., Siqueira-Neto, J. L., Freitas Lde, H. Jr., et al. (2010). The Leishmania amazonensis TRF (TTAGGG repeat-binding factor) homologue binds and co-localizes with telomeres. *BMC Microbiol.* 10:136. doi: 10.1186/1471-2180-10-136

de Lange, T. (2005). Shelterin: the protein complex that shapes and safeguards human telomeres. *Genes. Dev.* 19, 2100–2110. doi: 10.1101/gad.1346005

Diamond, L. S., Harlow, D. R., and Cunnick, C. C. (1978). A new medium for the axenic cultivation of *Entamoeba histolytica* and other *Entamoeba. Trans. R Soc. Trop. Med. Hyg.* 72, 431–432. doi: 10.1016/0035-9203(78)90144-X

Fairall, L., Chapman, L., Moss, H., de Lange, T., and Rhodes, D. (2001). Structure of the TRFH dimerization domain of the human telomeric proteins TRF1 and TRF2. *Mol. Cell* 8, 351–361. doi: 10.1016/S1097-2765(01)00321-5

Flotho, A., and Melchior, F. (2013). Sumoylation: a regulatory protein modification in health and disease. *Annu. Rev. Biochem.* 82, 357–385. doi: 10.1146/annurev-biochem-061909-093311

Foda, B. M., and Singh, U. (2015). Dimethylated H3K27 is a repressive epigenetic histone mark in the protist *Entamoeba histolytica* and is significantly enriched in genes silenced via the RNAi pathway. *J. Biol. Chem.* 290, 21114–21130. doi: 10.1074/jbc.M115.647263

Giraud-Panis, M. J., Pisano, S., Benarroch-Popivker, D., Pei, B., Le Du, M. H., and Gilson, E. (2013). One identity or more for telomeres? *Front. Oncol.* 3:48. doi: 10.3389/fonc.2013.00048

Goldman, R. D., Gruenbaum, Y., Moir, R. D., Shumaker, D. K., and Spann, T. P. (2002). Nuclear lamins: building blocks of nuclear architecture. *Genes. Dev.* 16, 533–547. doi: 10.1101/gad.960502

Gonzalo, S., and Eissenberg, J. C. (2016). Tying up loose ends: telomeres, genomic instability and lamins. *Curr. Opin. Genet. Dev.* 37, 109–118. doi: 10.1016/j.gde.2016.03.003

Guan, Y., Zhu, Q., Huang, D., Zhao, S., Jan Lo, L., and Peng, J. (2015). An equation to estimate the difference between theoretically predicted and SDS PAGE-displayed molecular weights for an acidic peptide. *Sci. Rep.* 5:13370. doi: 10.1038/srep13370

Hediger, F., Neumann, F. R., Van Houwe, G., Dubrana, K., and Gasser, S. M. (2002). Live imaging of telomeres: yKu and Sir proteins define redundant telomere-anchoring pathways in yeast. *Curr. Biol.* 12, 2076–2089. doi: 10.1016/S0960-9822(02)01338-6

Hilgarth, R. S., and Sarge, K. D. (2005). Detection of sumoylated proteins. *Methods Mol. Biol.* 301, 329–338. doi: 10.1385/1-59259-895-1:329

Hopp, T. P., and Woods, K. R. (1981). Prediction of protein antigenic determinants from amino acid sequences. *Proc. Natl. Acad. Sci. U.S.A.* 78, 3824–3828. doi: 10.1073/pnas.78.6.3824

Horvath, M. P. (2000–2013). "Evolution of telomere binding proteins," in Madame Curie Bioscience Database (Austin, TX: Landes Bioscience).

Hwang, M. G., Chung, I. K., Kang, B. G., and Cho, M. H. (2001). Sequence-specific binding property of *Arabidopsis thaliana* telomeric DNA binding protein 1 (AtTBP1). *FEBS Lett.* 503, 35–40. doi: 10.1016/S0014-5793(01)02685-0

Kumar, S., Stecher, G., and Tamura, K. (2016). MEGA7: molecular evolutionary genetics analysis version 7.0 for bigger datasets. *Mol. Biol. Evol.* 33, 1870–1874. doi: 10.1093/molbev/msw054

Li, B., Espinal, A., and Cross, G. A. (2005). Trypanosome telomeres are protected by a homologue of mammalian TRF2. *Mol. Cell Biol.* 25, 5011–5021. doi: 10.1128/MCB.25.12.5011-5021.2005

Linger, B. R., and Price, C. M. (2009). Conservation of telomere protein complexes: shuffling through evolution. *Crit. Rev. Biochem. Mol. Biol.* 44, 434–446. doi: 10.3109/10409230903307329

Lira, C. B., Giardini, M. A., Neto, J. L., Conte, F. F., and Cano, M. I. (2007). Telomere biology of trypanosomatids: beginning to answer some questions. *Trends Parasitol.* 23, 357–362. doi: 10.1016/j.pt.2007.06.005

Loftus, B., Anderson, I., Davies, R., Alsmark, U. C., Samuelson, J., Amedeo, P., et al. (2005). The genome of the protist parasite *Entamoeba histolytica. Nature* 433, 865–868. doi: 10.1038/nature03291

Lorenzi, H. A., Puiu, D., Miller, J. R., Brinkac, L. M., Amedeo, P., Hall, N., et al. (2010). New assembly, reannotation and analysis of the Entamoeba histolytica genome reveal new genomic features and protein content information. *PLoS Negl. Trop. Dis.* 4:e716. doi: 10.1371/journal.pntd.0000716

Lozano-Amado, D., Herrera-Solorio, A. M., Valdés, J., Alemán-Lazarini, L., Almaraz-Barrera Mde, J., Luna-Rivera, E., et al. (2016). Identification of repressive and active epigenetic marks and nuclear bodies in *Entamoeba histolytica. Parasit. Vectors* 9:19. doi: 10.1186/s13071-016-1298-7

Lue, N. F. (2010). Plasticity of telomere maintenance mechanisms in yeast. *Trends Biochem. Sci.* 35, 8–17. doi: 10.1016/j.tibs.2009.08.006

Lustig, A. J. (2016). Hypothesis: paralog formation from progenitor proteins and paralog mutagenesis spur the rapid evolution of telomere binding proteins. *Front. Genet.* 7:10. doi: 10.3389/fgene.2016.00010

Melville, S. E., Gerrard, C. S., and Blackwell, J. M. (1999). Multiple causes of size variation in the diploid megabase chromosomes of African tyrpanosomes. *Chromosome Res.* 7, 191–203. doi: 10.1023/A:1009247315947

Meneses, E., Cárdenas, H., Zárate, S., Brieba, L. G., Orozco, E., López-Camarillo, C., et al. (2010). The R2R3 Myb protein family in *Entamoeba histolytica. Gene* 455, 32–42. doi: 10.1016/j.gene.2010.02.004

Meyne, J., Ratliff, R. L., and Moyzis, R. K. (1989). Conservation of the human telomere sequence (TTAGGG)n among vertebrates. *Proc. Natl. Acad. Sci. U.S.A.* 86, 7049–7053. doi: 10.1073/pnas.86.18.7049

Moyzis, R. K., Buckingham, J. M., Cram, L. S., Dani, M., Deaven, L. L., Jones, M. D., et al. (1988). A highly conserved repetitive DNA sequence, (TTAGGG)n, present at the telomeres of human chromosomes. *Proc. Natl. Acad. Sci. U.S.A.* 85, 6622–6626. doi: 10.1073/pnas.85.18.6622

Olvera, A., Olvera, F., Vines, R. R., Recillas-Targa, F., Lizardi, P. M., Dhar, S., et al. (1997). Stable transfection of *Entamoeba histolytica* trophozoites by lipofection. *Arch. Med. Res.* 28, 49–51.

O'Sullivan, R. J., and Karlseder, J. (2010). Telomeres: protecting chromosomes against genome instability. *Nat. Rev. Mol. Cell Biol.* 11, 171–181. doi: 10.1038/nrm2848

Palm, W., and de Lange, T. (2008). How shelterin protects mammalian telomeres. *Annu. Rev. Genet.* 42, 301–334. doi: 10.1146/annurev.genet.41.110306.130350

Patarapotikul, J., and Langsley, G. (1988). Chromosome size polymorphism in Plasmodium falciparum can involve deletions of the subtelomeric pPFrep20 sequence. *Nucleic Acids Res.* 16, 4331–4340. doi: 10.1093/nar/16.10.4331

Royle, N. J., Foxon, J., Jeyapalan, J. N., Mendez-Bermudez, A., Novo, C. L., Williams, J., et al. (2008). Telomere length maintenance–an ALTernative mechanism. *Cytogenet. Genome Res.* 122, 281–291. doi: 10.1159/000167814

Saito-Nakano, Y., Yasuda, T., Nakada-Tsukui, K., Leippe, M., and Nozaki, T. (2004). Rab5-associated vacuoles play a unique role in phagocytosis of the enteric protozoan parasite *Entamoeba histolytica. J. Biol. Chem.* 279, 49497–49507. doi: 10.1074/jbc.M403987200

Schreiber, E., Matthias, P., Müller, M. M., and Schaffner, W. (1989). Rapid detection of octamer binding proteins with 'mini-extracts', prepared from a small number of cells. *Nucleic Acids Res.* 17:6419.

Schrumpfová, P. P., Vychodilová, I., Dvoráckova, M., Majerská, J., Dokládal, L., Schorová, S., et al. (2014). Telomere repeat binding proteins are functional components of Arabidopsis telomeres and interact with telomerase. *Plant J.* 77, 770–781. doi: 10.1111/tpj.12428

Segovia-Gamboa, N. C., Talamás-Rohana, P., Ángel-Martínez, A., Cázares-Raga, F. E., González-Robles, A., Hernández-Ramírez, V. I., et al. (2011). Differentiation of Entamoeba histolytica: a possible role for enolase. *Exp. Parasitol.* 129, 65–71. doi: 10.1016/j.exppara.2011.05.001

Tawari, B., Ali, I. K., Scott, C., Quail, M. A., Berriman, M., Hall, N., et al. (2008). Patterns of evolution in the unique tRNA gene arrays of the genus *Entamoeba. Mol. Biol. Evol.* 25, 187–198. doi: 10.1093/molbev/msm238

Walker, J. R., and Zhu, X. D. (2012). Post-translational modifications of TRF1 and TRF2 and their roles in telomere maintenance. *Mech. Ageing Dev.* 133, 421–434. doi: 10.1016/j.mad.2012.05.002

Watson, J. M., and Riha, K. (2010). Comparative biology of telomeres: where plants stand. *FEBS Lett.* 584, 3752–3759. doi: 10.1016/j.febslet.2010.06.017

Weber, C., Koutero, M., Dillies, M. A., Varet, H., Lopez-Camarillo, C., Coppée, J. Y., et al. (2016). Extensive transcriptome analysis correlates the plasticity of Entamoeba histolytica pathogenesis to rapid phenotype changes depending on the environment. *Sci. Rep.* 6:35852. doi: 10.1038/srep 35852

Willhoeft, U., and Tannich, E. (2000). Fluorescence microscopy and fluorescence *in situ* hybridization of *Entamoeba histolytica* nuclei to analyse mitosis and the localization of repetitive DNA. *Mol. Biochem. Parasitol.* 105, 291–296. doi: 10.1016/S0166-6851(99)00181-4

Yang, X., Figueiredo, L. M., Espinal, A., Okubo, E., and Li, B. (2009). RAP1 is essential for silencing telomeric variant surface glycoprotein genes in *Trypanosoma brucei. Cell* 137, 99–109. doi: 10.1016/j.cell.2009.01.037

Yu, J., Lan, J., Zhu, Y., Lai, X., and Huang, H. (2007). Sumoylation of TRF1 Is essential for its recruitment to ALT-associated PML bodies. *Blood* 110, 4169–4169. Available online at: http://www.bloodjournal.org/content/110/11/4169

3

Entamoeba histolytica Calreticulin Induces the Expression of Cytokines in Peripheral Blood Mononuclear Cells Isolated from Patients with Amebic Liver Abscess

Enrique Gonzalez Rivas, Cecilia Ximenez*, Miriam Enriqueta Nieves-Ramirez, Patricia Moran Silva, Oswaldo Partida-Rodríguez, Eric Hernandez Hernandez, Liliana Rojas Velázquez, Angelica Serrano Vázquez and Ulises Magaña Nuñez

Laboratorio de Inmunología, Unidad de Investigación de Medicina Experimental, Facultad de Medicina, Universidad Nacional Autónoma de México (UNAM), Ciudad de Mexico, Mexico

***Correspondence:**
Cecilia Ximénez
cximenez@unam.mx

Calreticulin (CRT) is a highly conserved protein in the endoplasmic reticulum that plays important roles in the regulation of key cellular functions. Little is known about the participation of *E. histolytica* CRT (*Eh*CRT) in the processes of pathogenicity or in the modulation of the host immune response. The aim of this study was to evaluate the role of CRT in the proliferation and the cytokine profile in peripheral blood mononuclear cells (PBMCs) from patients with amebic liver abscess (ALA) during the acute phase (AP-ALA) of the disease compared to patients during the resolution phase (R-ALA). The PBMCs from each participant were cocultured with *Eh*CRT and tested by the colorimetric method to evaluate their proliferation index (PI). The supernatants were subjected to an enzyme-linked immunosorbent assay (ELISA) to evaluate the concentration of cytokines. The mean values of all groups were compared using the independent *t*-test. When the PIs of individuals without diagnosis of liver abscess (NEG) were compared, there were no statistically significant differences in the proliferation of PBMCs between patients with AP-ALA and R-ALA when stimulated with *Eh*CRT or concanavalin A (ConA). However, the levels of interleukins [IL-6, IL-10, granulocyte colony stimulating factor (GCSF), and transforming growth factor β1 (TGFβ1)] were higher in patients with AP-ALA, whereas in patients with R-ALA, higher levels of interferon gamma (IFNγ) were detected. These results suggest that *Eh*CRT acts as a mitogen very similar to the activity of ConA. In addition, *Eh*CRT is an excellent immunogen for the specific activation of PBMCs, inducing the differential expression of ILs depending on the outcome of disease, determining the type of immune response: a Th2 cytokine profile during the acute phase and a Th1 profile during the resolution phase.

Keywords: amebic liver abscess, calreticulin, *Entamoeba histolytica*, mitogen, proliferation index, interleukins

INTRODUCTION

Infection with the enteric protozoan *E. histolytica* is one of the leading causes of death worldwide. The disease is a consequence of the parasite's abilities to invade the colon, causing amebic colitis. *E. histolytica* can disseminate to the liver via the portal venous system, resulting in amebic liver abscess (ALA). However, approximately 90% of infected people are asymptomatic cyst carriers (Haque et al., 2003). The molecular mechanisms by which this parasite causes invasive amebiasis are not fully understood. *E. histolytica* has adherence and cytotoxicity factors that are essential for its survival, but they are not directly responsible for ALA formation. It is known that the limitation and prevention of recurrent invasive amebiasis requires the development of an effective immune response. Thus, it is likely that the acute inflammatory response associated with *E. histolytica* infection is a key factor for the development of ALA (Chadee et al., 1985).

Parasite-specific immune responses are regulated by cytokines and chemokines that lead to the development of immunity, but these responses also contribute to infection, inducing pathogenesis and parasite persistence (Talvani et al., 2004). Little is known regarding the amebic signals that initiate an acute inflammatory response.

It has been reported that in mice infected with *E. histolytica,* host tissue damage is attributed primarily to the lectin activity of the galactose/*N*-acetyl-D-galactosamine (Gal/GalNAc) from *E. histolytica,* which promotes the accumulation of mononuclear cells, including neutrophils, inflammatory monocytes, and macrophages, at the site of infection (Blazquez et al., 2007). Intestinal epithelial cells infected with *E. histolytica in vitro* produce elevated levels of the cytokines, interleukin-8 (IL-8), growth-regulated protein alpha (GRO-α), granulocyte macrophage colony-stimulating factor (GMCSF), and IL-1 (Eckmann et al., 1995). Treatment of cultured human intestinal cells with the lectin Gal/GalNAc from pathogenic and nonpathogenic entamebas (*E. histolytica* and *E. dispar*) results in the secretion of chemoattractant and proinflammatory cytokines (Sharma et al., 2005), suggesting that these cells and cytokines also contribute to tissue damage, participating in the mechanisms of initiation, amplification, or limitation of the inflammatory processes during invasive amebiasis.

The identification of the mediators involved in leukocyte activation during infection by *E. histolytica* is of fundamental importance for understanding host responses in amebiasis. Cellular interactions and cytokines have been reported during amebic infections, and cytokines have been shown to be able to regulate monocyte function and increase the amebicidal activity of monocytes (Seydel et al., 2000; Lotter et al., 2013).

It is still not clear what other elements in the dynamics of host–parasite relationship define the outcome of infection, especially regarding the regulation of the immune response against *E. histolytica.*

To obtain further evidence about the relationships of immune cells with *E. histolytica*, other proteins have been studied to investigate the intracellular signals that promote the host immune response. Some examples include the cysteine proteinases 1 and 5 (CP1 and CP5) that breakdown IgA1 and IgA2 antibodies. These proteins cleave the Fc region that interacts with parasite surface receptors and mediates effector functions that can mask immunogenic surface molecules with inert Fab fragments, thus helping to prevent the parasite expulsion from the intestinal lumen (Garcia-Nieto et al., 2008).

The role of calreticulin (CRT) in host–parasite interactions has recently become a major area of research. The CRT genes from many parasites (*Trypanosoma, Leishmania, Entamoeba, Onchocerca, Schistosoma,* and *Haemonchus*) have been cloned and sequenced (Rokeach et al., 1994; Joshi et al., 1996; El-Gengehi et al., 2000; Marcelain et al., 2000; González et al., 2002; Suchitra and Joshi, 2005).

Although the functions of CRT are conserved in vertebrates, some CRT functions differ among parasites (Nakashi et al., 1998; Ferreira et al., 2004); parasite CRTs bind host C1q and inhibit C1q-dependent complement activation. The CRT of *Haemonchus contortus* binds host C-reactive protein and C1q (Naresha et al., 2009). The ecto-parasite *Amblyomma americanum* secretes CRT during feeding, suggesting that the anticoagulant ability of CRT may prevent blood clotting and allows the parasite to feed on the host and induce host antiparasite responses (Jaworski et al., 1995). The presence of CRT in the penetration gland cells of *Schistosoma* suggests that this molecule may be important for the host skin penetration (Khalife et al., 1994).

Previously, we reported the presence of CRT in *E. histolytica* (*Eh*CRT) and that this protein induces an important immunogenic response in the human host. More than 90% of patients with ALA develop high levels of serum antibodies against *Eh*CRT (González et al., 2002). We also reported the cloning of the CRT gene from *E. histolytica,* and the preparation of mono-specific antibodies against recombinant CRT. The immunohistochemical assays on trophozoites show that *Eh*CRT is in cytoplasmic vesicles and in vesicles that are in close contact with the inner cytoplasmic membrane (González et al., 2011). In addition, it was demonstrated that the CRT from both pathogenic *E. histolytica* and nonpathogenic *E. dispar* species specifically interact with human C1q molecules and inhibit the activation of the classical complement pathway (Ximénez et al., 2014). This activity is consistent with that reported by Vaithilingam et al. (2012). The trophozoites activated by the presence of jurkat cells clearly show the binding of C1q to CRT on the surface of the phagocytic mouths during the process of erythrophagocytosis.

However, the activation of the host immune response and the cytokine profile induced by *Eh*CRT have not yet been investigated.

In this study, we analyzed the proliferation and cytokine production of peripheral blood mononuclear cells (PBMCs) cultures isolated from ALA patients during the acute phase of the disease and from individuals who resolved ALA in order to characterize the cytokines profiles produced in response to *Eh*CRT.

METHODS

Ethics Statement

The present work was designed according to the guidelines for the management of human samples for experimental purposes as indicated in the Official Regulation NOM-12SSA3-2007 included in the General Health Law of Mexican Health Ministry. In addition, the project was approved by the Scientific and Ethics Committee of the Faculty of Medicine from the National Autonomous University of Mexico. Patients were informed about the purposes of the project, the sampling, and the potential risks during procedure, and the patients were invited to voluntarily participate by signing an informed consent letter.

Study Groups and Biological Samples

Patients with diagnosis of ALA admitted to the Internal Medicine, Gastroenterology, and Infectiology Services of the General Hospital of Mexico Dr. Eduaro Liciaga were recruited. These patients formed the group with acute phase amebic liver abscess (AP-ALA). The patients in the resolution phase of ALA (R-ALA) were recruited from a search of the archives of discharged patients from the General Hospital of Mexico, and they formed the ALA resolution group (R-ALA). Three fecal samples were collected from each patient from both groups at 1-week intervals after their hospitalization for microscopic examination for parasites. At the time of collection of the third sample, 10 ml of blood was drawn to evaluate serum antibodies against *E. histolytica* by enzyme-linked immunosorbent assay (ELISA), using an OD_{490nm} $\geq$0.5 as an indicator of a positive result (Morán et al., 2007). The remaining sample was used to isolate PBMCs.

A third group, named the negative control (NEG), was formed with clinically healthy individuals from the Blood Bank of the General Hospital of Mexico, with ELISA serum levels of antiamebic antibodies below the OD threshold (OD<0.5). Using the same protocol for ALA groups, three fecal samples and 10-ml blood samples were taken for microscopic examination and PBMC isolation, respectively. Ten individuals for the group were included.

Isolation and Culture of PBMC

The PBMCs were isolated from 10 ml peripheral blood samples collected from each participant in tubes with K2 ethylenediaminetetraacetic acid (EDTA) as anticoagulant (BD Vacutainer, Ref 368171). Cells were separated on a Ficoll-Hypaque gradient (Gibco, Life Technologies, Grand Island, NY, USA), and the PBMC pellet was separated and washed three times with phosphate-buffered saline PBS. After separation, PBMCs were centrifuged and resuspended in Roswell Park Memorial Institute medium RPMI culture medium supplemented with 10% fetal bovine serum. The cells (1×10^6 cells/ml) were incubated with r*Eh*CRT (5 μg/ml) at 37°C with 5% CO_2; concanavalin A (ConA) (Sigma Chemical St. Louis, MO USA) was used as a stimulating factor at 10 μg/ml for different periods of time (24, 48, 72, and 96 h). Each experiment was performed in duplicate. At each time point, the cultures were centrifuged for 10 min at 1,000 × g, and the supernatant was reserved for cytokine analysis.

Recombinant *Eh*CRT Production

Full-length r*Eh*CRT protein was expressed and purified as previously described (González et al., 2011). Briefly, the plasmid pBluescript-KS+ (pbKS+) was used to clone and express the 1,178 bp *Eh*crt gene (GB-EAL649855.1) (Loftus et al., 2005), which produces the full-length protein; it was subcloned into the prokaryotic expression vector pProEX HT-b (Gibco Life Technologies) to express the CRT protein with a six-histidine tag at the N-terminal end. Competent *Escherichia coli* BL21 cells were transformed with the recombinant plasmid. The expression of recombinant protein r*Eh*CRT was induced with a final concentration of 1 mM isopropyl-β-D-thiogalactoside. The QIAexpressionist system (Qiagen, Valencia, CA, USA) was used to purify the recombinant protein, and, briefly, the cells were harvested by centrifugation at 3,000 × g for 12 min, and the bacterial pellet was resuspended in 5 ml lysis buffer (8 M urea, 0.1 M NaH_2PO_4, and 0.1 M Tris-HCl, pH 8.0). The lysate was added to a 50% suspension of Ni-NTA agarose (Qiagen,). The mixture was passed through a filtration column, and the recombinant protein was eluted with 8 M-urea buffer pH 4.5. The selected fractions were dialyzed against 19 mM PBS. Protein concentration was determined by the Bradford method, and the quality was evaluated by 12% sodium dodecyl sulfate polyacrylamide gel electrophoresis (SDS–PAGE). The reactivity grade of the recombinant protein was tested against sera from patients with ALA and for anti-*E. coli* lipopolysaccharide antibody (LPS) antibody (ab211144, Abcam) by Western blot.

Proliferation Index (PI)

To obtain the PI at 24, 48, 72, and 96 h, 20 μl of 5 μg/ml [3-(4,5-dimethylthiazol-2-yl)-2,5-diphenyltetrazolium bromide] (MTT) (Sigma) was added to each well containing PBMCs incubated with r*Eh*CRT or ConA and incubated at 37°C for 1 h in a humidified incubator with 5% CO_2. After incubation, the plates were centrifuged at 1,000 × g for 10 min and the supernatant was discarded. The cells were resuspended in 300 μl dimethyl sulfoxide (Sigma) and the optical density (OD) was measured at 570 nm in an ELISA plate reader (EL × 800 BioTek). The proliferation index was calculated by [OD of test sample—OD of negative control/OD of negative control]. (Verma et al., 2010)

Cytokine Detection by ELISA

The supernatants of the PBMC cultures, treated with r*Eh*CRT, ConA, or without stimulus (RPMI-10% SFB), were tested for detection of interleukins IL-2, IL-4, IL-5, IL-6, IL-10, IL-12, IL-13, IL-17A, interferon gamma (IFNγ), tumor necrosis factor alpha (TNFα), granulocyte colony stimulating factor (GCSF), and transforming growth factor beta1 (TGFβ1) using a multianalytic ELISA array kit (MEH-003A, Qiagen), according to manufacturer's instructions. The concentrations of the cytokines are given in pg/ml and were calculated using the standard curve provided in the kit.

Statistical Analysis

All values are expressed as the means ± S.D. The student's *t* test for unpaired results was used for the evaluation of differences

TABLE 1 | Demographic characteristics of individuals in the AP-ALA, R-ALA, and healthy control (NEG) groups.

Groups	Age (range in years)	Male	Female	Total	ELISA (OD)
AP-ALA	39.11	9	1	10	0.87 ± 0.043
R-ALA	39.72	6	4	10	1.0 ± 0.025
NEG	47.62	7	3	10	0.15 ± 0.024

The antibodies against E. histolytica antigens present in all belonging to different studied groups were evaluated by ELISA. The data are expressed as the average OD ± SD in each group.

between cytokine concentrations in each group. Differences were statistically significant when $P \leq 0.05$.

RESULTS

Study Participants and *E. histolytica* Antibody Concentration

The demographic features of each group are shown in **Table 1**. Among all the individuals, the mean age was 39 ± 7 years old, and 70% were male and 30% were female. The microscopic examinations were negative in all samples. Results of ELISA assay are shown as OD $_{490nm}$ values, considering negative results when values were under the cut value of 0.520. The mean value for the negative group was 0.15, the AP-ALA group was 0.87, and the R-ALA group was 1.0.

Purification of r*Eh*CRT and PI

The purified r*Eh*CRT from *E. coli* appeared as a single band at 60 kDa on 12% SDS-PAGE after bromophenol blue staining (**Figure 1A**). The results indicate that r*Eh*CRT was a good immunogenic factor, and this was previously confirmed by the antibody production in animal models (rabbits and mice) (González et al., 2011). The r*Eh*CRT conserved its reactivity when it was tested as an antigen using serum from ALA patients in ELISA assays (**Table 1**) and in Western blots, and no reactivity was observed with anti-*E. coli* LPS antibody (**Figure 1B**).

The role of r*Eh*CRT as a costimulatory factor in the proliferation of PBMC was verified when cellular proliferation was measured by 3-[4,5-dimethylthiazol-2-yl]-2,5 diphenyl tetrazolium bromide (MTT) assays, comparing the stimulatory capacity of r*Eh*CRT vs. the mitogen activity of ConA. The differences in the PI values were not statistically significant for any time point when comparing between the NEG and ALA groups (AP-ALA, R-ALA) (**Figure 2**). However, at 72 h, we can see the highest PI (**Figure 3**) and the PI ≥ 1 is considered as positive proliferation (Verma et al., 2010).

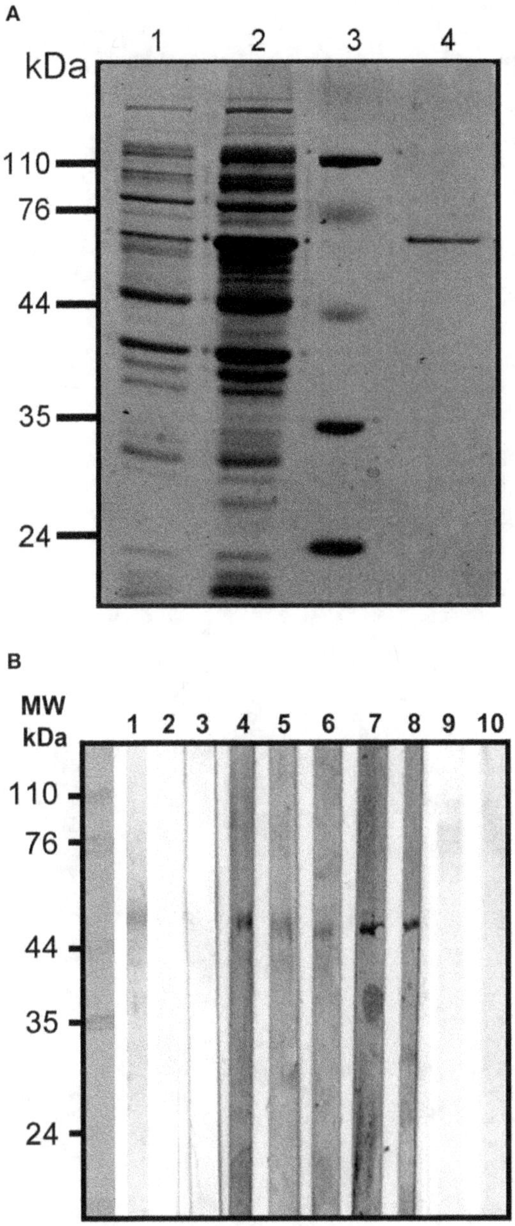

FIGURE 1 | (A) Purification under denaturing conditions of rEhCRT. Proteins were visualized by 12% SDS-PAGE and Coomassie staining; (1) cell lysate with plasmid, (2) cell lysate with plasmid after IPTG induction, (3) molecular weight, (4) rEhCRT eluid from Ni-NTA Agarose column, molecular weight marker are indicated in kilodaltons. **(B)** Westernblot of rEhCR. The reactivity of the rEhCRT was tested against sera from the different groups studied; (1) 5 μg of rEhCRT electrotransfered to NC membrane, (2–3) serum from control individuals (NEG), (4–6) serum of AP-ALA patients, (7–8) R-ALA patients, and (9–10) reactivity against *E. coli* -LPS antibody.

Detection of Cytokines in the Supernatants of PBMC Cultures

The concentrations of cytokines in PBMC samples obtained for sera from the ALA and NEG groups and treated with EhCRT were measured through ELISA only at 72 h (**Figure 4**). The pattern of pro-inflammatory cytokines from the AP-ALA and R-ALA groups were compared to the NEG group, who did not produce the mentioned cytokines in the absenceof EhCRT.

The trend of the data agrees with an overexpression of all interleukins analyzed in all groups.

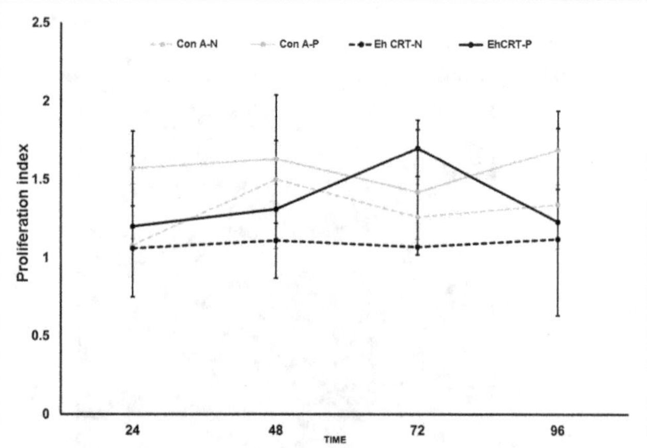

FIGURE 2 | Proliferation Index at different times, of PBMC cells obtained from control subjects (NEG) and ALA patients stimulated with rEhCRT or Con A.

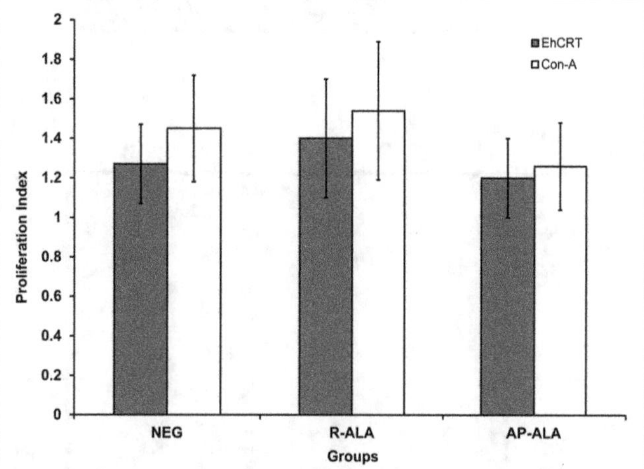

FIGURE 3 | Proliferation Index at 72 h post incubation of PBMC cells obtained from control subjects (NEG), AP-ALA or R-ALA patients with rEhCRT or Con A. PI ≥1 is considered as positive stimulus.

However, in the ALA groups, the overexpression was, in general, larger than in the negative group, and significant differences were measured in the expression of the following interleukins; IL-2, IL-5, IL-6, IL-10, IL-17, IFNγ, TNFα, GCSF, and TGFβ1 ($p = 0.0035, 0.0023, 0.019, 0.006, 0.0076, 0.0049, 0.0039, 0.0035, 0.0059$, respectively).

The comparisons of differential expressions of the interleukins between groups of AP-ALA and R-ALA are shown in **Figure 4**. We found differences in the overexpression of interleukins IL-2, IL-5, IL-6, IL-10, GCSF, and TGFβ1 ($p = 0.0067, 0.026, 0.0045, 0.0016, 0.0051, 0.0047$, respectively), which were higher in the AP-ALA group. In the R-ALA group, we observed higher overexpression of the interleukins IL-17, INFγ, and TNFα; however, statistically significant differences were detected only for INFγ ($p = 0.73, 0.0014, 0.096$).

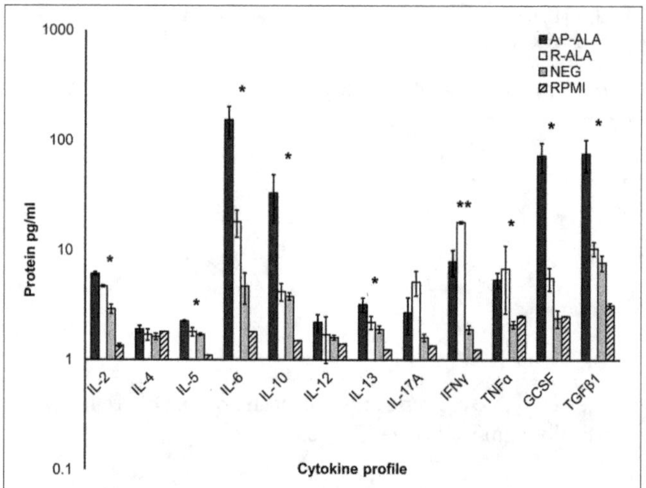

FIGURE 4 | Cytokine profile on PBMC cells stimulated with rEhCRT. The data shows the concentration of cytokines, obtained in the supernatant of PBMC cells of different studied groups (NEG, AP-ALA, and R-ALA) after 72 h of incubation and stimulated with rEhCRT or without stimulus (RPMI). The concentration of interleukins is expressed as pg/ml in a logarithmic scale. *$p \leq 0.005$, when compared groups of individuals (NEG) against the group of patients (ALA), **when compared AP-ALA against R-ALA groups.

DISCUSSION

The aim of this study was to examine the proliferation of PBMCs obtained from the blood of patients with AP-ALA and R-ALA stimulated *in vitro* with r*Eh*CRT or ConA and determine the cytokine profiles induced in the different groups. The responses of the PBMC show that *Eh*CRT is one of the many immunogenic proteins in *E. histolytica* that can induce activation and proliferation of PBMCs similarly to ConA. These results reinforce our previous observations that the *Eh*CRT is highly immunogenic in humans, mice, and rabbits (González et al., 2002, 2011).

When comparing the cytokine profiles between the AP-ALA and R-ALA groups in contrast with negative or PBMC without stimulus, it is clear that *Eh*CRT functions as a specific antigenic costimulator, inducing a different pattern of cytokines between different groups. This stimulatory action was specific because no reactivity with *E. coli* -LPS antibody was detected for the recombinant protein EhCRT (**Figure 1A**).

The expression levels of IL-2, IL-5, IL-6, IL-10, GCSF, and TGFβ1 were increased in patients with AP-ALA, while the expression levels of IL-17, INFγ, and TNFα were mainly upregulated in the R-ALA group. Nevertheless, there were statistically significant differences only for INFγ.

E. histolytica has different proteins that modulate the host immune response. The Gal/GalNAc-lectin induces the T cells to production of IL-2 and INFγ (Schain et al., 1992), whereas in macrophages, the amebicide activity of Gal/GalNAc-lectin induces the production of TNFα (Seguin et al., 1997). In dendritic cells, Gal/GalNAc-lectin favors a Th1 response in addition to inducing the production of major histocompatibility complex

(MHC) class II molecules, and the costimulatory molecules CD80, CD86, and CD40 (Ivory and Chadde, 2007).

Another protein called monocyte locomotion inhibitory factor (MLIF) is produced by *E. histolytica* in axenic cultures that induces the production of pro-inflammatory cytokines (IL-1β, IL-2, IL-5, IL-6, IFN-γ) and anti-inflammatory cytokines such as IL-10, as well as the low expression of chemokines CCL1, CCL4, and the receptor CCR1 in human monocytes (Rico et al., 2003; Utrera-Barillas et al., 2003).

In the group of patients with AP-ALA, the cytokines IL2, IL5, Il6, IL17A, IFNγ, and TNFα displayed an increase in their concentration and demonstrated that the immune response had a pro-inflammatory profile. This response has been observed in stimulation assays using Gal/GalNAc-lectin in intestinal cell cultures (Sharma et al., 2005) and in other parasitic diseases such as malaria (Vazquez et al., 2015). It is important to highlight the effect on IL2, IL6, IL-17, IFNγ, and TNFα, whose levels were the highest and overexpressed in comparison with the profile observed in the negative group.

Guo et al. (2011), demonstrated in an *Entamoeba histolytica* vaccination model that IL-17 provides protection to mice vaccinated with the recombinant LecA fragment of the Gal/GalNAc-lectin. Interestingly, the major source of IL-17 in these mice was the CD8 T cells, whereas CD4 T cells express elevated levels of IFN-γ. The authors suggest that IL-17 may enhance the protective functions of Th1 immune response.

These results lead us to propose that treatment of PBMC in culture with *Eh*CRT favors the production of IFNγ and increases the production of IL-17A, thus directing the cellular immune response to a Th1 Profile, in PMBCs obtained from R-ALA.

Our results agree with those published by Ghadirian and Denis (1992), who showed that IFNγ could activate mouse peritoneal macrophages, which, in turn, were able to eradicate the *E. histolytica* trophozoites from colon tissue *in vitro*. Studies in animal models (Seydel et al., 2000) and human infections (Haque et al., 2007) have established that amoeba-specific IFN-γ production is critically involved in the clearance of infection and in host protection. In addition, Meza et al. (2014) demonstrated that virgin T-cell differentiation into Th17 cells producing IL-17 occurred after the direct stimulation with other cytokines such as TGFβ, IL-6, and IL-1 in a murine model of infection with *Trypanosoma cruzi*. Moraes et al. (2015) reported that mononuclear cells collected from healthy individuals incubated with *E. histolytica* in culture induced the production of *IFNγ* and TGFβ, and that both had a beneficial effect on the modulation of the activity of these cells. Our results agree with data of Moraes regarding the effects on IFNγ. These cytokines are important in the control *E. histolytica* infection.

The R-ALA group showed an increase in the concentration of the cytokines IL-10 and TGFβ, which agrees with results of Bansal et al. (2005). These authors mention that, in addition to the production of these cytokines and the increased production of IL-4, a suppressive immune response was also induced in patients infected with *E. histolytica*, which, in turn, favored a symptomatic infection. The symptomatic group in Bansal et al. differs with our R-ALA group because the latter had no symptoms and they were all ALA with negative microscopic examinations and a resolved *E. histolytica* infection. In our opinion, this immunosuppressive effect is due to the direct stimulation of the PBMC by *Eh*CRT, and through autocrine, paracrine, and pleiotropic effects on cytokine production, which favored the increase in other types of cytokines such as IL-5, IL-6, and IL-13 capable of generating a Th2 immune response.

In addition, we found that the increased cytokine IL-10 in the AP-ALA group in our study was in contrast with the results reported by Bansal. These results suggest that IL-10 is an immunomodulator resulting in proinflammatory cytokine profiles that could promote immunosuppression in the R-ALA individuals. The effect attributed to IL-10 differs in other parasitic diseases such as *Leishmania donovani* (Andreani et al., 2015), *Trypanosoma cruzi* (Longhi et al., 2014), and *Giardia duodenalis* (Babaei et al., 2016). In these reports, a decrease in IL-10 was observed that favored the spread of parasites into the hepatic tissue.

On the contrary, the IL-10 level was increased in dysenteric and ALA patients (Utrera-Barillas et al., 2003; Bansal et al., 2005). These studies indicate that invasion of the colon and liver by *E. histolytica* elicits an anti-inflammatory immune response and may successfully suppress immune reaction to the amebae.

In summary, the ameba needs to balance IL-10 and the pro-inflammatory cytokine to allow establishment of infection. In contrast, peritoneal monocytes and macrophages exposed to lipopeptidophosphoglycan (LPPG) secreted TNF-α, IL-6, IL-8, IL-12, and IL-10 via TLR2 (Maldonaldo-Bernal et al., 2005). Thus, LPPG-driven signaling may activate a negative feedback loop that attenuates inflammatory responses.

Host protective immunity involves participation of both humoral and cellular responses; however, the mechanism involved in the immune evasion of *E. histolytica* is not clear. One of these mechanisms could be associated with the ability of parasites to modulate cytokine expression in the inflammatory process, which is initiated by expression of proinflammatory cytokines. *E. histolytica* infections induce a state of transient suppression of cell-mediated immunity in early stages of inflammation in amebic hepatic abscess, and a complex signaling system of cytokines is triggered by pathogen invasion (Eckmann et al., 1993; Romagnani, 2000).

CONCLUSIONS

The data obtained in this study confirmed that the *Eh*CRT behaves like an amebic immunogenic protein for humans and suggest that the *Eh*CRT participates in the specific stimulation of immune cells.

Our results suggest that the r*Eh*CRT can stimulate human PBMC proliferation independently of the presence of *E. histolytica* trophozoites, acting as a specific costimulator of the immune response like that induced by ConA. In addition, these results underline *Eh*CRT as a parasitic factor that can modulate the immune response, from the stimulation of proinflammatory cytokines to the immunosuppressive effects, depending on the progression of the ALA, thus inducing the development of a Th2 cytokine profile in the acute phase of disease and a Th1 profile once the individuals had resolved the ALA.

The functions of *Eh*CRT and its role in the pathogenesis of ALA need further research, particularly on the interaction with the cells of immune system and the induction of chemokines and cytokines regulators that hopefully will allow a better understanding of the pathogenesis of ALA.

AUTHOR CONTRIBUTIONS

CX conceptualized the manuscript. EG, MN-R, UM. PM, OP-R, EH, LR, and AS curated the data. CX, EG, MN-R, PM, OP-R, EH, LR, and AS performed the formal analysis. CX acquired the funding. EG, MN-R, and PM performed the investigation. MN-R, PM, AS, and UM provided the resources. EG, OP-R, and EH performed the software analysis. CX, EG, MN-R, and PM provided the supervision. CX, EG, MN-R, and PM executed the validation. CX, EG, MN-R, and PM wrote the original draft of the manuscript. CX, EG, MN-R, PM, OP-R, EH, UM, and AS wrote, reviewed and edited the manuscript.

FUNDING

We are grateful for the support provided by the following institutions: Grants: IN218214 from PAPIIT (DGAPA), Universidad Nacional Autónoma de México (UNAM), and 272601 from the Consejo Nacional de Ciencia y Tecniología (CONACyT).

ACKNOWLEDGMENTS

We thank Mario Nequiz-Avendaño for the axenic culture of *E. histolytica* (HM1:IMSS), and Marco Gudiño Zayas, for art design. LR-V, a doctoral student from the Programa de Doctorado en Ciencias Biomédicas, Universidad Nacional Autónoma de México (UNAM), is grateful for having received fellowship 239901 from CONACYT. We also appreciate the technical assistance of Martha Elena Zaragoza and Ma. de los Angeles Padilla, and the secretarial assistance of Mrs. Ma. Elena Ortiz.

REFERENCES

Andreani, G., Ouellet, M., Menasria, R., Gomez, A. M., Barat, T., and Tremblay, M. J. (2015). *Leishmania infantum* amastigotes trigger a subpopulation of human B cells with an immunoregulatory phenotype. *PLoS Negl. Trop. Dis.* 9:e0003543. doi: 10.1371/journal.pntd.0003543

Babaei, Z., Malihi, N., Zia-Ali, N., Sharifi, I., Mahommadi, M. A., Kagnoff, M. F. et al. (2016). Adaptative immune response in symptomatic and asymptomatic enteric protozoal infection: evidence for a determining role of parasite genetic heterogeneity in host immunity to human giardiasis. *Microbes Infect.* 18, 687–695. doi: 10.1016/j.micinf.2016.06.009

Bansal, D., Sehgal, R., Chawla, Y., Malla, N., and Mahajan, R. C. (2005). Cytokine mRNA expressions in symptomatic vs. *Asymptomatic amoebiasis patients. Parasite Immunol.* 27, 37–43. doi: 10.1111/j.1365-3024.2005.00739.x

Blazquez, S., Rigothier, M. C., Huerre, M., and Guillen, N. (2007). Initiation of inflammation and cell death during liver abscess formation by *Entamoeba histolytica* depends on activity of the galactose/N-acetyl-D-galactosamine lectin. *Int. J. Parasitol.* 37, 425–433. doi: 10.1016/j.ijpara.2006.10.008

Chadee, K., Meerovitch, E., and Moreau, F. (1985). *In vitro* and *in vivo* interaction between trophozoites of *Entamoeba histolytica* and gerbil lymphoid cells. *Infect. Immun.* 49, 828–832.

Eckmann, L., Jung, H. C., Schurer-Maly, C., Panja, A., Morzycka- Wroblewska, E., and Kagnoff, M. F. (1993). Differential cytokine expression of interleukin 8. *Gastroenterology* 105, 1689–1697. doi: 10.1016/0016-5085(93)91064-O

Eckmann, L., Reed, S. L., Smith, J. R., and Kagnoff, M. F. (1995). *Entamoeba histolytica* trophozoites induce an inflammatory cytokine response by cultured human cells through the paracrine action of cytolytically released interleukin-1α. *J. Clin. Invest.* 96, 1269–1719. doi: 10.1172/JCI118161

El-Gengehi, N., El-Ridi, R., Tawab, N. A., El-Demellawy, M., and Mangold, B. L. (2000). A *Schistosoma mansoni* 62 kDa band is identified as an irradiated vaccine T-cell antigen and characterized as calreticulin. *J. Parasitol.* 86, 993–1000. doi: 10.1645/0022-3395(2000)086[0993:ASMKBI]2.0.CO;2

Ferreira, V., Molina, M. C., Valck, C., Rojas, A., Aguilar, L., Ramírez, G., et al. (2004). Role of calreticulin from parasites in its interaction with vertebrate hosts. *Mol. Immunol.* 40, 1279–1291. doi: 10.1016/j.molimm.2003.11.018

Garcia-Nieto, R. M., Rico-Mata, R., Arias-Negrete, S., and Avila, E. E. (2008). Degradation of human secretory IgA1 and IgA2 by *Entamoeba histolytica* surface-associated proteolytic activity. *Parasitol. Int.* 57, l417–l423. doi: 10.1016/j.parint.2008.04.013

Ghadirian, E., and Denis, M. (1992). *In vivo* activation of macrophages by IFN-gamma to kill *Entamoeba histolytica* trophozoites *in vitro. Parasite Immunol.* 14, 397–404. doi: 10.1111/j.1365-3024.1992.tb00014.x

González, E., García de León, M. C., Meza, I., Ocadiz-Delgado, R., Gariglio, P., Silva-Olivares, A., et al. (2011). *Entamoeba histolytica* Calreticulin: an endoplasmic reticulum protein expressed by trophozoites into experimentally induced amoebic liver abscess. *Parasitol. Res.* 108, 439–449. doi: 10.1007/s00436-010-2085-6

González, E., Rico, G., Mendoza, G., Ramos, F., García, G., Morán, P., et al. (2002). Calreticulin-like molecule in trophozoites of *Entamoeba histolytica* HM1: IMSS. *Am. J. Trop. Med. Hyg.* 67, 636–639. doi: 10.4269/ajtmh.2002.67.636

Guo, X., Roberts, M. R., Becker, S. M., Podd, B., Zhang, Y., Chua, S. C., et al. (2011). Leptin signalling in intestinal epithelium mediates resistance to enteric infection by *Entamoeba histolytica. Mucosal. Immunol.* 4, 294–303. doi: 10.1038/mi.2010.76

Haque, R., Huston, C. D., Hughes, M., Houpt, E., and Petri, W. A. Jr. (2003). Current concepts: amebiasis. *N. Engl. J. Med.* 348, 1565–1573. doi: 10.1056/NEJMra022710

Haque, R., Mondal, D., Shu, J., Roy, S., Kabir, M., Davis, A. N., et al. (2007). Correlation of interferon-gamma production by peripheral blood mononuclear cells with childhood malnutrition and susceptibility to amebiasis. *Am. J. Trop. Med. Hyg.* 76, 340–344. doi: 10.4269/ajtmh.2007.76.340

Ivory, C. P. A., and Chadde, K. (2007). Activation of dendritic cells by the Gal-lectin of *Entamoeba histolytica* drives Th1 responses *in vitro* and *in vivo. Eur. J. Immunol.* 37, 385–394. doi: 10.1002/eji.200636476

Jaworski, D. C., Simmen, F. A., Lamoreaux, W., Coons, L. B., Muller, M. T., and Needham, G. R. (1995). A secreted calreticulin protein in ixoidid tick (*Amblyomma americanum*) saliva. *J. Insect Physiol.* 41, 369–375. doi: 10.1016/0022-1910(94)00107-R

Joshi, M., Pogue, G. P., Duncan, R. C., Lee, N. S., Singh, N. K., Atreya, C. D., et al. (1996). Isolation and characterization of *Leishmania donovani* calreticulin gene and its conservation of the RNA binding activity. *Mol. Biochem. Parasitol.* 81, 53–64. doi: 10.1016/0166-6851(96)02676-X

Khalife, J., Liu, J. L., Pierce, R., Porchet, E., Godin, C., and Capron, A. (1994). Characterization and localization of *Schistosoma mansoni* calreticulin Sm5. *Parasitol.* 108, 527–532. doi: 10.1017/S0031182000077398

Loftus, B., Anderson, I., Davies, R., Alsmark, U. C., Samuelson, J., Amedeo, P., et al. (2005). The genome of the protist parasite *Entamoeba histolytica. Nature* 433, 865–868. doi: 10.1038/nature03291

Longhi, S. A., Atienza, A., Perez Prados, G., Buying, A., Balouz, V., Buscaglia, C. A., et al. (2014). Cytokine production but lac of proliferation in peripheral blood mononuclear cells from chronic Chagas's disease cardiomyopathy patients in response to *T. cruzi* ribosomal P proteins. *PLoS Negl. Trop. Dis.* 8:e2906. doi: 10.1371/journal.pntd.0002906

Lotter, H., Helk, E., Bernin, H., Jacobs, T., Prehn, C., Adamski, J., et al. (2013). Testosterone increases susceptibility to amebic liver abscess in mice and mediates inhibition of IFNγ secretion in natural killer T cells. *PLoS ONE* 8:e55694. doi: 10.1371/journal.pone.0055694

Maldonaldo-Bernal, C., Kirschning, C. J., Rosenstein, Y., Rocha, L. M., Rios-Sarabia, N., Espinosa-Cantellano, M., et al. (2005). The innate immune response to *Entamoeba histolytica* lipopeptido phosphoglycan is mediated by toll-like receptors 2 and 4. *Parasite Immunol.* 27, 127–137. doi: 10.1111/j.1365-3024.2005.00754.x

Marcelain, K. A., Colombo, M. C., Molina, L., Ferreira, M., Lorca, J. C., Aguillón, J. C., et al. (2000). Development of an immunoenzymatic assay for the detection of human antibodies against *Tripanosoma cruzi* calreticulin, an immunodominant antigen. *Acta Tropica* 75, 291–300. doi: 10.1016/S0001-706X(00)00062-0

Meza, S. K., Kaneshima, E., de Oliveira, S., Gabriel, M., de Araujo, S., Gomes, M. L., et al. (2014). Comparative pathogenicity in Swiss mice of *Trypanosoma cruzi* IV from northern Brazil and *Trypanosoma cruzi* II from southern Brazil. *Exp. Parasitol.* 146, 34–42. doi: 10.1016/j.exppara.2014.08.014

Moraes, L. C., Franca, E. L., Pessoa, R. S., Fagundes, D. L., Hernandes, M. G., Ribeiro, V. P., et al. (2015). The effect of IFN-γ and TGF-β in the functional activity of mononuclear cells in the presence of *Entamoeba histolytica*. *Parasit Vec.* 8:413. doi: 10.1186/s13071-015-1028-6

Morán, P., Gómez, A., Valadez, A., Ramos, F., and González, E. (2007). "Amebic and pyogenic liver abscess: importance of differential diagnosis in endemic areas of amebiasis," in *5th European Congress on Tropical Medicine and International Health,* ed M. J. Boeree (Amsterdam), 57–64.

Nakashi, H. L., Pogue, G. P., Duncan, R. C., Joshi, M., Atreya, C. D., Lee, N. S., et al. (1998). Implications of calreticulin function in parasite biology. *Parasitol. Tdy* 14, 157–160. doi: 10.1016/S0169-4758(97)01180-0

Naresha, S., Suryawanshi, A., Agarwal, M., Sing, B. P., and Joshi, P. (2009). Mapping the complement C1q binding site in *Haemonchus contortus* calreticulin. *Mol. Biochem. Parasitol.* 166, 42–46. doi: 10.1016/j.molbiopara.2009.02.007

Rico, G., Leandro, E., Rojas, S., Jiménez, J. A., and Kretschmer, R. (2003). The monocyte locomotion inhibitory factor produced by *Entamoeba histolytica* inhibits induced nitric oxide production in human leukocytes. *Parasitol. Res.* 90, 264–267. doi: 10.1007/s00436-002-0780-7

Rokeach, L. A., Zimmerman, P. A., and Unnasch, T. R. (1994). Epitopes of *Onchocerca volvulus* RAL−1 antigen a member of the calreticulin family of proteins recognized by sera from patients with onchocerciasis. *Infect. Immun.* 62, 3696–3704. *PMCID:PMC*303020

Romagnani, S. (2000). T-cell subsets (Th1 versus Th2). *Ann. Allergy Asthma Immunol.* 85, 9–18. doi: 10.1016/S1081-1206(10)62426-X

Schain, D. C., Salata, R. A., and Raydin, J. I. (1992). Human T-lymphocyte proliferation lymphokine production and amebicidal activity elicited by the galactose-inhibitable adherence protein of *Entamoeba histolytica*. *Infect. Immun.* 60, 2143–2146.

Seguin, R., Mann, B. J., Keller, K., and Chadee, K. (1997). The tumor necrosis factor alpha-stimulating region of galactoses-inhibitable lectin of *Entamoeba histolytica* activates gamma interferon-primed macrophages for amebicidal activity mediated by nitric oxide. *Infect. Immun.* 65, 2522–2527.

Seydel, K. B., Smith, S. J., and Stanley, S. L. Jr. (2000). Innate immunity to amebic liver abscess is dependent on gamma interferon and nitric oxide in a murine model of disease. *Infect. Immun.* 68, 400–102. doi: 10.1128/IAI.68.1.400-402.2000

Sharma, M., Vohra, H., and Bhasin, D. (2005). Enhanced pro-inflammatory chemokine/cytokine response triggered by pathogenic *Entamoeba histolytica*: basis of invasive disease. *Parasitology* 131, 783–796. doi: 10.1017/S0031182005008541

Suchitra, S., and Joshi, P. (2005). Characterization of *Haemonchus contortus* calreticulin suggests its role in feeding and immune evasion by the parasite. *Biochim. Biophys. Acta* 1722, 293–303. doi: 10.1016/j.bbagen.2004.12.020

Talvani, A., Rocha, M. O., Ribeiro, A. L., Correa-Oliveira, R., and Teixeira, M. M. (2004). Chemokine receptor expression on the surface of peripheral blood mononuclear cells in chagas disease. *J. Infect. Dis.* 189, 214–220. doi: 10.1086/380803

Utrera-Barillas, D., Velazquez, J., Enciso, A., Cruz, S., Rico, G., Curiel-Quesada, E., et al. (2003). An anti-inflammatory oligopeptide produced by *Entamoeba histolytica* down-regulates the expression of pro-inflammatory chemokines. *Parasit. Immunol.* 25, 475–482. doi: 10.1111/j.1365-3024.2003.00657.x

Vaithilingam, A., Teixeira, J. E., Miller, P. J., Heron, B. T., and Huston, C. D. (2012). *Entamoeba histolytica* cell surface calreticulin binds human C1q and functions in amebic phagocytosis of host cells. *Infect. Immun.* 80, 2008–2018. doi: 10.1128/IAI.06287-11

Vazquez, B. P., Vazquez, T. P., Miguel, C. B., Rodríguez, W. F., and Méndez, M. T. (2015). Inflammatory responses and intestinal injury development during acute *Trypanosoma cruzi* infection are associated with the parasite load. *Parasit. Vec.* 8:206. doi: 10.1186/s13071-015-0811-8

Verma, A., Prasad, K. N., Singh, A. K., Nyati, K. K., Gupta, R. K., and Paliwal, V. M. (2010). Evaluation of the MTT lymphocyte proliferation assay for the diagnosis of neurocysticercosis. *J. Microbiol. Methods* 81, 175–178. doi: 10.1016/j.mimet.2010.03.001

Ximénez, C., González, E., Nieves, M. E., Silva-Olivares, A., Shibayama, M., Galindo-Gómez, S., et al. (2014). *Entamoeba histolytica* and *E. dispar* Calreticulin: inhibition of classical complement pathway and differences in the level of expression in amoebic liver abscess. *Biomed. Res. Int.* 2014:127453. doi: 10.1155/2014/127453

4

Reassessing the Role of *Entamoeba gingivalis* in Periodontitis

***Mark Bonner*[1], *Manuel Fresno*[2,3], *Núria Gironès*[2,3], *Nancy Guillén*[4,5] *and Julien Santi-Rocca*[6*]**

[1] International Institute of Periodontology, Victoriaville, QC, Canada, [2] Centro de Biología Molecular Severo Ochoa, Consejo Superior de Investigaciones Científicas, Universidad Autónoma de Madrid, Madrid, Spain, [3] Instituto de Investigación Sanitaria del Hospital Universitario de La Princesa, Madrid, Spain, [4] Institut Pasteur, Paris, France, [5] Centre National de la Recherche Scientifique, CNRS-ERL9195, Paris, France, [6] Science and Healthcare for Oral Welfare, Toulouse, France

Correspondence:
Julien Santi-Rocca
jsr@periodontitis.show

The protozoan *Entamoeba gingivalis* resides in the oral cavity and is frequently observed in the periodontal pockets of humans and pets. This species of *Entamoeba* is closely related to the human pathogen *Entamoeba histolytica*, the agent of amoebiasis. Although *E. gingivalis* is highly enriched in people with periodontitis (a disease in which inflammation and bone loss correlate with changes in the microbial flora), the potential role of this protozoan in oral infectious diseases is not known. Periodontitis affects half the adult population in the world, eventually leads to edentulism, and has been linked to other pathologies, like diabetes and cardiovascular diseases. As aging is a risk factor for the disorder, it is considered an inevitable physiological process, even though it can be prevented and cured. However, the impact of periodontitis on the patient's health and quality of life, as well as its economic burden, are underestimated. Commonly accepted models explain the progression from health to gingivitis and then periodontitis by a gradual change in the identity and proportion of bacterial microorganisms in the gingival crevices. Though not pathognomonic, inflammation is always present in periodontitis. The recruitment of leukocytes to inflamed gums and their passage to the periodontal pocket lumen are speculated to fuel both tissue destruction and the development of the flora. The individual contribution to the disease of each bacterial species is difficult to establish and the eventual role of protozoa in the fate of this disease has been ignored. Following recent scientific findings, we discuss the relevance of these data and propose that the status of *E. gingivalis* be reconsidered as a potential pathogen contributing to periodontitis.

Keywords: *Entamoeba gingivalis*, periodontitis, gingivitis, inflammation, parasitic infection, infectious disease

INTRODUCTION: A DISEASE WITH UNDERESTIMATED IMPACT

Periodontitis is a disease leading to alveolar bone destruction and eventually tooth loss. The prevalence of periodontitis is constant among the defined World Health Organization (WHO) regions, with around one person out of two between 35 and 44 years old (Petersen and Ogawa, 2005). This prevalence increases with age (Demmer and Papapanou, 2010). In the USA, between 2009 and 2012, 46% of adults aged 30 years or more suffer from periodontitis (Eke et al., 2015).

Periodontitis is a handicapping disease, for which the WHO calculated the loss of 3,518,002 DALYs (Disability-adjusted life years, a measure of disease burden as the loss of healthy life years) in 2015 in the world, meaning 0.132% of the worldwide DALYs (Organization, 2016), though the associated disability weight is low (0.007), reflecting only "minor bleeding of the gums from time to time, with mild discomfort" (Evaluation, 2016). Though periodontitis is linked to systemic diseases like diabetes (Nascimento et al., 2018) and ischemic stroke (Leira et al., 2017), the etiological link is difficult to demonstrate and the possible impact of periodontitis on other ailments is ignored for the calculation of DALYs.

The etiology of periodontitis is still unclear and it is classified by the WHO as a non-communicable disease. Some human genetic factors linked to periodontitis were demonstrated (Vieira and Albandar, 2014) and are still investigated to explain its prevalence in the global population, in conjunction with age (Demmer and Papapanou, 2010). Modifiable risk factors for the disease were also sought and some parameters have been identified: smoking (Eke et al., 2016), alcohol consumption (Wang et al., 2016), and poor oral hygiene (Lertpimonchai et al., 2017). Beyond pain from wounds, eventual edentulism, and defects in occlusion, the patients experience halitosis (Silva et al., 2017) and esthetic issues (Nieri et al., 2013). Altogether, these factors may account for their psychological and social distress (Lopez et al., 2012; Hsu et al., 2015; Dumitrescu, 2016; Reynolds and Duane, 2018).

Evolution toward gum disease goes through three stages (i) formation of dental plaque; (ii) gingivitis, which is an inflammation of the gums due to the dental plaque, and (iii) periodontitis, in which alveolar bone and fibers that hold the teeth in place are irreversibly damaged. The pathophysiology of the disease is harshly debated, but a consensus was reached about some key points. First, inflammation is compulsory and prior to bone loss, evidenced by pocket formation [reviewed in Van Dyke (2017)]. Second, the microbial flora in periodontal pockets differs from that observed in healthy sulci (Marsh, 1994). Last, plaque and calculi worsen prognosis (Löe et al., 1965). Consensual treatment in clinics is thus based on the mechanical and/or surgical removal of dental plaque, calculi, and damaged/inflamed tissues (Smiley et al., 2015). These paths lead to an inefficient solution dealing with late symptoms without considering the evoked causes of the disease. The keystone for the improvement of periodontitis management worldwide is a better knowledge of its pathophysiology.

Due to the important correlation of periodontitis with the presence of *Entamoeba gingivalis* in the oral cavity, here, we searched for the facts that can shed light on the question of whether *E. gingivalis* plays a role in the occurrence of the periodontitis. In this review, we summarize existing data on the biology of the amoeba *Entamoeba gingivalis* and on its potential role as an infectious agent in periodontitis. We aim at highlighting perspectives for new research on the pathophysiology and prophylaxis of this neglected disease.

MICROBIOLOGY OF PERIODONTITIS: THE BACTERIAL PARADIGM

Though the saliva contains low nutrient concentrations and antimicrobial defense systems [reviewed in van 'T Hof et al. (2014)], the healthy oral cavity houses a commensal microbiota, composed of bacterial communities [about 1,000 species across humans, Consortium (2012)], whereas the contribution of viruses, parasites, archaea, and fungi is still to be characterized. Microorganisms and oral mucosae maintain a mutualistic, resilient symbiotic relationship (Rosier et al., 2018). The bacterial ecosystem of healthy sulci is intriguingly similar between individuals and it comprises immotile bacilli and cocci, as seen in microscopy (Listgarten, 1976), with bacterial species differing from those encountered on the tongue (Aas et al., 2005; Consortium, 2012; Rogers and Bruce, 2012). At the tooth surface, in particular in the dental sulcus, nutrients coming from food and cellular debris accumulate and support the survival of bacteria that adhere and colonize the dental enamel. Bacterial flagella, pili, and wall proteins can recruit other bacteria, by co-aggregation (Kolenbrander and Celesk, 1983; Gibbons et al., 1988). Furthermore, the secretion of polysaccharides initiates the formation and organization of a scaffold (Jakubovics, 2010), while intercellular signaling molecules regulate biofilm development, in particular through a *quorum sensing* mechanism mediated by different types of messengers, as cyclic di-guanosine monophosphate or LuxS [reviewed in Marsh et al. (2011)]. This intra- and inter-species communication leads to coordination of activities and increases the chances of genetic material transfer. The resulting dental plaque is an organized biofilm, whose formation is not pathologic (Gibbons and Van Houte, 1973), though it was thought to be responsible for gingivitis and periodontitis (Schultz-Haudt et al., 1954).

Some bacteria are associated with periodontitis and this led to the proposal of a specific plaque explanation for the disease (Loesche, 1979). These bacteria group in clusters associated with disease progression (Socransky et al., 1998), reflecting the sequential colonization of the periodontal sulcus and pocket (Li et al., 2004; Feres et al., 2016). The "periodontopathogenic" red complex is comprised of anaerobic bacteria (*Aggregatibacter actinomycetemcomitans, Tannerella forsythia*, and *Porphyromonas gingivalis*), supporting the hypothesis of a gradual modification of the environment prior to and necessary for colonization by other bacterium types (Marsh, 2003; Darveau, 2010). However, *P. gingivalis* is present in some healthy patients (Socransky et al., 1998) and is not abundant, even in periodontitis (Moore et al., 1982), while this "keystone pathogen" provokes environmental changes in the sulcus promoting inflammation (Hajishengallis et al., 2011). Thus, *P. gingivalis* cannot be considered an etiological agent for periodontitis by itself, at least with respect to Koch's postulates.

Koch's postulates are the extreme case of Hill's criteria for causation (Hill, 1965) in which infection by a single etiologic agent is the unique parameter influencing the occurrence of the disease (Inglis, 2007). Thus, the quest for a single pathogen explaining the etiology of periodontitis by itself, following Koch's postulates, may be in vain. Contrariwise, periodontitis, as a biofilm disease (Schaudinn et al., 2009), may result from the integration of various causative parameters. Bacteria are among these parameters and the composition of the microbial communities accurately correlates with clinical outcome (Feres et al., 2016; Hunter et al., 2016). Indeed, some species can be efficiently used as markers for diagnosis (Meuric et al., 2017), re-opening ways for considerations about the use of bacterial identification–though in a multi-variate fashion–for epidemiology or treatment follow-up.

Beside changes in its composition, the bacterial community can harbor changes in its functions, generating a new equilibrium (dysbiosis) that is possible in the new dental plaque environment (Hajishengallis and Lamont, 2012). Bacterial entities collaborate and functional changes, such as synergism, are evidenced at the transcriptional level (Kirst et al., 2015; Yost et al., 2015; Deng et al., 2018). Nevertheless, the abundance of some bacterium species is not synonymous for their activity (Mark Welch et al., 2016), a fact compatible with the "keystone pathogen" theory and the role of *P. gingivalis* in shaping the ecology of the periodontal pocket. This ecology is impacted by the dysbiotic communities, as evidenced *in vitro* with deregulated host inflammatory responses (Yost et al., 2017; Herrero et al., 2018). The consequences of dysbiosis were also evidenced *in vivo* at the systemic level, with metabolic changes linked to diabetes (Branchereau et al., 2016; Blasco-Baque et al., 2017).

IMMUNO-PATHOLOGICAL PROCESSES TOWARD PERIODONTITIS

While the dental plaque stacks, mineralization leads to formation of tartar deposits, which can cause injury, as well as overhanging restorations or repetitive wounding. In parallel, the constant presence of bacterial components and the possible colonization by periodontopathogens can be sensed by the host and can cause chronic inflammation and an initial tissue lesion [reviewed in Kurgan and Kantarci (2018)]. The host takes part in fueling progression to disease by inflammation and active mediators of inflammation resolution improve the disease's outcome (Lee et al., 2016; Mizraji et al., 2018). Resident leukocytes and endothelial cells respond to bacterial biofilms: vascular permeability increases and interleukin 8 attracts neutrophils to the affected tissues (Tonetti et al., 1998). Neutrophils play a pivotal role in periodontitis (Ryder, 2010), producing reactive oxygen species (ROS), with probable impact at the systemic level [reviewed in Wang et al. (2017)]. While the early lesion progresses, other immune cells are recruited, including macrophages, lymphocytes, plasma cells, and mast cells. The inflammation can be visible at the microscopic level, where rete pegs–epithelial projections into the underlying connective tissue–form in the pocket epithelium and blood vessels proliferate [reviewed in Zoellner et al. (2002)], and at the macroscopic level, in particular by reddening and bleeding. Macrophages are predominant at this stage (Dennison and Van Dyke, 1997); they can derive from circulating monocytes produced in the spleen or be resident macrophages from embryonic origin, like Langerhans cells, with a possible different role during gum inflammation (Moughal et al., 1992). In established lesions, adaptive responses take place and lymphocytes are abundantly detected (Gemmell et al., 2007). Collagen fibers are increasingly altered, leading to a severe tissue remodeling and loosening of the pocket epithelium (Payne et al., 1975). Thus, greater amounts of dental plaque can accumulate in subgingival locations and aggravate gingivitis, which is considered reversible after elimination of the biofilm, in particular due to the absence of bone and periodontal ligament destruction (Ebersole et al., 2017).

Left untreated, gingivitis evolves to periodontitis, which is characterized by an inflammatory infiltrate composed of plasma cells, and by degradation of collagen fibers, loss of connective tissue, and bone destruction in an anaerobic environment (Mettraux et al., 1984). Periodontitis results in clinical attachment loss, i.e., the deeper positioning of the junction between the pocket epithelium and the cementum of the tooth root. The resulting volume below the gum forms the periodontal pocket, witnessing the breaking down of the initial epithelial attachment, the destruction of the connective tissues constituting the periodontal ligament, and the lysis of the alveolar bone. The sulcus depth–the distance between the free gingival margin and the epithelial attachment–is inferior to 3 mm in healthy or gingivitis sites. When superior to 3 mm, periodontitis is suspected and confirmed by inflammation (redness and swelling) and bleeding on probing.

During periodontitis, the balance between bone resorption and regeneration is displaced: Th17 cells induce osteoclastogenesis (Sato et al., 2006). Recently, it has been described that immunopathogenic Th17 lymphocytes [converted from Foxp3+ T cells; a recent review on T cell contribution to periodontitis in Kinane et al. (2017)] that cause bone damage in rheumatoid arthritis can also determine bone resorption and antimicrobial immunity in the oral cavity (Tsukasaki et al., 2018). In human periodontal lesions, Th17 lymphocytes are abundant (Hajishengallis, 2014) and the major source of IL-17. Foxp3+IL-17+ cells are found in the transition state. The generation of pathogenic exFoxp3+TH17 cells in the oral mucosa is dependent on IL-6, which is expressed by periodontal ligament fibroblasts in periodontitis and stimulated by bacterial PAMPs as LPS (Yamaji et al., 1995) through PRRs as TLR-2 and -4 (Sun et al., 2010; Makkawi et al., 2017). Furthermore, osteogenesis is impaired during periodontitis, while bone resorption by osteoclasts is promoted (Zhou et al., 2018), highlighting that not only immune mechanisms are involved in periodontitis pathophysiology. Beside the bacteria and human cells, some archaea, viruses, protozoa, and fungi are differentially present in healthy and diseased sites (Deng et al., 2017). The contributions of these different phenomena, as well as lysis by pathogens or other host immune cells, still need to be elucidated to solve the current paradigm of periodontitis physiopathology, in which only some of the players are visible in the game.

ENTAMOEBA GINGIVALIS AND PERIODONTAL INFECTIONS

Debate About the Presence of *Entamoeba gingivalis* During Periodontitis

Discovery of *Entamoeba gingivalis*

Though periodontitis was described since antiquity (Langsjoen, 1998), its association with parasites has been evidenced only a century ago. The first description of *Entamoeba gingivalis*–then named "*Amoebea gengivalis*"–was laconically performed in 1849 from dental plaque samples, mentioning amoebic movement and the presence of internal vesicles (Gros, 1849). Though free amoebae were described since 1755 (Rösel Von Rosenhof, 1755), *E. gingivalis* is the first amoeba which was found in humans. The pathogenic association of amoebae with humans was first documented in 1875, validating Koch's postulates in an animal model for the pathogen *Entamoeba histolytica*, then named "*Ameba coli*" (Lösch, 1875). The pathogenicity of *Entamoeba gingivalis* was questioned early (Kartulis, 1893) and the first systematic study associating it with periodontitis was preliminarily published in 1914 (Barrett, 1914): amoebae were detected in the totality of the 46 cases of pyorrhea (periodontitis) that were enrolled in the study. The authors later included 7 healthy individuals from the same group of patients in the "Insane Department of the Philadelphia Hospital" and claimed they could not detect amoebae in "the detritus collected around the neck of the teeth" (Smith and Barrett, 1915a). Furthermore, administration of emetine caused the withdrawal of amoebae and was followed by the cure of pyorrhea in 13 patients (Barrett, 1914). As emetine was thought to be a specific amoebicidal alkaloid with poor bactericidal effect, the etiological link between *Entamoeba gingivalis* and periodontitis was extrapolated and led Smith and Barrett to rename the disease "amoebic pyorrhea" (Barrett, 1914) or "oral endamebiasis" (Smith and Barrett, 1915b).

Rejection of Amoebic Etiology for Periodontitis

It is of epistemological importance to underline that systematic studies, some with a low number of participants, about the involvement of *Entamoeba gingivalis* in periodontitis were countered by specialist opinions without formal experimental proofs, as reported by Craig (Craig, 1916). This controversy led to an almost total abandon of the etiology- and emetine-based therapy, discrediting at the same time its original scientific background. Further statements about the non-permanent cure were made but were unsupported by scientific data, and incriminating relapses (Howitt, 1925). However, the possibility of re-infections was completely ignored and casts doubts about the understanding of both pathophysiology and epidemiology of the disease at that time. In parallel, a method for the culture of *E. gingivalis* was described, which allowed the study of the effects of emetine hydrochloride on the parasite: "emetine hydrochloride has, apparently, no very marked amoebicidal action *in vitro* against either of the strains of *E. gingivalis* used" (Howitt, 1925). However, in a single experiment were evaluated the minimum lethal concentration (MLC, around 116.5 μM, 1:16,600 dilution) and the subjectively determined minimal inhibitory concentration (MIC, around 38.5 μM, 1:50,000) were evaluated. It is noteworthy that the MLC obtained for the emetine-sensitive HM1:IMSS *E. histolytica* strain in a more recent study is higher than 100 μM, the IC_{50} is 29.9 μM, and the MIC is lower than 1 μM (Bansal et al., 2004). This underlines that the experimental methodology to study the effect of emetine on *E. gingivalis* was not accurate. The conclusions of this paper should thus be considered with caution because this *in vitro* study did not corroborate the results reported during the treatment of patients, as previously cited.

Entamoeba gingivalis Infections in the Genetic Era

After this controversy, only a few studies based on the microscopic detection of *E. gingivalis* were published, but almost all of them revealed a prevalence of the parasite close to 100% in advanced periodontal pockets (Fisher, 1927; Hinshaw and Simonton, 1928; Wantland and Wantland, 1960; Wantland and Lauer, 1970; Gottlieb and Miller, 1971; Keyes and Rams, 1983; Lange, 1984; Linke et al., 1989). In the cited publications, the prevalence of *E. gingivalis* in healthy sulci–when studied–ranged from 0 to 26%, suggesting possible errors in the identification of the amoeba. Development of gene amplification by polymerase chain reaction (PCR) and the sequencing of a gene of *E. gingivalis* (Yamamoto et al., 1995) opened ways for the molecular identification of the parasite and accurate epidemiological studies. The first study–using a long amplicon (1.4 kb) and a sub-optimal DNA purification protocol–revealed a prevalence of 6.25% (2 sites out of 32, from 8 patients) in gingivitis or periodontitis sites, without precision of either their relative number or grade; no amplification was obtained from 20 healthy sites (Kikuta et al., 1996). In the second study, 69.2% of periodontitis sites were positive in real-time PCR for *E. gingivalis*, while none of the 12 healthy sites included in the study were (Trim et al., 2011). A third study showed a prevalence of 80.6% (58/72) in periodontitis sites and 33.3% (11/33) in healthy sites by conventional PCR, with controls of PCR inhibition and matrix degradation (Bonner et al., 2014). Recently, transcriptomics revealed that *E. gingivalis* 18s rRNA sequence was detected in all (4/4) periodontal pockets and was less abundant in 60% (6/10), or undetected in 40% (4/10) of healthy sites (Deng et al., 2017). Furthermore, genetic variants of *E. gingivalis* have been identified (Cembranelli et al., 2013; Garcia et al., 2018b) and different levels of virulence reflected at the transcriptomic levels in genetically identical parasites (Santi-Rocca et al., 2008) may account for discrepancies in their molecular detection as compared with microscopy or clinical diagnoses. The new clinical characterization of periodontitis (Tonetti et al., 2018) will avoid further confusion about the definition of health and various disease grades, that may also be responsible for variability between the studies.

Altogether, these data suggest that *E. gingivalis* may be asymptomatically present in some sulci and may be associated with the disease after environmental changes, reminiscent of the intestinal pathogen *E. histolytica*.

Life Cycle of *E. gingivalis*

In most species of the genus *Entamoeba*, two cellular forms have been identified in nature: the cyst, which is the contaminant form found in the environment, and trophozoites, the vegetative cell able to divide, that initially derives from excystation of cysts ingested by the host. The survival of these *Entamoeba* species is ensured by their encystment in response to environmental changes (Mi-Ichi et al., 2016), permitting the survival in environments exposed to oxygen, like human stools, where identification of *Entamoeba* species is made by a simple morphological phenotyping that relies on the number of nuclei carried by the cyst. The sole *E. gingivalis* would not encyst, though cysts of *E. gingivalis* were reported in the literature at the beginning of the twentieth century (Chiavaro, 1914; Smith and Barrett, 1915b; Craig, 1916). However, it is now commonly accepted that *E. gingivalis* does not produce cysts, considering the absence of proof as a proof of absence. Nevertheless, the parasite *E. gingivalis* is essentially observed in periodontal pockets, suggesting that low oxygen levels are important for the survival of trophozoites, as in the case of *E. histolytica* and *E. dispar* [reviewed in Olivos-Garcia et al. (2016)]. Direct transmission of trophozoites to a new host would imply that they are resistant to oxygen, which raises questions about how *E. gingivalis* is transmitted in nature, and what ecological niche serves as a reservoir for this microorganism. Unfortunately, the complete life cycle of *E. gingivalis* is still missing and not addressed yet, hampering efficient prophylaxis.

In the closely-related specie *E. histolytica*, resistance to oxygen is modulated by interaction with bacteria (Varet et al., 2018), as well as virulence (Bracha and Mirelman, 1984; Galvan-Moroyoqui et al., 2008). The microbiota could be of major importance in switching from commensal to pathogenic forms and explain why only a minor part of *E. histolytica* intestinal infections are invasive and symptomatic. During periodontitis, bacterial virulence genes are strongly modulated (Deng et al., 2017) and the frequent and abundant detection of *E. gingivalis* in periodontitis pockets (Bonner et al., 2014) suggests and warns that interactions between constituents of the microbiota could be essential for their functions during the pathophysiology of the disease.

Ingestion of Human Cells by *E. gingivalis*

Entamoeba gingivalis resembles *E. histolytica* in several aspects: trophozoites measure about 30 μm, they are both endowed with mobility, and they ingest human cells and bacteria. The ability of *E. histolytica* to kill and phagocytose host cells correlates with parasite virulence and this amoeba is able to feed on human cells: erythrocytes, lymphocytes, and epithelial cells (Christy and Petri, 2011). Two mechanisms of cell killing and uptake have been discovered for *E. histolytica*: phagocytosis and trogocytosis (Ralston et al., 2014).

Phagocytosis is the phenomenon by which single cells ingest large volumes of material, like other cells or big particles; phagocytic cells include diverse unicellular entities as amoebae, but also macrophages and neutrophils that are cells from the immune system [a recent review in Niedergang and Grinstein (2018)]. In *E. histolytica*, phagocytosis is indispensable for its nutritional needs since this amoeba ingests bacteria in the intestinal lumen. Moreover, phagocytosis is correlated with virulence because *E. histolytica* kills human cells that are eventually phagocytosed. The current model is that *E. histolytica* first kills the host cells in a contact-dependent manner and then phagocytosis of dead cells takes place. However, live cells like bacteria and erythrocytes are also phagocytosed by *E. histolytica*.

In a recently-discovered second mechanism for cell damage, *E. histolytica* ingests fragments of live host cells in a nibbling-like process termed "trogocytosis" (Ralston et al., 2014). Though a specific AGC kinase1 was found exclusively involved in trogocytosis (Somlata and Nozaki, 2017), it seems premature to completely dissociate them from the phagocytic process. Furthermore, previous evidence has shown the existence of these structures during phagocytosis of epithelial and endothelial cells by *E. histolytica* [(Lejeune and Gicquaud, 1987; Nakada-Tsukui et al., 2009), Figure 2 in Faust et al. (2011)] and variability of phagocytic cup shape exist during phagocytosis (Tollis et al., 2010). It has been suggested that amoebic trogocytosis essentially concerns bits of live cells that are internalized, and phagocytosis is the process by which an entire cell is internalized (Ralston, 2015).

Phagocytosis of parts of human cells by *E. gingivalis* was reported almost a century ago (Child, 1926) but poorly studied since then. Some exceptions however existed and, thanks to video microscopy, the impressive process of cell ingestion by this amoeba has been highlighted (Lyons and Stanfield, 1989; Bonner et al., 2014). *Entamoeba gingivalis* is able to engulf one or more human cells at the time by a yet-undescribed mechanism (**Figure 1**). In the observed samples, cells around the amoebae present an altered cellular content, suggesting *E. gingivalis* can trigger signals leading to modification of human cells. As the only human cells observed in these samples were polymorphonuclear cells, and the literature mentions neutrophils are predominant in periodontal pockets, the target cells of amoebic phagocytosis may be the latter. The processes leading to the modifications in nuclear and cytoplasmic morphology in these cells remain to be defined and could be linked, for instance, to proteolytic activity of the amoebae and bacteria, or to a delayed/frustrated NETosis (Neutrophil extracellular traps). Whatever this process is, and whether the amoeba phagocytoses or trogocytosis, the cellular content of the neutrophils leads to one certain point: the first line of defense of cellular innate immunity against *E. gingivalis* and other organisms in the dysbiotic biofilm lacks its weapon (nuclei for NET formation and gene expression) and is thus unable to accomplish its functions.

Hot Topics About *E. gingivalis* Infections

The parasite *E. gingivalis* was identified for its amoeboid movement (Gros, 1849) and characteristics of its locomotion have not been studied since, unlike the closely-related species *E. histolytica* (Aguilar-Rojas et al., 2016). While observations in wet-mounted slides are possible, culture of the parasite is still a bottleneck for the study of *E. gingivalis* biology. Division events have not recently been documented and the whole life cycle is yet to be described.

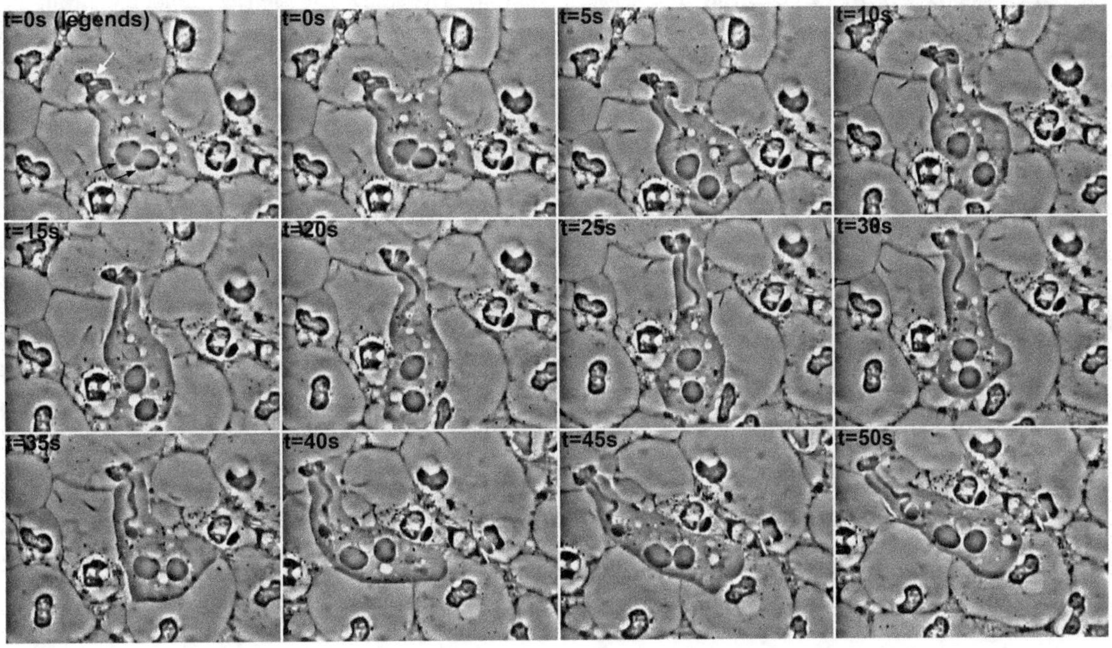

FIGURE 1 | Ingestion of material by an amoeba in a periodontal pocket. Pictures extracted every 5 s from a video-microscopy of saliva-mounted plaque from the deepest part of the periodontal pocket, at 1,000× magnification. In the first panel, the amoeba is pseudo colored in cyan; a black arrowhead indicates its nucleus with the typical peripheral chromatin, while the central karyosome is out of focus. The black arrows indicate food vacuoles. The white arrow designates the internal material (possibly a modified nucleus, perhaps with other subcellular structures) from a host cell (probably a leukocyte), whose ingestion has begun through a "channel," as already observed for trogocytosis and erythrophagocytosis in *E. histolytica*. After 30 s, a food vacuole begins to form at the extremity of the channel. It is noteworthy that the amoeba continues to emit pseudopods and to move during the process, and that it is surrounded by cells with nuclei of different shapes, or even lacking.

The genetic variability in the species *E. gingivalis* seems important (Garcia et al., 2018b) and the genetic distance between the ST1 and ST2 variants may indicate great differences in their biology, accounting for their probable association with different pathologies (Garcia et al., 2018a). As the genotyping of *E. gingivalis* is based on the only gene that has been sequenced, a greater genetic variability may be expected, and further epidemiological studies will precise if some subtypes colonize specific sulcus/pocket environments and, thus, correlate with different clinical outcomes.

The role of the microbiota cannot be ignored and the strong modulation of bacterial genes during periodontitis supports a dysbiotic environment that may impact and be impacted by *E. gingivalis* parasites. Transcriptomic studies will provide clues about these interactions and will rely on the identification of amoebic genetic material. This will be rendered possible by sequencing the *E. gingivalis* genome, probably after the axenic culture of the parasite.

The parasite *E. gingivalis* is more prevalent and more abundant in periodontal pockets, suggesting that this ecological niche is either propitious for its survival, or that the parasite induces changes leading to this environment. Further studies will have to take into consideration the physicochemical and biological characteristics of the periodontal pockets to allow relevant studies of the biology of the parasites, either *in vitro* or in animal models.

CONCLUSION

The absence of reliable animal models for infection by *E. gingivalis* after its axenic culture impedes the ability to conclude about its etiological role in periodontitis, with respect to Koch's postulates. However, recent advances in the field of periodontitis have introduced moderation about this vision, considering that keystone pathogens can participate in changing the environment and consequently in causing dysbiosis, without being the exclusive etiological agent of the disease. *Entamoeba gingivalis* can be an important agent in the pathophysiology of periodontitis and, since its presence is documented and undoubted, it cannot be ignored.

Interestingly, the natural diversity in the human host has allowed the identification of various components of periodontal infections: some pathological traits are preferentially associated with human genetic variants (Offenbacher et al., 2016) and the *P. gingivalis* paradigm may be only one of the possibilities or one of the steps of periodontitis pathophysiology. Indeed, evidence about the kinetics of periodontitis setup is scarce and other possible agents must be considered. First, the ST2 "kamaktli" variant, with a high genetic divergence from *E. gingivalis* ST1 (Garcia et al., 2018b) reminds us that strains of parasites may not be equally virulent or may not have the same tropism (Garcia et al., 2018a). Second, some transcripts from archaea species and viruses are differently abundant between the healthy and the diseased (Deng et al., 2017). In particular, herpes viruses are associated with periodontitis (Slots, 2015; Zhu et al., 2015; Li et al., 2017). Finally, another protozoan is present in some cases of human periodontitis: *Trichomonas tenax* (Marty et al., 2017). Further studies are needed to decipher the ecosystem of the different stages of the periodontal pockets, assigning roles for all of the detected biological entities, which can be opportunistic, neutral, pathogenic, or mutualistic with the organisms within the pocket, and which can have the same type of interactions with the host tissues. Interestingly, the host directly participates in the pathogenic process: osteogenesis is impaired during periodontitis, while bone resorption by osteoclasts is promoted (Zhou et al., 2018). Furthermore, inflammation has an important role in the disease, since active mediators of inflammation resolution improve the disease's outcome (Lee et al., 2016; Mizraji et al., 2018). The contributions of these different phenomena, as well as lysis by pathogens and host immune cells, still need to be elucidated.

All species of *Entamoeba* are not necessarily pathogenic and some of them are commensals (e.g., *E. dispar* or *E. coli*). The study of *E. gingivalis* biology during infection, in particular its virulence factors and pathogenic processes, will allow us to better understand the whole interactions in the ecosystem of the periodontal pockets and to determine the potential participation of *E. gingivalis* in the pathophysiogenesis of periodontitis. Further research should determine if it is taking part in the pathophysiology of periodontitis or just a *bona fide* marker of the disease. In addition, as the picture is getting more complex and the genetic susceptibility of patients shapes different microbiota (Offenbacher et al., 2016), what we call periodontitis might be a group of related diseases with comparable outcomes. Fundamental research must consider this variability to elucidate the pathophysiology of periodontal diseases and to implement efficient public health measures.

AUTHOR CONTRIBUTIONS

All authors contributed equally to the redaction of the manuscript, conceived, and directed by JS-R.

REFERENCES

Aas, J. A., Paster, B. J., Stokes, L. N., Olsen, I., and Dewhirst, F. E. (2005). Defining the normal bacterial flora of the oral cavity. *J. Clin. Microbiol.* 43, 5721–5732. doi: 10.1128/JCM.43.11.5721-5732.2005

Aguilar-Rojas, A., Olivo-Marin, J. C., and Guillen, N. (2016). The motility of *Entamoeba histolytica*: finding ways to understand intestinal amoebiasis. *Curr. Opin. Microbiol.* 34, 24–30. doi: 10.1016/j.mib.2016.07.016

Bansal, D., Sehgal, R., Chawla, Y., Mahajan, R. C., and Malla, N. (2004). *In vitro* activity of antiamoebic drugs against clinical isolates of *Entamoeba histolytica* and *Entamoeba dispar*. *Ann. Clin. Microbiol. Antimicrob.* 3:27. doi: 10.1186/1476-0711-3-27

Barrett, M. (1914). The protozoa of the mouth in relation to pyorrhea alveolaris. *Dent. Cosm.* 56, 948–953.

Blasco-Baque, V., Garidou, L., Pomie, C., Escoula, Q., Loubieres, P., Le Gall-David, S., et al. (2017). Periodontitis induced by *Porphyromonas gingivalis* drives periodontal microbiota dysbiosis and insulin resistance via an impaired adaptive immune response. *Gut* 66, 872–885. doi: 10.1136/gutjnl-2015-309897

Bonner, M., Amard, V., Bar-Pinatel, C., Charpentier, F., Chatard, J. M., Desmuyck, Y., et al. (2014). Detection of the amoeba *Entamoeba gingivalis* in periodontal pockets. *Parasite* 21:30. doi: 10.1051/parasite/2014029

Bracha, R., and Mirelman, D. (1984). Virulence of *Entamoeba histolytica* trophozoites. Effects of bacteria, microaerobic conditions, and metronidazole. *J. Exp. Med.* 160, 353–368. doi: 10.1084/jem.160.2.353

Branchereau, M., Reichardt, F., Loubieres, P., Marck, P., Waget, A., Azalbert, V., et al. (2016). Periodontal dysbiosis linked to periodontitis is associated with cardiometabolic adaptation to high-fat diet in mice. *Am. J. Physiol. Gastrointest. Liver Physiol.* 310, G1091–1101. doi: 10.1152/ajpgi.00424.2015

Cembranelli, S. B., Souto, F. O., Ferreira-Paim, K., Richinho, T. T., Nunes, P. L., Nascentes, G. A., et al. (2013). First evidence of genetic intraspecific variability and occurrence of *Entamoeba gingivalis* in HIV(+)/AIDS. *PLoS ONE* 8:e82864. doi: 10.1371/journal.pone.0082864

Chiavaro, A. (1914). Researches upon *Entamoeba buccalis*. *Dent. Rev.* 28, 1122–1135.

Child, H. J. (1926). Studies on the ingestion of leucocytes and on mitosis in *Endamoeba gingivalis*. *Univ. Calif. Publ. Zool.* 28, 251–284.

Christy, N. C., and Petri, W. A. Jr. (2011). Mechanisms of adherence, cytotoxicity and phagocytosis modulate the pathogenesis of *Entamoeba histolytica*. *Future Microbiol.* 6, 1501–1519. doi: 10.2217/fmb.11.120

Consortium, H. M. P. (2012). Structure, function and diversity of the healthy human microbiome. *Nature* 486, 207–214. doi: 10.1038/nature11234

Craig, C. F. (1916). Observations upon the Endamebae of the Mouth. I. *Endamoeba Gingivalis* (Buccalis). *J. Infect.Dis.* 18, 220–238. doi: 10.1093/infdis/18.2.220

Darveau, R. P. (2010). Periodontitis: a polymicrobial disruption of host homeostasis. *Nat. Rev. Microbiol.* 8, 481–490. doi: 10.1038/nrmicro2337

Demmer, R. T., and Papapanou, P. N. (2010). Epidemiologic patterns of chronic and aggressive periodontitis. *Periodontol. 2000* 53, 28–44. doi: 10.1111/j.1600-0757.2009.00326.x

Deng, Z. L., Szafranski, S. P., Jarek, M., Bhuju, S., and Wagner-Dobler, I. (2017). Dysbiosis in chronic periodontitis: key microbial players and interactions with the human host. *Sci. Rep.* 7:3703. doi: 10.1038/s41598-017-03804-8

Deng, Z. L., Sztajer, H., Jarek, M., Bhuju, S., and Wagner-Dobler, I. (2018). Worlds apart–transcriptome profiles of key oral microbes in the periodontal pocket compared to single laboratory culture reflect synergistic interactions. *Front. Microbiol.* 9:124. doi: 10.3389/fmicb.2018.00124

Dennison, D. K., and Van Dyke, T. E. (1997). The acute inflammatory response and the role of phagocytic cells in periodontal health and disease. *Periodontol. 2000* 14, 54–78. doi: 10.1111/j.1600-0757.1997.tb00192.x

Dumitrescu, A. L. (2016). Depression and inflammatory periodontal disease considerations-an interdisciplinary approach. *Front. Psychol.* 7:347. doi: 10.3389/fpsyg.2016.00347

Ebersole, J. L., Dawson, D. III, Emecen-Huja, P., Nagarajan, R., Howard, K., Grady, M. E., et al. (2017). The periodontal war: microbes and immunity. *Periodontol. 2000* 75, 52–115. doi: 10.1111/prd.12222

Eke, P. I., Dye, B. A., Wei, L., Slade, G. D., Thornton-Evans, G. O., Borgnakke, W. S., et al. (2015). Update on prevalence of periodontitis in adults in the United States: NHANES 2009 to 2012. *J. Periodontol.* 86, 611–622. doi: 10.1902/jop.2015.140520

Eke, P. I., Wei, L., Thornton-Evans, G. O., Borrell, L. N., Borgnakke, W. S., Dye, B., et al. (2016). Risk indicators for periodontitis in US adults: NHANES 2009 to 2012. *J. Periodontol.* 87, 1174–1185. doi: 10.1902/jop.2016.160013

Evaluation, I. F. H. M. A. (2016). *Global Burden of Disease Study 2015. Global Burden of Disease Study 2015 (GBD 2015) Disability Weights*. Seattle, WA. Available online at: http://ghdx.healthdata.org/record/global-burden-disease-study-2015-gbd-2015-disability-weights

Faust, D. M., Marquay Markiewicz, J., Santi-Rocca, J., and Guillen, N. (2011). New insights into host-pathogen interactions during *Entamoeba histolytica* liver infection. *Eur. J. Microbiol. Immunol.* 1, 10–18. doi: 10.1556/EuJMI.1.2011.1.4

Feres, M., Teles, F., Teles, R., Figueiredo, L. C., and Faveri, M. (2016). The subgingival periodontal microbiota of the aging mouth. *Periodontol. 2000* 72, 30–53. doi: 10.1111/prd.12136

Fisher, J. H. (1927). Pyorrhea alveolaris: the rôle of certain microörganisms found in the lesions. *Am. J. Pathol.* 3:169.

Galvan-Moroyoqui, J. M., Del Carmen Dominguez-Robles, M., Franco, E., and Meza, I. (2008). The interplay between Entamoeba and enteropathogenic bacteria modulates epithelial cell damage. *PLoS Negl. Trop. Dis.* 2:e266. doi: 10.1371/journal.pntd.0000266

Garcia, G., Ramos, F., Maldonado, J., Fernandez, A., Yanez, J., Hernandez, L., et al. (2018a). Prevalence of two *Entamoeba gingivalis* ST1 and ST2-kamaktli subtypes in the human oral cavity under various conditions. *Parasitol. Res.* 117, 2941–2948. doi: 10.1007/s00436-018-5990-8

Garcia, G., Ramos, F., Martinez-Hernandez, F., Hernandez, L., Yanez, J., and Gaytan, P. (2018b). A new subtype of *Entamoeba gingivalis*: "*E. gingivalis* ST2, kamaktli variant". *Parasitol. Res.* 117, 1277–1284. doi: 10.1007/s00436-018-5798-6

Gemmell, E., Yamazaki, K., and Seymour, G. J. (2007). The role of T cells in periodontal disease: homeostasis and autoimmunity. *Periodontol. 2000* 43, 14–40. doi: 10.1111/j.1600-0757.2006.00173.x

Gibbons, R. J., Hay, D. I., Cisar, J. O., and Clark, W. B. (1988). Adsorbed salivary proline-rich protein 1 and statherin: receptors for type 1 fimbriae of Actinomyces viscosus T14V-J1 on apatitic surfaces. *Infect. Immun.* 56, 2990–2993.

Gibbons, R. J., and Van Houte, J. (1973). On the formation of dental plaques. *J. Periodontol.* 44, 347–360. doi: 10.1902/jop.1973.44.6.347

Gottlieb, D. S., and Miller, L. H. (1971). *Entamoeba gingivalis* in periodontal disease. *J. Periodontol.* 42, 412–415. doi: 10.1902/jop.1971.42.7.412

Gros, G. (1849). Fragments d'helminthologie et de physiologie microscopique. *Bull. Soc. Impériale Nat. Moscou* 22, 549–573.

Hajishengallis, G. (2014). Immunomicrobial pathogenesis of periodontitis: keystones, pathobionts, and host response. *Trends Immunol.* 35, 3–11. doi: 10.1016/j.it.2013.09.001

Hajishengallis, G., and Lamont, R. J. (2012). Beyond the red complex and into more complexity: the polymicrobial synergy and dysbiosis (PSD) model of periodontal disease etiology. *Mol. Oral Microbiol.* 27, 409–419. doi: 10.1111/j.2041-1014.2012.00663.x

Hajishengallis, G., Liang, S., Payne, M. A., Hashim, A., Jotwani, R., Eskan, M. A., et al. (2011). Low-abundance biofilm species orchestrates inflammatory periodontal disease through the commensal microbiota and complement. *Cell Host Microb.* 10, 497–506. doi: 10.1016/j.chom.2011.10.006

Herrero, E. R., Fernandes, S., Verspecht, T., Ugarte-Berzal, E., Boon, N., Proost, P., et al. (2018). Dysbiotic biofilms deregulate the periodontal inflammatory response. *J. Dent. Res.* 97, 547–555. doi: 10.1177/0022034517752675

Hill, A. B. (1965). The environment and disease: association or causation? *Proc. R. Soc. Med.* 58, 295–300.

Hinshaw, H. C., and Simonton, F. (1928). The amoebas of the mouth in relation to incidence of pyorrhea, clinical symptoms, extent of lesions, and age of patients. *J. Dent. Res.* 8, 507–528. doi: 10.1177/00220345280080040501

Howitt, B. F. (1925). The cultivation of *Endamoeba gingivalis* (Gros). *Univ. Calif. Publ. Zool.* 28, 65–126.

Hsu, C. C., Hsu, Y. C., Chen, H. J., Lin, C. C., Chang, K. H., Lee, C. Y., et al. (2015). Association of periodontitis and subsequent depression: a nationwide population-based study. *Medicine* 94:e2347. doi: 10.1097/MD.0000000000002347

Hunter, M. C., Pozhitkov, A. E., and Noble, P. A. (2016). Microbial signatures of oral dysbiosis, periodontitis and edentulism revealed by Gene Meter methodology. *J. Microbiol. Methods* 131, 85–101. doi: 10.1016/j.mimet.2016.09.019

Inglis, T. J. (2007). Principia aetiologica: taking causality beyond Koch's postulates. *J. Med. Microbiol.* 56, 1419–1422. doi: 10.1099/jmm.0.47179-0

Jakubovics, N. S. (2010). Talk of the town: interspecies communication in oral biofilms. *Mol. Oral Microbiol.* 25, 4–14. doi: 10.1111/j.2041-1014.2009.00563.x

Kartulis, S. (1893). Muskelparasiten beim Menschen. *Z. Hyg. Infektionskr.* 13:2.

Keyes, P. H., and Rams, T. E. (1983). A rationale for management of periodontal diseases: rapid identification of microbial "therapeutic targets" with phase-contrast microscopy. *J. Am. Dent. Assoc.* 106, 803–812.

Kikuta, N., Yamamoto, A., and Goto, N. (1996). Detection and identification of Entamoeba gingivalis by specific amplification of rRNA gene. *Can. J. Microbiol.* 42, 1248–1251. doi: 10.1139/m96-161

Kinane, D. F., Stathopoulou, P. G., and Papapanou, P. N. (2017). Periodontal diseases. *Nat. Rev. Dis. Primers* 3:17038. doi: 10.1038/nrdp.2017.38

Kirst, M. E., Li, E. C., Alfant, B., Chi, Y. Y., Walker, C., Magnusson, I., et al. (2015). Dysbiosis and alterations in predicted functions of the subgingival microbiome in chronic periodontitis. *Appl. Environ. Microbiol.* 81, 783–793. doi: 10.1128/AEM.02712-14

Kolenbrander, P. E., and Celesk, R. A. (1983). Coaggregation of human oral cytophaga species and *Actinomyces israelii*. *Infect. Immun.* 40, 1178–1185.

Kurgan, S., and Kantarci, A. (2018). Molecular basis for immunohistochemical and inflammatory changes during progression of gingivitis to periodontitis. *Periodontol. 2000* 76, 51–67. doi: 10.1111/prd.12146

Lange, D. E. (1984). Microbiological aspects of periodontal diseases. *Zahnarztl. Mitt.* 74, 2420, 2422–2423, 2426–2427.

Langsjoen, O. (1998). "Diseases of the dentition," in *The Cambridge Encyclopedia of Human Paleopathology*, eds A. C. Aufderheide, and C. Rodríguez-Martín (Cambridge: University Press Cambridge), 393–412.

Lee, C. T., Teles, R., Kantarci, A., Chen, T., Mccafferty, J., Starr, J. R., et al. (2016). Resolvin E1 reverses experimental periodontitis and dysbiosis. *J. Immunol.* 197, 2796–2806. doi: 10.4049/jimmunol.1600859

Leira, Y., Seoane, J., Blanco, M., Rodriguez-Yanez, M., Takkouche, B., Blanco, J., et al. (2017). Association between periodontitis and ischemic stroke: a systematic review and meta-analysis. *Eur. J. Epidemiol.* 32, 43–53. doi: 10.1007/s10654-016-0170-6

Lejeune, A., and Gicquaud, C. (1987). Evidence for two mechanisms of human erythrocyte endocytosis by *Entamoeba histolytica*-like amoebae (Laredo strain). *Biol. Cell* 59, 239–245. doi: 10.1111/j.1768-322X.1987.tb00536.x

Lertpimonchai, A., Rattanasiri, S., Arj-Ong Vallibhakara, S., Attia, J., and Thakkinstian, A. (2017). The association between oral hygiene and periodontitis: a systematic review and meta-analysis. *Int. Dent. J.* 67, 332–343. doi: 10.1111/idj.12317

Li, F., Zhu, C., Deng, F. Y., Wong, M. C. M., Lu, H. X., and Feng, X. P. (2017). Herpesviruses in etiopathogenesis of aggressive periodontitis: a meta-analysis based on case-control studies. *PLoS ONE* 12:e0186373. doi: 10.1371/journal.pone.0186373

Li, J., Helmerhorst, E. J., Leone, C. W., Troxler, R. F., Yaskell, T., Haffajee, A. D., et al. (2004). Identification of early microbial colonizers in human dental biofilm. *J. Appl. Microbiol.* 97, 1311–1318. doi: 10.1111/j.1365-2672.2004.02420.x

Linke, H. A., Gannon, J. T., and Obin, J. N. (1989). Clinical survey of *Entamoeba gingivalis* by multiple sampling in patients with advanced periodontal disease. *Int. J. Parasitol.* 19, 803–808. doi: 10.1016/0020-7519(89)90069-6

Listgarten, M. A. (1976). Structure of the microbial flora associated with periodontal health and disease in man. A light and electron microscopic study. *J. Periodontol.* 47, 1–18. doi: 10.1902/jop.1976.47.1.1

Löe, H., Theilade, E., and Jensen, S. B. (1965). *Experimental gingivitis* in man. *J. Periodontol.* 36, 177–187. doi: 10.1902/jop.1965.36.3.177

Loesche, W. J. (1979). Clinical and microbiological aspects of chemotherapeutic agents used according to the specific plaque hypothesis. *J. Dent. Res.* 58, 2404–2412. doi: 10.1177/00220345790580120905

Lopez, R., Ramirez, V., Marro, P., and Baelum, V. (2012). Psychosocial distress and periodontitis in adolescents. *Oral Health Prev. Dent.* 10, 211–218. doi: 10.3290/j.ohpd.a28516

Lösch, F. (1875). Massenhafte Entwicklung von Amöben im Dickdarm. *Virchow. Arch.* 65, 196–211. doi: 10.1007/BF02028799

Lyons, T., and Stanfield, E. (1989). *Introduction to Protozoa and Fungi in Periodontal Infections: A Manual of Microbiological Diagnosis and Non-Surgical Treatment.* Ottawa, ON: Trevor Lyons.

Makkawi, H., Hoch, S., Burns, E., Hosur, K., Hajishengallis, G., Kirschning, C. J., et al. (2017). *Porphyromonas gingivalis* stimulates TLR2-PI3K signaling to escape immune clearance and induce bone resorption independently of MyD88. *Front. Cell. Infect. Microbiol.* 7:359. doi: 10.3389/fcimb.2017.00359

Mark Welch, J. L., Rossetti, B. J., Rieken, C. W., Dewhirst, F. E., and Borisy, G. G. (2016). Biogeography of a human oral microbiome at the micron scale. *Proc. Natl. Acad. Sci. U.S.A.* 113, E791–800. doi: 10.1073/pnas.1522149113

Marsh, P. D. (1994). Microbial ecology of dental plaque and its significance in health and disease. *Adv. Dent. Res.* 8, 263–271. doi: 10.1177/08959374940080022001

Marsh, P. D. (2003). Are dental diseases examples of ecological catastrophes? *Microbiology* 149, 279–294. doi: 10.1099/mic.0.26082-0

Marsh, P. D., Moter, A., and Devine, D. A. (2011). Dental plaque biofilms: communities, conflict and control. *Periodontol. 2000* 55, 16–35. doi: 10.1111/j.1600-0757.2009.00339.x

Marty, M., Lemaitre, M., Kemoun, P., Morrier, J. J., and Monsarrat, P. (2017). *Trichomonas tenax* and periodontal diseases: a concise review. *Parasitology* 144, 1417–1425. doi: 10.1017/S0031182017000701

Mettraux, G. R., Gusberti, F. A., and Graf, H. (1984). Oxygen tension (pO2) in untreated human periodontal pockets. *J. Periodontol.* 55, 516–521. doi: 10.1902/jop.1984.55.9.516

Meuric, V., Le Gall-David, S., Boyer, E., Acuna-Amador, L., Martin, B., Fong, S. B., et al. (2017). Signature of microbial dysbiosis in periodontitis. *Appl. Environ. Microbiol.* 83:e00462-17. doi: 10.1128/AEM.00462-17

Mi-Ichi, F., Yoshida, H., and Hamano, S. (2016). *Entamoeba Encystation*: new targets to prevent the transmission of Amebiasis. *PLoS Pathog.* 12:e1005845. doi: 10.1371/journal.ppat.1005845

Mizraji, G., Heyman, O., Van Dyke, T. E., and Wilensky, A. (2018). Resolvin D2 Restrains Th1 immunity and prevents alveolar bone loss in murine periodontitis. *Front. Immunol.* 9:785. doi: 10.3389/fimmu.2018.00785

Moore, W. E., Holdeman, L. V., Smibert, R. M., Hash, D. E., Burmeister, J. A., and Ranney, R. R. (1982). Bacteriology of severe periodontitis in young adult humans. *Infect. Immun.* 38, 1137–1148.

Moughal, N. A., Adonogianaki, E., and Kinane, D. F. (1992). Langerhans cell dynamics in human gingiva during experimentally induced inflammation. *J. Biol. Buccale* 20, 163–167.

Nakada-Tsukui, K., Okada, H., Mitra, B. N., and Nozaki, T. (2009). Phosphatidylinositol-phosphates mediate cytoskeletal reorganization during phagocytosis via a unique modular protein consisting of RhoGEF/DH and FYVE domains in the parasitic protozoon *Entamoeba histolytica*. *Cell. Microbiol.* 11, 1471–1491. doi: 10.1111/j.1462-5822.2009.01341.x

Nascimento, G. G., Leite, F. R. M., Vestergaard, P., Scheutz, F., and Lopez, R. (2018). Does diabetes increase the risk of periodontitis? A systematic review and meta-regression analysis of longitudinal prospective studies. *Acta Diabetol.* 55, 653–667. doi: 10.1007/s00592-018-1120-4

Niedergang, F., and Grinstein, S. (2018). How to build a phagosome: new concepts for an old process. *Curr. Opin. Cell Biol.* 50, 57–63. doi: 10.1016/j.ceb.2018.01.009

Nieri, M., Pini Prato, G. P., Giani, M., Magnani, N., Pagliaro, U., and Rotundo, R. (2013). Patient perceptions of buccal gingival recessions and requests for treatment. *J. Clin. Periodontol.* 40, 707–712. doi: 10.1111/jcpe.12114

Offenbacher, S., Divaris, K., Barros, S. P., Moss, K. L., Marchesan, J. T., Morelli, T., et al. (2016). Genome-wide association study of biologically informed periodontal complex traits offers novel insights into the genetic basis of periodontal disease. *Hum. Mol. Genet.* 25, 2113–2129. doi: 10.1093/hmg/ddw069

Olivos-Garcia, A., Saavedra, E., Nequiz, M., Santos, F., Luis-Garcia, E. R., Gudino, M., et al. (2016). The oxygen reduction pathway and heat shock stress response are both required for *Entamoeba histolytica* pathogenicity. *Curr. Genet.* 62, 295–300. doi: 10.1007/s00294-015-0543-5

Organization, W. H. (2016). *Global Health Estimates 2015: Deaths by Cause, Age, Sex, by Country and by Region, 2000–2015.* Geneva.

Payne, W. A., Page, R. C., Ogilvie, A. L., and Hall, W. B. (1975). Histopathologic features of the initial and early stages of experimental gingivitis in man. *J. Periodont. Res.* 10, 51–64. doi: 10.1111/j.1600-0765.1975.tb00008.x

Petersen, P. E., and Ogawa, H. (2005). Strengthening the prevention of periodontal disease: the WHO approach. *J. Periodontol.* 76, 2187–2193. doi: 10.1902/jop.2005.76.12.2187

Ralston, K. S. (2015). Chew on this: amoebic trogocytosis and host cell killing by *Entamoeba histolytica*. *Trends Parasitol.* 31, 442–452. doi: 10.1016/j.pt.2015.05.003

Ralston, K. S., Solga, M. D., Mackey-Lawrence, N. M., Somlata, Bhattacharya, A., and Petri, W. A. Jr. (2014). Trogocytosis by Entamoeba histolytica contributes to cell killing and tissue invasion. *Nature* 508, 526–530. doi: 10.1038/nature13242

Reynolds, I., and Duane, B. (2018). Periodontal disease has an impact on patients' quality of life. *Evid. Based Dent.* 19, 14–15. doi: 10.1038/sj.ebd.6401287

Rogers, G. B., and Bruce, K. D. (2012). Exploring the parallel development of microbial systems in neonates with cystic fibrosis. *MBio* 3:e00408–00412. doi: 10.1128/mBio.00408-12

Rösel Von Rosenhof, A. J. (1755). *Der Monatlich-Herausgegebenen Insecten-Belustigung.* Nürnberg: Fleischmann JJ.

Rosier, B. T., Marsh, P. D., and Mira, A. (2018). Resilience of the oral microbiota in health: mechanisms that prevent dysbiosis. *J. Dent. Res.* 97, 371–380. doi: 10.1177/0022034517742139

Ryder, M. I. (2010). Comparison of neutrophil functions in aggressive and chronic periodontitis. *Periodontol. 2000* 53, 124–137. doi: 10.1111/j.1600-0757.2009.00327.x

Santi-Rocca, J., Weber, C., Guigon, G., Sismeiro, O., Coppee, J. Y., and Guillen, N. (2008). The lysine- and glutamic acid-rich protein KERP1 plays a role in *Entamoeba histolytica* liver abscess pathogenesis. *Cell. Microbiol.* 10, 202–217. doi: 10.1111/j.1462-5822.2007.01030.x

Sato, K., Suematsu, A., Okamoto, K., Yamaguchi, A., Morishita, Y., Kadono, Y., et al. (2006). Th17 functions as an osteoclastogenic helper T cell subset that links T cell activation and bone destruction. *J. Exp. Med.* 203, 2673–2682. doi: 10.1084/jem.20061775

Schaudinn, C., Gorur, A., Keller, D., Sedghizadeh, P. P., and Costerton, J. W. (2009). Periodontitis: an archetypical biofilm disease. *J. Am. Dent. Assoc.* 140, 978–986. doi: 10.14219/jada.archive.2009.0307

Schultz-Haudt, S., Bruce, M. A., and Bibby, B. G. (1954). Bacterial factors in nonspecific gingivitis. *J. Dent. Res.* 33, 454–458. doi: 10.1177/00220345540330040301

Silva, M. F., Cademartori, M. G., Leite, F. R. M., Lopez, R., Demarco, F. F., and Nascimento, G. G. (2017). Is periodontitis associated with halitosis? A systematic review and meta-regression analysis. *J. Clin. Periodontol.* 44, 1003–1009. doi: 10.1111/jcpe.12786

Slots, J. (2015). Periodontal herpesviruses: prevalence, pathogenicity, systemic risk. *Periodontol. 2000* 69, 28–45. doi: 10.1111/prd.12085

Smiley, C. J., Tracy, S. L., Abt, E., Michalowicz, B. S., John, M. T., Gunsolley, J., et al. (2015). Evidence-based clinical practice guideline on the nonsurgical treatment of chronic periodontitis by means of scaling and root planing with or without adjuncts. *J. Am. Dent. Assoc.* 146, 525–535. doi: 10.1016/j.adaj.2015.01.026

Smith, A., and Barrett, M. (1915a). Emetin in the treatment of peridental suppurations. *Dent. Cosm.* 57:1201.

Smith, A. J., and Barrett, M. (1915b). The parasite of oral Endamebiasis, *Endameba gingivalis* (Gros). *J. Parasitol.* 1, 159–174.

Socransky, S. S., Haffajee, A. D., Cugini, M. A., Smith, C., and Kent, R. L. Jr. (1998). Microbial complexes in subgingival plaque. *J. Clin. Periodontol.* 25, 134–144. doi: 10.1111/j.1600-051X.1998.tb02419.x

Somlata, Nakada-Tsukui, K., and Nozaki, T. (2017). AGC family kinase 1 participates in trogocytosis but not in phagocytosis in *Entamoeba histolytica*. *Nat. Commun.* 8:101. doi: 10.1038/s41467-017-00199-y

Sun, Y., Shu, R., Li, C. L., and Zhang, M. Z. (2010). Gram-negative periodontal bacteria induce the activation of Toll-like receptors 2 and 4, and cytokine production in human periodontal ligament cells. *J. Periodontol.* 81, 1488–1496. doi: 10.1902/jop.2010.100004

Tollis, S., Dart, A. E., Tzircotis, G., and Endres, R. G. (2010). The zipper mechanism in phagocytosis: energetic requirements and variability in phagocytic cup shape. *BMC Syst. Biol.* 4:149. doi: 10.1186/1752-0509-4-149

Tonetti, M. S., Greenwell, H., and Kornman, K. S. (2018). Staging and grading of periodontitis: framework and proposal of a new classification and case definition. *J. Periodontol.* 89(Suppl. 1), S159–S172. doi: 10.1002/JPER.18-0006

Tonetti, M. S., Imboden, M. A., and Lang, N. P. (1998). Neutrophil migration into the gingival sulcus is associated with transepithelial gradients of interleukin-8 and ICAM-1. *J. Periodontol.* 69, 1139–1147. doi: 10.1902/jop.1998.69.10.1139

Trim, R. D., Skinner, M. A., Farone, M. B., Dubois, J. D., and Newsome, A. L. (2011). Use of PCR to detect *Entamoeba gingivalis* in diseased gingival pockets and demonstrate its absence in healthy gingival sites. *Parasitol. Res.* 109, 857–864. doi: 10.1007/s00436-011-2312-9

Tsukasaki, M., Komatsu, N., Nagashima, K., Nitta, T., Pluemsakunthai, W., Shukunami, C., et al. (2018). Host defense against oral microbiota by bone-damaging T cells. *Nat. Commun.* 9:701. doi: 10.1038/s41467-018-03147-6

Van Dyke, T. E. (2017). Pro-resolving mediators in the regulation of periodontal disease. *Mol. Aspects Med.* 58, 21–36. doi: 10.1016/j.mam.2017.04.006

van 'T Hof, W., Veerman, E. C., Nieuw Amerongen, A. V., and Ligtenberg, A. J. (2014). Antimicrobial defense systems in saliva. *Monogr. Oral Sci.* 24, 40–51. doi: 10.1159/000358783

Varet, H., Shaulov, Y., Sismeiro, O., Trebicz-Geffen, M., Legendre, R., Coppée, J.-Y., et al. (2018). Enteric bacteria boost defences against oxidative stress in *Entamoeba histolytica*. *Sci. Rep.* 8:9042. doi: 10.1038/s41598-018-27086-w

Vieira, A. R., and Albandar, J. M. (2014). Role of genetic factors in the pathogenesis of aggressive periodontitis. *Periodontol. 2000* 65, 92–106. doi: 10.1111/prd.12021

Wang, J., Lv, J., Wang, W., and Jiang, X. (2016). Alcohol consumption and risk of periodontitis: a meta-analysis. *J. Clin. Periodontol.* 43, 572–583. doi: 10.1111/jcpe.12556

Wang, Y., Andrukhov, O., and Rausch-Fan, X. (2017). Oxidative stress and antioxidant system in periodontitis. *Front. Physiol.* 8:910. doi: 10.3389/fphys.2017.00910

Wantland, W. W., and Lauer, D. (1970). Correlation of some oral hygiene variables with age, sex, and incidence of oral protozoa. *J. Dent. Res.* 49, 293–297. doi: 10.1177/00220345700490021601

Wantland, W. W., and Wantland, E. M. (1960). Incidence, ecology, and reproduction of oral protozoa. *J. Dent. Res.* 39:863. doi: 10.1177/00220345600390041801

Yamaji, Y., Kubota, T., Sasaguri, K., Sato, S., Suzuki, Y., Kumada, H., et al. (1995). Inflammatory cytokine gene expression in human periodontal ligament fibroblasts stimulated with bacterial lipopolysaccharides. *Infect. Immun.* 63, 3576–3581.

Yamamoto, A., Kikuta, N., Hashimoto, T., Oyaizu, H., and Goto, N. (1995). Nucleotide sequence of the SrRNA gene of *Entamoeba gingivalis*: applications for construction of a species-specific DNA probe and phylogenetic analysis. *Microbiol. Immunol.* 39, 185–192. doi: 10.1111/j.1348-0421.1995.tb02187.x

Yost, S., Duran-Pinedo, A. E., Krishnan, K., and Frias-Lopez, J. (2017). Potassium is a key signal in host-microbiome dysbiosis in periodontitis. *PLoS Pathog.* 13:e1006457. doi: 10.1371/journal.ppat.1006457

Yost, S., Duran-Pinedo, A. E., Teles, R., Krishnan, K., and Frias-Lopez, J. (2015). Functional signatures of oral dysbiosis during periodontitis progression revealed by microbial metatranscriptome analysis. *Genome Med.* 7:27. doi: 10.1186/s13073-015-0153-3

Zhou, R., Shen, L., Yang, C., Wang, L., Guo, H., Yang, P., et al. (2018). Periodontitis may restrain the mandibular bone healing via disturbing Osteogenic and Osteoclastic balance. *Inflammation* 41, 972–983. doi: 10.1007/s10753-018-0751-5

Zhu, C., Li, F., Wong, M. C., Feng, X. P., Lu, H. X., and Xu, W. (2015). Association between Herpesviruses and Chronic Periodontitis: a meta-analysis based on case-control studies. *PLoS ONE* 10:e0144319. doi: 10.1371/journal.pone.0144319

Zoellner, H., Chapple, C. C., and Hunter, N. (2002). Microvasculature in gingivitis and chronic periodontitis: disruption of vascular networks with protracted inflammation. *Microsc. Res. Tech.* 56, 15–31. doi: 10.1002/jemt.10009

5

Phosphatidylinositol Kinases and Phosphatases in *Entamoeba histolytica*

Kumiko Nakada-Tsukui [1*†], *Natsuki Watanabe* [1,2†], *Tomohiko Maehama* [3] *and Tomoyoshi Nozaki* [4*]

[1] *Department of Parasitology, National Institute of Infectious Diseases, Tokyo, Japan,* [2] *Graduate School of Life and Environmental Sciences, University of Tsukuba, Tsukuba, Japan,* [3] *Division of Molecular and Cellular Biology, Graduate School of Medicine, Kobe University, Kobe, Japan,* [4] *Department of Biomedical Chemistry, Graduate School of Medicine, The University of Tokyo, Tokyo, Japan*

Correspondence:
Kumiko Nakada-Tsukui
kumiko@nih.go.jp
Tomoyoshi Nozaki
nozaki@m.u-tokyo.ac.jp

† *These authors have contributed equally to this work*

Phosphatidylinositol (PtdIns) metabolism is indispensable in eukaryotes. Phosphoinositides (PIs) are phosphorylated derivatives of PtdIns and consist of seven species generated by reversible phosphorylation of the inositol moieties at the positions 3, 4, and 5. Each of the seven PIs has a unique subcellular and membrane domain distribution. In the enteric protozoan parasite *Entamoeba histolytica*, it has been previously shown that the PIs phosphatidylinositol 3-phosphate (PtdIns3P), PtdIns(4,5)P_2, and PtdIns(3,4,5)P_3 are localized to phagosomes/phagocytic cups, plasma membrane, and phagocytic cups, respectively. The localization of these PIs in *E. histolytica* is similar to that in mammalian cells, suggesting that PIs have orthologous functions in *E. histolytica*. In contrast, the conservation of the enzymes that metabolize PIs in this organism has not been well-documented. In this review, we summarized the full repertoire of the PI kinases and PI phosphatases found in *E. histolytica* via a genome-wide survey of the current genomic information. *E. histolytica* appears to have 10 PI kinases and 23 PI phosphatases. It has a panel of evolutionarily conserved enzymes that generate all the seven PI species. However, class II PI 3-kinases, type II PI 4-kinases, type III PI 5-phosphatases, and PI 4P-specific phosphatases are not present. Additionally, regulatory subunits of class I PI 3-kinases and type III PI 4-kinases have not been identified. Instead, homologs of class I PI 3-kinases and PTEN, a PI 3-phosphatase, exist as multiple isoforms, which likely reflects that elaborate signaling cascades mediated by PtdIns(3,4,5)P_3 are present in this organism. There are several enzymes that have the nuclear localization signal: one phosphatidylinositol phosphate (PIP) kinase, two PI 3-phosphatases, and one PI 5-phosphatase; this suggests that PI metabolism also has conserved roles related to nuclear functions in *E. histolytica*, as it does in model organisms.

Keywords: *Entamoeba histolytica*, phosphoinositide, kinase, phosphatase, signaling

1. INTRODUCTION

Phosphoinositides (PIs) are phosphorylated-phosphatidylinositol (PtdIns) derivatives and play pivotal roles in a variety of biological processes such as receptor-mediated signaling, vesicular traffic, cytoskeleton rearrangement, and regulation of channels and transporters (Sasaki et al., 2009; Balla, 2013). Spatiotemporal regulation of PI-mediated biological processes is achieved by interconversion of the phosphorylation states of PIs by specific kinases and phosphatases, followed by recruitment of PI-specific effectors. Phospholipids are ubiquitous in all three domains of life. Nevertheless, the complexity of PIs and enzymes that interconvert them appears to have increased in eukaryotes (Michell, 2008, 2011). It has been suggested that the PI metabolism developed in the last common eukaryotic ancestor (Michell, 2008) and diverged during eukaryotic evolution.

Human amebiasis is a common infection caused by the protozoan parasite *Entamoeba histolytica* in both developing and developed countries (Taniuchi et al., 2013; Lo et al., 2014; Ishikane et al., 2016), causing as far as 73,800 deaths annually (Lozano et al., 2012). The transmission usually occurs upon ingestion of water or food contaminated with *E. histolytica* cysts. The ingested cysts pass through the stomach and differentiate into trophozoites that colonize the colon. It is estimated that only 10–20% of individuals who are infected with *E. histolytica* develop symptoms (Gathiram and Jackson, 1985; Marie and Petri, 2014). The most common clinical manifestations in symptomatic cases are colitis and dysentery, and 5–10% of these are accompanied by invasive extraintestinal amebiasis, which is mostly amoebic liver abscess (Walsh, 1986).

Entamoeba histolytica belongs to the eukaryotic supergroup Amoebozoa, which is only distantly related to the eukaryotic model organisms in the Opisthokonta clade, including *Saccharomyces cerevisiae, Caenorhabditis elegans, Drosophila melanogaster,* and *Homo sapiens*. Various unique features of *E. histolytica* have been described due to its anaerobic/microaerophilic and parasitic life style, including metabolism of sulfur-containing amino acids, anaerobic energy generation, anti-oxidative stress mechanisms, and compartmentalization of sulfate activation to mitosomes, a unique mitochondria-related organelle (Ali and Nozaki, 2007; Müller et al., 2012; Makiuchi and Nozaki, 2014; Jeelani and Nozaki, 2016; Mi-Ichi et al., 2017; Pineda and Perdomo, 2017). Furthermore, the mechanisms regulating membrane trafficking in *E. histolytica* appear to be at least as complex as those found in higher eukaryotes. While most of the machineries underlying membrane-trafficking such as clathrin coats, coatomers, SNAREs, ESCRTs, and the retromer complex are conserved in *E. histolytica* (Nakada-Tsukui et al., 2005; Clark et al., 2007; Leung et al., 2008), unique evolutionary features in membrane trafficking are also apparent. For example, *E. histolytica* has numerous extremely diversified Rab small GTPases (104 genes) despite its unicellularity throughout its life cycle (Saito-Nakano et al., 2005; Nakada-Tsukui et al., 2010). In addition, a family of unique receptors that transport lysosomal hydrolase emerged in *Entamoeba* and related lineages during evolution (Furukawa et al., 2012, 2013; Nakada-Tsukui et al., 2012; Marumo et al., 2014). Although membrane trafficking in *E. histolytica* has been well-studied in the last few decades, *E. histolytica* PIs and PI metabolism are still relatively elusive despite the fact that they likely play critical roles in the physiology, especially in membrane trafficking, and pathogenicity of this organism (Raha et al., 1994, 1995; Giri et al., 1996; Makioka et al., 2001; Powell et al., 2006; Blazquez et al., 2008; Nakada-Tsukui et al., 2009; Byekova et al., 2010; Goldston et al., 2012; Koushik et al., 2013, 2014; López-Contreras et al., 2013; Lee et al., 2014; Bharadwaj et al., 2017). A previous genome-wide survey suggested that PI effectors found in other eukaryotes are not well-conserved in *E. histolytica* (Nakada-Tsukui et al., 2009). In this particular study, in order to better understand the level of conservation, elimination or diversification of the enzymes involved in the metabolism of *E. histolytica* PIs, we performed an extensive search for the potential kinases and phosphatases specific for the PIs found in the genome of this pathogen. Additionally, we summarized the known structural features and functions of similar enzymes in other organisms. To find and weigh the significance of possible homologs, we primarily used the E-values in the BLAST search. This was because *E. histolytica* homologs often differ in domain configurations and protein lengths to homologs in model organisms and the E-values better reflect both local and entire protein similarity. Such a comprehensive understanding of PI kinases and phosphatases will help us construct new hypotheses in future research.

Abbreviations: see **Supplementary Table S6**.

2. GENERAL OVERVIEW ON INTRACELLULAR LOCALIZATION AND ROLES OF PIs

2.1. Definition, Structure, Synthesis, Transport, and Localization of PIs

2.1.1. Definition, Structure, Synthesis, and Transport of PIs

PtdIns consists of a glycerol backbone with two covalently bound fatty acids at the stereospecifically numbered (*sn*)-1 and 2 positions, and a D-*myo*-inositol head group linked via the *sn*-3 phosphate of glycerol. Three hydroxyl groups of the D-*myo*-inositol head group (D3–5) are independently phosphorylated or dephosphorylated to form seven kinds of phosphorylated PtdIns (PIs) (**Figure 1**). PtdIns is synthesized in the endoplasmic reticulum (ER) from cytidine diphosphate diacylglycerol (CDP-DAG) and *myo*-inositol by PtdIns synthase (PIS) and transported to other cellular compartments either by vesicular transport or by PI transfer proteins (PITPs) (Di Paolo and De Camilli, 2006; Lev, 2010; Das and Nozaki, 2018). PtdInss are further metabolized to a variety of PIs on the membranes of these organelles (**Figure 1**).

2.1.2. Localization of PIs

PtdIns and PIs are concentrated at the cytosolic surface of the plasma membrane. Each PI type is enriched in a specific compartment(s) or sub-compartment(s) (Balla, 2013; Schink et al., 2016) (**Figure 2**). This disequilibrium in the type and distribution of PIs serves as a molecular tag to recruit specific effectors (Hammond and Balla, 2015; Várnai et al., 2017). In the model organisms, the distribution of PtdIns and PIs has been well-characterized. PtdIns4P and PtdIns(4,5)P_2 are enriched on the plasma membrane, where PtdIns(3,4)P_2 and PtdIns(3,4,5)P_3 are transiently generated *in situ* in response to extracellular stimuli or intracellular signaling (Di Paolo and De Camilli, 2006). PtdIns4P is enriched in the Golgi apparatus, where it regulates both intra-Golgi trafficking and the subsequent transport to the plasma membrane or the endosomal system (De Matteis et al., 2013). PtdIns3P is enriched in early endosomes and is known to trigger the recruitment of a number of effector proteins important for early endosomal identity and function (Di Paolo and De Camilli, 2006; Marat and Haucke, 2016; Schink et al., 2016). PtdIns(3,5)P_2, converted from PtdIns3P, accumulates in the multivesicular bodies (MVBs) and late endosomes/lysosomes as early endosomes mature (Marat and Haucke, 2016). PtdIns5P is present in the nucleus, plasma membrane, and endomembranes including autophagosomes (Hammond and Balla, 2015; Vicinanza et al., 2015; Várnai et al., 2017), and functions in cytoskeleton regulation, and stress signaling pathways (Viaud et al., 2014). Except for PtdIns(3,4)P_2 and PtdIns(3,5)P_2, nuclear localization of all the PIs has been reported (Ye and Ahn, 2008). Although PI metabolism in the nucleus is not fully understood, the involvement of nuclear PIs in transcription and chromatin remodeling in mammals, fly, yeast, and plant has been reported (Cheng and Shearn, 2004; Blind et al., 2012; Dieck et al., 2012; Shah et al., 2013; Poli et al., 2016).

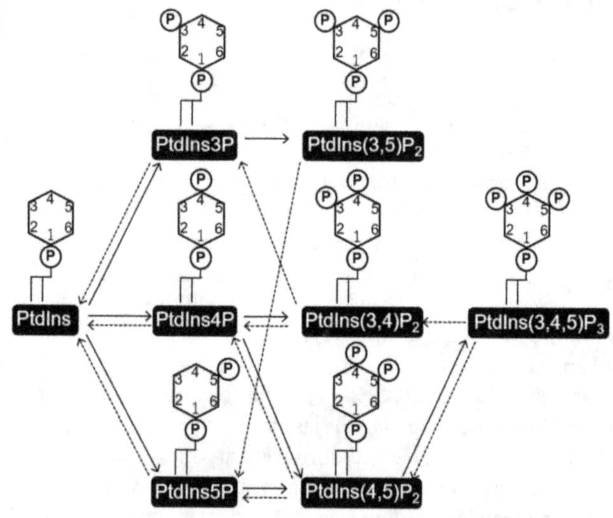

FIGURE 1 | Structures of phosphatidylinositol (PtdIns) and phosphoinositides (PI), and the routes of their interconversion. PtdIns consists of a glycerol backbone with two covalently attached fatty acids at the *sn-1* and *sn-2* positions, and a D-*myo*-inositol head group linked via the phosphate at the *sn-3* position. Three hydroxyl groups of the D-*myo*-inositol head group (D3-5) are independently phosphorylated or dephosphorylated to form the seven kinds of phosphorylated PtdIns, PIs. Solid and broken arrows indicate kinase and phosphate reactions, respectively.

2.2. Physiological Roles of PIs

2.2.1. Signaling via Phospholipase C-PtdIns(4,5)P_2 Breakdown

PIs are involved in signaling via two major pathways: as precursors of second messengers, and as regulators of various PI-specific effectors. The role of phospholipase C (PLC), which breaks down PtdIns(4,5)P_2 to inositol 1,4,5-trisphosphate[Ins(1,4,5)P_3] and DAG, in the receptor-mediated growth signal pathway was first demonstrated in the early '80s (Michell et al., 1981; Berridge, 1983; Nishizuka, 1984; Michell, 1995). The role of PI turnover and PI-mediated signaling in cell proliferation is well-established (Berridge, 1984, 1987). PI turnover has also been implicated in the upstream signaling of Ca^{2+} fluxes (Fain and Berridge, 1979). Given that the primary target of PLC is PtdIns(4,5)P_2 but not PtdIns (Berridge, 1983; Berridge et al., 1983; Creba et al., 1983), and Ins(1,4,5)P_3 is involved in Ca^{2+} release from the ER, PLC and PtdIns(4,5)P_2 indirectly affect the regulation of non-mitochondrial Ca^{2+} storage (Streb et al., 1983, 1984; Volpe et al., 1985). DAG activates the phospholipid-dependent kinase family, protein kinase C (PKC), and subsequently, the downstream signaling cascades (Nishizuka, 1984, 1995).

Ins(1,4,5)P_3-mediated calcium signaling is conserved in a wide range of eukaryotes (Plattner and Verkhratsky, 2013). Interestingly, Ins(1,4,5)P_3 can be generated by an alternative pathway independent of PLC, and many protists do not have orthologous genes for the canonical Ins(1,4,5)P_3 receptor, which regulates Ca^{2+} release from the ER (Kortholt et al., 2007; Plattner and Verkhratsky, 2013; Artemenko et al., 2014; Garcia et al., 2017). However, Ca^{2+} release by Ins(1,4,5)P_3 has been observed even in the organisms without an Ins(1,4,5)P_3 receptor. Besides, an orthologous gene has been identified in *Trypanosoma cruzi*, which is responsible for Chagas disease, suggesting some extent of conservation of the signaling pathway among eukaryotes (Hashimoto et al., 2013; Plattner and Verkhratsky, 2013).

2.2.2. Vesicular Traffic

PIs are involved in a variety of processes that involve vesicular trafficking, including secretion, recycling, endocytosis/phagocytosis, and autophagy (Frere et al., 2012; Balla, 2013; Swanson, 2014; Klinkert and Echard, 2016; Makowski et al., 2017; Wallroth and Haucke, 2018). A majority of secretory proteins are first transported into the ER lumen through the translocon on the ER membrane, then to the Golgi, where they are packaged into transport vesicles to be dispatched to endosomes or the plasma membrane. PtdIns4P, which is enriched in the Golgi, cooperatively works with PtdIns4P effectors such as GGA (Golgi-localized, gamma adaptin ear-containing, ARF-binding; a clathrin adaptor protein), Arf1, Ypt32p/Rab11 (small GTPase), and Sec2 (RabGEF) to form and target transport vesicles to the plasma membrane (De Matteis et al., 2013; Makowski et al., 2017). At the plasma membrane, PtdIns(4,5)P_2 cooperates with its effectors and promotes fusion of secretory vesicles with the plasma membrane (Li and Chin, 2003; Balla, 2013; Martin, 2015). PtdIns(4,5)P_2 at the plasma membrane is involved in the initiation of internalization processes such as endocytosis, micropinocytosis, and phagocytosis (Swanson, 2014; Wallroth and Haucke, 2018). During clathrin-mediated endocytosis, local synthesis of PtdIns(4,5)P_2 from PtdIns4P

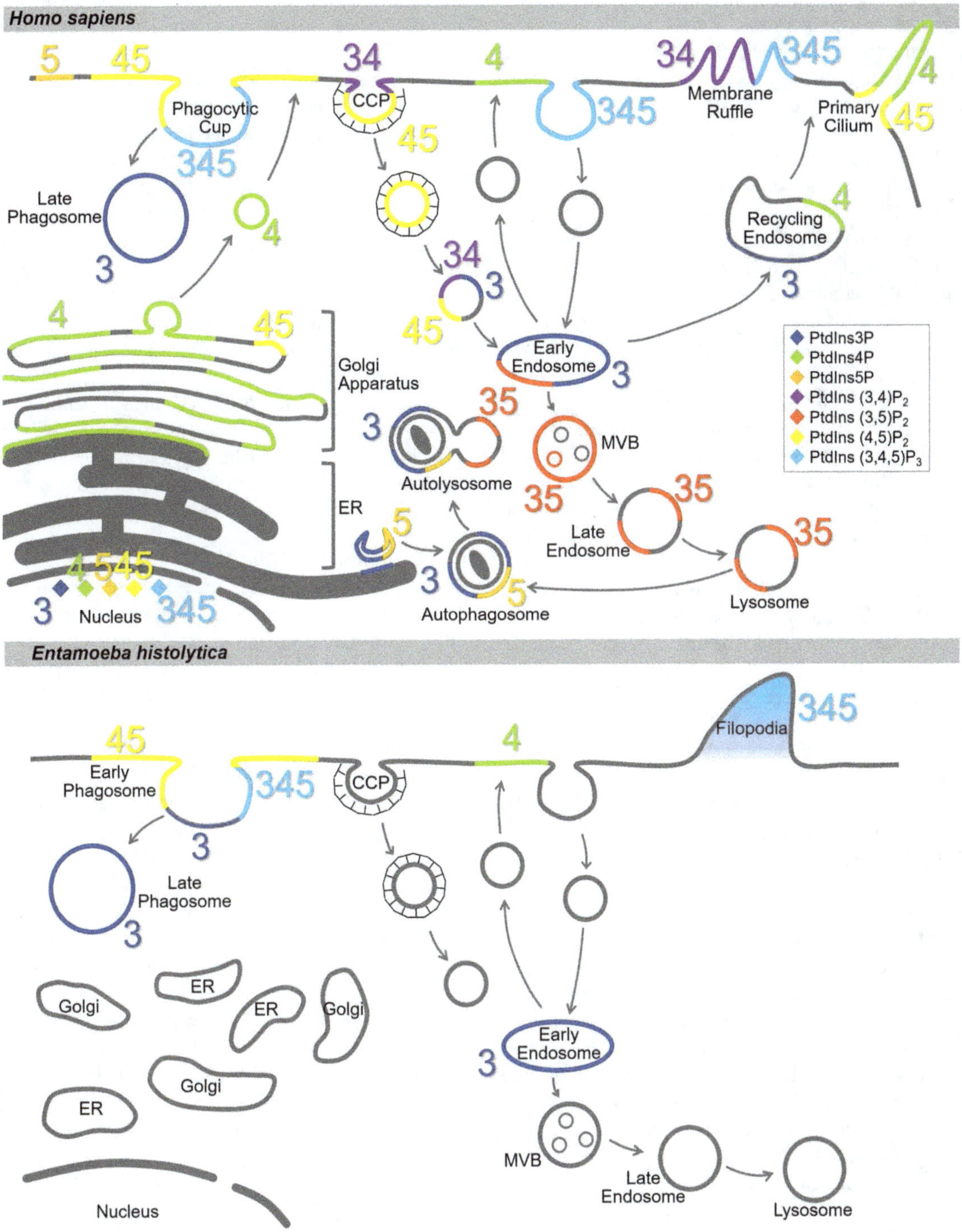

FIGURE 2 | Subcellular localization of PIs in *Homo sapiens* and *Entamoeba histolytica*. Schematic representation of subcellular localization of PIs in *H. sapiens* **(Upper)** and *E. histolytica* **(Lower)**. The seven PI species are depicted with different colors as indicated in the islet. Numbers 3, 4, and 5 depict the positions of phosphates in the PIs. Note that localization of the PIs in *E. histolytica* is largely elusive. CCP, clathrin-coated pit; MVB, multi vesicular body; ER, endoplasmic reticulum.

by PIP kinases initiates clathrin-coated pit (CCP) formation. Subsequent conversion of PtdIns(4,5)P_2 to PtdIns(3,4)P_2 is necessary for CCP maturation. It has been demonstrated that elimination of PtdIns(4,5)P_2, and generation of PtdIns(3,4)P_2 and PtdIns3P on CCPs by PI 5-phosphatases and PI 3-kinases are the key events for maturation of endosomes (Nakatsu et al., 2010). Generation of PtdIns4P on endosomes and recruitment of PtdIns4P effectors have been reported to be necessary for recycling the plasma membrane proteins (Henmi et al., 2016). Both macropinocytosis and phagocytosis depend on actin reorganization, in which PI metabolism is known to be involved (Yeung and Grinstein, 2007; Swanson, 2014). Briefly, local accumulation of PtdIns(4,5)P_2 stimulates actin rearrangement to form the phagocytic/macropinocytic cup. The accumulated PtdIns(4,5)P_2 is then removed from the cup via three different mechanisms: hydrolysis by PLC to generate Ins(1,4,5)P_3 and DAG, phosphorylation by PI 3-kinase to generate PtdIns(3,4,5)P_3, and dephosphorylation by PI 5-phosphatases (OCRL1 and INPP5B, see below sections) to generate PtdIns4P. Removal of PtdIns(4,5)P_2 from the cup causes actin dissociation and cup closure. On the nascent phagosomes, PtdIns3P accumulates by the action of type III PI 3-kinase and SHIP1/2 phosphatases. The generated PtdIns3P, alongside its effectors, engages in the early phase of phagosome/macropinosome maturation (Birkeland and Stenmark, 2004). In the later phase of the maturation, PtdIns3P is converted to PtdIns(3,5)P_2, which drives sorting of cargos, such as carboxypeptidase S in yeast, and EGF receptor in human, into MVBs in cooperation with the ESCRT (endosomal sorting complex required for transport) complex (Odorizzi et al., 1998; Whitley et al., 2003). Autophagy is a mechanism necessary for bulk breakdown of cytoplasmic proteins and organelles (Mizushima et al., 2011). The unique serine/threonine kinase ULK1 (unc-51-like kinase 1, Atg1 in yeast) is activated during autophagy, and it subsequently activates the class III PI 3-kinase Vps34 complex to generate PtdIns3P on the autophagic membrane. This, in turn, recruits a variety of proteins involved in autophagosome formation (Marat and Haucke, 2016). PtdIns(3,5)P_2 synthesis has been reported to be required at the later phase of autophagosome maturation (Ferguson et al., 2009; Zou et al., 2012; Al-Qusairi et al., 2013).

2.2.3. Cytoskeletal Rearrangement, Motility, and Regulation of Transporters

As mentioned above, PtdIns4P and PtdIns(4,5)P_2 are the major PIs on the plasma membrane, and PtdIns(3,4,5)P_3 is transiently generated to provide a temporary signal. The importance of PtdIns(4,5)P_2 has been well-established by a number of studies, and it has been shown that the level of PtdIns(4,5)P_2 on the plasma membrane changes. As discussed above, PtdIns(4,5)P_2 is involved in signal transduction and endocytosis/phagocytosis (see sections 2.2.1 and 2.2.2). PtdIns(4,5)P_2 is also involved in the regulation of actin cytoskeleton and membrane channel activity (Balla, 2013; Hille et al., 2015; Schink et al., 2016).

During chemotaxis, chemoattractants are recognized by G-protein-coupled receptors (GPCRs) on the plasma membrane. This interaction leads to dissociation of the Gα heterodimer, which in turn activates PI 3-kinase to generate PtdIns(3,4,5)P_3 from PtdIns(4,5)P_2 on the cytoplasmic side of the plasma membrane. Local accumulation of PtdIns(3,4,5)P_3 causes translocation of actin-binding proteins (ABP) that interact with PtdIns(3,4,5)P_3, and activates actin remodeling at the leading edge of the cell. On the contrary to these events at the leading edge, the PI 3-phosphatase PTEN (phosphatase and tensin homology located on chromosome 10), which converts PtdIns(3,4,5)P_3 to PtdIns(4.5)P_2 to cease the signal, has been shown to accumulate at the posterior side of the cell.

There are many ion channels regulated by PIs (Hilgemann and Ball, 1996; Hille et al., 2015). Kir2.2 is a member of the inwardly rectifying potassium channel family localized on the plasma membrane, and it is known to be activated upon interaction with PtdIns(4,5)P_2 (Hansen et al., 2011). Crystal structure analysis revealed that a direct interaction of PtdIns(4,5)P_2 with Kir2.2 induces a structural change on this channel. This, in turn, induces the channel to compress by pulling its cytoplasmic domain toward the potassium-selective pore on the membrane, shifting the channel to the active conformation (Rohács et al., 2003; Whorton and MacKinnon, 2011). Two possible advantages of PI dependence of ion channels have been suggested: (1) to achieve local activation of the channels depending on the lipid composition (i.e., no or decreased activity during synthesis and trafficking of the lipids to the target membrane) and (2) to swiftly regulate the channel activity by lipid modifying enzymes such as PLC, PI kinases, and PI phosphatases.

2.2.4. Nuclear Functions

Besides the various roles of PIs in the cytoplasm and the plasma membrane described above, PIs play indispensable roles in the nucleus. Localization of PIs, except for PtdIns(3,4)P_2 and PtdIns(3,5)P_2, in the nuclear matrix has been demonstrated (Payrastre et al., 1992; Vann et al., 1997; Tanaka et al., 1999; Gillooly et al., 2000; Clarke et al., 2001). Since the nuclear matrix is hydrophilic, it is not well-understood how PIs remain soluble in the nucleus (York, 2006). The significance of PtdIns(4,5)P_2 and PtdIns5P has been well-demonstrated (Irvine, 2003; Poli et al., 2016; Hamann and Blind, 2018). PtdIns(4,5)P_2 is involved in the transcriptional regulation and chromatin remodeling by interacting with histones (Yu et al., 1998; Cheng and Shearn, 2004; Shah et al., 2013). PtdIns(4,5)P_2 also regulates cell cycle and differentiation through DAG generated by PLC-induced hydrolysis (Clarke et al., 2001; Newton, 2010; Poli et al., 2013, 2014). Nuclear DAG accumulation is followed by translocation of PKC to the nucleus for the phosphorylation of the target proteins (Neri et al., 1998). PtdIns5P is known to interact with TAF3, a component of the TATA box-binding protein complex, TFIID, and the chromatin-associating protein ING2, to regulate transcription and chromatin remodeling (Shi et al., 2006; Bua et al., 2013; Stijf-Bultsma et al., 2015). Interestingly, nuclear PI metabolism is regulated independently from cytoplasmic PI metabolism (Lindsay et al., 2006).

2.3. Spatiotemporal Regulation of PI-Mediated Signaling

2.3.1. PI-Specific Binding Proteins

Spatiotemporal regulation of PI-mediated signaling occurs in a variety of biological processes by various PI-specific effectors and enzymes that mediate interconversion of PIs. The seven phosphorylated PI species are enriched on specific membrane regions in both the cytoplasm and nucleus (Balla, 2013), and specifically recognized by PI effectors. This specific recognition occurs through the interaction of the PI-specific binding domains

of the effector proteins with the head groups of PIs (**Figure 1**). All the distinct PI-binding domains, consisting of a total of 24, have already been reported (Várnai et al., 2017).

2.3.2. Major Players of PI Interconversion

Each PI interconversion reaction is regulated by specific kinases or phosphatases (**Figure 1**). In mammals, 18 PI interconversion reactions have been identified, and these reactions are mediated by 19 PI kinases and 28 PI phosphatases (**Supplementary Tables S1, S2**, Sasaki et al., 2009). PI 3-, PI 4-, and PIP kinases use PtdIns as a substrate to generate PtdIns3P, PtdIns4P, and PtdIns5P, respectively. Mono-phosphorylated PIs are further phosphorylated by PIP kinases to generate PtdIns(3,4)P_2, PtdIns(3,5)P_2, and PtdIns(4,5)P_2, which is further phosphorylated to generate PtdIns(3,4,5)P_3. Each PI is dephosphorylated by a series of PI phosphatases such as PI 3-phosphatases (PTEN, MTM) PI 4-phosphatases (INPP4, TMEM55), and PI 5-phosphatases (Synaptojanin, OCRL1, INPP5, SHIP). It has been suggested that unique expression and localization patterns of PI kinases and PI phosphatases influence the local accumulation of PIs (Balla, 2013; Schink et al., 2016).

3. PREVIOUS FINDINGS ON THE ROLE OF PIs IN *E. histolytica*

E. histolytica trophozoites have been reported to have phospholipid compositions similar to those of mammalian cells except for the unique ceramide, ceramide aminoethylphosphonate (CEAP), which constitutes ~15% of the total phospholipids (Aley et al., 1980). PI is a minor phospholipid component, constituting ~5% of all phospholipids (Aley et al., 1980). Similarly, PI content of intracellular vesicles and the plasma membrane is <5%. While the plasma membrane contains less phosphatidylcoline than other membranes, it has a high content (40%) of CEAP (Aley et al., 1980). The resistance of the plasma membrane of trophozoites to the intrinsic pore forming peptide, amoebapores, is attributable to CEAP (Andrä et al., 2004).

Several previous studies demonstrated that PIs are involved in pathogenesis related processes such as adhesion, secretion, and phagocytosis. When the amebic trophozoites adhere to host cells, Gal/GalNAc lectin serves as a major adhesion molecule and transduces the signals. It is composed of heavy (Hgl), intermediate (Igl), and light (Lgl) subunits, of which Igl and Lgl are GPI-anchored. The downstream cytosolic signals transmitted from the lectin have not been well-investigated except for one example (Hughes et al., 2003). However, it has been shown that PtdIns(4,5)P_2- and cholesterol-dependent enrichment of Gal/GalNAc lectin subunits to lipid rafts causes an increment of Ca^{2+} level followed by adhesion to the mammalian cell (Welter et al., 2011; Goldston et al., 2012). These results suggest involvement of PtdIns(4,5)P_2-mediated Ca^{2+} signaling during cell adhesion (Goldston et al., 2012).

Cysteine proteases (CPs) are the major virulence factors. They are secreted via the default brefeldin A-sensitive or unique brefeldin A-insensitive pathways, and Rab11B-dependent pathways (Manning-Cela et al., 2003; Mitra et al., 2007). In the model organisms, it has been established that Rab11 on the secretory vesicles, and Sec3 of the exocyst complex interact, leading to tethering of the Rab11 vesicles to the plasma membrane in a PtdIns(4,5)P_2-dependent manner (He et al., 2007; Zhang et al., 2008; Wu and Guo, 2015). The components of the exocyst complex including PtdIns(4,5)P_2-binding Sec3 and Exo70 are mostly conserved in *E. histolytica*. Thus, it is conceivable that PI-regulated secretion takes place in *E. histolytica*.

PIs are also involved in phagocytosis in *E. histolytica* as in mammals. Several studies in which amebic transformants that expressed PI-binding proteins fused with green fluorescent protein (GFP) or in which recombinant glutathione S-transferase (GST) were used as bioprobes demonstrated that PtdIns(4,5)P_2 were localized on the plasma membrane, while PtdIns(3,4,5)P_3 were localized on the extended pseudopodia, and phagocytic cups, and PtdIns3P on the phagocytic cups, nascent phagosomes, and internal vesicles (Powell et al., 2006; Nakada-Tsukui et al., 2009; Byekova et al., 2010; Koushik et al., 2013). Localization of PtdIns(3,4,5)P_3 and PtdIns3P is similar during *E. histolytica* phagocytosis and macrophage phagocytosis (Yeung and Grinstein, 2007). It has been recently shown that AGC kinases 1 and 2 that bind to PtdIns(3,4,5)P_3 or PtdIns(3,4)P_2 are localized to the contact site upon interaction with mammalian cells (Somlata et al., 2017). Interestingly, AGC kinases 1 and 2 have different localization patterns, although their apparent PtdIns specificities have been demonstrated with lipid overlay assay. AGC kinase 2 localizes to a tunnel-like structure proximal to the primary trogocytic cup and adjacent to the contact site on the plasma membrane during trogocytosis ("trogo" means "nibble" or "chew," and trogocytosis is the process of internalizing live cells by nibbling them). In contrast, AGC kinase 1 is confined to the intermediate part of the trogocytic tunnel. Such an observation has been made in *E. histolytica* but not in professional phagocytes of multicellular organisms, including mammals.

Cytoskeletons also play indispensable roles during phagocytosis and trogocytosis. EhRho1, which is involved in actin rearrangement via EhFormin1 and EhProfilin1 (Bharadwaj et al., 2018), has been shown to regulate membrane blebbing to initiate internalization of the prey through PI 3-kinases (Bharadwaj et al., 2017). Inducible expression of a constitutively active EhRho1 increased the PtdIns(3,4,5)P_3 level and reduced PtdIns(4,5)P_2 level, whereas expression of a dominant negative EhRho1 caused opposite effects (Bharadwaj et al., 2017). EhRho1 is considered to be orthologous to HsRhoA as the amino acid sequences of their ROCK-binding domains are 65% identical. Moreover, EhRho1 complements HsRhoA activity in HEK 293T cells (Bharadwaj et al., 2017). Interestingly, HsRhoA does not localize to the phagocytic cup in mammalian cells unlike EhRho1. Signaling transduced downstream of PtdIns3P in mammals appears to be different in *E. histolytica*, because *E. histolytica* does not seem to be equipped with the orthologs of known mammalian PtdIns3P effectors. Transformation of *E. histolytica* with GFP-fused human Hrs showed that PtdIns3P was concentrated on phagosomes, more specifically at the bottom of the phagocytic cup during the early phase of phagocytosis (prior to the closure of the phagosome) (Nakada-Tsukui et al., 2009). Two PtdIns3P-binding domains are known: Phox homology (PX) and Fab-1–YGL023–Vps27–EEA1 (FYVE) domains. *E. histolytica* apparently has two PX and twelve FYVE domain-containing proteins (Nakada-Tsukui et al., 2009; N. Watanabe, data not shown). It has been demonstrated that eleven out of the twelve *E. histolytica* FYVE domain-containing proteins (EhFPs) also have a RhoGEF domain, and one of EhFP (EhFP4) preferentially binds to PtdIns4P and localizes to the plasma membrane proximal to the phagosome that is not yet closed (Nakada-Tsukui et al., 2009). Surprisingly, the C-terminal domain instead of the FYVE domain of EhFP4 binds to PtdIns3P, PtdIns4P, and PtdIns5P (Nakada-Tsukui et al., 2009). In model organisms, phagosomal PtdIns3P has been shown to recruit FYVE domain-containing proteins, which are subsequently involved in maturation of the phagosomes. However, like RhoGEF, EhFP4 appears to be primarily involved in actin rearrangement during phagocytosis eventhough full length EhFP4 does not seem to recognize PtdIns3P. Additional PtdIns3P effectors on phagosomes, most likely to be PX domain-containing proteins, still remain elusive.

4. PI 3-KINASES

Phosphorylation of PtdIns and PIs is initially observed as conversion of PtdIns to PtdIns4P, and PtdIns4P to PtdIns(4,5)P_2 (Balla, 2013). The enzymes responsible for these activities are named PtdIns kinases and PI kinases, respectively. Currently, it is known that some enzymes can phosphorylate both PtdIns and PIs. The enzyme classification given in this review is based on the position of the hydroxyl group that the enzymes can phosphorylate.

PI 3-kinases phosphorylate the hydroxyl group at the D3 position of the inositol ring of PtdIns, PtdIns4P, and PtdIns(4,5)P_2 to generate PtdIns3P, PtdIns(3,4)P_2, and PtdIns (3,4,5)P_3, respectively. There are three subfamilies of PI 3-kinases: class I, II, and III (Sasaki et al., 2009). In general, class I enzymes preferentially generate PtdIns(3,4,5)P_3 from PtdIns(4,5)P_2. Class II enzymes mostly generate PtdIns(3,4)P_2 from PtdIns4P and also generate PtdIns3P from PtdIns. Class III enzymes almost exclusively generate PtdIns3P from PtdIns. In mammals, there are a total of 8 members of PI 3-kinases. All PI 3-kinases contain a "signature motif" consisting of the catalytic kinase domain, a helical domain, also called "lipid kinase unique (LKU) domain," and a membrane-binding C2 domain (Vanhaesebroeck et al., 2010a; Balla, 2013; Marat and Haucke, 2016). The class I to III classification of PI 3-kinases is mainly based on the presence of additional protein domains and their interactions with regulatory subunits. Class I enzymes have an adaptor binding domain (ABD), and regulatory subunit-binding and Ras binding domains (RBD). Class II enzymes have an N-terminal extension, which is involved in clathrin binding, and a C-terminal PX and extra C2 domains. It is of note that this PX domain in class II PI 3-kinase is known to preferentially bind to PtdIns(4,5)P_2 (Stahelin et al., 2006). These domains are involved in subcellular localization and activity of the enzyme, and downstream effector selection. The class I and class III enzymes have regulatory subunits which modulate localization and activity of these enzymes.

4.1. Class I PI 3-Kinase

4.1.1. General Description of Class I PI 3-Kinase

Class I PI 3-kinases predominantly produce PtdIns(3,4,5)P_3 from PtdIns(4,5)P_2. There are two kinds of class I PI 3-kinases based on their composition of catalytic and regulatory subunits. One of the three class IA catalytic subunits (p110α, β, and δ) associates with one of the five p85 class regulatory subunits (p85α, p85β, p55α, p55γ, and p50α), while the class IB catalytic subunit (p110γ) associates with one of the two P101/p87 class regulatory subunits (p101 and p87) (Vadas et al., 2011; Jean and Kiger, 2014) (**Figure 3**). In mammals, p110α and p110β are expressed ubiquitously, while p110δ and p110γ seem to be restricted to hematopoietic cells. The class IA catalytic subunits (p110α, β, and δ) are activated via receptor tyrosine kinases and generate PtdIns(3,4,5)P_3 at the plasma membrane. On the other hand, the p110β and p110γ catalytic subunits are activated downstream of the GPCR (Stephens et al., 1994; Stoyanov et al., 1995; Vanhaesebroeck et al., 2010a). PtdIns(3,4,5)P_3 generation causes recruitment of PI effectors, such as the protein kinase Akt, also named protein kinase B (PKB) (James et al., 1996; Ma et al., 2008; Rodgers et al., 2017). Activated Akt is involved in cell survival and metabolism via various cellular processes, including those that involve mammalian target of rapamycin complex-1 (mTORC1), the pro-apoptotic factor BAD, and FOXO transcription factors (Vanhaesebroeck et al., 2010a; Dibble and Cantley, 2015). Due to their crucial roles in cell growth and proliferation, dominant activating mutations of the class I PI 3-kinases are known to be associated with cancers, making PI 3-kinases potential drug targets (Vanhaesebroeck et al., 2010b).

4.1.2. Class I PI 3-Kinase of *E. histolytica*

In the *E. histolytica* genome (http://amoebadb.org/amoeba/), six potential catalytic subunits of class I PI 3-kinases were identified by probing the genome with the catalytic subunits of human class I PI 3-kinases as queries (NP_006209, NP_006210, AAH35683, and NP_005017, corresponding to p110α, β, γ, and δ, respectively). Independent of the query used, ten proteins were identified to share significant overall similarity, reflecting a possible redundancy among them (E-value $< 1 \times 10^{-10}$). Six of them have conserved domains, such as RBD, C2, LKU, and PI 3-kinase catalytic domains, but no protein with the ABD was identified (**Figure 3**; **Supplementary Table S1**). Four additional proteins were also identified during this survey: a class III PI 3-kinase (EHI_096560) and type III PI 4-kinase (EHI_148700) (see below), a catalytic domain-only protein (EHI_127850), and a protein that lacked the LKU domain (EHI_073560). As PI 3-kinase catalytic domain is also conserved in PI 3- and PI 4-kinases (Vogt et al., 2007), the identification of both class III PI 3-kinase and type III PI 4-kinase homologs during this search is understandable. In the present review, we tentatively designated the proteins that

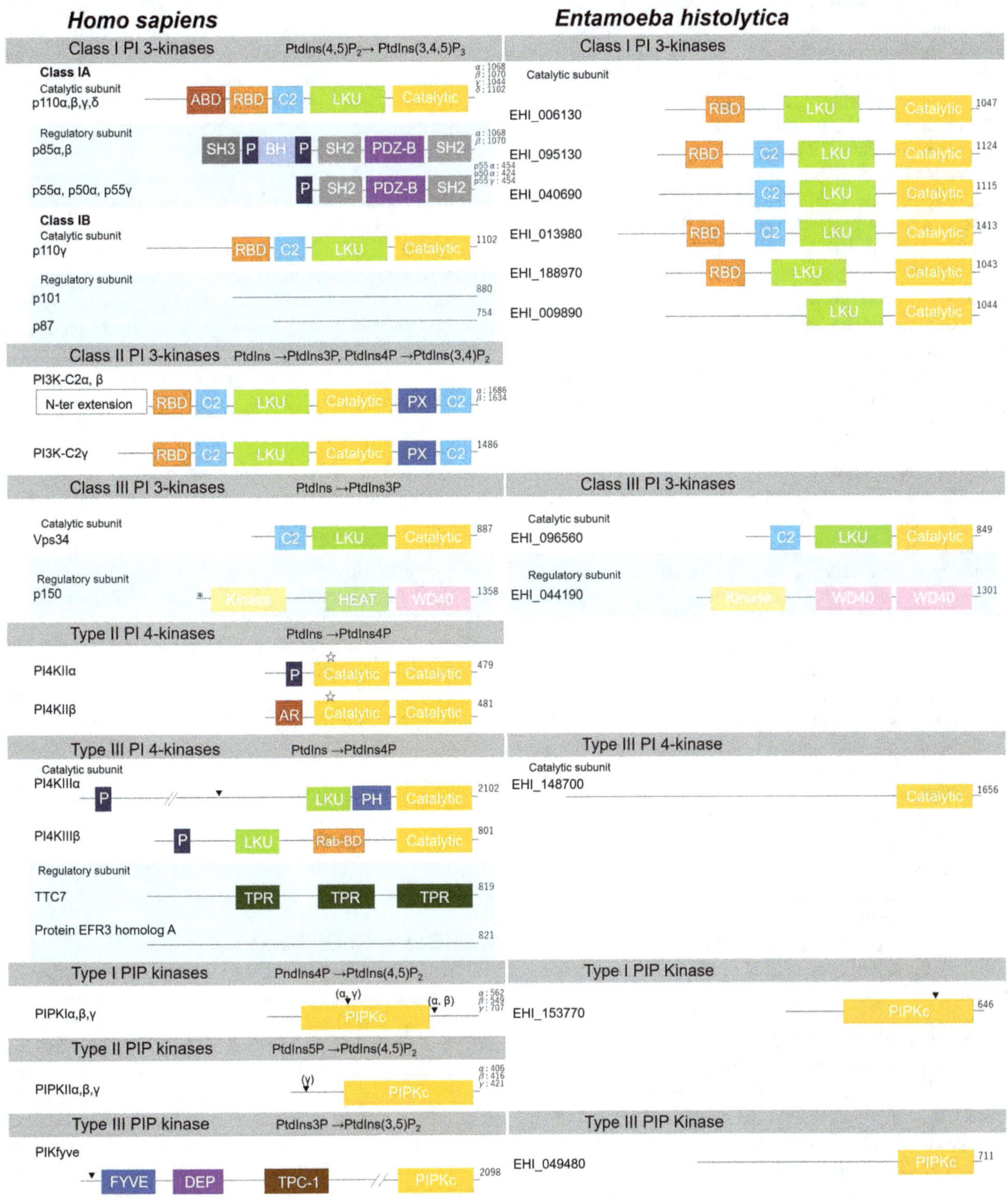

FIGURE 3 | Structural features of PI kinases of *H. sapiens* and *E. histolytica*. Structural features and domain organization of PI kinases, including their regulatory subunits are shown. Numbers showing at the end of the protein indicates amino acid length. ABD, adaptor binding domain; AR, acidic region; BH, Bcl Homology; C2,C2 domain; Catalytic, lipid kinase domain of PI 3- and PI 4-kinases; DEP, disheveled, Egl-10 and pleckstrin domain; FYVE, Fab1, YOTB, Vac1, and EEA1 domain; HEAT, Huntington, Elongation factor3, PR65/A, and TOR; Kinase, Ser/Thr kinase domain; LKU, lipid kinase unique domain; P, Proline-rich; PDZ-B, PDZ domain binding domain; PH, Pleckstrin-homology; PIPKc, kinase core domain of PIP kinases; PX, Phox homology; Rab-BD, Rab binding domain; RBD, Ras binding domain; SH2, Src homology 2; SH3, Src homology 3; TPC-1, T-complex 1 homology; TPR, tetratricopeptide repeat; WD40, WD40 repeat. Myristoylation, palmitoylation sites, and the nuclear localization signal are also depicted with "*", "☆", or "▼", respectively.

contain LKU and catalytic domains as class I PI 3-kinases, which excluded the four additional proteins mentioned above (**Figure 3**; **Supplementary Table S1**). Among the six class I PI 3-kinases, EHI_040690 showed a lower E-value to class II PI 3-kinase. The E-values with p110β and PI 3-kinase-C2α were 1×10^{-107} and 2×10^{-110}, respectively (**Supplementary Table S3** and N. Watanabe, data not shown). However, because it lacks the C-terminal domains and catalytic domain, we included this gene among the class I PI 3-kinases (also refer section 4.2.2). The six proteins with conserved RBD, C2, LKU, and PI 3-kinase catalytic domains cannot be further classified into p110α, β, γ, or δ, as none of them has the ABD and show only marginal E-value to the ABD-containing proteins p110α, β, or δ (**Supplementary Table S3**; **Supplementary Figure S4**). Furthermore, all potential class I PI 3-kinase catalytic subunit homologs showed the lowest E-value to p110β, but not for p110γ despite the fact that all the amebic homologs lack the ABD and structurally resemble p110γ (**Supplementary Table S3**). No homologs of the regulatory subunits that contain Src homology 2 (SH2) domain were identified in the *E. histolytica* genome database when p85α, β, p55α, p50α, and p55γ were used as the queries. Furthermore, only five proteins were predicted to have an SH2 domain and four of them were annotated as protein kinases, while the remaining protein was predicted to have a role in RNA stability and/or transcriptional regulation, with no possible link to PI 3-kinase regulatory subunits. These data suggest the possibility that the regulatory subunits of class I PI 3-kinase have been lost or replaced with a lineage-specific protein in *E. histolytica* during evolution. In *Saccharomyces cerevisiae,* class I and II PI 3-kinases are not conserved. *Dictyostelium discoideum* has catalytic but not regulatory subunits of three class I PI 3-kinases and lacks class II PI 3-kinases (Engelman et al., 2006). The catalytic subunits of *D. discoideum* class I PI 3-kinases also lack the ABD as in *E. histolytica.* Such lineage-specific modifications of the catalytic subunits and loss of the regulatory subunits of class I PI 3-kinases likely suggest divergence of PtdIns(3,4,5)P_3-mediated lipid signaling in eukaryotes. It should be noted that *E. histolytica* has six PtdIns(3,4,5)P_3 phosphatase homologs of PTEN, while there is only one PTEN gene in the human genome (see section 7.1).

4.2. Class II PI 3-Kinase

4.2.1. General Description of Class II PI 3-Kinase

Class II PI 3-kinases are monomeric enzymes that generate PtdIns(3,4)P_2 and PtdIns3P from PtdIns4P and PtdIns, respectively (Balla, 2013; Maffucci and Falasca, 2014). There are three subtypes: PI 3-kinase C2α, β, and γ, among which PI 3-kinase C2α and β have N-terminal extensions that are likely involved in autoinhibition and protein-protein interactions with clathrin (Marat and Haucke, 2016). Except for the N-terminal extensions, all class II PI 3-kinases contain one RBD, two C2, one LKU, one catalytic, and one PX domains. PI 3-kinase C2α and β isoforms are ubiquitously expressed, whereas the γ isoform is largely restricted to the liver. This class of PI 3-kinases does not have the regulatory subunit; however, they are regulated by interacting with proteins such as clathrin and Rab5 small GTPase. Clathrin associates with PI 3-kinase C2α and β isoforms through the N-terminal extension, and Rab5 interacts with the γ isoform via the RBD (Gaidarov et al., 2001, 2005; Braccini et al., 2015). Accumulating evidence suggests that class II PI 3-kinases are involved in the regulation of membrane trafficking from the plasma membrane via PtdIns(3,4)P_2 synthesis. PI 3-kinase C2α is involved in clathrin-mediated endocytosis by the formation of PtdIns(3,4)P_2, which constricts the membrane by recruiting PX and BAR domain-containing sorting nexin (SNX) SNX9 (Posor et al., 2013; Schöneberg et al., 2017). PI 3-kinase C2γ is recruited to endosomes as Rab5 effector for PtdIns(3,4)P_2 synthesis, which is indispensable for delayed and sustained activation of Akt2 in the liver (Braccini et al., 2015). It was also suggested that PI 3-kinase C2α and β also play a role in the regulation of intracellular PtdIns3P levels and directly or indirectly regulate membrane traffic and autophagy (Jean et al., 2012; Devereaux et al., 2013; Franco et al., 2014).

4.2.2. Class II PI 3-Kinase From *E. histolytica*

In *E. histolytica,* we concluded that there are no class II PI 3-kinases. When three human class II PI 3-kinases were used as queries, the best hits we obtained were the same proteins identified as class I PI 3-kinases (see above). As described above, because of the low similarity to class II PI 3-kinases in five out of six candidates and the absence of the PX domain in all the six, they were classified into class I PI 3-kinases. It is of note that EHI_040690 showed a lower E-value with PI3KC2α (2×10^{-110} with PI3KC2α and 1×10^{-107} with class I PI 3-kinase, p110β). Additionally, class II PI 3-kinases evolved after Metazoa, and another amoeboid organism, *D. discoideum,* lacks this class of PI 3-kinases (Engelman et al., 2006; Brown and Auger, 2011). According to these contexts, we decided to conclude that there are no class II PI 3-kinases in *E. histolytica.* However, the conservation of a gene showed low E-value with the class II PI 3-kinase, suggesting the possibility that some of the class I PI 3-kinases have a role similar to that of class II PI 3-kinases.

4.3. Class III PI 3-Kinase

4.3.1. General Description of Class III PI 3-Kinase

The human genome has one class III PI 3-kinase, vacuolar protein sorting (Vps) 34, which phosphorylates the D3-position of PtdIns. *Vps34* gene was first identified as a temperature-sensitive mutation that impairs the sorting of vacuolar hydrolases in yeast (Herman and Emr, 1990; Schu et al., 1993). Vps34 consists of one of each of the C2, LKU, and catalytic domains, and forms a dimer with the p150 regulatory subunit (Vps15 in yeast). p150 constitutively interacts with Vps34, and the myristoyl modification in its amino terminal links Vps34 to the membrane (Stack et al., 1993; Vanhaesebroeck et al., 2010a). Since Vps34 is the only PI 3-kinase in yeast, and also widely conserved in Eukaryota, Vps34 is considered to be the ancestral PI 3-kinase (Schu et al., 1993; Engelman et al., 2006; Brown and Auger, 2011). Vps34 participate in membrane trafficking, endocytosis, phagocytosis, and autophagy through the synthesis of PtdIns3P (Sasaki et al., 2009; Swanson, 2014; Wallroth and Haucke,

2018; also see section 2.2.2). In the endocytic pathway, early endosomes mature as PtdIns3P is synthesized *in situ*, subsequently recruiting Rab5 and Rab7 to early and late endosomes, respectively. Vps34 was identified as one of the mutual effectors of Rab5 and Rab7, involved in spatiotemporal generation of PtdIns3P on endosomal membranes (Christoforidis et al., 1999; Stein et al., 2003; Shin et al., 2005).

Vps34 has been shown to form two kinds of complexes that differ in localization and function (Marat and Haucke, 2016). Complex I consists of p150, and the mammalian orthologs of yeast Vps30, Atg14, and Atg38 (Beclin-1, ATG14L, and NRBF2, respectively). It is involved in autophagy (Itakura et al., 2008; Cao et al., 2014; Lu et al., 2014). In contrast, complex II consists of p150, Beclin-1, and UVRAG, which is the mammalian ortholog of yeast Vps38. Complex II is involved in the regulation of endosome and autophagosome maturation (Kihara et al., 2001; Matsunaga et al., 2009; Funderburk et al., 2010; Sun et al., 2010; Rostislavleva et al., 2015). It is also known that, in addition to its role in autophagy Vps34 functions as an amino acid sensor, and regulates mTORC1 activity and localization (Munson et al., 2015; Hong et al., 2017). These observations suggest multiple roles of Vps34 at the cross road of nutrient sensing and membrane trafficking. Vps34 is also involved in the negative regulation of autophagy through amino acid sensing (Furuya et al., 2005; Gulati and Thomas, 2007) and mTORC1 activation mediated by PtdIns3P-dependent recruitment of phospholipase D1 (PLD1) (Yoon et al., 2011; Bridges et al., 2012). Activated mTORC1 inhibits the autophagy-promoting activity of the Complex I by phosphorylating Atg14L in the complex (Yuan et al., 2013), while it activates the Complex II by phosphorylating UVRAG. Activation of the Complex II, in turn, leads to activation of Vps34 during the reformation of lysosomes from autophagosomes following recovery from starvation (Yu et al., 2010; Munson et al., 2015; Chen and Yu, 2017). Thus, Vps34-containing complexes are interactive and involved in eliciting opposite effects in the cell.

4.3.2. Class III PI 3-Kinase of *E. histolytica*

In *E. histolytica*, there are one of each Vps34 and p150 homolog (EHI_096560 and EHI_044190, respectively). Although neither their localization nor function have been demonstrated, roles of PtdIns3P are well-established as previously described (Powell et al., 2006; Nakada-Tsukui et al., 2009). During trogocytosis, which is ingestion by nibbling live mammalian cells (Ralston et al., 2014; Somlata et al., 2017), unclosed and nascent trogosomes are decorated with PtdIns3P. While localization of PtdIns3P to endosomes *per se* has not been well-documented, its localization to MVB-containing endosomes has been demonstrated (Nakada-Tsukui et al., 2009), suggesting a conserved role of PtdIns3P in the endocytic pathway in *E. histolytica*. It is conceivable that Vps34 is involved in the synthesis of PtdIns3P on trogosomes. *E. histolytica* has two TOR (EHI_155160 and EHI_169320) and two Atg8 homologs (EHI_130660 and EHI_172140). It is thus expected that *E. histolytica* Vps34 may also play a role in the response to starvation.

5. PI 4-KINASES

Among seven PtdIns isotypes, PtdIns(4,5)P_2 is the most abundant and well-studied in the context of PI turnover (see section 2.2.1). Since PI 4-kinase is one of the major enzymes responsible for producing the precursor of PtdIns(4,5)P_2, it plays a significant role by producing PtdIns4P (Wang et al., 2003; D'Angelo et al., 2008). Various roles have been suggested for PtdIns4P and PI 4-kinases, including signaling on the plasma membrane (Tan and Brill, 2014). Two types of PI 4-kinases are currently known in humans: type II and type III. Type I PI 4-kinase, which was initially identified in a bovine brain homogenate chromatography fraction that showed PI kinase activity has turned out to be identical to PI 3-kinase, and thus it is no longer referred (Whitman et al., 1988). The human genome encodes two isotypes of both type II and type III PI 4-kinase. Type II and III PI 4-kinases differ in their domain structure and sensitivity to wortmannin, since the former is insensitive unlike the latter.

5.1. Type II PI 4-Kinase

5.1.1. General Description of Type II PI 4-Kinase

Type II PI 4-kinases (PI4KII) contain a large lipid kinase domain that is separated by a long non-conserved insert. This structure is significantly different from that of type III PI 4-kinases (PI4KIII) whose catalytic domain consists of LKU and catalytic domains. It was inferred by phylogenetic analyses that type II PI 4-kinases are evolutionarily different from type III PI 4-kinases. Furthermore, type III PI 4-kinases share significant homology with the typical protein kinase PKA and PI 3-kinases (Minogue and Waugh, 2012). The catalytic domains of PI4KIIα and β are highly similar, but their N-terminal regions are divergent. The N-terminal proline-rich region (P) in PI4KIIα and acidic region (AR) in β have been shown to interact with AP-3 and AP-1 adaptor complexes, respectively (Salazar et al., 2005; Wieffer et al., 2013). Initially, PI 4-kinases were expected to have a role in the generation of PtdIns4P as a precursor of PtdIns(4,5)P_2, whereby they were thought to regulate signal transduction from the plasma membrane. However, it has recently been suggested that type II PI 4-kinases are mostly involved in the regulation of endomembrane sorting machinery. They do so mostly in the trans-Golgi network (TGN), which functions as a sorting hub. To date, there are four suggested roles of PI4KIIα and β during membrane trafficking: (1) cargo trafficking between the TGN and internal vesicles via interaction with adaptor proteins such as AP-1 and AP-3 (Wang et al., 2003; Salazar et al., 2005; Minogue et al., 2006; Wieffer et al., 2013); (2) synthesis of PtdIns4P on mature phagosomes/autophagosomes and regulation of fusion with lysosomes (Jeschke et al., 2015; Levin et al., 2017); (3) outbound traffic toward the plasma membrane (Husebye et al., 1990; Barylko et al., 2001; Xu et al., 2006); and (4) regulation of actin-dependent trafficking by interacting with actin regulatory proteins, such as RhoGEF1, and Wiskott-Aldrich Syndrome and SCAR homolog (WASH) complex components (Mössinger et al., 2012; Ryder et al., 2013; Gokhale et al., 2016). It has been shown in mammalian cells that the two isotypes of PI4KII are differently regulated due to differences in the regulatory proteins they interact with. Both PI4KII isotypes are palmitoylated at the CCPCC motif in the catalytic domain; however, only PI4KIIβ has the ability to bind to HSP90, and the interaction is disrupted upon stimulation by epidermal and platelet-derived growth factors (Jung et al., 2011). This association with HSP90 enables stabilization of the lipid-modified PI4KIIβ in the cytosol by preventing its proteasomal degradation (Jung et al., 2011). Such elaborate mechanisms enable isotype-specific regulation of PI4KII.

5.1.2. Type II PI 4-Kinase of *E. histolytica*

In *E. histolytica*, no ortholog with the E-value $< 1 \times 10^{-4}$ was identified by using human type II PI 4-kinases as a query in the BLAST search. It has been reported that a majority of parasitic protists including *Trypanosoma*, *Leishmania*, *Trichomonas vaginalis*, *Giardia lamblia*, and *E. histolytica*, apparently lack type II PI 4-kinases (Brown and Auger, 2011). However, apicomplexans such as *Plasmodium* exceptionally conserve a type II PI 4-kinase. Fungal and apicomplexan type II PI 4-kinase orthologs are closely related to those found in metazoans and plants, respectively. This observation is consistent with the current understanding of the evolution scheme that fungi are closely related to metazoans, and Apicomplexa acquired a plant-associated enzyme together with the plastid-like apicoplast by endosymbios (Baldauf and Palmer, 1993; McFadden, 2000). Although *Entamoeba* appears to lack type II PI 4-kinases, there is a possibility that *Entamoeba* and other organisms that lack type II PI 4-kinase may have a novel type of PI 4-kinase that is yet to be identified.

5.2. Type III PI 4-Kinase

5.2.1. General Description of Type III PI 4-Kinase

Type III PI 4-kinases contain a continuous (uninterrupted) catalytic domain like PI 3-kinases, and both kinase types similarly show wortmannin sensitivity. Different from type II PI 4-kinases, the type III enzymes have a lipid kinase unique (LKU) domain, which is conserved among PI 3-kinases (Balla, 2013). As described above, the primary role of type III PI 4-kinases is generation of PtdIns4P, a precursor of PtdIns(4,5)P_2, at the plasma membrane. PI4KIIIα has been shown to be recruited to the plasma membrane by interacting with two binding proteins, EFR3B and TTC7B, which are the mammalian homologs of yeast Efr3 and Ypp1 (Baird et al., 2008, see below). Additionally, knocking down PI4KIIIα causes reduction in PtdIns4P and PtdIns(4,5)P_2 level at the plasma membrane (Nakatsu et al., 2012). Notably, in the PI4KIIIα knockout mouse embryonic fibroblast (MEF) cells, the total cellular level of PtdIns(4,5)P_2 did not change due to the compensatory upregulation of PIPKIβ and γ, which also generate PtdIns(4,5)P_2 from PtdIns4P. However, the level of PtdIns(4,5)P_2 in the internal vesicles increased in the PI4KIIIα-knockout MEF cells. Several plasma membrane proteins such as M1 muscarinic receptor, and myristoylated/palmitoylated N-terminal anchor of LCK have been demonstrated to be concentrated in the internal vesicles where PtdIns(4,5)P_2 is also enriched. These results suggest that PI4KIIIα gives unique properties to the plasma membrane, and thus lack of PI4KIIIα perturbs the membrane identity (Nakatsu et al., 2012).

Of two isotypes in humans, PI4KIIIα contains a bipartite nuclear localization sequence (NLS) and PH domain (Heilmeyer et al., 2003). In contrast, PI4KIIIβ does not have either of these domains; however, it contains several stretches rich in basic amino acids and leucine-rich sequences that can potentially serve as nuclear localization and export signals, overall suggesting their nuclear localization (Heilmeyer et al., 2003). Both PI4KIIIs have indeed been detected in the nucleus, and the yeast homolog of PI4KIIIβ, Pik1p, has been shown to shuttle between the cytosol and nucleus, suggesting its contribution to the PI pools in the nuclear speckles (Garcia-Bustos et al., 1994; de Graaf et al., 2002; Heilmeyer et al., 2003; Demmel et al., 2008; Mellman et al., 2008; Barlow et al., 2010). PI4KIIIβ plays a role as Rab11 effector, and participate in the recruitment of Rab11 to the Golgi and TGN (de Graaf et al., 2004). The crystal structures of PI4KIIIβ, Rab11, and Rab11 effector FIP3 revealed that PI4KIIIβ-Rab11 binding is independent of the kinase activity of PI4KIIIβ, which suggests a role of PI4KIIIβ other than PI phosphorylation (Burke et al., 2014). While type II PI 4-kinases are palmitoylated, type III PI 4-kinases are soluble and present in the cytosol. For membrane association, they interact with other proteins that have membrane affinity. PI4KIIIα has been shown to bind to TTC7 and EFR3 (Baird et al., 2008; Nakatsu et al., 2012). These proteins function as a scaffold for PI4KIIIα (Wu et al., 2014). For instance, EFR3 binds to acidic phospholipids, whereby it recruits the enzyme complex to the plasma membrane (Nakatsu et al., 2012). On the other hand, PIK4IIIβ binds to neuronal calcium sensor 1 (NCS-1), acyl-CoA-binding domain containing protein 3 (ACBD3), 14–3–3, and ADP-ribosylation factor 1 (Arf1) (Zhao et al., 2001; Hausser et al., 2006; Hsu et al., 2010; Sasaki et al., 2012; Klima et al., 2016). NCS-1 is a myristoylated calcium binding protein involved in membrane recruitment and activation of PI4KIIIβ. ACBD3 is a Golgi adaptor protein involved in the recruitment of PI4KIIIβ to the Golgi. Arf1 is a Golgi-localized small GTPase and its activation enhances binding and activity of PI4KIIIβ. 14–3–3 is a phosphoserine/threonine-binding protein. It binds to protein kinase D-phosphorylated PI4KIIIβ and this interaction stabilizes PI4KIIIβ activity. These binding proteins are the key regulators of type III PI 4-kinases.

5.2.2. Type III PI 4-Kinase of *E. histolytica*

Entamoeba histolytica has only one homolog of PI4KIIIα and PI4KIIIβ (EHI_148700). As described above, *E. histolytica* does not have a type II PI 4-kinases, and EHI_148700 is the only potential PI 4-kinase in this organism. NLS search did not indicate presence of NLS on EHI_1478700 (http://nls-mapper.iab.keio.ac.jp/cgi-bin/NLS_Mapper_form.cgi) (Heilmeyer et al., 2003; Kosugi et al., 2009). Considering the analogy of *E. histolytica* to other organisms and also the fact that its type I PIP kinase is predicted to have NLS (see section 6.1.2 below), it is reasonable to speculate that *E. histolytica* also has a PtdIns4P pool in the nucleus. If so, as described above for PI4KIIIβ, basic amino acid-stretches and leucine-rich sequences in EHI_148700 may function as a nuclear localization signal. This potential *E. histolytica* type III PI 4-kinase is a soluble protein and predicted to associate with the plasma membrane through its binding proteins. However, no orthologs for the known PI4KIIIα-binding proteins TTC7 and EFR3 have been identified with an E-value lower than 1×10^{-10}. EHI_118850 has been identified during a similarity search using human TTC7 as the query, and thus the two proteins are thought to be homologs. However, although TTC7 has three tetratricopeptide repeat (TPR) domains, EHI_118850 has two. No homologs of human/yeast ERF3 have been identified in *E. histolytica*; however, one should note that human and yeast ERF3 share only low (19.4%) amino acid homology according to Clustal Omega alignment, and no DNA similarity was detected by BLAST search. Murine homologs of EFR3 and TTC7 were identified from the PI4KIIIα immunoprecipitates of mouse brain extract (Nakatsu et al., 2012). Thus, biochemical approaches must be pursued in *E. histolytica* for the identification of its proteins that are functionally homologous to TTC7 and ERF3. It is also worth mentioning that type III PI4K of *P. falciparum* has been exploited for the development of antimalarials (McNamara et al., 2013; Kandepedu et al., 2018).

6. PHOSPHATIDYLINOSITOL PHOSPHATE KINASES (PIP KINASES)

PIP kinases have a unique catalytic domain that is not homologous to any other known lipid or protein kinases. There are three types of PIP kinases based on the substrate specificities. Type I and II PIP kinases generate PtdIns(4,5)P_2 from PtdIns4P and PtdIns5P, respectively. Type III PIP kinases generate PtdIns(3,5)P_2 form PtdIns3P. The only recognizable domain present in all PIPKs is the highly conserved kinase core domain (PIPKc) (Sasaki et al., 2009; Balla, 2013).

6.1. Type I PIP Kinase

6.1.1. General Description of Type I PIP Kinase (PIP 5-Kinase)

Three type I PIP kinases (PIPKI) have been identified in humans: PIPKIα, β, and γ. The *PIPKIγ* mRNA transcript has been shown to be alternatively spliced to encode multiple forms of PIPKIγ isoforms: PIPKIγ-i1 to 6 (Ishihara et al., 1998; Giudici et al., 2004; Schill and Anderson, 2009; Xia et al., 2011). All PIPKI isoforms share a central kinase core (PIPKc) domain with 80% amino acid homology (Ishihara et al., 1998). The C-terminal part of the PIPKc domain contains a 25 amino acid activation loop that is critical for both the substrate specificity and subcellular targeting of PIPKs (Kunz et al., 2000, 2002; Liu et al., 2016). PIPKIs are the major PtdIns(4,5)P_2-generating enzymes, which phosphorylate the hydroxyl group at the D5 position of the inositol ring of PtdIns4P, and have a wide variety of roles relating to PtdIns(4,5)P_2 synthesis (Rameh et al., 1997). Since one of the major roles of PtdIns(4,5)P_2 is the actin-mediated processes, PIPKIs are also indispensable for the actin dynamics. In fact, yeast has a single PIPKI, Mss4p, and the *mss4* mutant showed a phenotype similar to actin deficiency (Desrivières et al., 1998; Homma et al., 1998). In mammals, PIPKIs have also been shown to be involved in actin dynamics and membrane activities by generating PtdIns(4,5)P_2 from PtdIns4P, and the specific role of each PIPK seems to vary depending on their expression levels and the cell type (Balla, 2013). PIPKIs are widely distributed in the cell, and each isoform shows a unique localization pattern, whereby it regulates a specialized (compartmentalized) pool of PtdIns(4,5)P_2 (Doughman et al., 2003; Tan et al., 2015). PIPKIγi1–3 and 5 have been shown to be localized on the plasma membrane (Balla, 2013), while PIPKIγi2 is also localized in the recycling endosomes and focal adhesions (Di Paolo et al., 2002; Ling et al., 2002). It has been also shown that PIPKIα and β are targeted to autolysosomes (Rong et al., 2012). Additionally, it has been independently demonstrated that PIPKIα and PIPKIγi4 are found in nuclear speckles (Li et al., 2013), and PIPKIβ accumulates at the perinuclear regions (Doughman et al., 2003). PIPKIs apparently play redundant roles, and only a single copy of PIPKIγ is sufficient to support the development and growth of mice to the adulthood (Volpicelli-Daley et al., 2010). All three PIPKI isozymes have been linked to endosomal traffic (Galiano et al., 2002; Shinozaki-Narikawa et al., 2006). PIPKIα and β are known to initiate lysosomal reformation during autophagy (Yu et al., 2010; Rong et al., 2012; Chen and Yu, 2017). PIPKIα and γ are also implicated in chemotaxis (Lacalle et al., 2007; Lokuta et al., 2007). PIPKIγi1 is involved in the generation of pools of PtdIns(4,5)P_2 for Ins(1,4,5)P_3, which regulates calcium release in histamine-stimulated HeLa cells (Wang et al., 2004). PIPKIα has been shown to be involved in pre-mRNA processing in association with non-canonical poly(A) polymerase, Star-PAP, which is specifically stimulated by PtdIns(4,5)P_2 (Mellman et al., 2008).

Activation of PIPKI differs from that of type II PIP kinase (PIPKII). PIPKI activity is stimulated by phosphatidic acid (PA) (Jenkins et al., 1994). Phospholipase D (PLD) and diacylglycerol kinase produce PA and are thought to be involved in the activation of PIPKIs (Tolias et al., 1998; Honda et al., 1999; Divecha et al., 2000). In mammals, two PLD isotypes use PtdIns(4,5)P_2 as a cofactor (Cockcroft, 2001), and thus, locally accumulated PIPKI and PLD mutually activate each other through their products, which results in a positive feedback loop (Mahankali et al., 2015). It has been shown that Arf6, a small GTPase which regulates membrane traffic, recruits PLD2 to membrane ruffles and stimulates PIPKI activity (Skippen et al., 2002). PLD1 is involved in initiation of autophagy by stimulating the PIPKI activity to generate necessary PtdIns(4,5)P_2 pool for the formation of the isolation membrane (Jenkins and Frohman, 2005; Dall'Armi et al., 2010; Fan et al., 2011; He et al., 2013).

6.1.2. Type I PIP Kinase (PIP 5-Kinase) of *E. histolytica*

In *E. histolytica*, only one possible ortholog (EHI_153770) with the E-value of $< 1 \times 10^{-10}$ was found (E-value, 1×10^{-38}) by using three *H. sapiens* type I PIP kinases (PIPKI) (NP_001129110, AAH30587, and NP_001287778) as queries. EHI_153770 has a PIPKc domain based on pfam search. Furthermore, human and yeast PIPKIs, PIPKIβ (NP_001265182) and Mss4p (BAA02869), respectively, were identified with the corresponding E-values of 8×10^{-39} and 5×10^{-37}, when EHI_153770 was used as a query to search for a human or yeast ortholog, respectively. Since no PIPKII ortholog has been identified in *E. histolytica* (see below section 6.2.2), EHI_153770 likely has a major role in PtdIns(4,5)P_2 generation from PtdIns4P. This single type I PIP kinase should have a wide variety of roles in *E. histolytica*. It is of note that the NLS is conserved in EHI_153770 and the putative PLD of *E. histolytica* also has an NLS (K. Das, data not shown). Sharma and colleagues recentrly demonstrated of EHI_15377 (Sharma et al., 2019).

6.2. Type II PIP Kinase

6.2.1. General Description of Type II PIP Kinase (PIP 4-Kinase)

Type II PIP kinase is the oldest PIP kinase identified among the others. However, the role of this class of enzymes is not as well-understood as that of type I PIP kinases (Boronenkov and Anderson, 1995; Divecha et al., 1995). Although PIPKII was initially thought to be responsible for generation of PtdIns(4,5)P_2 from PtdIns5P, this enzyme is currently considered to play a role in the regulation of the PtdIns5P levels (Clarke et al., 2010). Three PIPKII isotypes, PIPKIIα, β, and γ, are known, all of which contain the conserved PIPKc kinase domain bisected in the center by a non-conserved inserted sequence (Loijens et al., 1996; Itoh et al., 1998; Sasaki et al., 2009). All three PIPKIIs contain the ~25 amino acid activation loop at the C-terminal part of the PIPKc domain as in PIPKIs (Sasaki et al., 2009). PIPKII α, β, and γ isotypes differ in their relative enzymatic activities in the order listed, with α being the most active (Clarke et al., 2008; Bultsma et al., 2010). It was speculated that the weak forms of PIPKII (β and γ) dimerize with the strong enzyme PIPKIIα and serve as adaptor proteins that bring it to specific membrane compartments (Clarke et al., 2010). Nuclear localization of PIPKIIα and PIPKIIβ has been reported (Bultsma et al., 2010; Wang et al., 2010). PIPKIIβ, which lacks an NLS, is targeted to the nucleus by a unique nuclear localization sequence consisting of an acidic α helix present in its unique insertion region in the kinase domain (Ciruela et al., 2000; Bunce et al., 2008). In contrast, PIPKIIγ has been detected in the ER by immunochemistry and subcellular fractionation, and also in other compartments of the endomembrane system (Itoh et al., 1998; Clarke et al., 2009).

Type II PIP kinase does not seem to play a role in the regulation of actin dynamics, as human type II PIP kinase failed to rescue yeast mss4 (type I PIP kinase) deficiency (Homma et al., 1998; Ishihara et al., 1998). It has been shown that PIPKIIα is involved in the formation and secretion of alpha granules in platelets (Rozenvayn and Flaumenhaft, 2001, 2003; Schulze et al., 2006). PIPKIIβ knockout mice show increased insulin sensitivity, likely through enhanced Akt activity (Carricaburu et al., 2003; Lamia et al., 2004). This is tentatively explained by slow degradation of PtdIns(3,4,5)P_3 in the knockout mice; however, the molecular basis remains elusive. The hypothesis that an excess amount of PtdIns5P inhibits phosphatase activity has been rejected (Campbell et al., 2003; Schaletzky et al., 2003). It has been shown that increasing the PtdIns5P level by overexpressing a bacterial PtdIns(4,5)$P_2$4-phosphatase (IpgD) enhanced Akt activity (Pendaries et al., 2006). It has also been shown that nuclear PIPKIIβ is involved in nuclear stress response. For instance, UV irradiation induces phosphorylation of Ser236 in PIPKIIβ, and this phosphorylation inactivates PIPKIIα kinase-activity, which is associated with PIPKIIβ and accumulation of PtdIns5P (Jones et al., 2006; Bultsma et al., 2010; Wang et al., 2010) (also see section 2.2.4).

6.2.2. Type II PIP Kinase (PIP 4-Kinase) of *E. histolytica*

The *E. histolytica* genome was found to encode one possible PIPKI with a reasonable E-value of 6×10^{-26} when three human PIPKII isotypes were used as queries in BLAST search. This protein (EHI_153770) was identified as a top hit with a lower E-value of 6×10^{-37} when PIPKI was used as a query, as described above. Because of this higher similarity to PIPKIs, EHI_153770 is categorized as a PIPKI.

6.3. Type III PIP Kinase

6.3.1. General Description of Type III PIP Kinase (PIP 5-Kinase)

Type III PIP kinases (PIPKIII) phosphorylate PtdIns3P to PtdIns(3,5)P_2, which is one of the least abundant PIs (Hasegawa et al., 2017). PIPKIII was initially found in yeast by a genetic screening for defects in nuclear segregation (Yamamoto et al., 1995). A PIPKIII-deficient yeast line showed enlargement of vacuoles and retardation in vacuole delivery of hydrolases, such as carboxypeptidase Y (CPY) (Gary et al., 1998). This observation suggests the primary effect of PIPKIII deficiency is on membrane trafficking. PIPKIII is a large protein of >2000 amino acids and contains the C-terminal catalytic domain of PIPKc, which is similar to that of PIPKI and PIPKII. Distinct from other PIP kinases, PIPKIIIs have multiple domains in humans: FYVE (Fab1p, YOTB, Vac1p, and EEA1), DEP (disheveled, Egl-10, and pleckstrin), and TCP-1 (t-complex polypeptide-1) domains (Sasaki et al., 2009; Balla, 2013).These domains are involved in PtdIns3P binding, membrane association, and actin/tubulin binding, respectively (Cabezas et al., 2006). As PtdIns(3,5)P_2 has a critical role in endosome/lysosome biogenesis, PtdIns3P, which is highly used in endocytic pathways, is converted to PtdIns(3,5)P_2 by PIPKIII on endosomes to initiate MVB formation (Odorizzi et al., 1998). PIPKIII deficiency in mammalian cells has also been shown to cause massive vacuolization (enlarged endosomes) due to defective MVB formation (Ikonomov et al., 2003). PIPKIIIs are involved in a variety of membrane traffic pathways and signaling, such as retrograde transport of cation-independent mannose 6-phosphate receptor and sortilin, lysosomal localization and activity of mTORC1, and autophagosome-lysosome fusion (Rutherford et al., 2006; Zhang et al., 2007; Bridges et al., 2012; Hasegawa et al., 2016; Jin et al., 2016). It is of note that suppression of PIPKIII hampered phagosome maturation but did not inhibit acidification of lysosomes in macrophages (Kim et al., 2014). Additionally, PIPKIIIs are involved in nutrient (or macromolecule) import via vacuoles (Krishna et al., 2016). PIPKIII thus plays multiple roles by tightly regulating PtdIns3P and PtdIns(3,5)P_2 concentrations in vesicular trafficking. In mammals and yeast, PIPKIIIs are known to form a complex with the Sac1-related PI phosphatase, Fig4/Sac3, and a scaffold protein, Vac14/ArPIKfyve. In yeast, PIPKIII is also known to interact with the WD domain protein Atg18 and Vac7 (Duex et al., 2006; Chow et al., 2007; Sbrissa et al., 2007; Botelho et al., 2008; Jin et al., 2008). Deletion of Fig4/Sac3 and Vac14/ArPIKfyve reduces PtdIns(3,5)P_2 level (Gary et al., 1998, 2002; Bonangelino et al., 2002; Dove et al., 2002; Rudge et al., 2004; Duex et al., 2006; Zhang et al., 2007; Zolov et al., 2012). Thus, PIPKIII activation and stabilization is also regulated by the associated proteins, such as phosphatases and scaffold proteins in the complex, to tightly control the PtdIns(3,5)P_2 level.

6.3.2. Type III PIP Kinase of *E. histolytica*

A genome survey of *E. histolytica* by a BLAST search with *H. sapiens* PIPKIII as the query identified one ortholog candidate (EHI_049480). EHI_049480 shows similarities to human PIPKI and PIPKIII with the E-values of 5×10^{-4} and 4×10^{-45}, respectively. EHI_049480 is considerably smaller than the potential human homolog, and has not been predicted to contain any additional domains such as FYVE. However, based on the highest similarity between the catalytic domains of EHI_049480 and human PIPKIII, we tentatively annotated EHI_049480 as a *E. histolytica* PIPKIII. Additionally, a BLASTP search against the *H. sapiens* and *S. cerevisiae* genomes with EHI_049480 as the query identified PIPKIII and Fab1 with the E-values of 2×10^{-45} and 9×10^{-40}, respectively.

We further searched for other PIPKIII complex components such as Vac7, Vac14, Atg18, and Fig4 (the yeast homolog of the mammalian Sac3). Potential orthologs for Atg18 and Fig4 were identified with the E-values of 1×10^{-20} and 1×10^{-34}, respectively. This possible Fig4 ortholog showed a lower E-value with Sac1 (1×10^{-82}). Thus, it is reasonable to tentatively assign this protein as a Sac1 ortholog, although it is not possible to specifically categorize Sac1 among Sac orthologs (see section 10). A human ortholog of Atg18 (WIPI), which is a WD repeat-containing protein that interacts with phosphoinositides, recognizes PtdIns3P on the nascent autophagosome and recruits the lipidation machinery to the autophagosome for LC3. However, the role of WIPI in PtdIns(3,5)P_2 metabolism remains unknown. It is unknown whether *E. histolytica* has PtdIns(3,5)P_2 metabolic pathways similar to other organisms. However, conservation of ESCRT and MVB, and the localization of PtdIns3P on phagosomes indicate that PtdIn(3,5)P_2-mediated vesicular trafficking is also conserved in *E. histolytica*. We failed to identify potential Vac7 and Vac14 homologs with an E-value $< 1 \times 10^{-1}$. As 19 HEAT repeat-containing proteins are present in the *E. histolytica* genome, it is possible that some of them function in lieu of Vac14.

7. PI 3-PHOSPHATASES

PI phosphatases are also important regulators of PI signaling. Because identification of lipid kinases and PLC-mediated second messengers had a significant impact, studies on phosphatase activity in the early '80s was largely focused on Ins(1,4,5)P_3 decomposition. A number of inositol phosphatases and PI phosphatases were identified and characterized (Majerus et al., 1986). In the '90s, it was revealed that mutations in PI phosphatases are responsible for human genetic disorders, including Oculo-Cerebro-Renal Syndrome of Lowe (OCRL), human X-linked centromyotubular myopathy, and Charcot-Marie-Tooth disease type 4B. OCRL1, myotubularin-related (MTMR) 1, and MTMR2 were identified as the genes responsible for the above-mentioned human genetic disorders, respectively (Attree et al., 1992; Myers et al., 1997; Maehama and Dixon, 1998, 1999; Blondeau et al., 2000; Taylor et al., 2000; Kim S. A. et al., 2002). One of the most studied PI phosphatases, PTEN, was identified as a tumor suppressor gene (Maehama and Dixon, 1998). Similar to PI kinases, classification of PI phosphatases is primarily based on the position of the hydroxyl group that they dephosphorylate. The human and yeast genomes are known to encode twenty-eight and six PI phosphatases, respectively (Odorizzi et al., 2000; Sasaki et al., 2009).

PI 3-phosphatases are categorized into two groups based on substrate specificities. One group includes PTEN, TPTE (transmembrane phosphatase with tensin homology), and TPIP (TPTE and PTEN homologs inositol lipid phosphatase), while the other group includes myotubularins (MTMs). Since TPTEs have no phosphatase activity, and their functional role remains unclear, they are not discussed in this review. However, TPTE has been reported to be associated with cancers. For instance, it has been demonstrated that TPTE is upregulated in prostate cancer, and autoantibody production against TPTE is observed in lung cancer (Walker et al., 2001; Tapparel et al., 2003; Bansal et al., 2015; Kuemmel et al., 2015). PTEN and TPIP have similar catalytic domains but differ in substrate specificity. PTEN removes the phosphate moiety at D3 position of PtdIns(3,4,5)P_3 and PtdIns(3,4)P_2, while TPIPs dephosphorylate any of the 3′-phosphorylated inositides at D3 position (Walker et al., 2001; Malek et al., 2017). On the other hand, MTMs remove the D3 phosphate from PtdIns(3,5)P_2 and PtdIns3P. The catalytic center of both groups of PI 3-phosphatases contains the CX_5R motif, which is also found in protein tyrosine phosphatases (Hsu and Mao, 2015).

7.1. PTEN and TPIP

7.1.1. General Descriptions of PTEN and TPIP

PTEN was initially identified as a tumor suppressor gene located on chromosome 10 (Li et al., 1997; Steck et al., 1997; Maehama and Dixon, 1998). It is among the most frequently mutated genes in various cancers in humans (Guldberg et al., 1997; Li et al., 1997; Steck et al., 1997; Tashiro et al., 1997; Cairns et al., 1998; Kohno et al., 1998; Maehama, 2007), and in hereditary cancer predisposition syndromes, such as Cowden disease (Myers et al., 1997; Furnari et al., 1998). Human TPIP was bioinformatically identified as a protein encoded by PTEN-related genes (Walker et al., 2001). PTEN consists of a protein tyrosine phosphatase (PTP)-related lipid phosphatase domain, a C2 domain, two PEST (proline, glutamine, serine, threonine) sequences, and a PDZ domain (**Figure 4**). The C2 domain is known to be involved in lipid binding and protein stability. PEST sequences are known to enhance proteolytic sensitivity, and the PDZ domain is involved in protein-protein interactions (Maehama, 2007; Sasaki et al., 2009; Balla, 2013). The human genome encodes three isotypes of TPIP, and only two of them have an N-terminal transmembrane domain (**Figure 4**). PTEN and TPIP have a CX_5R motif-containing PTP-related lipid phosphatase domain, whose core sequence is CKAGKGR and CKGGKGR, respectively. This domain forms the catalytic cleft of PTEN, and it is wider than the corresponding domain of protein tyrosine phosphatases. This allows the bulky PtdIns(3,4,5)P_3 head group to access the active center of the enzyme (Lee et al., 1999). The principal role of PTEN is to cease the cell proliferation signal by inactivating Akt though dephosphorylation of PtdIns(3,4,5)P_3, whereby it serves as a tumor suppressor.

PTEN is predominantly localized to the cytosol, and also dynamically associated with the plasma membrane, where it hydrolyzes PtdIns(3,4,5)P_3 (Billcliff and Lowe, 2014). Although PTEN lacks an NLS, it also localizes to the nucleus and plays important roles in chromosome stability by directly interacting with centromere specific binding protein C (CENP-C), DNA repair by interacting with p53 and Rad51, and cell cycle regulation by interacting with APC and MAP kinases (Freeman et al., 2003; Chung and Eng, 2005; Chung et al., 2006; Tang and Eng, 2006a,b; Shen et al., 2007; Trotman et al., 2007; Song et al., 2011). This nuclear translocation depends on the cytoplasmic localization signal and ubiquitination (Denning et al., 2007; Trotman et al., 2007; Wang et al., 2007; Drinjakovic et al., 2010). Mutations in the N-terminal cytoplasmic localization signal, which is found in familial Cowden disease patients, increases nuclear localization (Denning et al., 2007). Mono-ubiquitination of K13 and K298 serves as the nuclear translocation signal, while poly-ubiquitination causes degradation of PTEN (Trotman et al., 2007; Wang et al., 2007; Drinjakovic et al., 2010). PTEN has also been shown to participate in phagocytosis, autophagy and determination of cell polarity through dephosphorylation of PtdIns(3,4,5)P_3 (Arico et al., 2001; Kim J.S et al., 2002; Martin-Belmonte et al., 2007). In contrast, the physiological role of TPIP is not well-understood. TPIPα and γ both have the transmembrane domain unlike TPIPβ. Accordingly, they are localized on internal membranes, whereas TPIPβ remains in the cytosol (Walker et al., 2001).

7.1.2. PTEN and TPIP of *E. histolytica*

The *E. histolytica* genome potentially encodes six PTEN orthologs with E-values $< 1 \times 10^{-10}$ to the human PTEN (**Figure 4; Supplementary Table S2; Supplementary Figure S5**). Domain search by pfam showed that these six PTEN orthologs contain the CX_5R motif-containing phosphatase domain. Furthermore, the same protein candidates were detected when the three human TPIP isoforms were used as queries. The E-values against TPIP were around 1×10^{-16}-10^{-17}, which is higher than those against PTEN (**Supplementary Table S2**). Thus, we concluded that they are likely PTEN orthologs. Furthermore, five out of the six orthologs have a CX_5R motif identical to that found in PTEN (CKAGKGR). The CX_5R sequence of the remaining ortholog (EHI_131070) is CLAGRGR. Three of the *E. histolytica* PTEN orthologs also had a C2 domain. PTENs commonly have the cytosol localization signal (**Supplementary Figure S2**) (Denning et al., 2007). Among the three C2 domain-containing candidates, all six consensus amino acids of the cytosol localization signal are conserved in EHI_131070, and all but one amino acid are also conserved in EHI_197010 and EHI_098450 (**Supplementary Figure S2**). In the three *E. histolytica* PTEN candidates, which lack the C2 domain, only a few residues are conserved (four in EHI_010360, EHI_054460; three in EHI_041900) (**Supplementary Figure S2**). All the three candidates have lysine or tyrosine instead of phenylalanine that is found in the amino acid 22 position of human PTEN. It has been shown that F21A mutation causes nuclear localization of PTEN, which in turn fails to activate Akt even though the phosphatase activity is retained (Denning et al., 2007). Thus, it is not clear if the three *E. histolytica* PTEN candidates which lack the C2 domain have functional cytosol localization signals. According to the gene expression profile, two of the PTEN homologs, EHI_197010 and EHI_098450, are actively transcribed (**Supplementary Figure S1**). Both of them have a C2 domain and the cytosol localization signal.

7.2. Myotubularin (MTM)

7.2.1. General Description of MTM

The human myotubularin (MTM) family consists of 15 members [MTM1 and MTM related (MTMR) 1–14]. As in PTEN, the CX_5R motif of their phosphatase domain is overall well-conserved. Among the 15 MTMs, six of them (MTMR5 and MTMR9–13) substituted the conserved cysteine and arginine residues within the CX_5R motif with other amino acids, and thus these MTMs are catalytically inactive (Laporte et al., 2003; Hnia et al., 2012; Hsu and Mao, 2015). The CX_5R motif in MTMs (CXXGWDR) is slightly different from that in PTEN (CKAGKGR). While PTEN prefers PtdIns(3,4,5)P_3 and PtdIns(3,4)P_2 as substrates, MTMs preferentially dephosphorylate PtdIns3P and PtdIns(3,5)P_2. MTMs are categorized into six groups based on their domain configurations and catalytic activity: MTM1 and MTMR1–2; MTMR3–4; MTMR6–8; MTMR14; MTMR5 and 13; and MTMR9–12 (**Figure 4**). In all MTMs, except for MTMR14, the PH-GRAM (pleckstrin homology-glucosyltransferase, Rab-like GTPase activator and myotubularin) domain is conserved. This domain is involved in PI binding. Additionally, they all have an active or inactive catalytic core, and coiled-coil domain, which is involved in homo- or hetero- dimerization. In addition, some members have the C-terminal PDZ binding sequence and FYVE domain. The N-terminal DENN and C-terminal PH domains are conserved in two of the catalytically inactive MTM members, MTMR5 and MTMR13. Although all the catalytically inactive members (MTMR5 and MTMR9–13) lack an active phosphatase domain, they can heterodimerize with active MTMs, whereby inactive MTMs likely regulate the activity and localization of active MTMs (Kim et al., 2003; Mochizuki and Majerus, 2003; Lorenzo et al., 2006). The role of MTMs and their preferred substrates [PtdIns3P and PtdIns(3,5)P_2] in endocytosis and membrane traffic have been well-characterized (Robinson and Dixon, 2006; Hohendahl et al., 2016). Besides these, MTMs have been suggested to have other roles in cellular processes, including cell proliferation and differentiation, autophagy, phagocytosis, organelle positioning, cytokinesis, cytoskeletal rearrangement, and cell junction dynamics (Hnia et al., 2012; Lawlor et al.,

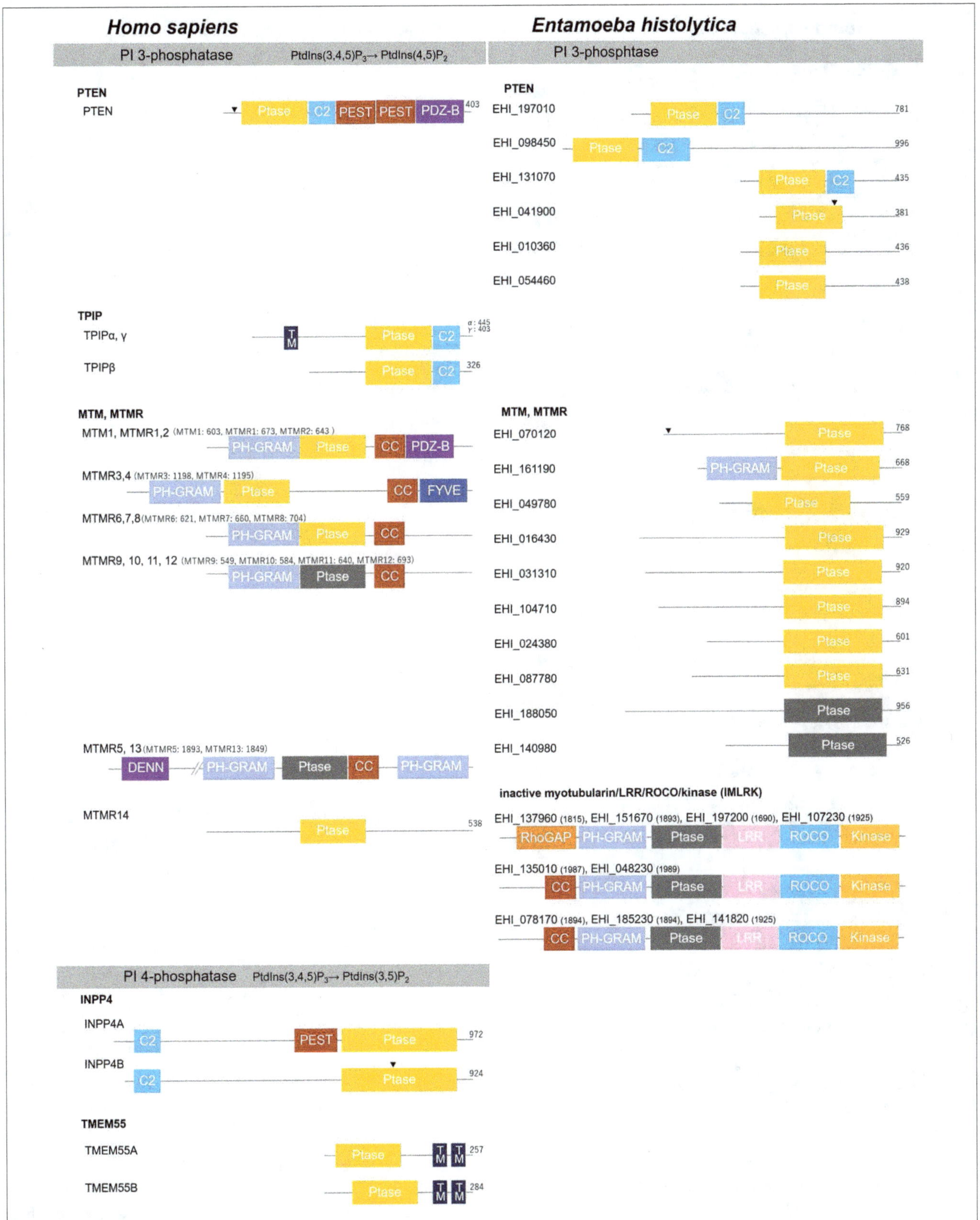

FIGURE 4 | Continued

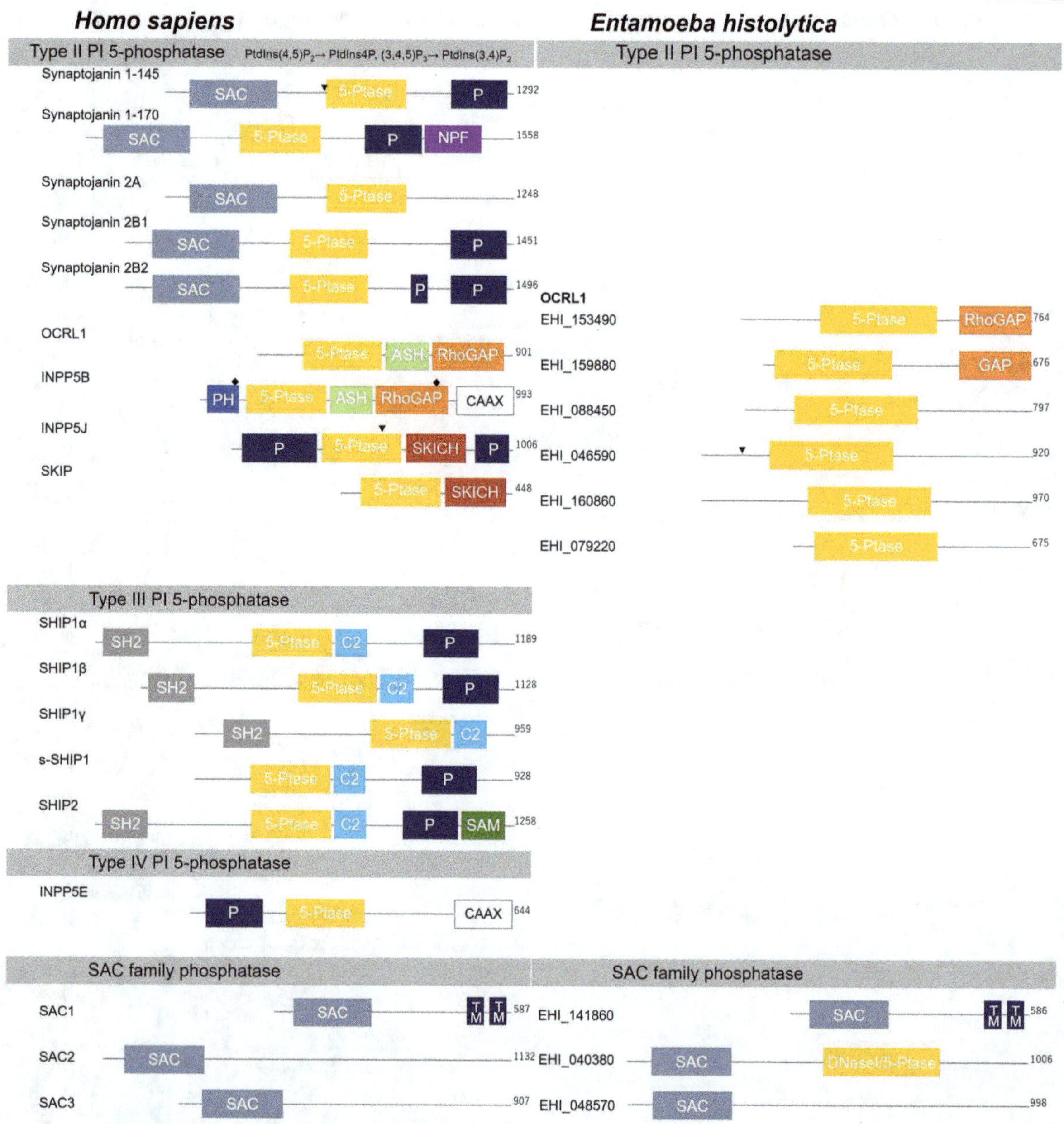

FIGURE 4 | Structural features of PI phosphatases of *H. sapiens* and *E. histolytica*. Structural features and domain organization of the PI phosphatases are shown. Numbers showing at the end of the protein or after the name of the protein indicates amino acid length. 5-Ptase, PI 5-phosphatase domain; ASH, ASPM-SPD2-hydin; C2, C2 domain; CAAX, CAAX motif; CC, coiled coil domain; DENN, differentially expressed in normal vs. neoplastic; DNaseI, DNase I-like domain; FYVE, Fab1, YOTB, Vac1, and EEA1 domain; GRAM, glucosyltransferases Rab-like GTPase activators and myotubularins; GAP, GTPase-activating domain; kinase, protein kinase domain; LRR, leucine-rich repeats; NPF, asparagine- proline-phenylalanine repeats; P, Proline-rich; PDZ-B, PDZ domain binding domain; PEST, Proline, glutamine, serine, threonine; PH, Pleckstrin-homology; (Ptase; gray), inactive Ptase domain; (Ptase; yellow), active CX5R motif containing PI 3- or PI 4-phosphatase domain; ROCO, comprised of a ROC (Ras of complex proteins) and COR (C-terminal of ROC) region; SAC, Sac domain; SAM, sterile alpha motif; SH2, Src homology 2; SKICH, SKIP carboxylhomology; TM, transmembrane domain. Clathrin-binding domain and the nuclear localization signal are also labeled with "♦" and "▼", respectively.

2016). It is of note that some of the cellular functions performed by MTMs depend on the tissue-specific expression patterns of their binding proteins and do not involve a phosphatase activity. For instance, disrupting the interaction between MTM1 and its intermediate filament, desmin, causes the formation of desmin aggregates, and this impairment is associated with myofibrillar myopathies and cardiomyopathies (Hnia et al., 2011).

7.2.2. MTM of *E. histolytica*

Genome-wide survey against the *E. histolytica* genome using human MTM1, MTMR3, 5, 6, 9, or 14 as the query identified an identical set of 11 proteins with E-values $< 1 \times 10^{-58}$. We concluded that 10 out of these 11 potential homologs are *E. histolytica* MTM orthologs by pfam search, because they contain a myotubularin-like phosphatase domain (**Figure 4**;

Supplementary Tables S1, S4). All of them, except EHI_140980 and EHI_188050, contain the conserved catalytic domain. The phosphatase domains of these two exceptions conserved the cysteine residue in their C(S/T)DGWDR motifs, but arginine is replaced with serine or isoleucine (CRNGWDS and CIDGTGI, respectively). Although *E. histolytica* MTMs appear to have a simpler domain organization, they also are thought to heterodimerize as in model organisms given that the genome contains both active and inactive MTMs. Among all the PI phosphatases in *E. histolytica*, MTMs are the most diverged ones.

It should be noted that Amoebozoa supergroup members exclusively have a protein family that contain multiple inactive myotubularin domains. These proteins have been designated as inactive myotubularin/LRR/ROCO/kinase (IMLRK) proteins (Kerk and Moorhead, 2010). Nine IMLRK proteins have previously been identified in the *E. histolytica* genome by the FFAS03 (Fold and Function Assignment System) sequence: profile method and the HHPred [Hidden Markov Model (HMM)-HMM structure prediction] profile: profile method (Kerk and Moorhead, 2010). The *D. discoideum* homologs of IMLRKs, Pats1 and GbpC, have been identified as a cytokinesis-related protein and cGMP-binding protein, respectively (Goldberg et al., 2002; Abysalh et al., 2003). Since both *D. discoideum* IMLRK homologs are involved in cytoskeleton-related processes such as cytokinesis and chemotaxis, *E. histolytica* IMLRKs may also be involved in the similar processes (Bosgraaf et al., 2002, 2005; Abysalh et al., 2003; Lewis, 2009). However, it is not clear why *E. histolytica* has inactive myotubularin domains, and more IMLRK proteins than *D. discoideum* (nine vs. two, respectively).

8. PI 4-PHOSPHATASES

Dissimilar to PI 3- and PI 5-phosphatases, which belong to multiple families of enzymes, PI 4-phosphatases consist of only four proteins. All members of human PI 4-phosphatases have the CX_5R motif in the catalytic domain. There are two groups of PI 4-phosphatases: inositol polyphosphate-4-phosphatase (INPP4) and transmembrane protein 55 (TMEM55) (**Figure 4**). INPP4 dephosphorylates PtdIns(3,4)P_2, and TMEM55 dephosphorylates PtdIns(4,5)P_2. No PI 4-phosphatases that use PtdIns(3,4,5)P_3 as a substrate have been identified yet. *E. histolytica* has no homologs of PI 4-phosphatases in this class. Here, we will discuss only the general aspects of PI 4-phosphatases.

8.1. INPP4

Two INPP4 proteins have been identified in the human genome and named INPP4A and B. They both contain a conserved catalytic domain and N-terminal C2 domain; however only INPP4A contains the PEST sequence (Sasaki et al., 2009; Balla, 2013) (**Figure 4**). The C2 domains of these proteins show different binding specificities. The C2 domain of INPP4A preferentially binds to PtdIns(3,4)P_2, PtdIns3P, phosphatidylserine, and calcium (Ivetac et al., 2005, 2009; Shearn and Norris, 2007), while that of INPP4B prefers phosphatidic acid and PtdIns(3,4,5)P_3 (Ferron and Vacher, 2006). INPP4A is cleaved and inactivated by calpain via recognition of the PEST sequence in INPP4A (Norris et al., 1995), as shown in platelets stimulated with thrombin and calcium ionophores (Norris et al., 1997). INPP4A is known to be localized in recycling and early endosomes in resting cells and translocated to the plasma membrane upon serum stimulation (Ivetac et al., 2005). In contrast, INPP4B has been shown to be localized diffusely in the cytoplasm. INPP4A is involved in the regulation of membrane traffic, which is consistent with its endosomal localization. It has been shown that INPP4A is activated by Rab5, and knocking down Rab5 inhibits transferrin uptake (Shin et al., 2005). On the other hand, overexpression of INPP4A suppresses the enlarged endosome morphology caused by PtdIns3P deficiency in INPP4A knock-out MEF cells (Ivetac et al., 2009), suggesting that INPP4A produces PtdIns3P from PtdIns(3,4)P_2. A significant role of INPP4A in the generation of PtdIns3P to recruit SNX9 and actin polymerization machineries during clathrin-mediated endocytosis has also been reported (Malek et al., 2017). No potential orthologous genes with the E-value $< 1 \times 10^{-1}$ have been identified in *E. histolytica*.

8.2. TMEM55

TMEM55 (transmembrane protein 55), which was named after the transmembrane regions it contains, was originally identified based on its homology to the virulence factor of *Burkholderia pseudomallei*, BopB, a putative phosphatase that contains a CX_5R motif (Ungewickell et al., 2005). There are two isotypes of TMEM55, termed TMEM55A and B. They both consist of a CX_5R motif-containing phosphatase domain and two putative transmembrane domains at the C-terminus (Rynkiewicz et al., 2012). Based on *in vitro* and *in vivo* observations, TMEM55 specifically hydrolyzes the D4 phosphate of PtdIns(4,5)P_2. Both TMEM55A and TMEM55B show cytosolic and late endosomal membrane localization (Ungewickell et al., 2005). Overexpression of TMEM55A enhances EGFR degradation induced by EGF stimulation, suggesting that TMEM55A is involved in the endocytic and recycling pathways (Ungewickell et al., 2005). Additionally, TMEM55A has been reported to be involved in macrophage phagocytosis (Morioka et al., 2018). On the other hand, TMEM55B translocates from the cytosol to the nucleus and increases the PtdIns5P level in response to DNA damage (Zou et al., 2007). This upregulation of PtdIns5P in the nucleus is accompanied by activation of ING2 (Gozani et al., 2003) and enhanced p53-mediated cell death (Zou et al., 2007). In *E. histolytica*, no potential orthologous genes with the E-value $< 1 \times 10^{-1}$ have been identified. It is possible that *E. histolytica* utilizes Sac phosphatase (see below) for dephosphorylation of the D4 position of PIs.

9. PI 5-PHOSPHATASES

Inositol polyphosphate 5-phosphatases (INPP5s) have an inositol 5-phosphatase (5-Ptase) domain that contains two signature motifs (F/Y)WXGDXN(F/Y)R and P(A/S)(W/Y)(C/T)DR(I/V)L(W/Y) separated by ~60–75 residues (Majerus et al., 1999). INPP5s are Mg^{2+}-dependent enzymes and share homology with apurinic/apyrimidinic family of endonucleases (Whisstock et al., 2000). There are four classes of PI 5-phosphatases (types I–IV). However, the type I enzyme (INPP5A) does not have lipid phosphatase activity, and dephosphorylate Ins(1,4,5)P_3 and Ins(1,3,4,5)P_4 (Laxminarayan et al., 1993, 1994; De Smedt et al., 1994). Type II PI 5-phosphatases include the synaptojanins OCRL1, INPP5B, INPP5J, and SKIP. The type III enzymes are two SHIPs, namely SHIP1 and 2. Interestingly, there is only one type IV PI 5-phosphatase, named INPP5E. Because *E. histolytica* has a low conservation of PI 5-phosphatases, we will describe the search result at the end of this section. However, the enzyme Sac can act as a PI 5-phosphatase. Although it does not contain the 5-Ptase domain, it contains the CX_5R motif-containing phosphatase domain (CKAGRSR). As described below, like PTEN, it differs from PI 5-phosphatases in its active center configuration and substrate specificity.

9.1. Type II PI 5-Phosphatase

There are five kinds of type II PI 5-phosphatases, such as synaptojanins, OCRL1, INPP5B, INPP5J, and SKIP. They differ in structure and function.

9.1.1. General Description of Synaptojanins

There are two synaptojanins in mammals, and each of them has multiple splice variants (McPherson et al., 1996). All the synaptojanins have a conserved 5-Ptase catalytic domain and N-terminal Sac domain. The Sac domain also has inositol phosphatase activity. The domain configuration of the C-terminal region varies in each splice form (**Figure 4**). Most synaptojanin splice forms encode proteins that contain a proline-rich (P) region, and SYNJ1-170 additionally has an asparagine-proline-phenylalanine (NPF) repeat. NPF repeat is involved in the association of these proteins with the endocytic protein Eps15 (Haffner et al., 1997). SYNJ2A is ubiquitously expressed, and SYNJ1-170 shows a broad tissue distribution. Interestingly, SYNJ1-145, SYNEJ2B1, and SYNEJ2B2 are highly expressed in the brain, and SYNEJ2B1 and 2 are also abundant in the testis (Nemoto et al., 2001). The 5-Ptase domain of all SYNJ1 and 2 proteins enables them to dephosphorylate Ins(1,4,5)P_3, Ins(1,3,4,5)P_4, PtdIns(4,5)P_2, and PtdIns(3,4,5)P_3 at the D5 position (McPherson et al., 1996; Sakisaka et al., 1997). Furthermore, the Sac domain of Synaptojanins enable them to dephosphorylate PtdIns3P, PtdIns4P and PtdIns(3,5)P_2 (Guo et al., 1999). Sac domain has been suggested to use the product generated by the PI 5-phosphatase domain to finally generate PtdIns (Guo et al., 1999; Nemoto et al., 2001). SYNJ1 has been found to be involved in synaptic vesicle exocytosis and recycling (McPherson et al., 1996). Additionally, synaptojanins have a critical role in the fate determination of clathrin-coated vesicles (CCVs). Knocking out SYNJ1 in the mouse caused accumulation of endocytosed CCVs and poor recycling of vesicles into the fusion-competent synaptic vesicle pool (Kim W. T. et al., 2002). Consequently, it caused neurological defects, and death after birth (Cremona et al., 1999). Synaptojanins are involved in endocytosis and synaptic vesicle recycling in concert with a variety of binding proteins such as endocytic proteins amphiphysin, endophilin syndapin/pacsin, and intersectin/Dap160 (McPherson et al., 1996; Bauerfeind et al., 1997; de Heuvel et al., 1997; Ringstad et al., 1997; Roos and Kelly, 1998; Qualmann et al., 1999). Also, the C-terminal NPF region of SYNJ1-170 enables the interaction with the EH (Eps15 homology) domain of Eps15, ear domain of the α-adaptin component of the adaptor protein (AP) 2 complex, and N-terminal domain of the clathrin heavy chain (Barbieri et al., 2001; Krauss et al., 2006).

9.1.2. General Descriptions of OCRL1 and INPP5B

OCRL1 was originally identified as a protein responsible for the *X*-linked human disease OCRL. It shares a high amino acid sequence homology (45%) with INPP5B (Attree et al., 1992; Jefferson and Majerus, 1995; Speed et al., 1995; Matzaris et al., 1998). OCRL1 and INPP5B consist of a PH domain, 5-Ptase domain, ASH (ASPM, SPD2, hydin) domain, and RhoGAP domain. Only OCRL1 has two clathrin binding domains (CB), and only INPP5B has a C-terminal CAAX extension for prenylation of the cysteine residue (Jefferson and Majerus, 1995). These two proteins are the only RhoGAP domain-containing PI 5-phosphatases in the human and mouse (Jefferson and Majerus, 1995; Speed et al., 1995; Matzaris et al., 1998; Lowe, 2005). However, their RhoGAP domains appear to lack the catalytic activity because of amino acid substitutions at the catalytic region (Peck et al., 2002). Even though these domains lack a catalytic activity, RhoGAP domain of OCRL1 can interact with Rac1, Cdc42, ARF1, and ARF6 (Faucherre et al., 2003; Lichter-Konecki et al., 2006; Erdmann et al., 2007; Choudhury et al., 2009). OCRL1 prefer PtdIns(4,5)P_2, Ins(1,4,5)P_3, Ins(1,3,4,5)P_4, and PtdIns(3,4,5)P_3 as dephosphorylation substrates (Zhang et al., 1995; Schmid et al., 2004). OCRL1 can also dephosphorylate PtdIns(3,5)P_2 (Schmid et al., 2004). On the other hand, INPP5B can remove the D5 phosphate of PtdIns(4,5)P_2, PtdIns(3,4,5)P_3, Ins(1,4,5)P_3, and Ins(1,3,4,5)P_4 with comparable efficiencies, but it is ineffective in the dephosphorylation of PtdIns(3,5)P_2 (Jefferson and Majerus, 1995; Schmid et al., 2004). OCRL1 is involved in the regulation of vesicular trafficking between endosomes and the TGN (Choudhury et al., 2005). This is in line with OCRL1's localization on the TGN, early endosomes, membrane ruffles, and clathrin-coated trafficking intermediates (Olivos-Glander et al., 1995; Dressman et al., 2000; Ungewickell et al., 2004; Choudhury et al., 2005; Faucherre et al., 2005; Erdmann et al., 2007). OCRL1 deficiency causes abnormal cytoskeletal reorganization (Suchy and Nussbaum, 2002; Faucherre et al., 2005). This is not only due to perturbation of the functions exerted by the RhoGAP-like domain, but also due to perturbed modulation of PtdIns(4,5)P_2 levels, suggesting the importance of OCRL1 in PtdIns(4,5)P_2 homeostasis. INPP5B is associated with the Golgi apparatus, ER exit sites, and Rab (Williams et al., 2007). Its localization is affected by interactions with Rab proteins (Vyas et al., 2000; Shin et al., 2005; Williams et al., 2007). These data suggest that INPP5B is involved in the early secretory pathway.

9.1.3. General Descriptions of INPP5J and SKIP

INPP5J and SKIP (skeletal muscle- and kidney-enriched inositol polyphosphate phosphatase) have been identified by virtue of two conserved consensus motifs characteristic of PI 5-phosphatases

(Mochizuki and Takenawa, 1999; Gurung et al., 2003). INPP5J is also called proline-rich inositol polyphosphate 5-phosphatase (PIPP) because of the two proline-rich regions at the N- and C- terminal of the protein. The N-terminal proline-rich region of INPP5J contains a putative SH3-binding motif (PRSPSR) and six 14–3–3 binding motifs (Gurung et al., 2003), and a SKICH (SKIP carboxyl homology) domain which mediates localization to the plasma membrane (Ooms et al., 2006). The C-terminus of the 5-Ptase domain is overall conserved in both INPP5J and SKIP. INPP5J removes the D5 phosphate of PtdIns(4,5)P_2, PtdIns(3,4,5)P_3, Ins(1,4,5)P_3, and Ins(1,3,4,5)P_4, while SKIP prefers PtdIns(3,4,5)P_3, but can also dephosphorylate PtdIns(4,5)P_2, Ins(1,4,5)P_3, and Ins(1,3,4,5)P_4 (Ijuin and Takenawa, 2003). INPP5J and SKIP are localized on the plasma membrane, and also in the TGN and ER of resting cells, respectively. Following insulin stimulation, SKIP translocates to the plasma membrane via the SKICH domain (Gurung et al., 2003). Both enzymes are considered to regulate Akt activation by negatively regulating PtdIns(3,4,5)P_3 (Ijuin and Takenawa, 2003; Ooms et al., 2006). Furthermore, SKIP participates in insulin response by regulating GULT4 translocation and glucose uptake in skeletal muscle.

9.2. Type III PI 5-Phosphatase

Type III PI 5-phosphatases, termed SHIP (SH2-containing inositol phosphatase), consists of SHIP1 and SHIP2. SHIP1 has several splice variants: a full-length isoform (SHIP1α) and shorter isoforms (SHIP1β, SHIP1γ, and s-SHIP1) (Lucas and Rohrschneider, 1999; Tu et al., 2001). SHIP1 was originally identified as a binding protein of several adaptor proteins such as Shc, Grab2, and DOK (Liu et al., 1994), and immunoreceptor tyrosine-based inhibitory (ITIM) or activation (ITAM) motifs of immune receptors (Osborne et al., 1996; Kimura et al., 1997). Both enzymes are composed of an N-terminal SH2 domain, a 5-Ptase catalytic domain followed by a C2 domain, and an NPXY motif. All SHIP isoforms except for SHIP1γ contain a C-terminal proline-rich domain. SHIP2 has a sterile alpha (SAM) motif at the C-terminus of the proline rich region. SHIP1 is exclusively expressed in hematopoietic and spermatogenic lineages, whereas SHIP2 expression is ubiquitous (Liu et al., 1998). SHIP1 isoforms hydrolyze the D5 phosphate of both PtdIns(3,4,5)P_3 and Ins(1,3,4,5)P_4, whereas SHIP2 activity appears to be more specific for PtdIns(3,4,5)P_3 (Wisniewski et al., 1999). SHIP1 is involved in myeloid cell homeostasis, chemotaxis, bone metabolism, and mast cell activation (Helgason et al., 1998; Huber et al., 1998; Liu et al., 1999; Jiang et al., 2005; Nishio et al., 2007). SHIP2 is involved in the negative regulation of insulin-mediated cellular response (Wada et al., 2001; Kaisaki et al., 2004; Sleeman et al., 2005). These phenotypes are explicable given the high level of PtdIns(3,4,5)P_3 in the cells, also pointing to the pivotal role of SHIPs in PtdIns(3,4,5)P_3-mediated signaling.

9.3. Type IV PI 5-Phosphatase

There is only one type IV PI 5-phosphatase, which is also called INPP5E, 72-kDa polyphosphate 5-phosphatase, or Pharbin (Kisseleva et al., 2000; Kong et al., 2000). INPP5E consists of the C-terminal farnesylation CAAX motif and the central 5-phosphatase domain, flanked by an N-terminal proline-rich region. PtdIns(4,5)P_2, PtdIns(3,4,5)P_3, and PtdIns(3,5)P_2 have been reported to be substrates of INPP5E (Kisseleva et al., 2000; Kong et al., 2000). Notably, INPP5E has the highest affinity to PtdIns(3,4,5)P_3 and shows ten times higher affinity for PtdIns(3,4,5)P_3 than SHIP (Kisseleva et al., 2000). It localizes to the cytosol, and Golgi in proliferating cells (Kong et al., 2000). In macrophages, INPP5E localizes to the phagocytic cup and regulates FcγR1-mediated, but not complement receptor 3-mediated, phagocytosis (Horan et al., 2007). In adipocytes, INPP5E has been shown to hydrolyze PtdIns(3,5)P_2 to PtdIns3P and enhance GULT4 translocation; however, insulin signaling does not decrease upon INPP5E overexpression (Kong et al., 2000). Importantly, INPP5E also plays a critical role in ciliopathies (Bielas et al., 2009; Jacoby et al., 2009). The primary cilium is a microtubule-based organelle, which forms protrusions on the plasma membrane and functions as a sensor for the environmental factors such as light, chemicals, and mechanical stress (Goetz and Anderson, 2010). Additionally, primary cilia are central in hedgehog signaling, which is a major pathway involved in the structural organization of the body, organogenesis, and tumorigenesis (Elliott and Brugmann, 2019). PtdIns4P and PtdIns(4,5)P_2 have been shown to be localized on the primary cilium membrane and ciliary base, respectively. This position-specific PI distribution pattern is maintained by INPP5E localized at the primary cilium (Chávez et al., 2015; Garcia-Gonzalo et al., 2015). Disrupting the PI compartmentalization pattern or increasing the PtdIns(4,5)P_2 level in the primary cilium causes cilial accumulation of Tulp3, which contains a PtdIns(4,5)P_2-binding domain. In turn, Tulp3's binding proteins, Gpr161 and IFT-A, are recruited to the primary cilium. Gpr161 is a negative regulator of the hedgehog signaling, and IFT-A is a flagellar transporting protein, respectively. Accumulation of this complex has been shown to perturb hedgehog signaling from the primary cilium. This observation emphasizes the significance of PI metabolism in cell physiology (Nakatsu, 2015).

9.4. PI 5-Phosphatases of *E. histolytica*

The possible *E. histolytica* PI 5-phosphatases all have a simple domain configuration: a 5-phosphatase domain alone or together with one more domain (**Figure 4**). PI 5-phosphatases have divergent and specialized roles in the human. For instance, synaptojanins are involved in neurotransmitter secretion, while SHIPs participate in hematopoietic cell signaling. Thus, the simplification of 5-phosphatases in *E. histolytica* may indicate the importance of IP5-phosphatase in multicellularity, and also the possibility of *E. histolytica* having only the ancestral type of PI 5-phosphatases.

Six candidate proteins showed E-values lower than 1×10^{-30} when searched with human OCRL1 as the query (AAB03839). One candidate, EHI_153490, has the 5-Ptase and RhoGAP domains, and the other protein, EHI_159880, contains the 5-Ptase and GAP domains. They both lack the C-terminus CAAX motif conserved in INPP5B. The apparent similarity in domain configurations suggests that these two proteins may have homologous roles to those of OCRL1. The rest of the hits (four) only have the 5-Ptase domain

(**Supplementary Figure S3**) and showed only low levels of E-values to OCRL1 (**Supplementary Table S5**). Searching with type III and type IV PI 5-phosphatases detected the six candidates with higher E-values. Based on this result, we tentatively assigned the four proteins as type II PI 5-phosphatases homologous to OCRL1 (**Figure 4**; **Supplementary Table S2**). When searched with synaptojanin1 and synaptojanin2, nine candidates with E-values lower than 1×10^{-25} were detected. Six of them are identical to the above mentioned OCRL1 homologs and showed lower E-values to OCRL1. Other three candidates have a SAC domain, and thus they are considered as SAC homologs (see section 10). EHI_040380, as one of these SAC domain-containing proteins, was found to also harbor a DNase I domain by InterPro analysis (https://www.ebi.ac.uk/interpro/). The domain is classified in the endonuclease/exonuclease/phosphatase superfamily (IPR036691). As mentioned above, the 5-Ptase domain shares homology to the apurinic/apyrimidinic family of endonucleases (Whisstock et al., 2000), but EHI_040380 lacks the residues critical for the 5-Ptase activity (**Supplementary Figure S3**). Consequently, we classified this domain as "SAC with DNase I or 5-Ptase" domain (**Figure 4**). If this protein has a IP 5-phosphatase activity, it may act as synaptojanin in *E. histolytica*.

10. Sac FAMILY PHOSPHATASES

10.1. General Description of Sac

The first member of Sac (suppressor of actin), Sac1, was originally discovered in yeast by two independent genetic suppressor screens, which searched for the genes that rescued either actin cytoskeleton defects (Novick et al., 1989) or secretion defects caused by *sec14* mutation (Cleves et al., 1989). The catalytic domain of the Sac family phosphatases conserves the CX_5R motif, which is commonly found in protein and PI phosphatases. According to the crystal structure, configuration of Sac1 catalytic center has a unique feature compared with PTEN and MTMs (Lee et al., 1999; Begley et al., 2003, 2006; Manford et al., 2010). The catalytic cysteine is oriented away from the conserved arginine in Sac1, while the corresponding residue in PTEN and MTMs faces toward the arginine and generates a narrow active center. This observation suggests that Sac1's catalytic center probably undergoes a conformational change during the catalysis. This premise appears to agree with the fact that Sac1 is an allosteric enzyme, and its activity is stimulated by anionic phospholipids (Zhong et al., 2012). The Sac domain is also found in synaptojanins (see section 9.1). It is responsible for the removal of phosphate from D3, D4, and/or D5 positions of various PIs, and thus, Sac is considered to be a PI phosphatase with broad specificity. Sac1 dephosphorylates PtdIns3P, PtdIns4P, and PtdIns(3,5)P_2, but not PtdIns(4,5)P_2 (Nemoto et al., 2000), and Sac2 acts on D5 position of PtdIns(4,5)P_2 and PtdIns(3,4,5)P_3 (Minagawa et al., 2001), whereas Sac3 hydrolyzes only PtdIns(3,5)P_2 (Botelho et al., 2008). Sac1 is mostly localized on the ER and shuttles between the Golgi and ER. The C-terminus of Sac1 mediates an association with the COPI complex via a conserved KXKXX motif and this association induces the retrieval of Sac1 to the ER (Blagoveshchenskaya et al., 2008). Sac1 preferentially utilizes PtdIns4P as its substrate, and mutations that downregulate Sac1 cause the cellular PtdIns4P levels to increase in yeast and mammals (Guo et al., 1999; Nemoto et al., 2000). Sac1 has been also shown to be involved in the maintenance of the plasma membrane PtdIns4P levels at the ER-plasma membrane junctions (Stefan et al., 2011). Sac2 is a mammalian-specific negative regulator of the Akt pathway (Trivedi et al., 2007), and involved in the endocytic pathway as a PI 4-phosphatase (Nakatsu et al., 2015). Sac3 is important for the regulation of the endocytic pathway given that it regulates PtdIns(3,5)P_2 levels. Sac3 deficiency causes PtdIns(3,5)P_2 levels to increase and impairs late-endosome to lysosome transition. It is also involved in the regulation of PIPKIII enzymatic activity (see section 6.3.1).

10.2. Sac of *E. histolytica*

In the *E. histolytica* genome database, three proteins (EHI_141860, EHI_040380, EHI_048570) showed E-values lower than 1×10^{-10} with human Sac1 in a blastp search. These proteins were also detected when Sac2 and Sac3 were used as queries, and the E-values were lower than those obtained with Sac1. Therefore, these three proteins seem to be homologous to the human Sac1. EHI_141860 has the highest homology to the human Sac1, conserves the two transmembrane domains (**Figure 4**), and thus, it is considered to be the *E. histolytica* Sac1 ortholog. EHI_141860 also has the C-terminal COPI complex binding motif, KXKXX. As mentioned above, EHI_040380 has a DNaseI domain. Since 5-Ptase domain shares homology to the apurinic/apyrimidinic family of endonucleases (Whisstock et al., 2000), there is a possibility that this protein functions like synaptojanin. However, as the domain in EHI_040380 lacks the residues critical for the active center of PI 5-phosphatase (**Supplementary Figure S3**), we classified it as "SAC with DNase I or PI 5-phosphatase" domain (**Figure 4**). Nevertheless, further experimental evidence on its PI 5-phosphatase potential is necessary. Since *E. histolytica* appears to lack PI 4-phosphatases (see section 8), Sac orthologs may act as PI 4-phosphatase in this organism.

11. POSSIBLE PATHWAY-DEPENDENT COORDINATED REGULATION OF KEY PI METABOLIZING ENZYMES

11.1. Biosynthetic, Secretory, and Exocytotic Pathways

While a majority of interconversion steps between specific PIs are catalyzed by >1 enzymes, some steps are catalyzed by a single enzyme encoded by a single gene, which may suggest the significance of the enzyme. Furthermore, mRNA expression levels, inferred by transcriptomic analyses, often suggest biological importance of the enzyme(s) for the reaction under given conditions. In the biosynthetic and secretory pathways, the PtdIns4P level is maintained in an organelle specific fashion: low in the ER and high in the Golgi, by the coordinated action of PI 4-kinases, PI4KIIα and PI4KIIIβ, and

Sac1 (Blumental-Perry et al., 2006; Graham and Burd, 2011; Bajaj Pahuja et al., 2015). *E. histolytica* possesses only one PI 4-kinase, EHI_148700, which is most likely involved in this pathway. Role of Sac1 to maintain the low PtdIns4P level in the ER was shown (Bajaj Pahuja et al., 2015). It is conceivable to assume a single two transmembrane domain-containing PI-phosphatase Sac, EHI_141860, likely plays important role to maintain the low PtdIns4P level in the Golgi to regulate biosynthetic and secretory pathways. The transcriptome data also suggest the robust expression (**Supplementary Figure S1**) and thus the significance of EHI_141860.

Since clathrin-mediated trafficking machinery for the exocytic pathway is well-conserved in this organism (Clark et al., 2007), PtdIns4P is likely used in the Golgi apparatus as a key signaling molecule to recruit effector molecules, such as clathrin binding proteins AP, Arf, and Rab11for cargo selection and packaging. Following the generation of transport vesicles in the Golgi, PtdIns4P on the PtdIns4P-rich transport vesicles is replaced with sterol by oxysterol binding protein (OSBP), to form sterol-rich vesicles (Schink et al., 2016). This exchange is necessary to recruit exocyst complex onto the transfer vesicles and also function as sterol transfer mechanism from the ER to the plasma membrane (Schink et al., 2016). It remains elusive if this mechanism also works in *E. histolytica*, although its genome encodes 2-4 possible OSBP (Das and Nozaki, 2018).

At the plasma membrane, PtdIns(4,5)P_2 generated from PtdIns4P by single type I PIP kinase, EHI_153770, likely determines the site of exocytosis, where the exocyst complex mediates a release of the content of the sterol-rich secretory vesicles. Sec3 and Exo70 of the exocyst complex are known PtdIns(4,5)P_2 effectors on secretory vesicles. On the plasma membrane, Syntaxin-1, CAPS, Munc13-1/2, and Synaptotagmin-1 involved in the fusion of transport vesicles and the plasma membrane, leading to secretion (Martin, 2015). *E. histolytica* conserves a homolog of Syntaxin (EHI_052830, E-value 1×10^{-18}), Sec3 (EHI_148590, E-value 9×10^{-6}), and Exo70 (EHI_142040, E-value 2×10^{-8}). The functionality of the apparently conserved basic amino acids implicated for PtdIns(4,5)P_2 binding should be verified for the amebic homolog (Martin, 2015; K. Nakada-Tsukui data not shown).

11.2. Endocytic Pathways

In the clathrin-dependent endocytic pathway, AP complex connects membrane cargo receptors and clathrin via PtdIns(4,5)P_2 by recognizing the cytoplasmic region of the cargo receptors and PtdIns(4,5)P_2. In this process, single type I PIP kinase, EHI_153770, is necessary to synthesize PtdIns(4,5)P_2 from PtdIns4P. During the scission of the vesicles from the plasma membrane, generation of PtdIns(3,4)P_2 from PtdIns4P by class II PI 3-kinase is necessary to recruit SNX9 (sorting nexin that recognizes membrane curvature and PIs) in mammals. However, *E. histolytica* does not possess either PX-domain containing class II PI 3-kinases or BAR domain containing SNXs, e.g., SNX9. However, it is conceivable that one or some of six class I PI 3-kinases also have PtdIns4P 3-kinase activity and some of putative SNXs lacking BAR domain have ability to recognize PIs (N. Watanabe et al., data not shown). Therefore, it is expected that as enclosed endosomes mature after closure, PtdIns(4,5)P_2 is subsequently dephosphorylated into PtdIns and then further phosphorylated to PtdIns3P by the action of type III PI 3-kinase, Vps34, which is present in *E. histolytica* as a single protein. In mammals, a series of dephosphorylation reactions involving PtdIns(4,5)P_2 are regulated by OCRL1 and Sac2 (Nakatsu et al., 2015) and Synaptojanins (Cremona et al., 1999). Since Synaptojanins, which contain PI 5-phosphatase and PI 4-phosphatase domains, are not conserved in *E. histolytica*, the most highly transcribed PI 5-phosphatase, EHI_160860, out of 6 type II PI 5-phosphatases, and one of two transmembrane lacking Sac proteins, EHI_040380 and EHI_048570, are likely involved in this process (**Figure 4; Supplementary Figure S1**).

11.3. Phago- and Trogocytic Pathways

During phagocytosis, one single type I PIP-kinase, EHI_153770, and/or one or more of six class I PI 3-kinases are likely involved in local enrichment of PtdIns(4,5)P_2 and PtdIns(3,4,5)P_3 from PtdIns4P in response to the signal from a not-yet-identified ligand receptor (most likely galatose/N-acetylgalactosamine specific lectin) for phagocytosis at the plasma membrane. Based on the mRNA expression levels, five out of 6 class I PI 3-kinase genes appear to be abundantly expressed at similar levels and thus, it is not clear which is predominantly involved in this process (**Supplementary Figure S1**). In mammalian THP-1 cells, isoform-specific roles of class I PI 3-kinases were reported: p110α is involved in FcγR-mediated phagocytosis and oxidative burst mediated by PMA or opsonized zymosan, but not in CR3-mediated phagocytosis (Lee et al., 2007). On the other hand, p110β is involved in Rab5 recruitment and activation during phagosome maturation, while p110δ is involved in adhesion to VCAM-1 (Kurosu and Katada, 2001; Ferreira et al., 2006; Thi et al., 2012; Whitecross and Anderson, 2017).

In *E. histolytica*, two different modes of ingestion for target uptake, phagocytosis and trogocytosis, have been observed, and they have been shown to be regulated by different AGC kinases in an isotype-specific manner. It is conceivable that different receptors and class I PI 3-kinases are differentially involved in these processes. Elucidation of the isoform-specific involvement of class I PI 3-kinases in trogocytosis and phagocytosis shall be important to understand the pathogenesis of *E. histolytica*.

On the enclosed phagosomes, PtdIns(4,5)P_2 and PtdIns(3,4,5)P_3 are, as also seen in endocytosis, dephosphorylated to PtdIns by PI-phosphatases and then phosphorylated again to form PtdIns3P by class III PI 3-kinase, such as OCRL1, NPP5B, SHIP, INPP5E, TMEM55a, myotubularin, Sac2, and Vps34, in mammals (Cox et al., 2001; Ai et al., 2006; Horan et al., 2007; Neukomm et al., 2011; Bohdanowicz et al., 2012; Levin et al., 2017; Morioka et al., 2018). Similarly, conversion of PIs on the *E. histolyica* phagosomes is expected to proceed in a similar but possibly modified fashion. Among a number of type II PI 5-phosphatases, Sacs, myotubularins, and type III PI 3-kinase, we assume the following members are likely involved in this process. Among eight myotubularins that appear to be catalytically active, three isotypes, EHI_016430, EHI_104710, and,

EHI_024380, show relatively high expression and are likely involved in this maturation process. Once phagosomes are decorated with PtdIns3P, PtdIns3P is further phosphorylated to PtdIns(3,5)P_2 as phagosomes are further maturated. While in mammals, PIKfyve is involved in this process, type III PIP-kinase lacking FYVE domain, EHI_049480, may be responsible for this reaction in *E. histolytica.* As described above (section 6.3.1), type III PIP-kinases form complex with Sac phosphatase and scaffold proteins (Sbrissa et al., 2007; Botelho et al., 2008; Jin et al., 2008). Since two Sacs lacking the transmembrane domain, EHI_040380 and EHI_048570, are present in *E. histolytica*, it is possible that one of them forms complex with EHI_049480, similar to mammalian Sac3, while the other independently works in endocytic and phagocytic pathways similar to mammalian Sac2 (Nakatsu et al., 2015; Levin et al., 2017).

11.4. Motility

In the regulation of cell motility, local accumulation of PtdIns(4,5)P_2 and PtdIns(3,4,5)P_3 at the leading edge is the key initial event. Similar to phagocytosis, type I PIP-kinase, EHI_153770, and some of six type I PI 3-kinases are likely involved in this process. Also, dephosphorylation of PtdIns(3,4,5)P_3 by PI 3-phosphatases, PTEN, and PI 5-phosphatase, SHIP, at the side and the rear of the cell is known to be indispensable to regulate local accumulation of the lipid signal in mammals. In *E. histolytica*, some of six PTEN homologs and six PI 5-phosphatases are likely involved in this process. Among three of six amebic PTENs that contain C2 domain and the putative cytosol localization signal (see section 7.1.2), two showed significantly higher expression levels than four other PTEN isotypes (**Supplementary Figure S1**). Altogether, these data suggest that these two PTENs, EHI_197010 and EHI_098450, may be involved in the formation and maintenance of cellular polarity in *E. histolytica.*

11.5. Nuclear Functions

It is conceivable that PI kinases and PIP phosphatases that contain the nuclear localization signal have specific roles in the nucleus such as chromatin regulation and transcription. Such PI kinases and PIP phosphatases include type I PIP-kinase, EHI_153770; PTEN, EHI_041900; MTM, EHI_070120; and PI 5-phosphatase, EHI_046590. Also, PTENs that lack the cytosol localization signal, EHI_041900, EHI_010360, and EHI_054460, may also be involved in nuclear functions.

12. CONCLUSION AND FUTURE PERSPECTIVE

One of the hallmarks of *E. histolytica* as an invasive eukaryotic pathogen is its extremely active cell motility accompanied with elaborate cytoskeletal rearrangement and membrane traffic. To enable such activities, spaciotemporal regulation of PI-mediated signaling that controls transient association with effector molecules is indispensable and accomplished via concerted regulation of PI metabolism. The *E. histolytica* genome encodes the majority of PI kinases and PI phosphatases conserved in model organisms. Strikingly, significant diversity of PI 3-kinases and PI 3-phosphatases was observed in *E. histolytica,* as represented by a higher level of complexity of class I PI 3-kinases, PTEN, MTM/MTMR, and IMLRKs in this unicellular eukaryote relative to human, which has a 100 times larger genome. The dependence of *E. histolytica* on the complexity of the D3 phosphate metabolism emphasizes the significance of PtdIns(3,4,5)P_3-centric pathways for pathogenesis and physiology of *E. histolytica.*

On the other hand, the regulatory subunit of PI kinases, except for class III PI 3-kinase, was not identified, suggesting that their regulatory mechanisms had been gained only in higher eukaryotes or had differently evolved in *E. histolytica* in a lineage-specific fashion. The latter was also observed as an example with PI 4-kinase regulator EFR3 which is not conserved between the yeast and human. PtdIns4P metabolism also appears to have uniquely evolved in *E. histolytica.* No PtdIns4P-specific phosphatases that show similarity to the canonical enzymes are conserved in *E. histolytica.* It harbors only one PIP kinase, type I PIP kinase, which generate PtdIns(4,5)P_2 from PtdIns4P. PtdIns4P is known as one of the major PIs and is important as it is the precursor of the most abundant PI, PtdIns(4,5)P_2. Since PtdIns(4,5)P_2 is indispensable for the regulation of actin cytoskeleton-dependent processes, which is vital for the pathogenesis of the amoeba, type I PIP kinase appears to be a rational drug target. Uniquely expanded gene families, such as class I PI 3-kinases and PTENs, may also be potential drug target. However, multiple enzymes may have a redundant role as shown for mammalian PIPKI (see section 6.1.1).

Besides expansion, certain families of PI kinases and PI phosphatases in *E. histolytica* are structurally unique in the sense that they have simpler domain configurations, especially type III PIP kinases and PI phosphatases, relative to their human counterparts with a exceptions such as inactive myotubularin/LRR/ROCO/kinase (IMLRK). Lineage-specific expansions of PIP phosphatases are found in particular for OCRL1 type II PI 5-phosphatase and IMLRK, some of which should be listed in the roster of rational drug targets once their functions are determined.

Extremely higher expression levels of two PTEN and one PI 5-phosphatase genes relative to other genes involved in PI metabolism may reflect the importance of phosphatases rather than kinases in stopping the PI signals. PTEN has also been reported to function as a protein phosphatase, and thus, it is also possible that the high expression of PTEN is because it has roles other than PI signaling (Shinde and Maddika, 2016; Wozniak et al., 2017).

Furthermore, it has recently been demonstrated that besides the phosphorylation status, type pf the acyl-chains in the lipids are important in the regulation of lipid functions (Choy et al., 2017). In mammals, the predominant type found in PIs is 1-stearoyl-2-arachidonoyl (18:0/20:4)

(Traynor-Kaplan et al., 2017). This acyl chain type is generated by lysocardiolipin acyltransferase (LYCAT) (Imae et al., 2012), whose deficiency persturbes PI-mediated-membrane traffic (Bone et al., 2017). Mechanisms underlying such acyl-dependent regulation of PI signaling and downstream cascades are just about to unveil in the lipid research field and should be explored in amebiasis research. Furthermore, a new family of lipid transport proteins that mediate the regulation of PI metabolisms in both the cytoplasm and the nucleus have been described (Das and Nozaki, 2018). It may also be of interest that several PI kinases and PI phosphatases as well as several PI species are localized in the nucleus. However, PI metabolism and physiological roles of PI in the nucleus is poorly understood.

AUTHOR CONTRIBUTIONS

All authors listed have made a substantial, direct and intellectual contribution to the work, and approved it for publication.

FUNDING

This work was supported in part by a grant for Research on Emerging and Re-emerging Infectious Diseases from Japan Agency for Medical Research and Development (AMED) (JP18fk0108046 and JP19fk0108046 to TN; JP18fk0108049 and JP19fk0108049 to KN-T), a grant for US-Japan Cooperative Medical Science Program from AMED (JP17jk0210018 to KN-T), grants from Japan Ministry of Education, Culture, Sports, Science, and Technology (MEXT)/Japan Society for the Promotion of Science (JSPS) (KAKENHI JP17K19416, and JP18H02650 to TN; JP16K08766, JP18H02650, and JP19H03463 to KN-T), a grant from the National Center for Global Health and Medicine (29–2013 to TN), and a grant from Science and Technology Research Partnership for Sustainable Development (SATREPS) from AMED and Japan International Cooperation Agency (JICA) to TN.

SUPPLEMENTARY MATERIAL

Supplementary Figure S1 (Image 1) | Expression levels of PI kinases and PI phosphatases in *E. histolytica* trophozoites. Relative expression levels of indicated PI kinase and PI phosphatase genes of the HM-1:IMSS cl6 reference strain during *in vitro* cultivation. Signal intensity was normalized against the transcript of RNA polymerase II gene. Two bars represent the data from two independent experiments (Husain et al., 2011; Penuliar et al., 2015).

Supplementary Figure S2 (Image 2) | Cytosolic localization signal in human and *E. histolytica* PTEN. The cytosol localization signal of human PTEN was aligned with the corresponding region of *E. histolytica* PTEN orthologs. Green underlines depict the key amino acids for the signal and the amino acids conserved in PTENs from human and *E. histolytica* are indicated with green boxes.

Supplementary Figure S3 (Image 3) | Conservation of consensus amino acid sequences in PI 5-phosphatases. Amino acids of two consensus regions of PI 5-phosphatases, human OCRL1 and *E. histolytica* orthologs. Gray boxes indicate conserved amino acids.

Supplementary Figure S4 (1–4) (Images 4–7) | Multiple alignment of class I PI 3-kinases. LKU domain and catalytic core are indicated by green and yellow bar, respectively.

Supplementary Figure S5 (1–3) (Images 8–10) | Multiple alignment of PTEN. Catalytic core is indicated by yellow bar.

Supplementary Table S1 (Tab 1 in Table 1) | Potential PI kinase orthologs in *E. histolytica*. *H. sapiens* enzymes used as queries, and E-values are shown.

Supplementary Table S2 (Tab 2 in Table 1) | Potential PI phosphatase orthologs in *E. histolytica*. *H. sapiens* enzymes used as queries, and E-values are also shown.

Supplementary Table S3 (Tab 3 in Table 1) | Similarity between *H. sapiens* and *E. histolytica* class I PI 3-kinases. *H. sapiens* isotypes used as queries, and E-values are also shown.

Supplementary Table S4 (Tab 4 in Table 1) | Similarity between *H. sapiens* and *E. histolytica* MTM and MTMRs. *H. sapiens* isotypes used as queries, and E-values are also shown.

Supplementary Table S5 (Tab 5 in Table 1) | Similarity between *H. sapiens* and *E. histolytica* PI 5-phosphatases.

Supplementary Table S6 (Tab 6 in Table 1) | Abbreviation list.

REFERENCES

Abysalh, J. C., Kuchnicki, L. L., and Larochelle, D. A. (2003). The identification of pats1, a novel gene locus required for cytokinesis in *Dictyostelium discoideum*. *Mol. Biol. Cell* 14, 14–25. doi: 10.1091/mbc.e02-06-0335

Ai, J., Maturu, A., Johnson, W., Wang, Y., Marsh, C. B., and Tridandapani, S. (2006). The inositolphosphatase SHIP-2 down-regulates FcgammaR-mediated phagocytosis in murinemacrophages independently of SHIP-1. *Blood* 107, 813–820. doi: 10.1182/blood-2005-05-1841

Aley, S. B., Scott, W. A., and Cohn, Z. A. (1980). Plasma membrane of *Entamoeba histolytica*. *J. Exp. Med.* 152, 391–404. doi: 10.1084/jem.152.2.391

Ali, V., and Nozaki, T. (2007). Current therapeutics, their problems, and sulfur-containing-amino-acid metabolism as a novel target against infections by "amitochondriate" protozoan parasites. *Clin. Microbiol. Rev.* 20, 164–187. doi: 10.1128/CMR.00019-06

Al-Qusairi, L., Prokic, I., Amoasii, L., Kretz, C., Messaddeq, N., Mandel, J. L., et al. (2013). Lack of myotubularin (MTM1) leads to muscle hypotrophy through unbalanced regulation of the autophagy and ubiquitin-proteasome pathways. *FASEB J.* 27, 3384–3394. doi: 10.1096/fj.12-220947

Andrä, J., Berninghausen, O., and Leippe, M. (2004). Membrane lipid composition protects *Entamoeba histolytica* from self-destruction by its pore-forming toxins. *FEBS Lett.* 564, 109–115. doi: 10.1016/S0014-5793(04)00324-2

Arico, S., Petiot, A., Bauvy, C., Dubbelhuis, P. F., Meijer, A. J., Codogno, P., et al. (2001). The tumor suppressor PTEN positively regulates macroautophagy by inhibiting the phosphatidylinositol 3-kinase/protein kinase B pathway. *J. Biol. Chem.* 276, 35243–35246. doi: 10.1074/jbc.C100319200

Artemenko, Y., Lampert, T. J., and Devreotes, P. N. (2014). Moving towards a paradigm: common mechanisms of chemotactic signaling in *Dictyostelium* and mammalian leukocytes. *Cell Mol. Life Sci.* 71, 3711–3747. doi: 10.1007/s00018-014-1638-8

Attree, O., Olivos, I. M., Okabe, I., Bailey, L. C., Nelson, D. L., Lewis, R. A., et al. (1992). The Lowe's oculocerebrorenal syndrome gene encodes a protein highly homologous to inositol polyphosphate-5-phosphatase. *Nature* 358, 239–242. doi: 10.1038/358239a0

Baird, D., Stefan, C., Audhya, A., Weys, S., and Emr, S. D. (2008). Assembly of the PtdIns 4-kinase Stt4 complex at the plasma membrane requires Ypp1 and Efr3. *J. Cell Biol.* 183, 1061–1074. doi: 10.1083/jcb.200804003

Bajaj Pahuja, K., Wang, J., Blagoveshchenskaya, A., Lim, L., Madhusudhan, M. S., Mayinger, P., et al. (2015). Phosphoregulatory protein 14-3-3 facilitates SAC1 transport from the endoplasmic reticulum. *Proc. Natl. Acad. Sci. U.S.A.* 112, E3199–E3206. doi: 10.1073/pnas.1509119112

Baldauf, S. L., and Palmer, J. D. (1993). Animals and fungi are each other's closest relatives: congruent evidence from multiple proteins. *Proc. Natl. Acad. Sci. U.S.A.* 90, 11558–11562. doi: 10.1073/pnas.90.24.11558

Balla, T. (2013). Phosphoinositides: tiny lipids with giant impact on cell regulation. *Physiol. Rev.* 93, 1019–1137. doi: 10.1152/physrev.00028.2012

Bansal, N., Mishra, P. J., Stein, M., DiPaola, R. S., and Bertino, J. R. (2015). Axl receptor tyrosine kinase is up-regulated in metformin resistant prostate cancer cells. *Oncotarget* 6, 15321–15331. doi: 10.18632/oncotarget.4148

Barbieri, M. A., Heath, C. M., Peters, E. M., Wells, A., Davis, J. N., and Stahl, P. D. (2001). Phosphatidylinositol-4-phosphate 5-kinase-1beta is essential for epidermal growth factor receptor-mediated endocytosis. *J. Biol. Chem.* 276, 47212–47216. doi: 10.1074/jbc.C100490200

Barlow, C. A., Laishram, R. S., and Anderson, R. A. (2010). Nuclear phosphoinositides: a signaling enigma wrapped in a compartmental conundrum. *Trends Cell Biol.* 20, 25–35. doi: 10.1016/j.tcb.2009.09.009

Barylko, B., Gerber, S. H., Binns, D. D., Grichine, N., Khvotchev, M., Südhof, T. C., et al. (2001). A novel family of phosphatidylinositol 4-kinases conserved from yeast to humans. *J. Biol. Chem.* 276, 7705–7708. doi: 10.1074/jbc.C000861200

Bauerfeind, R., Takei, K., and De Camilli, P. (1997). Amphiphysin I is associated with coated endocytic intermediates and undergoes stimulation-dependent dephosphorylation in nerve terminals. *J. Biol. Chem.* 272, 30984–30992. doi: 10.1074/jbc.272.49.30984

Begley, M. J., Taylor, G. S., Brock, M. A., Ghosh, P., Woods, V. L., and Dixon, J. E. (2006). Molecular basis for substrate recognition by MTMR2, a myotubularin family phosphoinositide phosphatase. *Proc. Natl. Acad. Sci. U.S.A.* 103, 927–932. doi: 10.1073/pnas.0510006103

Begley, M. J., Taylor, G. S., Kim, S. A., Veine, D. M., Dixon, J. E., and Stuckey, J. A. (2003). Crystal structure of a phosphoinositide phosphatase, MTMR2: insights into myotubular myopathy and Charcot-Marie-Tooth syndrome. *Mol. Cell* 12, 1391–1402. doi: 10.1016/S1097-2765(03)00486-6

Berridge, M. J. (1983). Rapid accumulation of inositol trisphosphate reveals that agonists hydrolyze polyphosphoinositides instead of phosphatidylinositol. *Biochem. J.* 212, 849–858. doi: 10.1042/bj2120849

Berridge, M. J. (1984). Inositol trisphosphate and diacylglycerol as second messengers. *Biochem. J.* 220, 345–360. doi: 10.1042/bj2200345

Berridge, M. J. (1987). Inositol trisphosphate and diacylglycerol: two interacting second messengers. *Annu. Rev. Biochem.* 56, 159–193. doi: 10.1146/annurev.bi.56.070187.001111

Berridge, M. J., Dawson, R. M., Downes, C. P., Heslop, J. P., and Irvine, R. F. (1983). Changes in the levelsof inositol phosphates after agonist-dependent hydrolysis of membrane phosphoinositides. *Biochem. J.* 212, 473–482. doi: 10.1042/bj2120473

Bharadwaj, R., Arya, R., Shahid Mansuri, M., Bhattacharya, S., and Bhattacharya, A. (2017). EhRho1 regulates plasma membrane blebbing through PI 3-kinase in *Entamoeba histolytica*. *Cell Microbiol.* 19:e12751. doi: 10.1111/cmi.12751

Bharadwaj, R., Sharma, S., Janhawi, Arya, R., Bhattacharya, S., and Bhattacharya, A. (2018). EhRho1 regulates phagocytosis by modulating actin dynamics through EhFormin1 and EhProfilin1 in *Entamoeba histolytica*. *Cell Microbiol.* 20:e12851. doi: 10.1111/cmi.12851

Bielas, S. L., Silhavy, J. L., Brancati, F., Kisseleva, M. V., Al-Gazali, L., Sztriha, L., et al. (2009). Mutations in INPP5E, encoding inositol polyphosphate-5-phosphatase E, link phosphatidyl inositol signaling to the ciliopathies. *Nat. Genet.* 41, 1032–1036. doi: 10.1038/ng.423

Billcliff, P. G., and Lowe, M. (2014). Inositol lipid phosphatases in membrane trafficking and human disease. *Biochem. J.* 461, 159–175. doi: 10.1042/BJ20140361

Birkeland, H. C., and Stenmark, H. (2004). Protein targeting to endosomes and phagosomes via FYVE and PX domains. *Curr. Top. Microbiol. Immunol.* 282, 89–115. doi: 10.1007/978-3-642-18805-3_4

Blagoveshchenskaya, A., Cheong, F. Y., Rohde, H. M., Glover, G., Knödler, A., Nicolson, T., et al. (2008). Integration of Golgi trafficking and growth factor signaling by the lipid phosphatase SAC1. *J. Cell Biol.* 180, 803–812. doi: 10.1083/jcb.200708109

Blazquez, S., Guigon, G., Weber, C., Syan, S., Sismeiro, O., Coppée, J. Y., et al. (2008). Chemotaxis of *Entamoeba histolytica* towards the pro-inflammatory cytokine TNF is based on PI3K signalling, cytoskeleton reorganization and the Galactose/N-acetylgalactosamine lectin activity. *Cell Microbiol.* 10, 1676–1686. doi: 10.1111/j.1462-5822.2008.01158.x

Blind, R. D., Suzawa, M., and Ingraham, H. A. (2012). Direct modification and activation of a nuclear receptor-PIP2 complex by the inositol lipid kinase IPMK. *Sci. Signal.* J5:ra44. doi: 10.1126/scisignal.2003111

Blondeau, F., Laporte, J., Bodin, S., Superti-Furga, G., Payrastre, B., and Mandel, J. L. (2000). Myotubularin, a phosphatase deficient in myotubular myopathy, acts on phosphatidylinositol 3-kinase and phosphatidylinositol 3-phosphate pathway. *Hum. Mol. Genet.* 9, 2223–2229. doi: 10.1093/oxfordjournals.hmg.a018913

Blumental-Perry, A., Haney, C. J., Weixel, K. M., Watkins, S. C., Weisz, O. A., and Aridor, M. (2006). Phosphatidylinositol 4-phosphate formation at ER exit sites regulates ER export. *Dev. Cell* 11, 671–682. doi: 10.1016/j.devcel.2006.09.001

Bohdanowicz, M., Balkin, D. M., De Camilli, P., and Grinstein, S. (2012). Recruitment of OCRL andInpp5B to phagosomes by Rab5 and APPL1 depletes phosphoinositides and attenuates Akt signaling. *Mol. Biol. Cell* 23, 176–187. doi: 10.1091/mbc.e11-06-0489

Bonangelino, C. J., Nau, J. J., Duex, J. E., Brinkman, M., Wurmser, A. E., Gary, J. D., et al. (2002). Osmotic stress-induced increase of phosphatidylinositol 3,5-bisphosphate requires Vac14p, an activator of the lipid kinase Fab1p. *J. Cell Biol.* 156, 1015–1028. doi: 10.1083/jcb.200201002

Bone, L. N., Dayam, R. M., Lee, M., Kono, N., Fairn, G. D., Arai, H., et al. (2017). The acyltransferase LYCAT controls specific phosphoinositides and related membrane traffic. *Mol. Biol. Cell* 28, 161–172. doi: 10.1091/mbc.e16-09-0668

Boronenkov, I. V., and Anderson, R. A. (1995). The sequence of phosphatidylinositol-4-phosphate 5-kinase defines a novel family of lipid kinases. *J. Biol. Chem.* 270, 2881–2284. doi: 10.1074/jbc.270.7.2881

Bosgraaf, L., Russcher, H., Smith, J. L., Wessels, D., Soll, D. R., and Van Haastert, P. J. (2002). A novel cGMP signalling pathway mediating myosin phosphorylation and chemotaxis in *Dictyostelium*. *EMBO J.* 21, 4560–4570. doi: 10.1093/emboj/cdf438

Bosgraaf, L., Waijer, A., Engel, R., Visser, A. J., Wessels, D., Soll, D., et al. (2005). RasGEF-containing proteins GbpC and GbpD have differential effects on cell polarity and chemotaxis in *Dictyostelium*. *J. Cell Sci.* 118, 1899–18910. doi: 10.1242/jcs.02317

Botelho, R. J., Efe, J. A., Teis, D., and Emr, S. D. (2008). Assembly of a Fab1 phosphoinositide kinase signaling complex requires the Fig4 phosphoinositide phosphatase. *Mol. Biol. Cell* 19, 4273–4286. doi: 10.1091/mbc.e08-04-0405

Braccini, L., Ciraolo, E., Campa, C. C., Perino, A., Longo, D. L., Tibolla, G., et al. (2015). PI3K-C2γ is a Rab5 effector selectively controlling endosomal Akt2 activation downstream of insulin signalling. *Nat. Commun.* 6:7400. doi: 10.1038/ncomms8400

Bridges, D., Ma, J. T., Park, S., Inoki, K., Weisman, L. S., and Saltiel, A. R. (2012). Phosphatidylinositol 3,5-bisphosphate plays a role in the activation and subcellular localization of mechanistic target of rapamycin 1. *Mol. Biol. Cell* 23, 2955–2962. doi: 10.1091/mbc.e11-12-1034

Brown, J. R., and Auger, K. R. (2011). Phylogenomics of phosphoinositide lipid kinases: perspectives on the evolution of second messenger signaling and drug discovery. *BMC Evol. Biol.* 11:4. doi: 10.1186/1471-2148-11-4

Bua, D. J., Martin, G. M., Binda, O., and Gozani, O. (2013). Nuclear phosphatidylinositol-5-phosphate regulates ING2 stability at discrete chromatin targets in response to DNA damage. *Sci. Rep.* 3:2137. doi: 10.1038/srep02137

Bultsma, Y., Keune, W. J., and Divecha, N. (2010). PIP4Kbeta interacts with and modulates nuclear localization of the high-activity PtdIns5P-4-kinase isoform PIP4Kalpha. *Biochem. J.* 430, 223–235. doi: 10.1042/BJ20100341

Bunce, M. W., Boronenkov, I. V., and Anderson, R. A. (2008). Coordinated activation of the nuclear ubiquitin ligase Cul3-SPOP by the generation of phosphatidylinositol 5-phosphate. *J. Biol. Chem.* 283, 8678–8686. doi: 10.1074/jbc.M710222200

Burke, J. E., Inglis, A. J., Perisic, O., Masson, G. R., McLaughlin, S. H., Rutaganira, F., et al. (2014). Structures of PI4KIIIβ complexes show simultaneous recruitment of Rab11 and its effectors. *Science* 344, 1035–1038. doi: 10.1126/science.1253397

Byekova, Y. A., Powell, R. R., Welter, B. H., and Temesvari, L. A. (2010). Localization of phosphatidylinositol (3,4,5)-trisphosphate to phagosomes in *Entamoeba histolytica* achieved using glutathione S-transferase- and green fluorescent protein-tagged lipid biosensors. *Infect. Immun.* 78, 125–137. doi: 10.1128/IAI.00719-09

Cabezas, A., Pattni, K., and Stenmark, H. (2006). Cloning and subcellular localization of a human phosphatidylinositol 3-phosphate 5-kinase, PIKfyve/Fab1. *Gene* 371, 34–41. doi: 10.1016/j.gene.2005.11.009

Cairns, P., Evron, E., Okami, K., Halachmi, N., Esteller, M., Herman, J. G., et al. (1998). Point mutation and homozygous deletion of PTEN/MMAC1 in primary bladder cancers. *Oncogene* 16, 3215–3218. doi: 10.1038/sj.onc.1201855

Campbell, R. B., Liu, F., and Ross, A. H. (2003). Allosteric activation of PTEN phosphatase byphosphatidylinositol 4,5-bisphosphate. *J. Biol. Chem.* 278, 33617–33620. doi: 10.1074/jbc.C300296200

Cao, Y., Wang, Y., Abi Saab, W. F., Yang, F., Pessin, J. E., and Backer, J. M. (2014). NRBF2 regulates macroautophagy as a component of Vps34 Complex I. *Biochem. J.* 461, 315–322. doi: 10.1042/BJ20140515

Carricaburu, V., Lamia, K. A., Lo, E., Favereaux, L., Payrastre, B., Cantley, L. C., et al. (2003). The phosphatidylinositol (PI)-5-phosphate 4-kinase type II enzyme controls insulin signaling by regulating PI-3,4,5-trisphosphate degradation. *Proc. Natl. Acad. Sci. U.S.A.* 100, 9867–9872. doi: 10.1073/pnas.1734038100

Chávez, M., Ena, S., Van Sande, J., de Kerchove d'Exaerde, A., Schurmans, S., and Schiffmann, S. N. (2015). Modulation of ciliary phosphoinositide content regulates trafficking and sonic hedgehog signaling output. *Dev. Cell* 34, 338–350. doi: 10.1016/j.devcel.2015.06.016

Chen, Y., and Yu, L. (2017). Recent progress in autophagic lysosome reformation. *Traffic* 18, 358–361. doi: 10.1111/tra.12484

Cheng, M. K., and Shearn, A. (2004). The direct interaction between ASH2, a *Drosophila* trithorax group protein, and SKTL, a nuclear phosphatidylinositol 4-phosphate 5-kinase, implies a role for phosphatidylinositol 4,5-bisphosphate in maintaining transcriptionally active chromatin. *Genetics* 167, 1213–1223. doi: 10.1534/genetics.103.018721

Choudhury, R., Diao, A., Zhang, F., Eisenberg, E., Saint-Pol, A., Williams, C., et al. (2005). Lowe syndrome protein OCRL1 interacts with clathrin and regulates protein trafficking between endosomes and the trans-Golgi network. *Mol. Biol. Cell* 16, 3467–3479. doi: 10.1091/mbc.e05-02-0120

Choudhury, R., Noakes, C. J., McKenzie, E., Kox, C., and Lowe, M. (2009). Differential clathrin binding and subcellular localization of OCRL1 splice isoforms. *J. Biol. Chem.* 284, 9965–9973. doi: 10.1074/jbc.M807442200

Chow, C. Y., Zhang, Y., Dowling, J. J., Jin, N., Adamska, M., Shiga, K., et al. (2007). Mutation of FIG4 causes neurodegeneration in the pale tremor mouse and patients with CMT4J. *Nature* 448, 68–72. doi: 10.1038/nature05876

Choy, C. H., Han, B. K., and Botelho, R. J. (2017). Phosphoinositide diversity, distribution, and effector function: stepping out of the box. *BioEssays* 39:1700121. doi: 10.1002/bies.201700121

Christoforidis, S., Miaczynska, M., Ashman, K., Wilm, M., Zhao, L., Yip, S. C., et al. (1999). Phosphatidylinositol-3-OH kinases are Rab5 effectors. *Nat. Cell Biol.* 1, 249–252. doi: 10.1038/12075

Chung, J. H., and Eng, C. (2005). Nuclear-cytoplasmic partitioning of phosphatase and tensin homologue deleted on chromosome 10 (PTEN) differentially regulates the cell cycle and apoptosis. *Cancer Res.* 65, 8096–8100. doi: 10.1158/0008-5472.CAN-05-1888

Chung, J. H., Ostrowski, M. C., Romigh, T., Minaguchi, T., Waite, K. A., and Eng, C. (2006). The ERK1/2 pathway modulates nuclear PTEN-mediated cell cycle arrest by cyclin D1 transcriptional regulation. *Hum. Mol. Genet.* 15, 2553–2559. doi: 10.1093/hmg/ddl177

Ciruela, A., Hinchliffe, K. A., Divecha, N., and Irvine, R. F. (2000). Nuclear targeting of the beta isoform of type II phosphatidylinositol phosphate kinase (phosphatidylinositol 5-phosphate 4-kinase) by its alpha-helix 7. *Biochem. J.* 346(Pt 3), 587–591. doi: 10.1042/bj3460587

Clark, C. G., Alsmark, U. C., Tazreiter, M., Saito-Nakano, Y., Ali, V., Marion, S., et al. (2007). Structure and content of the *Entamoeba histolytica* genome. *Adv. Parasitol.* 65, 51–190. doi: 10.1016/S0065-308X(07) 65002-7

Clarke, J. H., Emson, P. C., and Irvine, R. F. (2008). Localization of phosphatidylinositol phosphate kinase IIgamma in kidney to a membrane trafficking compartment within specialized cells of the nephron. *Am. J. Physiol. Renal. Physiol.* 295, F1422–1430. doi: 10.1152/ajprenal.903 10.2008

Clarke, J. H., Emson, P. C., and Irvine, R. F. (2009). Distribution and neuronal expression of phosphatidylinositol phosphate kinase IIgamma in the mouse brain. *J. Comp. Neurol.* 517, 296–312. doi: 10.1002/cne.22161

Clarke, J. H., Letcher, A. J., D'santos, C. S., Halstead, J. R., Irvine, R. F., and Divecha, N. (2001). Inositol lipids are regulated during cell cycle progression in the nuclei of murine erythroleukaemia cells. *Biochem. J.* 357(Pt 3), 905–910. doi: 10.1042/bj3570905

Clarke, J. H., Wang, M., and Irvine, R. F. (2010). Localization, regulation and function of type II phosphatidylinositol 5-phosphate 4-kinases. *Adv. Enzyme Regul.* 50, 12–18. doi: 10.1016/j.advenzreg.2009.10.006

Cleves, A. E., Novick, P. J., and Bankaitis, V. A. (1989). Mutations in the SAC1 gene suppress defects in yeast Golgi and yeast actin function. *J. Cell Biol.* 109(6 Pt 1), 2939–2950. doi: 10.1083/jcb.109.6.2939

Cockcroft, S. (2001). Signalling roles of mammalian phospholipase D1 and D2. *Cell. Mol. Life Sci.* 58, 1674–1687. doi: 10.1007/PL00000805

Cox, D., Dale, B. M., Kashiwada, M., Helgason, C. D., and Greenberg, S. (2001). A regulatory role for Src homology 2 domain-containing inositol 5'-phosphatase (SHIP) in phagocytosis mediated by Fc gamma receptors and complement receptor 3 (alpha(M) beta(2);CD11b/CD18). *J. Exp. Med.* 193, 61–71. doi: 10.1084/jem.193.1.61

Creba, J. A., Downes, C. P., Hawkins, P. T., Brewster, G., Michell, R. H., and Kirk, C. J. (1983). Rapid breakdown of phosphatidylinositol 4-phosphate and phosphatidylinositol 4,5-bisphosphate in rat hepatocytes stimulated by vasopressin and other Ca2-mobilizing hormones. *Biochem. J.* 212, 733–747. doi: 10.1042/bj2120733

Cremona, O., Di Paolo, G., Wenk, M. R., Lüthi, A., Kim, W. T., Takei, K., et al. (1999). Essential role of phosphoinositide metabolism in synaptic vesicle recycling. *Cell* 99, 179–188. doi: 10.1016/S0092-8674(00)81649-9

Dall'Armi, C., Hurtado-Lorenzo, A., Tian, H., Morel, E., Nezu, A., Chan, R. B., et al. (2010). The phospholipase D1 pathway modulates macroautophagy. *Nat. Commun.* 1:142. doi: 10.1038/ncomms1144

D'Angelo, G., Vicinanza, M., Di Campli, A., and DeMatteis, M. A. (2008). The multiple roles of PtdIns(4)P – not just the precursor of PtdIns(4,5)P2. *J. Cell Sci.* 21(Pt 12), 1955–1963. doi: 10.1242/jcs.023630

Das, K., and Nozaki, T. (2018). Non-vesicular lipid transport machinery in *Entamoeba histolytica*. *Front. Cell Infect. Microbiol.* 8:315. doi: 10.3389/fcimb.2018.00315

de Graaf, P., Klapisz, E. E., Schulz, T. K., Cremers, A. F., Verkleij, A. J., and van Bergen en Henegouwen, P. M. (2002). Nuclear localization of phosphatidylinositol 4-kinase beta. *J. Cell Sci.* 115(Pt 8), 1769–1775.

de Graaf, P., Zwart, W. T., van Dijken, R. A., Deneka, M., Schulz, T. K., Geijsen, N., et al. (2004). Phosphatidylinositol 4-kinase beta is critical for functional association of rab11 with the Golgi complex. *Mol. Biol. Cell* 15, 2038–2047. doi: 10.1091/mbc.e03-12-0862

de Heuvel, E., Bell, A. W., Ramjaun, A. R., Wong, K., Sossin, W. S., and McPherson, P. S. (1997). Identification of the major synaptojanin-binding proteins in brain. *J. Biol. Chem.* 272, 8710–8716. doi: 10.1074/jbc.272.13.8710

De Matteis, M. A., Wilson, C., and D'Angelo, G. (2013). Phosphatidylinositol-4-phosphate: the Golgi and beyond. *Bioessays* 35, 612–622. doi: 10.1002/bies.201200180

De Smedt, F., Verjans, B., Mailleux, P., and Erneux, C. (1994). Cloning and expression of human brain type I inositol 1,4,5-trisphosphate 5-phosphatase. High levels of mRNA in cerebellar Purkinje cells. *FEBS Lett.* 347, 69–72. doi: 10.1016/0014-5793(94)00509-5

Demmel, L., Beck, M., Klose, C., Schlaitz, A. L., Gloor, Y., Hsu, P. P., et al. (2008). Nucleocytoplasmic shuttling of the Golgi phosphatidylinositol 4-kinase Pik1 is regulated by 14-3-3 proteins and coordinates Golgi function with cell growth. *Mol. Biol. Cell* 19, 1046–1061. doi: 10.1091/mbc.e07-02-0134

Denning, G., Jean-Joseph, B., Prince, C., Durden, D. L., and Vogt, P. K. (2007). A short N-terminal sequence of PTEN controls cytoplasmic localization and is required for suppression of cell growth. *Oncogene* 26, 3930–3940. doi: 10.1038/sj.onc.1210175

Desrivières, S., Cooke, F. T., Parker, P. J., and Hall, M. N. (1998). MSS4, a phosphatidylinositol-4-phosphate 5-kinase required for organization of the actin cytoskeleton in *Saccharomyces cerevisiae*. *J. Biol. Chem.* 273, 15787–15793. doi: 10.1074/jbc.273.25.15787

Devereaux, K., Dall'Armi, C., Alcazar-Roman, A., Ogasawara, Y., Zhou, X., Wang, F., et al. (2013). Regulation of mammalian autophagy by class II and III PI 3-kinases through PI3P synthesis. *PLoS ONE* 8:e76405. doi: 10.1371/journal.pone.0076405

Di Paolo, G., and De Camilli, P. (2006). Phosphoinositides in cell regulation and membrane dynamics. *Nature* 443, 651–657. doi: 10.1038/nature05185

Di Paolo, G., Pellegrini, L., Letinic, K., Cestra, G., Zoncu, R., Voronov, S., et al. (2002). Recruitment and regulation of phosphatidylinositol phosphate kinase type 1 gamma by the FERM domain of talin. *Nature* 420, 85–89. doi: 10.1038/nature01147

Dibble, C. C., and Cantley, L. C. (2015). Regulation of mTORC1 by PI3K signaling. *Trends Cell Biol.* 25, 545–555. doi: 10.1016/j.tcb.2015.06.002

Dieck, C. B., Boss, W. F., and Perera, I. Y. (2012). A role for phosphoinositides in regulating plant nuclear functions. *Front. Plant Sci.* 3:50. doi: 10.3389/fpls.2012.00050

Divecha, N., Roefs, M., Halstead, J. R., D'Andrea, S., Fernandez-Borga, M., Oomen, L., et al. (2000). Interaction of the type I alpha PIPkinase with phospholipase D: a role for the local generation of phosphatidylinositol 4, 5-bisphosphate in the regulation of PLD2 activity. *EMBO J.* 19, 5440–5449. doi: 10.1093/emboj/19.20.5440

Divecha, N., Truong, O., Hsuan, J. J., Hinchliffe, K. A., and Irvine, R. F. (1995). The cloning and sequence of the C isoform of PtdIns4P 5-kinase. *Biochem. J.* 309(Pt 3), 715–719. doi: 10.1042/bj3090715

Doughman, R. L., Firestone, A. J., and Anderson, R. A. (2003). Phosphatidylinositol phosphate kinases put PI4,5P(2) in its place. *J. Membr. Biol.* 194, 77–89. doi: 10.1007/s00232-003-2027-7

Dove, S. K., McEwen, R. K., Mayes, A., Hughes, D. C., Beggs, J. D., and Michell, R. H. (2002). Vac14 controls PtdIns(3,5)P(2) synthesis and Fab1-dependent protein trafficking to the multivesicular body. *Curr. Biol.* 12, 885–893. doi: 10.1016/S0960-9822(02)00891-6

Dressman, M. A., Olivos-Glander, I. M., Nussbaum, R. L., and Suchy, S. F. (2000). Ocrl1, a PtdIns(4,5)P(2) 5-phosphatase, is localized to the trans-Golgi network of fibroblasts and epithelial cells. *J. Histochem. Cytochem.* 48, 179–190. doi: 10.1177/002215540004800203

Drinjakovic, J., Jung, H., Campbell, D. S., Strochlic, L., Dwivedy, A., and Holt, C. E. (2010). E3 ligase Nedd4 promotes axon branching by downregulating PTEN. *Neuron* 65, 341–357. doi: 10.1016/j.neuron.2010.01.017

Duex, J. E., Nau, J. J., Kauffman, E. J., and Weisman, L. S. (2006). Phosphoinositide 5-phosphatase Fig4p is required for both acute rise and subsequent fall in stress-induced phosphatidylinositol 3,5-bisphosphate levels. *Eukaryot. Cell* 5, 723–731. doi: 10.1128/EC.5.4.723-731.2006

Elliott, K. H., and Brugmann, S. A. (2019). Sending mixed signals: cilia-dependent signaling during development and disease. *Dev. Biol.* 447, 28–41. doi: 10.1016/j.ydbio.2018.03.007

Engelman, J. A., Luo, J., and Cantley, L. C. (2006). The evolution of phosphatidylinositol 3-kinases as regulators of growth and metabolism. *Nat. Rev. Genet.* 7, 606–619. doi: 10.1038/nrg1879

Erdmann, K. S., Mao, Y., McCrea, H. J., Zoncu, R., Lee, S., Paradise, S., et al. (2007). A role of the Lowe syndrome protein OCRL in early steps of the endocytic pathway. *Dev. Cell* 13, 377–379. doi: 10.1016/j.devcel.2007.08.004

Fain, J. N., and Berridge, M. J. (1979). Relationship between phosphatidylinositol synthesis and recovery of 5-hydroxytryptamine-responsive Ca^{2+} flux in blowfly salivary glands. *Biochem. J.* 180, 655–661. doi: 10.1042/bj1800655

Fan, W., Nassiri, A., and Zhong, Q. (2011). Autophagosome targeting and membrane curvature sensing by Barkor/Atg14(L). *Proc. Natl. Acad. Sci. U.S.A.* 108, 7769–7774. doi: 10.1073/pnas.1016472108

Faucherre, A., Desbois, P., Nagano, F., Satre, V., Lunardi, J., Gacon, G., et al. (2005). Lowe syndrome protein Ocrl1 is translocated to membrane ruffles upon Rac GTPase activation: a new perspective on Lowe syndrome pathophysiology. *Hum. Mol. Genet.* 14, 1441–1448. doi: 10.1093/hmg/ddi153

Faucherre, A., Desbois, P., Satre, V., Lunardi, J., Dorseuil, O., and Gacon, G. (2003). Lowe syndrome protein OCRL1 interacts with Rac GTPase in the trans-Golgi network. *Hum. Mol. Genet.* 12, 2449–2456. doi: 10.1093/hmg/ddg250

Ferguson, C. J., Lenk, G. M., and Meisler, M. H. (2009). Defective autophagy in neurons and astrocytes from mice deficient in PI(3,5)P2. *Hum. Mol. Genet.* 18, 4868–4878. doi: 10.1093/hmg/ddp460

Ferreira, A. M., Isaacs, H., Hayflick, J. S., Rogers, K. A., and Sandig, M. (2006). The p110delta isoform of PI3K differentially regulates beta1 and beta2 integrin-mediated monocyte adhesion and spreading and modulates diapedesis. *Microcirculation* 13, 439–456. doi: 10.1080/10739680600776062

Ferron, M., and Vacher, J. (2006). Characterization of the murine Inpp4b gene and identification of a novel isoform. *Gene* 376, 152–156. doi: 10.1016/j.gene.2006.02.022

Franco, I., Gulluni, F., Campa, C. C., Costa, C., Margaria, J. P., Ciraolo, E., et al. (2014). PI3K class II α controls spatially restricted endosomal PtdIns3P and Rab11 activation to promote primary cilium function. *Dev. Cell* 28, 647–658. doi: 10.1016/j.devcel.2014.01.022

Freeman, D. J., Li, A. G., Wei, G., Li, H. H., Kertesz, N., Lesche, R., et al. (2003). PTEN tumor suppressor regulates p53 protein levels and activity through phosphatase-dependent and -independent mechanisms. *Cancer Cell* 3, 117–130. doi: 10.1016/S1535-6108(03)00021-7

Frere, S. G., Chang-Ileto, B., and Di Paolo, G. (2012). Role of phosphoinositides at the neuronal synapse. *Subcell. Biochem.* 59, 131–175. doi: 10.1007/978-94-007-3015-1_5

Funderburk, S. F., Wang, Q. J., and Yue, Z. (2010). The Beclin 1-VPS34 complex–at the crossroads of autophagy and beyond. *Trends Cell Biol.* 20, 355–362. doi: 10.1016/j.tcb.2010.03.002

Furnari, F. B., Huang, H. J., and Cavenee, W. K. (1998). The phosphoinositol phosphatase activity of PTEN mediates a serum-sensitive G1 growth arrest in glioma cells. *Cancer Res.* 58, 5002–5008.

Furukawa, A., Nakada-Tsukui, K., and Nozaki, T. (2012). Novel transmembrane receptor involved in phagosome transport of lysozymes and β-hexosaminidase in the enteric protozoan *Entamoeba histolytica*. *PLoS Pathog.* 8:e1002539. doi: 10.1371/journal.ppat.1002539

Furukawa, A., Nakada-Tsukui, K., and Nozaki, T. (2013). Cysteine protease-binding protein family 6 mediates the trafficking of amylases to phagosomes in the enteric protozoan *Entamoeba histolytica*. *Infect. Immun.* 81, 1820–1829. doi: 10.1128/IAI.00915-12

Furuya, N., Yu, J., Byfield, M., Pattingre, S., and Levine, B. (2005). The evolutionarily conserved domain of Beclin 1 is required for Vps34 binding, autophagy and tumor suppressor function. *Autophagy* 1, 46–52. doi: 10.4161/auto.1.1.1542

Gaidarov, I., Smith, M. E., Domin, J., and Keen, J. H. (2001). The class II phosphoinositide 3-kinase C2alpha is activated by clathrin and regulates clathrin-mediated membrane trafficking. *Mol. Cell* 7, 443–449. doi: 10.1016/S1097-2765(01)00191-5

Gaidarov, I., Zhao, Y., and Keen, J. H. (2005). Individual phosphoinositide 3-kinase C2alpha domain activities independently regulate clathrin function. *J. Biol. Chem.* 280, 40766–40772. doi: 10.1074/jbc.M507731200

Galiano, F. J., Ulug, E. T., and Davis, J. N. (2002). Overexpression of murine phosphatidylinositol 4-phosphate 5-kinase type I beta disrupts a phosphatidylinositol 4,5 bisphosphate regulated endosomal pathway. *J. Cell Biochem.* 85, 131–145. doi: 10.1002/jcb.10100

Garcia, C. R. S., Alves, E., Pereira, P. H. S., Bartlett, P. J., Thomas, A. P., Mikoshiba, K., et al. (2017). InsP3 signaling in apicomplexan parasites. *Curr. Top. Med. Chem.* 17, 2158–2165. doi: 10.2174/1568026617666170130121042

Garcia-Bustos, J. F., Marini, F., Stevenson, I., Frei, C., and Hall, M. N. (1994). PIK1, an essential phosphatidylinositol 4-kinase associated with the yeast nucleus. *EMBO J.* 13, 2352–2361. doi: 10.1002/j.1460-2075.1994.tb06519.x

Garcia-Gonzalo, F. R., Phua, S. C., Roberson, E. C., Garcia, G. 3rd, Abedin, M., Schurmans, S., et al. (2015). Phosphoinositides regulate ciliary protein trafficking to modulate hedgehog signaling. *Dev. Cell* 34, 400–409. doi: 10.1016/j.devcel.2015.08.001

Gary, J. D., Sato, T. K., Stefan, C. J., Bonangelino, C. J., Weisman, L. S., and Emr, S. D. (2002). Regulation of Fab1 phosphatidylinositol 3-phosphate 5-kinase pathway by Vac7 protein and Fig4, a polyphosphoinositide phosphatase family member. *Mol. Biol. Cell* 13, 1238–1251. doi: 10.1091/mbc.01-10-0498

Gary, J. D., Wurmser, A. E., Bonangelino, C. J., Weisman, L. S., and Emr, S. D. (1998). Fab1p is essential for PtdIns(3)P 5-kinase activity and the maintenance of vacuolar size and membrane homeostasis. *J. Cell Biol.* 143, 65–79. doi: 10.1083/jcb.143.1.65

Gathiram, V., and Jackson, T. F. (1985). Frequency distribution of *Entamoeba histolytica* zymodemes in a rural South African population. *Lancet* 1, 719–721. doi: 10.1016/S0140-6736(85)91263-2

Gillooly, D. J., Morrow, I. C., Lindsay, M., Gould, R., Bryant, N. J., Gaullier, J. M., et al. (2000). Localization of phosphatidylinositol 3-phosphate in yeast and mammalian cells. *EMBO J.* 19, 4577–4588. doi: 10.1093/emboj/19.17.4577

Giri, B., Raha, S., Bhattacharyya, B., Biswas, S., and Biswas, B. B. (1996). Relative importance of inositol (1,4,5) trisphosphate and inositol (1,3,4,5) tetrakisphosphate in *Entamoeba histolytica*. *FEBS Lett.* 393, 109–112. doi: 10.1016/0014-5793(96)00866-6

Giudici, M. L., Emson, P. C., and Irvine, R. F. (2004). A novel neuronal-specific splice variant of Type I phosphatidylinositol 4-phosphate 5-kinase isoform gamma. *Biochem J.* 379, 489–496. doi: 10.1042/bj20031394

Goetz, S. C., and Anderson, K. V. (2010). The primary cilium: a signalling centre during vertebrate development. *Nat. Rev. Genet.* 11, 331–344. doi: 10.1038/nrg2774

Gokhale, A., Ryder, P. V., Zlatic, S. A., and Faundez, V. (2016). Identification of the interactome of a palmitoylated membrane protein, phosphatidylinositol 4-kinase type II alpha. *Methods Mol. Biol.* 1376, 35–42. doi: 10.1007/978-1-4939-3170-5_4

Goldberg, J. M., Bosgraaf, L., Van Haastert, P. J., and Smith, J. L. (2002). Identification of four candidate cGMP targets in *Dictyostelium*. *Proc. Natl. Acad. Sci. U.S.A.* 99, 6749–6754. doi: 10.1073/pnas.102167299

Goldston, A. M., Powell, R. R., Koushik, A. B., and Temesvari, L. A. (2012). Exposure to host ligands correlates with colocalization of Gal/GalNAc lectin subunits in lipid rafts and phosphatidylinositol (4,5)-bisphosphate signaling in *Entamoeba histolytica*. *Eukaryot. Cell* 11, 743–751. doi: 10.1128/EC.00054-12

Gozani, O., Karuman, P., Jones, D. R., Ivanov, D., Cha, J., Lugovskoy, A. A., et al. (2003). The PHD finger of the chromatin-associated protein ING2 functions as a nuclear phosphoinositide receptor. *Cell* 114, 99–111. doi: 10.1016/S0092-8674(03)00480-X

Graham, T. R., and Burd, C. G. (2011). Coordination of Golgi functions by phosphatidylinositol 4-kinases. *Trends Cell Biol.* 21, 113–121. doi: 10.1016/j.tcb.2010.10.002

Gulati, P., and Thomas, G. (2007). Nutrient sensing in the mTOR/S6K1 signalling pathway. *Biochem. Soc. Trans.* 35, 236–238. doi: 10.1042/BST0350236

Guldberg, P., thor Straten, P., Birck, A., Ahrenkiel, V., Kirkin, A. F., and Zeuthen, J. (1997). Disruption of the MMAC1/PTEN gene by deletion or mutation is a frequent event in malignant melanoma. *Cancer Res.* 57, 3660–3663.

Guo, S., Stolz, L. E., Lemrow, S. M., and York, J. D. (1999). SAC1-like domains of yeast SAC1, INP52, and INP53 and of human synaptojanin encode polyphosphoinositide phosphatases. *J. Biol. Chem.* 274, 12990–12995. doi: 10.1074/jbc.274.19.12990

Gurung, R., Tan, A., Ooms, L. M., McGrath, M. J., Huysmans, R. D., Munday, A. D., et al. (2003). Identification of a novel domain in two mammalian inositol-polyphosphate 5-phosphatases that mediates membrane ruffle localization. The inositol 5-phosphatase skip localizes to the endoplasmic reticulum and translocates to membrane ruffles following epidermal growth factor stimulation. *J. Biol. Chem.* 278, 11376–11385. doi: 10.1074/jbc.M209991200

Haffner, C., Takei, K., Chen, H., Ringstad, N., Hudson, A., Butler, M. H., et al. (1997). Synaptojanin 1: localization on coated endocytic intermediates in nerve terminals and interaction of its 170 kDa isoform with Eps15. *FEBS Lett.* 419, 175–180. doi: 10.1016/S0014-5793(97)01451-8

Hamann, B. L., and Blind, R. D. (2018). Nuclear phosphoinositide regulation of chromatin. *J. Cell Physiol.* 233, 107–123. doi: 10.1002/jcp.25886

Hammond, G. R., and Balla, T. (2015). Polyphosphoinositide binding domains: key to inositol lipid biology. *Biochim. Biophys. Acta* 1851, 746–758. doi: 10.1016/j.bbalip.2015.02.013

Hansen, S. B., Tao, X., and MacKinnon, R. (2011). Structural basis of PIP2 activation of the classical inward rectifier K^+ channel Kir2.2. *Nature* 477, 495–498. doi: 10.1038/nature10370

Hasegawa, J., Iwamoto, R., Otomo, T., Nezu, A., Hamasaki, M., and Yoshimori, T. (2016). Autophagosome-lysosome fusion in neurons requires INPP5E, a protein associated with Joubert syndrome. *EMBO J.* 35, 1853–1867. doi: 10.15252/embj.201593148

Hasegawa, J., Strunk, B. S., and Weisman, L. S. (2017). PI5P and PI(3,5)P(2): minor, but essential phosphoinositides. *Cell Struct. Funct.* 42, 49–60. doi: 10.1247/csf.17003

Hashimoto, M., Enomoto, M., Morales, J., Kurebayashi, N., Sakurai, T., Hashimoto, T., et al. (2013). Inositol 1,4,5-trisphosphate receptor regulates replication, differentiation, infectivity and virulence of the parasitic protist *Trypanosoma cruzi*. *Mol. Microbiol.* 87, 1133–1150. doi: 10.1111/mmi.12155

Hausser, A., Link, G., Hoene, M., Russo, C., Selchow, O., and Pfizenmaier, K. (2006). Phospho-specific binding of 14-3-3 proteins to phosphatidylinositol 4-kinase III beta protects from dephosphorylation and stabilizes lipid kinase activity. *J. Cell Sci.* 119(Pt 17), 3613–3621. doi: 10.1242/jcs.03104

He, B., Xi, F., Zhang, X., Zhang, J., and Guo, W. (2007). Exo70 interacts with phospholipids and mediates the targeting of the exocyst to the plasma membrane. *EMBO J.* 26, 4053–4065. doi: 10.1038/sj.emboj.7601834

He, S., Ni, D., Ma, B., Lee, J. H., Zhang, T., Ghozalli, I., et al. (2013). PtdIns(3)P-bound UVRAG coordinates Golgi-ER retrograde and Atg9 transport by differential interactions with the ER tether and the beclin 1 complex. *Nat. Cell Biol.* 15, 1206–1219. doi: 10.1038/ncb2848

Heilmeyer, L. M. Jr., Vereb, G. Jr., Vereb, G., Kakuk, A., and Szivák, I. (2003). Mammalian phosphatidylinositol 4-kinases. *IUBMB Life* 55, 59–65. doi: 10.1080/1521654031000090896

Helgason, C. D., Damen, J. E., Rosten, P., Grewal, R., Sorensen, P., Chappel, S. M., et al. (1998). Targeted disruption of SHIP leads to hemopoietic perturbations, lung pathology, and a shortened life span. *Genes Dev.* 12, 1610–1620. doi: 10.1101/gad.12.11.1610

Henmi, Y., Morikawa, Y., Oe, N., Ikeda, N., Fujita, A., Takei, K., et al. (2016). PtdIns4KIIα generates endosomal PtdIns(4)P and is required for receptor sorting at early endosomes. *Mol. Biol. Cell* 27, 990–1001. doi: 10.1091/mbc.E15-08-0564

Herman, P. K., and Emr, S. D. (1990). Characterization of VPS34, a gene required for vacuolar protein sorting and vacuole segregation in Saccharomyces cerevisiae. *Mol. Cell Biol.* 10, 6742–6754. doi: 10.1128/MCB.10.12.6742

Hilgemann, D. W., and Ball, R. (1996). Regulation of cardiac Na^+, Ca^{2+} exchange and KATP potassium channels by PIP2. *Science* 273, 956–959. doi: 10.1126/science.273.5277.956

Hille, B., Dickson, E. J., Kruse, M., Vivas, O., and Suh, B. C. (2015). Phosphoinositides regulate ion channels. *Biochim. Biophys. Acta* 1851, 844–856. doi: 10.1016/j.bbalip.2014.09.010

Hnia, K., Tronchère, H., Tomczak, K. K., Amoasii, L., Schultz, P., Beggs, A. H., et al. (2011). Myotubularin controls desmin intermediate filament architecture and mitochondrial dynamics in human and mouse skeletal muscle. *J. Clin. Invest.* 121, 70–85. doi: 10.1172/JCI44021

Hnia, K., Vaccari, I., Bolino, A., and Laporte, J. (2012). Myotubularin phosphoinositide phosphatases: cellular functions and disease pathophysiology. *Trends Mol. Med.* 18, 317–327. doi: 10.1016/j.molmed.2012.04.004

Hohendahl, A., Roux, A., and Galli, V. (2016). Structural insights into the centronuclear myopathy-associated functions of BIN1 and dynamin 2. *J. Struct. Biol.* 196, 37–47. doi: 10.1016/j.jsb.2016.06.015

Homma, K., Terui, S., Minemura, M., Qadota, H., Anraku, Y., Kanaho, Y., et al. (1998). Phosphatidylinositol-4-phosphate 5-kinase localized on the plasma membrane is essential for yeast cell morphogenesis. *J. Biol. Chem.* 273, 15779–15786. doi: 10.1074/jbc.273.25.15779

Honda, A., Nogami, M., Yokozeki, T., Yamazaki, M., Nakamura, H., Watanabe, H., et al. (1999). Phosphatidylinositol 4-phosphate 5-kinase alpha is a downstream effector of the small G protein ARF6 in membrane ruffle formation. *Cell* 99, 521–532. doi: 10.1016/S0092-8674(00)81540-8

Hong, Z., Pedersen, N. M., Wang, L., Torgersen, M. L., Stenmark, H., and Raiborg, C. (2017). PtdIns3P controls mTORC1 signaling through lysosomal positioning. *J. Cell Biol.* 216, 4217–4233. doi: 10.1083/jcb.201611073

Horan, K. A., Watanabe, K., Kong, A. M., Bailey, C. G., Rasko, J. E., Sasaki, T., et al. (2007). Regulation of FcgammaR-stimulated phagocytosis by the 72-kDa inositol polyphosphate 5-phosphatase: SHIP1, but not the 72-kDa 5-phosphatase, regulates complement receptor 3 mediated phagocytosis by differential recruitment of these 5-phosphatases to the phagocytic cup. *Blood* 110, 4480–4491. doi: 10.1182/blood-2007-02-073874

Hsu, F., and Mao, Y. (2015). The structure of phosphoinositide phosphatases: Insights into substrate specificity and catalysis. *Biochim. Biophys. Acta* 1851, 698–710. doi: 10.1016/j.bbalip.2014.09.015

Hsu, N. Y., Ilnytska, O., Belov, G., Santiana, M., Chen, Y. H., Takvorian, P. M., et al. (2010). Viral reorganization of the secretory pathway generates distinct organelles for RNA replication. *Cell* 141, 799–811. doi: 10.1016/j.cell.2010.03.050

Huber, M., Helgason, C. D., Damen, J. E., Liu, L., Humphries, R. K., and Krystal, G. (1998). The src homology 2-containing inositol phosphatase (SHIP) is the gatekeeper of mast cell degranulation. *Proc. Natl. Acad. Sci. U.S.A.* 95, 11330–11335. doi: 10.1073/pnas.95.19.11330

Hughes, M. A., Lee, C. W., Holm, C. F., Ghosh, S., Mills, A., Lockhart, L. A., et al. (2003). Identification of Entamoeba histolytica thiol-specific antioxidant as a GalNAc lectin-associated protein. *Mol. Biochem. Parasitol.* 127, 113–120. doi: 10.1016/S0166-6851(02)00326-2

Husain, A., Jeelani, G., Sato, D., and Nozaki, T. (2011). Global analysis of gene expression in response to L-Cysteine deprivation in the anaerobic protozoan parasite *Entamoeba histolytica*. *BMC Genomics* 12:275. doi: 10.1186/1471-2164-12-275

Husebye, E. S., Letcher, A. J., Lander, D. J., and Flatmark, T. (1990). Purification and kinetic properties of a membrane-bound phosphatidylinositol kinase of the bovine adrenal medulla. *Biochim. Biophys. Acta* 1042, 330–337. doi: 10.1016/0005-2760(90)90161-P

Ijuin, T., and Takenawa, T. (2003). SKIP negatively regulates insulin-induced GLUT4 translocation and membrane ruffle formation. *Mol. Cell Biol.* 23, 1209–1220. doi: 10.1128/MCB.23.4.1209-1220.2003

Ikonomov, O. C., Sbrissa, D., Foti, M., Carpentier, J. L., and Shisheva, A. (2003). PIKfyve controls fluid phase endocytosis but not recycling/degradation of endocytosed receptors or sorting of procathepsin D by regulating multivesicular body morphogenesis. *Mol. Biol. Cell* 14, 4581–4591. doi: 10.1091/mbc.e03-04-0222

Imae, R., Inoue, T., Nakasaki, Y., Uchida, Y., Ohba, Y., Kono, N., et al. (2012). LYCAT, a homologue of *C. elegans* acl-8, acl-9, and acl-10, determines the fatty acid composition of phosphatidylinositol in mice. *J. Lipid Res.* 53, 335–347. doi: 10.1194/jlr.M018655

Irvine, R. F. (2003). Nuclear lipid signalling. *Nat. Rev. Mol. Cell Biol.* 4, 349–360. doi: 10.1038/nrm1100

Ishihara, H., Shibasaki, Y., Kizuki, N., Wada, T., Yazaki, Y., Asano, T., et al. (1998). Type I phosphatidylinositol-4-phosphate 5-kinases. Cloning of the third isoform and deletion/substitution analysis of members of this novel lipid kinase family. *J. Biol. Chem.* 273, 8741–8748. doi: 10.1074/jbc.273.15.8741

Ishikane, M., Arima, Y., Kanayama, A., Takahashi, T., Yamagishi, T., Yahata, Y., et al. (2016). Epidemiology of domestically acquired amebiasis in Japan, 2000-2013. *Am. J. Trop. Med. Hyg.* 94, 1008–1014. doi: 10.4269/ajtmh.15-0560

Itakura, E., Kishi, C., Inoue, K., and Mizushima, N. (2008). Beclin 1 forms two distinct phosphatidylinositol 3-kinase complexes with mammalian Atg14 and UVRAG. *Mol. Biol. Cell* 19, 5360–5372. doi: 10.1091/mbc.e08-01-0080

Itoh, T., Ijuin, T., and Takenawa, T. (1998). A novel phosphatidylinositol-5-phosphate 4-kinase (phosphatidylinositol-phosphate kinase IIgamma) is phosphorylated in the endoplasmic reticulum in response to mitogenic signals. *J. Biol. Chem.* 273, 20292–20299. doi: 10.1074/jbc.273.32.20292

Ivetac, I., Gurung, R., Hakim, S., Horan, K. A., Sheffield, D. A., Binge, L. C., et al. (2009). Regulation of PI(3)K/Akt signalling and cellular transformation by inositol polyphosphate 4-phosphatase-1. *EMBO Rep.* 10, 487–493. doi: 10.1038/embor.2009.28

Ivetac, I., Munday, A. D., Kisseleva, M. V., Zhang, X. M., Luff, S., Tiganis, T., et al. (2005). The type Ialpha inositol polyphosphate 4-phosphatase generates and terminates phosphoinositide 3-kinase signals on endosomes and the plasma membrane. *Mol. Biol. Cell* 16, 2218–2233. doi: 10.1091/mbc.e04-09-0799

Jacoby, M., Cox, J. J., Gayral, S., Hampshire, D. J., Ayub, M., Blockmans, M., et al. (2009). INPP5E mutations cause primary cilium signaling defects, ciliary instability and ciliopathies in human and mouse. *Nat. Genet.* 41, 1027–1031. doi: 10.1038/ng.427

James, S. R., Downes, C. P., Gigg, R., Grove, S. J., Holmes, A. B., and Alessi, D. R. (1996). Specific binding of the Akt-1 protein kinase to phosphatidylinositol 3,4,5-trisphosphate without subsequent activation. *Biochem. J.* 315(Pt 3), 709–713. doi: 10.1042/bj3150709

Jean, S., Cox, S., Schmidt, E. J., Robinson, F. L., and Kiger, A. (2012). Sbf/MTMR13 coordinates PI(3)P and Rab21 regulation in endocytic control of cellular remodeling. *Mol. Biol. Cell* 23, 2723–2740. doi: 10.1091/mbc.e12-05-0375

Jean, S., and Kiger, A. A. (2014). Classes of phosphoinositide 3-kinases at a glance. *J. Cell Sci.* 127(Pt 5), 923–928. doi: 10.1242/jcs.093773

Jeelani, G., and Nozaki, T. (2016). *Entamoeba* thiol-based redox metabolism: a potential target for drug development. *Mol. Biochem. Parasitol.* 206, 39–45. doi: 10.1016/j.molbiopara.2016.01.004

Jefferson, A. B., and Majerus, P. W. (1995). Properties of type II inositol polyphosphate 5-phosphatase. *J. Biol. Chem.* 270, 9370–9377. doi: 10.1074/jbc.270.16.9370

Jenkins, G. H., Fisette, P. L., and Anderson, R. A. (1994). Type I phosphatidylinositol 4-phosphate 5-kinase isoforms are specifically stimulated by phosphatidic acid. *J. Biol. Chem.* 269, 11547–11554.

Jenkins, G. M., and Frohman, M. A. (2005). Phospholipase D: a lipid centric review. *Cell Mol. Life. Sci.* 62, 2305–2316. doi: 10.1007/s00018-005-5195-z

Jeschke, A., Zehethofer, N., Lindner, B., Krupp, J., Schwudke, D., Haneburger, I., et al. (2015). Phosphatidylinositol 4-phosphate and phosphatidylinositol 3-phosphate regulate phagolysosome biogenesis. *Proc. Nat. Acad. Sci. U.S.A.* 112, 4636–4641. doi: 10.1073/pnas.1423456112

Jiang, Y., Zhao, J., Liao, E. Y., Dai, R. C., Wu, X. P., and Genant, H. K. (2005). Application of micro-CT assessment of 3-D bone microstructure in preclinical and clinical studies. *J. Bone Miner Metab.* 23(Suppl.), 122–131. doi: 10.1007/BF03026336

Jin, N., Chow, C. Y., Liu, L., Zolov, S. N., Bronson, R., Davisson, M., et al. (2008). VAC14 nucleates a protein complex essential for the acute interconversion of PI3P and PI(3,5)P(2) in yeast and mouse. *EMBO J.* 27, 3221–3234. doi: 10.1038/emboj.2008.248

Jin, N., Lang, M. J., and Weisman, L. S. (2016). Phosphatidylinositol 3,5-bisphosphate: regulation of cellular events in space and time. *Biochem. Soc. Trans.* 44, 177–184. doi: 10.1042/BST20150174

Jones, D. R., Bultsma, Y., Keune, W. J., Halstead, J. R., Elouarrat, D., Mohammed, S., et al. (2006). Nuclear PtdIns5P as a transducer of stress signaling: an *in vivo* role for PIP4Kbeta. *Mol. Cell* 23, 685–695. doi: 10.1016/j.molcel.2006.07.014

Jung, G., Barylko, B., Lu, D., Shu, H., Yin, H., and Albanesi, J. P. (2011). Stabilization of phosphatidylinositol 4-kinase type II beta by interaction with Hsp90. *J. Biol. Chem.* 286, 12775–12784. doi: 10.1074/jbc.M110.178616

Kaisaki, P. J., Delépine, M., Woon, P. Y., Sebag-Montefiore, L., Wilder, S. P., Menzel, S., et al. (2004). Polymorphisms in type II SH2 domain-containing inositol 5-phosphatase (INPPL1, SHIP2) are associated with physiological abnormalities of the metabolic syndrome. *Diabetes* 53, 1900–1904. doi: 10.2337/diabetes.53.7.1900

Kandepedu, N., Gonzàlez Cabrera, D., Eedubilli, S., Taylor, D., Brunschwig, C., Gibhard, L., et al. (2018). Identification, characterization, and optimization of 2,8-disubstituted-1,5-naphthyridines as novel *Plasmodium falciparum* phosphatidylinositol-4-kinase inhibitors with *in vivo* efficacy in a humanized mouse model of malaria. *J. Med. Chem.* 61, 5692–5703. doi: 10.1021/acs.jmedchem.8b00648

Kerk, D., and Moorhead, G. B. (2010). A phylogenetic survey of myotubularin genes of eukaryotes: distribution, protein structure, evolution, and gene expression. *BMC Evol. Biol.* 10:196. doi: 10.1186/1471-2148-10-196

Kihara, A., Noda, T., Ishihara, N., and Ohsumi, Y. (2001). Two distinct Vps34 phosphatidylinositol 3-kinase complexes function in autophagy and carboxypeptidase Y sorting in *Saccharomyces cerevisiae*. *J. Cell Biol.* 152, 519–530. doi: 10.1083/jcb.152.3.519

Kim, G. H., Dayam, R. M., Prashar, A., Terebiznik, M., and Botelho, R. J. (2014). PIKfyve inhibition interferes with phagosome and endosome maturation in macrophages. *Traffic* 15, 1143–1163. doi: 10.1111/tra.12199

Kim, J. S., Peng, X., De, P. K., Geahlen, R. L., and Durden, D. L. (2002). PTEN controls immunoreceptor (immunoreceptor tyrosine-based activation motif) signaling and the activation of Rac. *Blood* 99, 694–697. doi: 10.1182/blood.V99.2.694

Kim, S. A., Taylor, G. S., Torgersen, K. M., and Dixon, J. E. (2002). Myotubularin and MTMR2, phosphatidylinositol 3-phosphatases mutated in myotubular myopathy and type 4B Charcot-Marie-Tooth disease. *J. Biol. Chem.* 277, 4526–4531. doi: 10.1074/jbc.M111087200

Kim, S. A., Vacratsis, P. O., Firestein, R., Cleary, M. L., and Dixon, J. E. (2003). Regulation of myotubularin-related (MTMR)2 phosphatidylinositol phosphatase by MTMR5, a catalytically inactive phosphatase. *Proc. Natl. Acad. Sci. U.S.A.* 100, 4492–4497. doi: 10.1073/pnas.0431052100

Kim, W. T., Chang, S., Daniell, L., Cremona, O., Di Paolo, G., and De Camilli, P. (2002). Delayed reentry of recycling vesicles into the fusion-competent synaptic vesicle pool in synaptojanin 1 knockout mice. *Proc. Natl. Acad. Sci. U.S.A.* 99, 17143–17148. doi: 10.1073/pnas.222657399

Kimura, T., Sakamoto, H., Appella, E., and Siraganian, R. P. (1997). The negative signaling molecule SH2 domain-containing inositol-polyphosphate 5-phosphatase (SHIP) binds to the tyrosine-phosphorylated beta subunit of the high affinity IgE receptor. *J. Biol. Chem.* 272, 13991–13996. doi: 10.1074/jbc.272.21.13991

Kisseleva, M. V., Wilson, M. P., and Majerus, P. W. (2000). The isolation and characterization of a cDNA encoding phospholipid-specific inositol polyphosphate 5-phosphatase. *J. Biol. Chem.* 275, 20110–20116. doi: 10.1074/jbc.M910119199

Klima, M., Tóth, D. J., Hexnerova, R., Baumlova, A., Chalupska, D., Tykvart, J., et al. (2016). Structural insights and *in vitro* reconstitution of membrane targeting and activation of human PI4KB by the ACBD3 protein. *Sci. Rep.* 6:23641 doi: 10.1038/srep23641

Klinkert, K., and Echard, A. (2016). Rab35 GTPase: a central regulator of phosphoinositides and F-actin in endocytic recycling and beyond. *Traffic* 17, 1063–1077. doi: 10.1111/tra.12422

Kohno, T., Takahashi, M., Manda, R., and Yokota, J. (1998). Inactivation of the PTEN/MMAC1/TEP1 gene in human lung cancers. *Genes Chromosomes Cancer* 22, 152–156. doi: 10.1002/(SICI)1098-2264(199806)22:2<152::AID-GCC10>3.0.CO;2-S

Kong, A. M., Speed, C. J., O'Malley, C. J., Layton, M. J., Meehan, T., Loveland, K. L., et al. (2000). Cloning and characterization of a 72-kDa inositol-polyphosphate 5-phosphatase localized to the Golgi network. *J. Biol. Chem.* 275, 24052–24064. doi: 10.1074/jbc.M000874200

Kortholt, A., King, J. S., Keizer-Gunnink, I., Harwood, A. J., and Van Haastert, P. J. (2007). Phospholipase C regulation of phosphatidylinositol 3,4,5-trisphosphate-mediated chemotaxis. *Mol. Biol. Cell* 18, 4772–4779. doi: 10.1091/mbc.e07-05-0407

Kosugi, S., Hasebe, M., Tomita, M., and Yanagawa, H. (2009). Systematic identification of cell cycle-dependent yeast nucleocytoplasmic shuttling proteins by prediction of composite motifs. *Proc. Natl. Acad. Sci. U.S.A.* 106, 10171–10176. doi: 10.1073/pnas.0900604106

Koushik, A. B., Powell, R. R., and Temesvari, L. A. (2013). Localization of phosphatidylinositol 4,5-bisphosphate to lipid rafts and uroids in the human protozoan parasite *Entamoeba histolytica*. *Infect. Immun.* 81, 2145–2155. doi: 10.1128/IAI.00040-13

Koushik, A. B., Welter, B. H., Rock, M. L., and Temesvari, L. A. (2014). A genome wide overexpression screen identifies genes involved in the phosphatidylinositol 3-kinase pathway in the human protozoan parasite *Entamoeba histolytica*. *Eukaryot. Cell* 13, 401–411. doi: 10.1128/EC.00329-13

Krauss, M., Kukhtina, V., Pechstein, A., and Haucke, V. (2006). Stimulation of phosphatidylinositol kinase type I-mediated phosphatidylinositol (4,5)-bisphosphate synthesis by AP-2mu-cargo complexes. *Proc. Natl. Acad. Sci. U.S.A.* 103, 11934–11939. doi: 10.1073/pnas.0510306103

Krishna, S., Palm, W., Lee, Y., Yang, W., Bandyopadhyay, U., Xu, H., et al. (2016). PIKfyve regulates vacuole maturation and nutrient recovery following engulfment. *Dev. Cell* 38, 536–547. doi: 10.1016/j.devcel.2016.08.001

Kuemmel, A., Simon, P., Breitkreuz, A., Röhlig, J., Luxemburger, U., Elsäßer, A., et al. (2015). Humoral immune responses of lung cancer patients against the Transmembrane Phosphatase with TEnsin homology (TPTE). *Lung Cancer* 90, 334–341. doi: 10.1016/j.lungcan.2015.07.012

Kunz, J., Fuelling, A., Kolbe, L., and Anderson, R. A. (2002). Stereo-specific substrate recognition by phosphatidylinositol phosphate kinases is swapped by changing a single amino acid residue. *J. Biol. Chem.* 277, 5611–5619. doi: 10.1074/jbc.M110775200

Kunz, J., Wilson, M. P., Kisseleva, M., Hurley, J. H., Majerus, P. W., and Anderson, R. A. (2000). The activation loop of phosphatidylinositol phosphate kinases determines signaling specificity. *Mol. Cell* 5, 1–11. doi: 10.1016/S1097-2765(00)80398-6

Kurosu, H., and Katada, T. (2001). Association of phosphatidylinositol 3-kinase composed of p110beta-catalytic and p85-regulatory subunits with the small GTPase Rab5. *J. Biochem.* 130, 73–78. doi: 10.1093/oxfordjournals.jbchem.a002964

Lacalle, R. A., Peregil, R. M., Albar, J. P., Merino, E., Martínez-A, C., Mérida, I., et al. (2007). Type I phosphatidylinositol 4-phosphate 5-kinase controls neutrophil polarity and directional movement. *J. Cell Biol.* 179, 1539–1553. doi: 10.1083/jcb.200705044

Lamia, K. A., Peroni, O. D., Kim, Y. B., Rameh, L. E., Kahn, B. B., and Cantley, L. C. (2004). Increased insulin sensitivity and reduced adiposity in phosphatidylinositol 5-phosphate 4-kinase beta-/- mice. *Mol. Cell Biol.* 24, 5080–5087. doi: 10.1128/MCB.24.11.5080-5087.2004

Laporte, J., Bedez, F., Bolino, A., and Mandel, J. L. (2003). Myotubularins, a large disease-associated family of cooperating catalytically active and inactive phosphoinositides phosphatases. *Hum. Mol. Genet.* 12(Spec No. 2), R285–R292. doi: 10.1093/hmg/ddg273

Lawlor, M. W., Beggs, A. H., Buj-Bello, A., Childers, M. K., Dowling, J. J., James, E. S., et al. (2016). Skeletal muscle pathology in X-linked myotubular myopathy: review with cross-species comparisons. *J. Neuropathol. Exp. Neurol.* 75, 102–110. doi: 10.1093/jnen/nlv020

Laxminarayan, K. M., Chan, B. K., Tetaz, T., Bird, P. I., and Mitchell, C. A. (1994). Characterization of a cDNA encoding the 43-kDa membrane-associated inositol-polyphosphate 5-phosphatase. *J. Biol. Chem.* 269, 17305–17310.

Laxminarayan, K. M., Matzaris, M., Speed, C. J., and Mitchell, C. A. (1993). Purification and characterization of a 43-kDa membrane-associated inositol polyphosphate 5-phosphatase from human placenta. *J. Biol. Chem.* 268, 4968–4974.

Lee, J. O., Yang, H., Georgescu, M. M., Di Cristofano, A., Maehama, T., Shi, Y., et al. (1999). Crystal structure of the PTEN tumor suppressor: implications for its phosphoinositide phosphatase activity and membrane association. *Cell* 99, 323–334. doi: 10.1016/S0092-8674(00)81663-3

Lee, J. S., Nauseef, W. M., Moeenrezakhanlou, A., Sly, L. M., Noubir, S., Leidal, K. G., et al. (2007). Monocyte p110 alpha phosphatidylinositol 3-kinase regulates phagocytosis, the phagocyte oxidase, and cytokine production. *J. Leukoc. Biol.* 81, 1548–1561. doi: 10.1189/jlb.0906564

Lee, Y. A., Kim, K. A., Min, A., and Shin, M. H. (2014). Amoebic PI3K and PKC is required for Jurkat T cell death induced by *Entamoeba histolytica*. *Korean J. Parasitol.* 52, 355–365. doi: 10.3347/kjp.2014.52.4.355

Leung, K. F., Dacks, J. B., and Field, M. C. (2008). Evolution of the multivesicular body ESCRT machinery; retention across the eukaryotic lineage. *Traffic* 9, 1698–1716. doi: 10.1111/j.1600-0854.2008.00797.x

Lev, S. (2010). Non-vesicular lipid transport by lipid-transfer proteins and beyond. *Nat. Rev. Mol. Cell Biol.* 11, 739–750. doi: 10.1038/nrm2971

Levin, R., Hammond, G. R., Balla, T., De Camilli, P., Fairn, G. D., and Grinstein, S. (2017). Multiphasic dynamics of phosphatidylinositol 4-phosphate during phagocytosis. *Mol. Biol. Cell* 28, 128–140. doi: 10.1091/mbc.e16-06-0451

Lewis, P. A. (2009). The function of ROCO proteins in health and disease. *Biol. Cell* 101, 183–191. doi: 10.1042/BC20080053

Li, J., Yen, C., Liaw, D., Podsypanina, K., Bose, S., Wang, S. I., et al. (1997). PTEN, a putative protein tyrosine phosphatase gene mutated in human brain, breast, and prostate cancer. *Science* 275, 1943–1947. doi: 10.1126/science.275.5308.1943

Li, L., and Chin, L. S. (2003). The molecular machinery of synaptic vesicle exocytosis. *Cell Mol. Life Sci.* 60, 942–960. doi: 10.1007/s00018-003-2240-7

Li, W., Laishram, R. S., and Anderson, R. A. (2013). The novel poly(A) polymerase Star-PAP is a signal-regulated switch at the 3'-end of mRNAs. *Adv. Biol. Regul.* 53, 64–76. doi: 10.1016/j.jbior.2012.10.004

Lichter-Konecki, U., Farber, L. W., Cronin, J. S., Suchy, S. F., and Nussbaum, R. L. (2006). The effect of missense mutations in the RhoGAP-homology domain on ocrl1 function. *Mol. Genet. Metab.* 89, 121–128. doi: 10.1016/j.ymgme.2006.04.005

Lindsay, Y., McCoull, D., Davidson, L., Leslie, N. R., Fairservice, A., Gray, A., et al. (2006). Localization of agonist-sensitive PtdIns(3,4,5)P3 reveals a nuclear pool that is insensitive to PTEN expression. *J. Cell Sci.* 119, 5160–5168. doi: 10.1242/jcs.000133

Ling, K., Doughman, R. L., Firestone, A. J., Bunce, M. W., and Anderson, R. A. (2002). Type I gamma phosphatidylinositol phosphate kinase targets and regulates focal adhesions. *Nature* 420, 89–93. doi: 10.1038/nature01082

Liu, A., Sui, D., Wu, D., and Hu, J. (2016). The activation loop of PIP5K functions as a membrane sensor essential for lipid substrate processing. *Sci. Adv.* 2:e1600925. doi: 10.1126/sciadv.1600925

Liu, L., Damen, J. E., Cutler, R. L., and Krystal, G. (1994). Multiple cytokines stimulate the binding of a common 145-kilodalton protein to Shc at the Grb2 recognition site of Shc. *Mol. Cell Biol.* 14, 6926–6935. doi: 10.1128/MCB.14.10.6926

Liu, Q., Sasaki, T., Kozieradzki, I., Wakeham, A., Itie, A., Dumont, D. J., et al. (1999). SHIP is a negative regulator of growth factor receptor-mediated PKB/Akt activation and myeloid cell survival. *Genes Dev.* 13, 786–791. doi: 10.1101/gad.13.7.786

Liu, Q., Shalaby, F., Jones, J., Bouchard, D., and Dumont, D. J. (1998). The SH2-containing inositol polyphosphate 5-phosphatase, ship, is expressed during hematopoiesis and spermatogenesis. *Blood* 91, 2753–2759.

Lo, Y. C., Ji, D. D., and Hung, C. C. (2014). Prevalent and incident HIV diagnoses among *Entamoeba histolytica*-infected adult males: a changing epidemiology associated with sexual transmission–Taiwan, 2006-2013. *PLoS Negl. Trop. Dis.* 8:e3222. doi: 10.1371/journal.pntd.0003222

Loijens, J. C., Boronenkov, I. V., Parker, G. J., and Anderson, R. A. (1996). The phosphatidylinositol 4-phosphate 5-kinase family. *Adv. Enzyme Regul.* 36, 115–140. doi: 10.1016/0065-2571(95)00005-4

Lokuta, M. A., Senetar, M. A., Bennin, D. A., Nuzzi, P. A., Chan, K. T., Ott, V. L., et al. (2007). Type Igamma PIP kinase is a novel uropod component that regulates rear retraction during neutrophil chemotaxis. *Mol. Biol. Cell* 18, 5069–5080. doi: 10.1091/mbc.e07-05-0428

López-Contreras, L., Hernández-Ramírez, V. I., Flores-García, Y., Chávez-Munguía, B., and Talamás-Rohana, P. (2013). Src and PI3 K inhibitors affect the virulence factors of *Entamoeba histolytica*. *Parasitology* 140, 202–209. doi: 10.1017/S0031182012001540

Lorenzo, O., Urbé, S., and Clague, M. J. (2006). Systematic analysis of myotubularins: heteromeric interactions, subcellular localisation and endosome related functions. *J. Cell Sci.* 119, 2953–2959. doi: 10.1242/jcs.03040

Lowe, M. (2005). Structure and function of the Lowe syndrome protein OCRL1. *Traffic* 6, 711–719. doi: 10.1111/j.1600-0854.2005.00311.x

Lozano, R., Naghavi, M., Foreman, K., Lim, S., Shibuya, K., Aboyans, V., et al. (2012). Global and regional mortality from 235 causes of death for 20 age groups in 1990 and 2010: a systematic analysis for the Global Burden of Disease Study 2010. *Lancet* 380, 2095–2128. doi: 10.1016/S0140-6736(12) 61728-0

Lu, J., He, L., Behrends, C., Araki, M., Araki, K., Jun Wang, Q., et al. (2014). NRBF2 regulates autophagy and prevents liver injury by modulating Atg14L-linked phosphatidylinositol-3 kinase III activity. *Nat. Commun.* 5:3920. doi: 10.1038/ncomms4920

Lucas, D. M., and Rohrschneider, L. R. (1999). A novel spliced form of SH2-containing inositol phosphatase is expressed during myeloid development. *Blood* 93, 1922–1933.

Ma, K., Cheung, S. M., Marshall, A. J., and Duronio, V. (2008). PI(3,4,5)P3 and PI(3,4)P2 levels correlate with PKB/akt phosphorylation at Thr308 and Ser473, respectively; PI(3,4)P2 levels determine PKB activity. *Cell Signal.* 20, 684–694. doi: 10.1016/j.cellsig.2007.12.004

Maehama, T. (2007). PTEN: its deregulation and tumorigenesis. *Biol. Pharm. Bull.* 30, 1624–1627. doi: 10.1248/bpb.30.1624

Maehama, T., and Dixon, J. E. (1998). The tumor suppressor, PTEN/MMAC1, dephosphorylates the lipid second messenger, phosphatidylinositol 3,4,5-trisphosphate. *J. Biol. Chem.* 273, 13375–13378. doi: 10.1074/jbc.273.22.13375

Maehama, T., and Dixon, J. E. (1999). PTEN: a tumour suppressor that functions as a phospholipid phosphatase. *Trends Cell Biol.* 9, 125–128. doi: 10.1016/S0962-8924(99)01519-6

Maffucci, T., and Falasca, M. (2014). New insight into the intracellular roles of class II phosphoinositide 3-kinases. *Biochem. Soc. Trans.* 42, 1378–1382. doi: 10.1042/BST20140140

Mahankali, M., Alter, G., and Gomez-Cambronero, J. (2015). Mechanism of enzymatic reaction and protein-protein interactions of PLD from a 3D structural model. *Cell Signal.* 27, 69–81. doi: 10.1016/j.cellsig.2014.09.008

Majerus, P. W., Connolly, T. M., Deckmyn, H., Ross, T. S., Bross, T. E., Ishii, H., et al. (1986). The metabolism of phosphoinositide-derived messenger molecules. *Science* 234, 1519–1526. doi: 10.1126/science.3024320

Majerus, P. W., Kisseleva, M. V., and Norris, F. A. (1999). The role of phosphatases in inositol signaling reactions. *J. Biol. Chem.* 274, 10669–10672. doi: 10.1074/jbc.274.16.10669

Makioka, A., Kumagai, M., Ohtomo, H., Kobayashi, S., and Takeuchi, T. (2001). Inhibition of encystation of *Entamoeba invadens* by wortmannin. *Parasitol. Res.* 87, 371–375. doi: 10.1007/s004360000339

Makiuchi, T., and Nozaki, T. (2014). Highly divergent mitochondrion-related organelles in anaerobic parasitic protozoa. *Biochimie* 100, 3–17. doi: 10.1016/j.biochi.2013.11.018

Makowski, S. L., Tran, T. T., and Field, S. J. (2017). Emerging themes of regulation at the Golgi. *Curr. Opin. Cell Biol.* 45, 17–23. doi: 10.1016/j.ceb.2017.01.004

Malek, M., Kielkowska, A., Chessa, T., Anderson, K. E., Barneda, D., Pir, P., et al. (2017). PTEN regulates PI(3,4)P(2) signaling downstream of class I PI3K. *Mol. Cell* 68, 566–580.e10. doi: 10.1016/j.molcel.2017.09.024

Manford, A., Xia, T., Saxena, A. K., Stefan, C., Hu, F., Emr, S. D., et al. (2010). Crystal structure of the yeast Sac1: implications for its phosphoinositide phosphatase function. *EMBO J.* 9, 1489–1498. doi: 10.1038/emboj.2010.57

Manning-Cela, R., Marquez, C., Franco, Talamás-Rohana, P., and Meza, I. (2003). BFA-sensitive and insensitive exocytic pathways in *Entamoeba histolytica* trophozoites: their relationship to pathogenesis. *Cell. Microbiol.* 5, 921–932. doi: 10.1046/j.1462-5822.2003.00332.x

Marat, A. L., and Haucke, V. (2016). Phosphatidylinositol 3-phosphates-at the interface between cell signalling and membrane traffic. *EMBO J.* 35, 561–579. doi: 10.15252/embj.201593564

Marie, C., and Petri, W. A. Jr. (2014). Regulation of virulence of *Entamoeba histolytica*. *Annu. Rev. Microbiol.* 68, 493–520. doi: 10.1146/annurev-micro-091313-103550

Martin, T. F. (2015). PI(4,5)P2-binding effector proteins for vesicle exocytosis. *Biochim. Biophys. Acta* 1851, 785–793. doi: 10.1016/j.bbalip.2014.09.017

Martin-Belmonte, F., Gassama, A., Datta, A., Yu, W., Rescher, U., Gerke, V., et al. (2007). PTEN-mediated apical segregation of phosphoinositides controls epithelial morphogenesis through Cdc42. *Cell* 128, 383–397. doi: 10.1016/j.cell.2006.11.051

Marumo, K., Nakada-Tsukui, K., Tomii, K., and Nozaki, T. (2014). Ligand heterogeneity of the cysteine protease binding protein family in the parasitic protist *Entamoeba histolytica*. *Int. J. Parasitol.* 44, 625–635. doi: 10.1016/j.ijpara.2014.04.008

Matsunaga, K., Saitoh, T., Tabata, K., Omori, H., Satoh, T., Kurotori, N., et al. (2009). Two Beclin 1-binding proteins, Atg14L and Rubicon, reciprocally regulate autophagy at different stages. *Nat. Cell Biol.* 11, 385–396. doi: 10.1038/ncb1846

Matzaris, M., O'Malley, C. J., Badger, A., Speed, C. J., Bird, P. I., and Mitchell, C. A. (1998). Distinct membrane and cytosolic forms of inositol polyphosphate 5-phosphatase II. Efficient membrane localization requires two discrete domains. *J. Biol. Chem.* 273, 8256–8267. doi: 10.1074/jbc.273.14.8256

McFadden, G. I. (2000). Mergers and acquisitions: malaria and the great chloroplastheist. *Genome Biol.* 1:REVIEWS1026. doi: 10.1186/gb-2000-1-4-reviews1026

McNamara, C. W., Lee, M. C., Lim, C. S., Lim, S. H., Roland, J., Simon, O., et al. (2013). Targeting *Plasmodium* PI(4)K to eliminate malaria. *Nature* 504, 248–253. doi: 10.1038/nature12782

McPherson, P. S., Garcia, E. P., Slepnev, V. I., David, C., Zhang, X., Grabs, D., et al. (1996). A presynaptic inositol-5-phosphatase. *Nature* 379, 353–357. doi: 10.1038/379353a0

Mellman, D. L., Gonzales, M. L., Song, C., Barlow, C. A., Wang, P., Kendziorski, C., et al. (2008). A PtdIns4,5P2-regulated nuclear poly(A) polymerase controls expression of select mRNAs. *Nature* 451, 1013–1017. doi: 10.1038/nature06666

Michell, B. (1995). Early steps along the road to inositol-lipid-based signalling. *Trends Biochem. Sci.* 20, 326–329. doi: 10.1016/S0968-0004(00)89061-1

Michell, R. H. (2008). Inositol derivatives: evolution and functions. *Nat. Rev. Mol. Cell. Biol.* 9, 151–161. doi: 10.1038/nrm2334

Michell, R. H. (2011). Inositol and its derivatives: their evolution and functions. *Adv. Enzyme Regul.* 51, 84–90. doi: 10.1016/j.advenzreg.2010.10.002

Michell, R. H., Kirk, C. J., Jones, L. M., Downes, C. P., and Creba, J. A. (1981). The stimulation of inositol lipid metabolism that accompanies calcium mobilization in stimulated cells: defined characteristics and unanswered questions. *Philos. Trans. R. Soc. Lond. B. Biol. Sci.* 296, 123–138. doi: 10.1098/rstb.1981.0177

Mi-Ichi, F., Miyamoto, T., and Yoshida, H. (2017). Uniqueness of *Entamoeba* sulfur metabolism: sulfolipid metabolism that plays pleiotropic roles in the parasitic life cycle. *Mol. Microbiol.* 106, 479–491. doi: 10.1111/mmi.13827

Minagawa, T., Ijuin, T., Mochizuki, Y., and Takenawa, T. (2001). Identification and characterization of a sac domain-containing phosphoinositide 5-phosphatase. *J. Biol. Chem.* 276, 22011–22015. doi: 10.1074/jbc.M101579200

Minogue, S., and Waugh, M. G. (2012). The phosphatidylinositol 4-kinases: don't call it a comeback. *Subcell. Biochem.* 58, 1–24. doi: 10.1007/978-94-007-3012-0_1

Minogue, S., Waugh, M. G., De Matteis, M. A., Stephens, D. J., Berditchevski, F., and Hsuan, J. J. (2006). Phosphatidylinositol 4-kinase is required for endosomal trafficking and degradation of the EGF receptor. *J. Cell Sci.* 119(Pt 3), 571–581. doi: 10.1242/jcs.02752

Mitra, B. N., Saito-Nakano, Y., Nakada-Tsukui, K., Sato, D., and Nozaki, T. (2007). Rab11B small GTPase regulates secretion of cysteine proteases in the enteric protozoan parasite *Entamoeba histolytica*. *Cell. Microbiol.* 9, 2112–2125. doi: 10.1111/j.1462-5822.2007.00941.x

Mizushima, N., Yoshimori, T., and Ohsumi, Y. (2011). The role of Atg proteins in autophagosome formation. *Annu. Rev. Cell Dev. Biol.* 27, 107–132. doi: 10.1146/annurev-cellbio-092910-154005

Mochizuki, Y., and Majerus, P. W. (2003). Characterization of myotubularin-related protein 7 and its binding partner, myotubularin-related protein 9. *Proc. Natl. Acad. Sci. U.S.A.* 100, 9768–9773. doi: 10.1073/pnas.1333958100

Mochizuki, Y., and Takenawa, T. (1999). Novel inositol polyphosphate 5-phosphatase localizes at membrane ruffles. *J. Biol. Chem.* 274, 36790–36795.

Morioka, S., Nigorikawa, K., Okada, E., Tanaka, Y., Kasuu, Y., Yamada, M., et al. (2018). TMEM55a localizes to macrophage phagosomes to downregulate phagocytosis. *J. Cell Sci.* 131:jcs213272. doi: 10.1242/jcs.213272

Mössinger, J., Wieffer, M., Krause, E., Freund, C., Gerth, F., Krauss, M., et al. (2012). Phosphatidylinositol 4-kinase IIα function at endosomes is regulated by the ubiquitin ligase Itch. *EMBO Rep.* 13, 1087–1094. doi: 10.1038/embor.2012.164

Müller, M., Mentel, M., van Hellemond, J. J., Henze, K., Woehle, C., Gould, S. B., et al. (2012). Biochemistry and evolution of anaerobic energy metabolism in eukaryotes. *Microbiol. Mol. Biol. Rev.* 76, 444–495. doi: 10.1128/MMBR.05024-11

Munson, M. J., Allen, G. F., Toth, R., Campbell, D. G., Lucocq, J. M., and Ganley, I. G. (2015). mTOR activates the VPS34-UVRAG complex to regulate autolysosomal tubulation and cell survival. *EMBO J.* 34, 2272–2290. doi: 10.15252/embj.201590992

Myers, M. P., Stolarov, J. P., Eng, C., Li, J., Wang, S. I., Wigler, M. H., et al. (1997). P-TEN, the tumor suppressor from human chromosome 10q23, is a dual-specificity phosphatase. *Proc. Natl. Acad. Sci. U.S.A.* 94, 9052–9057. doi: 10.1073/pnas.94.17.9052

Nakada-Tsukui, K., Okada, H., Mitra, B. N., and Nozaki, T. (2009). Phosphatidylinositol-phosphates mediate cytoskeletal reorganization during phagocytosis via a unique modular protein consisting of RhoGEF/DH and FYVE domains in the parasitic protozoon *Entamoeba histolytica*. *Cell. Microbiol.* 11, 1471–1491. doi: 10.1111/j.1462-5822.2009.01341.x

Nakada-Tsukui, K., Saito-Nakano, Y., Ali, V., and Nozaki, T. (2005). A retromer like complex is a novel Rab7 effector that is involved in the transport of the virulence factor cysteine protease in the enteric protozoan parasite *Entamoeba histolytica*. *Mol. Biol. Cell* 16, 5294–5303. doi: 10.1091/mbc.e05-04-0283

Nakada-Tsukui, K., Saito-Nakano, Y., Husain, A., and Nozaki, T. (2010). Conservation and function of Rab small GTPases in *Entamoeba*: annotation of *E. invadens* Rab and its use for the understanding of Entamoeba biology. *Exp. Parasitol.* 126, 337–347. doi: 10.1016/j.exppara.2010.04.014

Nakada-Tsukui, K., Tsuboi, K., Furukawa, A., Yamada, Y., and Nozaki, T. (2012). A novel class of cysteine protease receptors that mediate lysosomal transport. *Cell. Microbiol.* 14, 1299–1317. doi: 10.1111/j.1462-5822.2012.01800.x

Nakatsu, F. (2015). A phosphoinositide code for primary cilia. *Dev. Cell* 34, 379–380. doi: 10.1016/j.devcel.2015.08.008

Nakatsu, F., Baskin, J. M., Chung, J., Tanner, L. B., Shui, G., Lee, S. Y., et al. (2012). PtdIns4P synthesis by PI4KIIIα at the plasma membrane and its impact on plasma membrane identity. *J. Cell Biol.* 199, 1003–1016. doi: 10.1083/jcb.201206095

Nakatsu, F., Messa, M., Nández, R., Czapla, H., Zou, Y., Strittmatter, S. M., et al. (2015). Sac2/INPP5F is an inositol 4-phosphatase that functions in the endocytic pathway. *J. Cell Biol.* 209, 85–95. doi: 10.1083/jcb.201409064

Nakatsu, F., Perera, R. M., Lucast, L., Zoncu, R., Domin, J., Gertler, F. B., et al. (2010). The inositol 5-phosphatase SHIP2 regulates endocytic clathrin-coated pit dynamics. *J. Cell Biol.* 190, 307–315. doi: 10.1083/jcb.201005018

Nemoto, Y., Kearns, B. G., Wenk, M. R., Chen, H., Mori, K., Alb, J. G. Jr., et al. (2000). Functional characterization of a mammalian Sac1 and mutants exhibiting substrate-specific defects in phosphoinositide phosphatase activity. *J. Biol Chem.* 275, 34293–34305. doi: 10.1074/jbc.M003923200

Nemoto, Y., Wenk, M. R., Watanabe, M., Daniell, L., Murakami, T., Ringstad, N., et al. (2001). Identification and characterization of a synaptojanin 2 splice isoform predominantly expressed in nerve terminals. *J. Biol. Chem.* 276, 41133–41142. doi: 10.1074/jbc.M106404200

Neri, L. M., Borgatti, P., Capitani, S., and Martelli, A. M. (1998). Nuclear diacylglycerol produced by phosphoinositide-specific phospholipase C is responsible for nuclear translocation of protein kinase C-alpha. *J. Biol. Chem.* 273:29738–29744. doi: 10.1074/jbc.273.45.29738

Neukomm, L. J., Nicot, A. S., Kinchen, J. M., Almendinger, J., Pinto, S. M., Zeng, S., et al. (2011). The phosphoinositide phosphatase MTM-1 regulates apoptotic cell corpse clearance through CED-5-CED-12 in *C. elegans*. *Development* 138, 2003–2014. doi: 10.1242/dev.060012

Newton, A. C. (2010). Protein kinase C: poised to signal. *Am. J. Physiol. Endocrinol. Metab.* 298, E395–E402. doi: 10.1152/ajpendo.00477.2009

Nishio, M., Watanabe, K., Sasaki, J., Taya, C., Takasuga, S., Iizuka, R., et al. (2007). Control of cell polarity and motility by the PtdIns(3,4,5)P3 phosphatase SHIP1. *Nat. Cell Biol.* 9, 36–44. doi: 10.1038/ncb1515

Nishizuka, Y. (1984). The role of protein kinase C in cell surface signal transduction and tumour promotion. *Nature* 308, 693–698. doi: 10.1038/308693a0

Nishizuka, Y. (1995). Protein kinase C and lipid signaling for sustained cellular responses. *FASEB J.* 9, 484–496. doi: 10.1096/fasebj.9.7.7737456

Norris, F. A., Atkins, R. C., and Majerus, P. W. (1997). Inositol polyphosphate 4-phosphatase is inactivated by calpain-mediated proteolysis in stimulated human platelets. *J. Biol. Chem.* 272, 10987–10989. doi: 10.1074/jbc.272.17.10987

Norris, F. A., Auethavekiat, V., and Majerus, P. W. (1995). The isolation and characterization of cDNA encoding human and rat brain inositol polyphosphate 4-phosphatase. *J. Biol. Chem.* 270, 16128–16133. doi: 10.1074/jbc.270.27.16128

Novick, P., Osmond, B. C., and Botstein, D. (1989). Suppressors of yeast actin mutations. *Genetics* 121, 659–674.

Odorizzi, G., Babst, M., and Emr, S. D. (1998). Fab1p PtdIns(3)P 5-kinase function essential for protein sorting in the multivesicular body. *Cell* 95, 847–858. doi: 10.1016/S0092-8674(00)81707-9

Odorizzi, G., Babst, M., and Emr, S. D. (2000). Phosphoinositide signaling and the regulation of membrane trafficking in yeast. *Trends Biochem. Sci.* 25, 229–235. doi: 10.1016/S0968-0004(00)01543-7

Olivos-Glander, I. M., Jänne, P. A., and Nussbaum, R. L. (1995). The oculocerebrorenal syndrome gene product is a 105-kD protein localized to the Golgi complex. *Am. J. Hum. Genet.* 57, 817–823.

Ooms, L. M., Fedele, C. G., Astle, M. V., Ivetac, I., Cheung, V., Pearson, R. B., et al. (2006). The inositol polyphosphate 5-phosphatase, PIPP, Is a novel regulator of phosphoinositide 3-kinase-dependent neurite elongation. *Mol. Biol. Cell* 17, 607–622. doi: 10.1091/mbc.e05-05-0469

Osborne, M. A., Zenner, G., Lubinus, M., Zhang, X., Songyang, Z., Cantley, L. C., et al. (1996). The inositol 5'-phosphatase SHIP binds to immunoreceptor signaling motifs and responds to high affinity IgE receptor aggregation. *J. Biol. Chem.* 271, 29271–29278. doi: 10.1074/jbc.271.46.29271

Payrastre, B., Nievers, M., Boonstra, J., Breton, M., Verkleij, A. J., and Van Bergen en Henegouwen, P. M. (1992). A differential location of phosphoinositide kinases, diacylglycerol kinase, and phospholipase C in the nuclear matrix. *J. Biol Chem.* 267, 5078–5084.

Peck, J., Douglas, G. 4th, Wu, C. H., and Burbelo, P. D. (2002). Human RhoGAP domain-containing proteins: structure, function and evolutionary relationships. *FEBS Lett.* 528, 27–34. doi: 10.1016/S0014-5793(02)03331-8

Pendaries, C., Tronchère, H., Arbibe, L., Mounier, J., Gozani, O., Cantley, L., et al. (2006). PtdIns5P activates the host cell PI 3-kinase/Akt pathway during *Shigella flexneri* infection. *EMBO J.* 25, 1024–1034. doi: 10.1038/sj.emboj.7601001

Penuliar, G. M., Nakada-Tsukui, K., and Nozaki, T. (2015). Phenotypic and transcriptional profiling in *Entamoeba histolytica* reveal costs to fitness and adaptive responses associated with metronidazole resistance. *Front. Microbiol.* 6:354. doi: 10.3389/fmicb.2015.00354

Pineda, E., and Perdomo, D. (2017). *Entamoeba histolytica* under oxidative stress: what countermeasure mechanisms are in place? *Cells* 6:E44. doi: 10.3390/cells6040044

Plattner, H., and Verkhratsky, A. (2013). Ca^{2+} signalling early in evolution–all but primitive. *J. Cell Sci.* 126(Pt 10), 2141–2150. doi: 10.1242/jcs.127449

Poli, A., Billi, A. M., Mongiorgi, S., Ratti, S., McCubrey, J. A., Suh, P. G., et al. (2016). Nuclear phosphatidylinositol signaling: focus on phosphatidylinositol phosphate kinases and phospholipases C. *J. Cell Physiol.* 231, 1645–1655. doi: 10.1002/jcp.25273

Poli, A., Faenza, I., Chiarini, F., Matteucci, A., McCubrey, J. A., and Cocco, L. (2013). K562 cell proliferation is modulated by PLCβ1 through a PKCα-mediated pathway. *Cell Cycle* 12, 1713–1721. doi: 10.4161/cc.24806

Poli, A., Mongiorgi, S., Cocco, L., and Follo, M. Y. (2014). Protein kinase C involvement in cell cycle modulation. *Biochem. Soc. Trans.* 42, 1471–1476. doi: 10.1042/BST20140128

Posor, Y., Eichhorn-Gruenig, M., Puchkov, D., Schöneberg, J., Ullrich, A., Lampe, A., et al. (2013). Spatiotemporal control of endocytosis by phosphatidylinositol-3,4-bisphosphate. *Nature* 499, 233–237. doi: 10.1038/nature12360

Powell, R. R., Welter, B. H., Hwu, R., Bowersox, B., Attaway, C., and Temesvari, L. A. (2006). *Entamoeba histolytica*: FYVE-finger domains, phosphatidylinositol 3-phosphate biosensors, associate with phagosomes but not fluid filled endosomes. *Exp. Parasitol.* 112, 221–231. doi: 10.1016/j.exppara.2005.11.013

Qualmann, B., Roos, J., DiGregorio, P. J., and Kelly, R. B. (1999). Syndapin I, a synaptic dynamin-binding protein that associates with the neural Wiskott-Aldrich syndrome protein. *Mol. Biol. Cell* 10, 501–513. doi: 10.1091/mbc.10.2.501

Raha, S., Dalal, B., Biswas, S., and Biswas, B. B. (1994). Myo-inositol trisphosphate-mediated calcium release from internal stores of *Entamoeba histolytica*. *Mol. Biochem. Parasitol.* 65, 63–71. doi: 10.1016/0166-6851(94)90115-5

Raha, S., Giri, B., Bhattacharyya, B., and Biswas, B. B. (1995). Inositol(1,3,4,5) tetrakisphosphate plays an important role in calcium mobilization from *Entamoeba histolytica*. *FEBS Lett.* 362, 316–318. doi: 10.1016/0014-5793(95)00265-B

Ralston, K. S., Solga, M. D., Mackey-Lawrence, N. M., Somlata, Bhattacharya, A., and Petri, W. A. Jr. (2014). Trogocytosis by *Entamoeba histolytica* contributes to cell killing and tissue invasion. *Nature* 508, 526–530. doi: 10.1038/nature13242

Rameh, L. E., Tolias, K. F., Duckworth, B. C., and Cantley, L. C. (1997). A new pathway for synthesis of phosphatidylinositol-4,5-bisphosphate. *Nature* 390, 192–196. doi: 10.1038/36621

Ringstad, N., Nemoto, Y., and De Camilli, P. (1997). The SH3p4/Sh3p8/SH3p13 protein family: binding partners for synaptojanin and dynamin via a Grb2-like Src homology 3 domain. *Proc. Natl. Acad. Sci. U.S.A.* 94, 8569–8574. doi: 10.1073/pnas.94.16.8569

Robinson, F. L., and Dixon, J. E. (2006). Myotubularin phosphatases: policing 3-phosphoinositides. *Trends Cell Biol.* 16, 403–412. doi: 10.1016/j.tcb.2006.06.001

Rodgers, S. J., Ferguson, D. T., Mitchell, C. A, and Ooms, L. M. (2017). Regulation of PI3K effector signalling in cancer by the phosphoinositide phosphatases. *Biosci. Rep.* 37:BSR20160432. doi: 10.1042/BSR20160432

Rohács, T., Lopes, C. M., Jin, T., Ramdya, P. P., Molnár, Z., and Logothetis, D. E. (2003). Specificity of activation by phosphoinositides determines lipid regulation of Kir channels. *Proc. Natl. Acad. Sci. U.S.A.* 100, 745–750. doi: 10.1073/pnas.0236364100

Rong, Y., Liu, M., Ma, L., Du, W., Zhang, H., Tian, Y., et al. (2012). Clathrin and phosphatidylinositol-4,5-bisphosphate regulate autophagic lysosome reformation. *Nat. Cell Biol.* 14, 924–934. doi: 10.1038/ncb2557

Roos, J., and Kelly, R. B. (1998). Dap160, a neural-specific Eps15 homology and multiple SH3 domain-containing protein that interacts with *Drosophila* dynamin. *J. Biol. Chem.* 273, 19108–19119. doi: 10.1074/jbc.273.30.19108

Rostislavleva, K., Soler, N., Ohashi, Y., Zhang, L., Pardon, E., Burke, J. E., et al. (2015). Structure and flexibility of the endosomal Vps34 complex reveals the basis of its function on membranes. *Science* 350:aac7365. doi: 10.1126/science.aac7365

Rozenvayn, N., and Flaumenhaft, R. (2001). Phosphatidylinositol 4,5-bisphosphate mediates Ca^{2+}-induced platelet alpha-granule secretion: evidence for type II phosphatidylinositol 5-phosphate 4-kinase function. *J. Biol. Chem.* 276, 22410–22419. doi: 10.1074/jbc.M008184200

Rozenvayn, N., and Flaumenhaft, R. (2003). Protein kinase C mediates translocation of type II phosphatidylinositol 5-phosphate 4-kinase required for platelet alpha-granule secretion. *J. Biol. Chem.* 278, 8126–8134. doi: 10.1074/jbc.M206493200

Rudge, S. A., Anderson, D. M., and Emr, S. D. (2004). Vacuole size control: regulation of PtdIns(3,5)P2 levels by the vacuole-associated Vac14-Fig4 complex, a PtdIns(3,5)P2-specific phosphatase. *Mol. Biol. Cell* 15, 24–36. doi: 10.1091/mbc.e03-05-0297

Rutherford, A. C., Traer, C., Wassmer, T., Pattni, K., Bujny, M. V., Carlton, J. G., et al. (2006). The mammalian phosphatidylinositol 3-phosphate 5-kinase (PIKfyve) regulates endosome-to-TGN retrograde transport. *J. Cell Sci.* 119(Pt 19), 3944–3957. doi: 10.1242/jcs.03153

Ryder, P. V., Vistein, R., Gokhale, A., Seaman, M. N., Puthenveedu, M. A., and Faundez, V. (2013). The WASH complex, an endosomal Arp2/3 activator, interacts with the Hermansky-Pudlak syndrome complex BLOC-1 and its cargo phosphatidylinositol-4-kinase type IIα. *Mol. Biol. Cell* 24, 2269–2284. doi: 10.1091/mbc.e13-02-0088

Rynkiewicz, N. K., Liu, H. J., Balamatsias, D., and Mitchell, C. A. (2012). INPP4A/INPP4B and P-Rex proteins: related but different? *Adv. Biol. Regul.* 52, 265–279. doi: 10.1016/j.advenzreg.2011.09.001

Saito-Nakano, Y., Loftus, B. J., Hall, N., and Nozaki, T. (2005). The diversity of Rab GTPases in *Entamoeba histolytica*. *Exp. Parasitol.* 110, 244–252. doi: 10.1016/j.exppara.2005.02.021

Sakisaka, T., Itoh, T., Miura, K., and Takenawa, T. (1997). Phosphatidylinositol 4,5-bisphosphate phosphatase regulates the rearrangement of actin filaments. *Mol. Cell. Biol.* 17, 3841–3849. doi: 10.1128/MCB.17.7.3841

Salazar, G., Craige, B., Wainer, B. H., Guo, J., De Camilli, P., and Faundez, V. (2005). Phosphatidylinositol-4-kinase type II alpha is a component of adaptor protein-3-derived vesicles. *Mol. Biol. Cell* 16, 3692–3704. doi: 10.1091/mbc.e05-01-0020

Sasaki, J., Ishikawa, K., Arita, M., and Taniguchi, K. (2012). ACBD3-mediated recruitment of PI4KB to picornavirus RNA replication sites. *EMBO J.* 31, 754–766. doi: 10.1038/emboj.2011.429

Sasaki, T., Takasuga, S., Sasaki, J., Kofuji, S., Eguchi, S., Yamazaki, M., et al. (2009). Mammalian phosphoinositide kinases and phosphatases. *Prog. Lipid. Res.* 48, 307–343. doi: 10.1016/j.plipres.2009.06.001

Sbrissa, D., Ikonomov, O. C., Fu, Z., Ijuin, T., Gruenberg, J., Takenawa, T., et al. (2007). Core protein machinery for mammalian phosphatidylinositol 3,5-bisphosphate synthesis and turnover that regulates the progression of endosomal transport. Novel Sac phosphatase joins the ArPIKfyve-PIKfyve complex. *J. Biol. Chem.* 282, 23878–23891. doi: 10.1074/jbc.M611678200

Schaletzky, J., Dove, S. K., Short, B., Lorenzo, O., Clague, M. J., and Barr, F. A. (2003). Phosphatidylinositol-5-phosphate activates. *Curr. Biol.* 13, 504–509. doi: 10.1016/S0960-9822(03)00132-5

Schill, N. J., and Anderson, R. A. (2009). Two novel phosphatidylinositol-4-phosphate 5-kinase type I gamma splice variants expressed in human cells display distinctive cellular targeting. *Biochem. J.* 422, 473–482. doi: 10.1042/BJ20090638

Schink, K. O., Tan, K. W., and Stenmark, H. (2016). Phosphoinositides in control of membrane dynamics. *Annu. Rev. Cell. Dev. Biol.* 32, 143–171. doi: 10.1146/annurev-cellbio-111315-125349

Schmid, A. C., Wise, H. M., Mitchell, C. A., Nussbaum, R., and Woscholski, R. (2004). Type II phosphoinositide 5-phosphatases have unique sensitivities towards fatty acid composition and head group phosphorylation. *FEBS Lett.* 576, 9–13. doi: 10.1016/j.febslet.2004.08.052

Schöneberg, J., Lehmann, M., Ullrich, A., Posor, Y., Lo, W. T., Lichtner, G., et al. (2017). Lipid-mediated PX-BAR domain recruitment couples local membrane constriction to endocytic vesicle fission. *Nat. Commun.* 8:15873. doi: 10.1038/ncomms15873

Schu, P. V., Takegawa, K., Fry, M. J., Stack, J. H., Waterfield, M. D., and Emr, S. D. (1993). Phosphatidylinositol 3-kinase encoded by yeast VPS34 gene essential for protein sorting. *Science* 260, 88–91. doi: 10.1126/science.8385367

Schulze, H., Korpal, M., Hurov, J., Kim, S. W., Zhang, J., Cantley, L. C., et al. (2006). Characterization of the megakaryocyte demarcation membrane system and its role in thrombopoiesis. *Blood* 107, 3868–3875. doi: 10.1182/blood-2005-07-2755

Shah, Z. H., Jones, D. R., Sommer, L., Foulger, R., Bultsma, Y., D'Santos, C., et al. (2013). Nuclear phosphoinositides and their impact on nuclear functions. *FEBS J.* 280, 6295–6310. doi: 10.1111/febs.12543

Sharma, S., Bhattacharya, S., and Bhattacharya, A. (2019). PtdIns(4,5)P(2) is generated by a novel phosphatidylinositol 4-phosphate 5-kinase in the protist parasite *Entamoeba histolytica*. *FEBS. J.* doi: 10.1111/febs.14804 [Epub ahead of print].

Shearn, C. T., and Norris, F. A. (2007). Biochemical characterization of the type I inositol polyphosphate 4-phosphatase C2 domain. *Biochem. Biophys. Res. Commun.* 356, 255–259. doi: 10.1016/j.bbrc.2007.02.115

Shen, W. H., Balajee, A. S., Wang, J., Wu, H., Eng, C., Pandolfi, P. P., et al. (2007). Essential role for nuclear PTEN in maintaining chromosomal integrity. *Cell* 128, 157–170. doi: 10.1016/j.cell.2006.11.042

Shi, X., Hong, T., Walter, K. L., Ewalt, M., Michishita, E., Hung, T., et al. (2006). ING2 PHD domain links histoneH3 lysine 4 methylation to active gene repression. *Nature* 442, 96–99. doi: 10.1038/nature04835

Shin, H. W., Hayashi, M., Christoforidis, S., Lacas-Gervais, S., Hoepfner, S., Wenk, M. R., et al. (2005). An enzymatic cascade of Rab5 effectors regulates phosphoinositide turnover in the endocytic pathway. *J. Cell Biol.* 170, 607–618. doi: 10.1083/jcb.200505128

Shinde, S. R., and Maddika, S. (2016). PTEN modulates EGFR late endocytic trafficking and degradation by dephosphorylating Rab7. *Nat. Commun.* 7:10689. doi: 10.1038/ncomms10689

Shinozaki-Narikawa, N., Kodama, T., and Shibasaki, Y. (2006). Cooperation of phosphoinositides and BAR domain proteins in endosomal tubulation. *Traffic* 7, 1539–1550. doi: 10.1111/j.1600-0854.2006.00480.x

Skippen, A., Jones, D. H., Morgan, C. P., Li, M., and Cockcroft, S. (2002). Mechanism of ADP ribosylation factor-stimulated phosphatidylinositol 4,5-bisphosphate synthesis in HL60 cells. *J. Biol. Chem.* 277, 5823–5831. doi: 10.1074/jbc.M110274200

Sleeman, M. W., Wortley, K. E., Lai, K. M., Gowen, L. C., Kintner, J., Kline, W. O., et al. (2005). Absence of the lipid phosphatase SHIP2 confers resistance to dietary obesity. *Nat. Med.* 11, 199–205. doi: 10.1038/nm1178

Somlata, Nakada-Tsukui, K., and Nozaki, T. (2017). AGC family kinase 1 participates in trogocytosis but not in phagocytosis in *Entamoeba histolytica*. *Nat. Commun.* 8:101. doi: 10.1038/s41467-017-00199-y

Song, M. S., Carracedo, A., Salmena, L., Song, S. J., Egia, A., Malumbres, M., et al. (2011). Nuclear PTEN regulates the APC-CDH1 tumor-suppressive complex in a phosphatase-independent manner. *Cell* 144, 187–199. doi: 10.1016/j.cell.2010.12.020

Speed, C. J., Matzaris, M., Bird, P. I., and Mitchell, C. A. (1995). Tissue distribution and intracellular localisation of the 75-kDa inositol polyphosphate 5-phosphatase. *Eur. J. Biochem.* 234, 216–224. doi: 10.1111/j.1432-1033.1995.216_c.x

Stack, J. H., Herman, P. K., Schu, P. V., and Emr, S. D. (1993). A membrane-associated complex containing the Vps15 protein kinase and the Vps34 PI 3-kinase is essential for protein sorting to the yeast lysosome-like vacuole. *EMBO J.* 12, 2195–2204. doi: 10.1002/j.1460-2075.1993.tb05867.x

Stahelin, R. V., Karathanassis, D., Bruzik, K. S., Waterfield, M. D., Bravo, J., Williams, R. L., et al. (2006). Structural and membrane binding analysis of the Phox homology domain of phosphoinositide 3-kinase-C2alpha. *J. Biol. Chem.* 281, 39396–39406. doi: 10.1074/jbc.M607079200

Steck, P. A., Pershouse, M. A., Jasser, S. A., Yung, W. K., Lin, H., Ligon, A. H., et al. (1997). Identification of a candidate tumour suppressor gene, MMAC1, at chromosome 10q23.3 that is mutated in multiple advanced cancers. *Nat. Genet.* 15, 356–362. doi: 10.1038/ng0497-356

Stefan, C. J., Manford, A. G., Baird, D., Yamada-Hanff, J., Mao, Y., and Emr, S. D. (2011). Osh proteins regulate phosphoinositide metabolism at ER-plasma membrane contact sites. *Cell* 144, 389–401. doi: 10.1016/j.cell.2010.12.034

Stein, M. P., Feng, Y., Cooper, K. L., Welford, A. M., and Wandinger-Ness, A. (2003). Human VPS34 and p150 are Rab7 interacting partners. *Traffic* 4, 754–771. doi: 10.1034/j.1600-0854.2003.00133.x

Stephens, L., Smrcka, A., Cooke, F. T., Jackson, T. R., Sternweis, P. C., and Hawkins, P. T. (1994). A novel phosphoinositide 3 kinase activity in myeloid-derived cells is activated by G protein beta gamma subunits. *Cell* 77, 83–93. doi: 10.1016/0092-8674(94)90237-2

Stijf-Bultsma, Y., Sommer, L., Tauber, M., Baalbaki, M., Giardoglou, P., Jones, D. R., et al. (2015). The basal transcription complex component TAF3 transduces changes in nuclear phosphoinositides into transcriptional output. *Mol. Cell* 58, 453–467. doi: 10.1016/j.molcel.2015.03.009

Stoyanov, B., Volinia, S., Hanck, T., Rubio, I., Loubtchenkov, M., Malek, D., et al. (1995). Cloning and characterization of a G protein-activated human phosphoinositide-3 kinase. *Science* 269, 690–693. doi: 10.1126/science.7624799

Streb, H., Bayerdörffer, E., Haase, W., Irvine, R. F., and Schulz, I. (1984). Effect of inositol-1,4,5-trisphosphate on isolated subcellular fractions of rat pancreas. *J. Membr. Biol.* 81, 241–253. doi: 10.1007/BF01868717

Streb, H., Irvine, R. F., Berridge, M. J., and Schulz, I. (1983). Release of Ca^{2+} from a nonmitochondrial intracellular store in pancreatic acinar cells by inositol-1,4,5-trisphosphate. *Nature* 306, 67–69. doi: 10.1038/306067a0

Suchy, S. F., and Nussbaum, R. L. (2002). The deficiency of PIP2 5-phosphatase in Lowe syndrome affects actin polymerization. *Am. J. Hum. Genet.* 71, 1420–1427. doi: 10.1086/344517

Sun, Q., Westphal, W., Wong, K. N., Tan, I., and Zhong, Q. (2010). Rubicon controls endosome maturation as a Rab7 effector. *Proc. Natl. Acad. Sci. U.S.A.* 107, 19338–19343. doi: 10.1073/pnas.1010554107

Swanson, J. A. (2014). Phosphoinositides and engulfment. *Cell. Microbiol.* 16, 1473–1483. doi: 10.1111/cmi.12334

Tan, J., and Brill, J. A. (2014). Cinderella story: PI4P goes from precursor to key signaling molecule. *Crit. Rev. Biochem. Mol. Biol.* 49, 33–58. doi: 10.3109/10409238.2013.853024

Tan, X., Thapa, N., Choi, S., and Anderson, R. A. (2015). Emerging roles of PtdIns(4,5)P2—beyond the plasma membrane. *J. Cell Sci.* 128, 4047–4056. doi: 10.1242/jcs.175208

Tanaka, K., Horiguchi, K., Yoshida, T., Takeda, M., Fujisawa, H., Takeuchi, K., et al. (1999). Evidence that a phosphatidylinositol 3,4,5-trisphosphate-binding protein can function in nucleus. *J. Biol. Chem.* 274, 3919–3922. doi: 10.1074/jbc.274.7.3919

Tang, Y., and Eng, C. (2006a). PTEN autoregulates its expression by stabilization of p53 in a phosphatase-independent manner. *Cancer Res.* 66, 36–42. doi: 10.1158/0008-5472.CAN-05-1557

Tang, Y., and Eng, C. (2006b). p53 down-regulates phosphatase and tensin homologue deleted on chromosome 10 protein stability partially through caspase-mediated degradation in cells with proteasome dysfunction. *Cancer Res.* 66, 6139–6148. doi: 10.1158/0008-5472.CAN-06-0772

Taniuchi, M., Sobuz, S. U., Begum, S., Platts-Mills, J. A., Liu, J., Yang, Z., et al. (2013). Etiology of diarrhea in Bangladeshi infants in the first year of life analyzed using molecular methods. *J. Infect. Dis.* 208, 1794–1802. doi: 10.1093/infdis/jit507

Tapparel, C., Reymond, A., Girardet, C., Guillou, L., Lyle, R., Lamon, C., et al. (2003). The TPTE gene family: cellular expression, subcellular localization and alternative splicing. *Gene* 323, 189–199. doi: 10.1016/j.gene.2003.09.038

Tashiro, H., Blazes, M. S., Wu, R., Cho, K. R., Bose, S., Wang, S. I., et al. (1997). Mutations in PTEN are frequent in endometrial carcinoma but rare in other common gynecological malignancies. *Cancer Res.* 57, 3935–3940.

Taylor, G. S., Maehama, T., and Dixon, J. E. (2000). Myotubularin, a protein tyrosine phosphatase mutated in myotubular myopathy, dephosphorylates the lipid second messenger, phosphatidylinositol 3-phosphate. *Proc. Natl. Acad. Sci. U.S.A.* 97, 8910–8915. doi: 10.1073/pnas.160255697

Thi, E. P., Lambertz, U., and Reiner, N. E. (2012). Class IA phosphatidylinositol 3-kinase p110α regulates phagosome maturation. *PLoS ONE* 7:e43668. doi: 10.1371/journal.pone.0043668

Tolias, K. F., Couvillon, A. D., Cantley, L. C., and Carpenter, C. L. (1998). Characterization of a Rac1- and RhoGDI-associated lipid kinase signaling complex. *Mol. Cell. Biol.* 18, 762–770. doi: 10.1128/MCB.18.2.762

Traynor-Kaplan, A., Kruse, M., Dickson, E. J., Dai, G., Vivas, O., Yu, H., et al. (2017). Fatty-acyl chain profiles of cellular phosphoinositides. *Biochim. Biophys. Acta* 1862, 513–522. doi: 10.1016/j.bbalip.2017.02.002

Trivedi, C. M., Luo, Y., Yin, Z., Zhang, M., Zhu, W., Wang, T., et al. (2007). Hdac2 regulates the cardiac hypertrophic response by modulating Gsk3 beta activity. *Nat. Med.* 13, 324–331. doi: 10.1038/nm1552

Trotman, L. C., Wang, X., Alimonti, A., Chen, Z., Teruya-Feldstein, J., Yang, H., et al. (2007). Ubiquitination regulates PTEN nuclear import and tumor suppression. *Cell* 128, 141–156. doi: 10.1016/j.cell.2006.11.040

Tu, Z., Ninos, J. M., Ma, Z., Wang, J. W., Lemos, M. P., Desponts, C., et al. (2001). Embryonic and hematopoietic stem cells express a novel SH2-containing inositol 5'-phosphatase isoform that partners with the Grb2 adapter protein. *Blood* 98, 2028–2038. doi: 10.1182/blood.V98.7.2028

Ungewickell, A., Hugge, C., Kisseleva, M., Chang, S. C., Zou, J., Feng, Y., et al. (2005). The identification and characterization of two phosphatidylinositol-4,5-bisphosphate 4-phosphatases. *Proc. Natl. Acad. Sci. U.S.A.* 102, 18854–18859. doi: 10.1073/pnas.0509740102

Ungewickell, A., Ward, M. E., Ungewickell, E., and Majerus, P. W. (2004). The inositol polyphosphate 5-phosphatase Ocrl associates with endosomes that are partially coated with clathrin. *Proc. Natl. Acad. Sci. U.S.A.* 101, 13501–13506. doi: 10.1073/pnas.0405664101

Vadas, O., Burke, J. E., Zhang, X., Berndt, A., and Williams, R. L. (2011). Structural basis for activation and inhibition of class I phosphoinositide 3-kinases. *Sci. Signal* 4:re2. doi: 10.1126/scisignal.2002165

Vanhaesebroeck, B., Guillermet-Guibert, J., Graupera, M., and Bilanges, B. (2010a). The emerging mechanisms of isoform-specific PI3K signalling. *Nat. Rev. Mol. Cell. Biol.* 11, 329–341. doi: 10.1038/nrm2882

Vanhaesebroeck, B., Vogt, P. K., and Rommel, C. (2010b). PI3K: from the bench to the clinic and back. *Curr. Top. Microbiol. Immunol.* 347, 1–19. doi: 10.1007/82_2010_65

Vann, L. R., Wooding, F. B, Irvine, R. F., and Divecha, N. (1997). Metabolism and possible compartmentalization of inositol lipids in isolated rat-liver nuclei. *Biochem. J.* 327, 569–576. doi: 10.1042/bj3270569

Várnai, P., Gulyás, G., Tóth, D. J., Sohn, M., Sengupta, N., and Balla, T. (2017). Quantifying lipid changes in various membrane compartments using lipid binding protein domains. *Cell Calcium.* 64, 72–82. doi: 10.1016/j.ceca.2016.12.008

Viaud, J., Boal, F., Tronchère, H., Gaits-Iacovoni, F., and Payrastre, B. (2014). Phosphatidylinositol 5-phosphate: a nuclear stress lipid and a tuner of membranes and cytoskeleton dynamics. *Bioessays* 36, 260–272. doi: 10.1002/bies.201300132

Vicinanza, M., Korolchuk, V. I., Ashkenazi, A., Puri, C., Menzies, F. M., Clarke, J. H., et al. (2015). PI(5)P regulates autophagosome biogenesis. *Mol. Cell* 57, 219–234. doi: 10.1016/j.molcel.2014.12.007

Vogt, P. K., Kang, S., Elsliger, M. A., and Gymnopoulos, M. (2007). Cancer-specific mutations in phosphatidylinositol 3-kinase. *Trends Biochem. Sci.* 32, 342–349. doi: 10.1016/j.tibs.2007.05.005

Volpe, P., Salviati, G., Di Virgilio, F., and Pozzan, T. (1985). Inositol 1,4,5-trisphosphate induces calcium release from sarcoplasmic reticulum of skeletal muscle. *Nature* 316, 347–349. doi: 10.1038/316347a0

Volpicelli-Daley, L. A., Lucast, L., Gong, L. W., Liu, L., Sasaki, J., Sasaki, T., et al. (2010). Phosphatidylinositol-4-phosphate 5-kinases and phosphatidylinositol 4,5-bisphosphate synthesis in the brain. *J. Biol. Chem.* 285, 28708–28714. doi: 10.1074/jbc.M110.132191

Vyas, P., Norris, F. A., Joseph, R., Majerus, P. W., and Orkin, S. H. (2000). Inositol polyphosphate 4-phosphatase type I regulates cell growth downstream of transcription factor GATA-1. *Proc. Natl. Acad. Sci. U.S.A.* 97, 13696–13701. doi: 10.1073/pnas.250476397

Wada, T., Sasaoka, T., Funaki, M., Hori, H., Murakami, S., Ishiki, M., et al. (2001). Overexpression of SH2-containing inositol phosphatase 2 results in negative regulation of insulin-induced metabolic actions in 3T3-L1 adipocytes via its 5'-phosphatase catalytic activity. *Mol. Cell. Biol.* 21, 1633–1646. doi: 10.1128/MCB.21.5.1633-1646.2001

Walker, S. M., Downes, C. P., and Leslie, N. R. (2001). TPIP: a novel phosphoinositide 3-phosphatase. *Biochem. J.* 360(Pt 2), 277–283. doi: 10.1042/bj3600277

Wallroth, A., and Haucke, V. (2018). Phosphoinositide conversion in endocytosis and the endolysosomal system. *J. Biol. Chem.* 293, 1526–1535. doi: 10.1074/jbc.R117.000629

Walsh, J. A. (1986). Problems in recognition and diagnosis of amebiasis: estimation of the global magnitude of morbidity and mortality. *Rev. Infect. Dis.* 8, 228–238. doi: 10.1093/clinids/8.2.228

Wang, M., Bond, N. J., Letcher, A. J., Richardson, J. P., Lilley, K. S., Irvine, R. F., et al. (2010). Genomic tagging reveals a random association of endogenous PtdIns5P 4-kinases IIalpha and IIbeta and a partial nuclear localization of the IIalpha isoform. *Biochem. J.* 430, 215–221. doi: 10.1042/BJ20100340

Wang, X., Trotman, L. C., Koppie, T., Alimonti, A., Chen, Z., Gao, Z., et al. (2007). NEDD4-1 is aproto-oncogenic ubiquitin ligase for PTEN. *Cell* 128, 129–139. doi: 10.1016/j.cell.2006.11.039

Wang, Y. J., Li, W. H., Wang, J., Xu, K., Dong, P., Luo, X., et al. (2004). Critical role of PIP5KIγ87 in InsP3-mediated Ca^{2+} signaling. *J. Cell Biol.* 167, 1005–1010. doi: 10.1083/jcb.200408008

Wang, Y. J., Wang, J., Sun, H. Q., Martinez, M., Sun, Y. X., Macia, E., et al. (2003). Phosphatidylinositol 4 phosphate regulates targeting of clathrin adaptor AP-1 complexes to the Golgi. *Cell* 114, 299–310. doi: 10.1016/S0092-8674(03)00603-2

Welter, B. H., Goldston, A. M., and Temesvari, L. A. (2011). Localisation to lipid rafts correlates with increased function of the Gal/GalNAc lectin in the human protozoan parasite, *Entamoeba histolytica*. *Int. J. Parasitol.* 41, 1409–1419. doi: 10.1016/j.ijpara.2011.10.003

Whisstock, J. C., Romero, S., Gurung, R., Nandurkar, H., Ooms, L. M., Bottomley, S. P., et al. (2000). The inositol polyphosphate 5-phosphatases and the apurinic/apyrimidinic base excision repair endonucleases share a common mechanism for catalysis. *J. Biol. Chem.* 275, 37055–37061. doi: 10.1074/jbc.M006244200

Whitecross, D. E., and Anderson, D. H. (2017). Identification of the binding sites on Rab5 and p110beta phosphatidylinositol 3-kinase. *Sci. Rep.* 7:16194. doi: 10.1038/s41598-017-16029-6

Whitley, P., Reaves, B. J., Hashimoto, M., Riley, A. M., Potter, B. V., and Holman, G. D. (2003). Identification of mammalian Vps24p as an effector of phosphatidylinositol 3,5-bisphosphate-dependent endosome compartmentalization. *J. Biol. Chem.* 278, 38786–38795. doi: 10.1074/jbc.M306864200

Whitman, M., Downes, C. P., Keeler, M., Keller, T., and Cantley, L. (1988). Type I phosphatidylinositol kinase makes a novel inositol phospholipid, phosphatidylinositol-3-phosphate. *Nature* 332, 644–646. doi: 10.1038/332644a0

Whorton, M. R., and MacKinnon, R. (2011). Crystal structure of the mammalian GIRK2 K^+ channel and gating regulation by G proteins, PIP2, and sodium. *Cell* 147, 199–208. doi: 10.1016/j.cell.2011.07.046

Wieffer, M., Cibrián Uhalte, E., Posor, Y., Otten, C., Branz, K., Schütz, I., et al. (2013). PI4K2β/AP-1-based TGN-endosomal sorting regulates Wnt signaling. *Curr. Biol.* 23, 2185–2190. doi: 10.1016/j.cub.2013.09.017

Williams, C., Choudhury, R., McKenzie, E., and Lowe, M. (2007). Targeting of the type II inositol polyphosphate 5-phosphatase INPP5B to the early secretory pathway. *J. Cell Sci.* 120(Pt 22), 3941–3951. doi: 10.1242/jcs.014423

Wisniewski, D., Strife, A., Swendeman, S., Erdjument-Bromage, H., Geromanos, S., Kavanaugh, W. M., et al. (1999). A novel SH2-containing phosphatidylinositol 3,4,5-trisphosphate 5-phosphatase (SHIP2) is constitutively tyrosine phosphorylated and associated with src homologous and collagen gene (SHC) in chronic myelogenous leukemia progenitor cells. *Blood* 93, 2707–2720.

Wozniak, D. J., Kajdacsy-Balla, A., Macias, V., Ball-Kell, S., Zenner, M. L., Bie, W., et al. (2017). PTEN is a protein phosphatase that targets active PTK6 and inhibits PTK6 oncogenic signaling in prostate cancer. *Nat. Commun.* 8:1508. doi: 10.1038/s41467-017-01574-5

Wu, B., and Guo, W. (2015). The exocyst at a glance. *J. Cell Sci.* 128, 2957–2964. doi: 10.1242/jcs.156398

Wu, C. Y., Lin, M. W., Wu, D. C., Huang, Y. B., Huang, H. T., and Chen, C. L. (2014). The role of phosphoinositide-regulated actin reorganization in chemotaxis and cell migration. *Br. J. Pharmacol.* 171, 5541–5554. doi: 10.1111/bph.12777

Xia, Y., Irvine, R. F., and Giudici, M. L. (2011). Phosphatidylinositol 4-phosphate 5-kinase Iγ_v6, a new splice variant found in rodents and humans. *Biochem. Biophys. Res. Commun.* 411, 416–420. doi: 10.1016/j.bbrc.2011.06.168

Xu, Z., Huang, G., and Kandror, K. V. (2006). Phosphatidylinositol 4-kinase type IIalpha is targeted specifically to cellugyrin-positive glucose transporter 4 vesicles. *Mol. Endocrinol.* 20, 2890–2897. doi: 10.1210/me.2006-0193

Yamamoto, A., DeWald, D. B., Boronenkov, I. V., Anderson, R. A., Emr, S. D., and Koshland, D. (1995). Novel PI(4)P 5-kinase homologue, Fab1p, essential for normal vacuole function and morphology in yeast. *Mol. Biol. Cell* 6, 525–539. doi: 10.1091/mbc.6.5.525

Ye, K., and Ahn, J. Y. (2008). Nuclear phosphoinositide signaling. *Front. Biosci.* 13, 340–348. doi: 10.2741/2699

Yeung, T., and Grinstein, S. (2007). Lipid signaling and the modulation of surface charge during phagocytosis. *Immunol. Rev.* 219, 17–36. doi: 10.1111/j.1600-065X.2007.00546.x

Yoon, M. S., Du, G., Backer, J. M., Frohman, M. A., and Chen, J. (2011). Class III PI-3-kinase activates phospholipase D in an amino acid-sensing mTORC1 pathway. *J. Cell Biol.* 195, 435–447. doi: 10.1083/jcb.2011 07033

York, J. D. (2006). Regulation of nuclear processes by inositol polyphosphates. *Biochim. Biophys. Acta* 1761, 552–559. doi: 10.1016/j.bbalip.2006.04.014

Yu, H., Fukami, K., Watanabe, Y., Ozaki, C., and Takenawa, T. (1998). Phosphatidylinositol 4,5-bisphosphate reverses the inhibition of RNA transcription caused by histone H1. *Eur. J. Biochem.* 251, 281–287. doi: 10.1046/j.1432-1327.1998.2510281.x

Yu, L., McPhee, C. K., Zheng, L., Mardones, G. A., Rong, Y., Peng, J., et al. (2010). Termination of autophagy and reformation of lysosomes regulated by mTOR. *Nature* 465, 942–946. doi: 10.1038/nature09076

Yuan, H. X., Russell, R. C., and Guan, K. L. (2013). Regulation of PIK3C3/VPS34 complexes by MTOR in nutrient stress-induced autophagy. *Autophagy* 9, 1983–1995. doi: 10.4161/auto.26058

Zhang, X., Jefferson, A. B., Auethavekiat, V., and Majerus, P. W. (1995). The protein deficient in Lowe syndrome is a phosphatidylinositol-4,5-bisphosphate 5-phosphatase. *Proc. Natl. Acad. Sci. U.S.A.* 92, 4853–4856. doi: 10.1073/pnas.92.11.4853

Zhang, X., Orlando, K., He, B., Xi, F., Zhang, J., Zajac, A., et al. (2008). Membrane association and functional regulation of Sec3 by phospholipids and Cdc42. *J. Cell Biol.* 180, 145–158. doi: 10.1083/jcb.200704128

Zhang, Y., Zolov, S. N., Chow, C. Y., Slutsky, S. G., Richardson, S. C., Piper, R. C., et al. (2007). Loss of Vac14, a regulator of the signaling lipid phosphatidylinositol 3,5-bisphosphate, results in neurodegeneration in mice. *Proc. Natl. Acad. Sci. U.S.A.* 104, 17518–17523. doi: 10.1073/pnas.0702275104

Zhao, X., Várnai, P., Tuymetova, G., Balla, A., Tóth, Z. E., Oker-Blom, C., et al. (2001). Interaction of neuronal calcium sensor-1 (NCS-1) with phosphatidylinositol 4-kinase beta stimulates lipid kinase activity and affects membrane trafficking in COS-7 cells. *J. Biol. Chem.* 276, 40183–40189. doi: 10.1074/jbc.M104048200

Zhong, S., Hsu, F., Stefan, C. J., Wu, X., Patel, A., Cosgrove, M. S., et al. (2012). Allosteric activation of the phosphoinositide phosphatase Sac1 by anionic phospholipids. *Biochemistry* 51, 3170–3177. doi: 10.1021/bi300086c

Zolov, S. N., Bridges, D., Zhang, Y., Lee, W. W., Riehle, E., Verma, R., et al. (2012). *In vivo*, Pikfyve generates PI(3,5)P2, which serves as both a signaling lipid and the major precursor for PI5P. *Proc. Natl. Acad. Sci. U S A.* 109, 17472–17477. doi: 10.1073/pnas.1203106109

Zou, J., Marjanovic, J., Kisseleva, M. V., Wilson, M., and Majerus, P. W. (2007). Type I phosphatidylinositol-4,5-bisphosphate 4-phosphatase regulates stress-induced apoptosis. *Proc. Natl. Acad. Sci. U.S.A.* 104, 16834–16839. doi: 10.1073/pnas.0708189104

Zou, J., Zhang, C., Marjanovic, J., Kisseleva, M. V., Majerus, P. W., and Wilson, M. P. (2012). Myotubularin-related protein (MTMR) 9 determines the enzymatic activity, substrate specificity, and role in autophagy of MTMR8. *Proc. Natl. Acad. Sci. U.S.A.* 109, 9539–9544. doi: 10.1073/pnas.1207021109

6

Entamoeba histolytica Cyclooxygenase-Like Protein Regulates Cysteine Protease Expression and Virulence

Preeti Shahi, France Moreau and Kris Chadee*

Department of Microbiology, Immunology and Infectious Diseases, Snyder Institute for Chronic Diseases, University of Calgary, Calgary, AB, Canada

***Correspondence:**
Kris Chadee
kchadee@ucalgary.ca

The intestinal protozoan parasite *Entamoeba histolytica* (*Eh*) causes amebiasis associated with severe diarrhea and/or liver abscess. *Eh* pathogenesis is multifactorial requiring both parasite virulent molecules and host-induced innate immune responses. *Eh*-induced host pro-inflammatory responses plays a critical role in disease pathogenesis by causing damage to tissues allowing parasites access to systemic sites. *Eh* cyclooxygenase (*Eh*Cox) derived prostaglandin E_2 stimulates the chemokine IL-8 from mucosal epithelial cells that recruits neutrophils to the site of infection to exacerbate disease. At present, it is not known how *Eh*Cox is regulated or whether it affects the expression of other proteins in *Eh*. In this study, we found that gene silencing of *Eh*Cox (*EhCoxgs*) markedly increased endogenous cysteine protease (CP) protein expression and virulence without altering CP gene transcripts. Live virulent *Eh* pretreated with arachidonic acid substrate to enhance PGE_2 production or aspirin to inhibit *Eh*Cox enzyme activity or addition of exogenous PGE_2 to *Eh* had no effect on *Eh*CP activity. Increased CP enzyme activity in *EhCoxgs* was stable and significantly enhanced erythrophagocytosis, cytopathic effects on colonic epithelial cells and elicited pro-inflammatory cytokines in mice colonic loops. Acute infection with *EhCoxgs* in colonic loops increased inflammation associated with high levels of myeloperoxidase activity. This study has identified *Eh*Cox protein as one of the important endogenous regulators of cysteine protease activity. Alterations of CP activity in response to Cox gene silencing may be a negative feedback mechanism in *Eh* to limit proteolytic activity during colonization that can inadvertently trigger inflammation in the gut.

Keywords: *Entamoeba histolytica*, parasites, cox like protein, cysteine protease, actinin like protein, virulence, pro-inflammatory cytokines

INTRODUCTION

Entamoeba histolytica (*Eh*) is an invasive extracellular protozoan parasite responsible for amebic colitis and liver abscess (World Health Organization, 1998). It is one of the major cause of severe diarrhea in areas of poor sanitation and nutrition particularly in tropical and developing countries. While the majority of *Eh* infection remains asymptomatic, about 10% of infection converts to an invasive phenotype where *Eh* invades the mucosal epithelium resulting in 100,000 death/year (World Health Organization, 1997; Stanley, 2003).

The host innate immune status and parasite virulence factors play major roles in disease pathogenesis (Faust and Guillen, 2012; Verkerke et al., 2012; Marie and Petri, 2014; Nozaki and Bhattacharya, 2015). The host immune response during *Eh* invasion of the colonic mucosa is characterized by increased levels of pro-inflammatory cytokines that recruits inflammatory cells including macrophages and neutrophils (Seydel et al., 1997; Mortimer and Chadee, 2010; Nakada-Tsukui and Nozaki, 2016) to the site of infection. The major *Eh* virulent factors identified to date are the galactose/N-acetyl-D-galactosamine (Gal/GalNAc) lectin (Gal-lectin), cysteine proteinases, amoebapore, and prostaglandin E_2 (Moonah et al., 2013; Marie and Petri, 2014).

Prostaglandins are lipid mediators synthesize from arachidonic acid through cyclooxygenase and are associated with various diarrheal disease including bacterial and inflammatory bowel diseases (Ahrenstedt et al., 1994; Alcantara et al., 2001; Resta-Lenert and Barrett, 2002). We have shown that *Eh* synthesizes PGE_2 through a cyclooxygenase like enzyme as confirmed by gas chromatography/mass spectrometry analysis (Belley and Chadee, 2000). Surprisingly, *Eh*PGE_2 was not immunosuppressive to reduce host defenses but rather, PGE_2 bound EP4 receptors on colonic epithelial cells and stimulated the potent neutrophil chemoattractant, IL-8 mRNA expression and protein production. In addition, *Eh*PGE_2 also altered tight junction proteins and increased ion permeability that led to diarrhea in intestinal amebiasis (Lejeune et al., 2011). Even though *Eh* produces high levels of PGE_2 in the presence of arachidonic acid the parasite can also stimulate host cells such as macrophages and colonic epithelial cell to produce PGE_2 as part of the pro-inflammatory response elicited by the parasite (Stenson et al., 2001; Sanchez-Ramirez et al., 2004). *Eh*Cox encodes a functional cyclooxygenase enzyme as evidenced by Cox enzymatic assays. An unusual aspect is that *Eh*Cox is primitive and has little homology to other Cox proteins from mammalian cells and some eukaryotes. At present, the biological function of *Eh*Cox other than being an enzyme that catalyzes the production of PGE_2 in *Eh* is not known.

In this study, we made the seminal observation that silencing *Eh*Cox enhanced cysteine protease protein expression and enzyme activity independent of *Eh*Cox-induced PGE_2 production. These results suggest that increased cysteine protease activity in *EhCoxgs* is linked to increase parasite-induced inflammation and pathogenicity. These findings increase our understanding on the molecular basis of pathogenicity in *Eh* and how dissimilar enzymes can regulate their activity in the parasite.

MATERIALS AND METHODS

Reagent

E64, leupeptin, aprotinin, and Nonidet P-40 detergent were obtained from Sigma-Aldrich. Z-VVR-AMC substrate was purchased from Enzo Life Sciences. The Z-Arg-Arg-pNA.2 HCl substrate was purchased from Bachem. Mouse monoclonal anti-actin clone C4 antibody was purchased from MP Biomedical, LLC. Antibodies to *Eh*CP4 and the CP inhibitors WRR483 and WRR605 were a kind gift from Dr. Sharon Reed, University of California, San Diego. *Eh*CP5 and *Eh*Cox1 like antibodies were generated in rabbits using recombinant proteins expressed in *E. coli* (Belley and Chadee, 2000). Ubiquitin antibody (P4D1) was from Cell Signaling Technology and cycloheximide from Sigma-Aldrich.

Cultivation and Harvesting of *E. histolytica*

G3 *Eh* were grown axenically in TYI-S-33 medium at 37°C. After 72 h, logarithmic-growth-phase *Eh* cultures were harvested by chilling on ice for 9 min, pelleted at 200 g, and washed two times with PBS. For the detection of proteins and enzymatic activity, *Eh* lysate was prepared by using three cycles of freeze-thawlysis and proteins quantified by the bicinchoninic acid protein assay, using bovine serum albumin as protein standard (#23225, Thermo Scientific). *Eh* secretory protein (SP) were prepared as described previously (Lidell et al., 2006). Briefly, secreted components were collected from mid-log phase *Eh* incubated in Hanks' balanced salt solution (Invitrogen) for 2 h at 37°C at a final concentration of 2×10^7 *Eh* per ml. Following incubation, *Eh* was removed by centrifugation at 10,000 × g for 10 min. Secretory proteins were quantified by the bicinchoninic acid protein assay. To quantify the growth of control and *EhCoxgs,* 2.5×10^5 log phase *Eh* were inoculated in 14 ml TYI-S-33 medium and the number of parasites counted every 24 h using a hemocytometer.

Cloning of the *Eh*Cox-Like Gene

*Eh*Cox-like gene (Acc No. AF208390) 500 bp long 5′ end of protein-coding region was amplified by PCR from cDNA using specific primer containing stu1 and sac1 restriction sites (**Table 1**). The PCR product was sub cloned using the pGEM-T Easy vector system (Promega) and then digested with the restriction enzymes, stu1 and sac1. The digested DNA insert was cloned into StuI- and SacI-digested pSAP2-gunma (kind gift from Dr. Tomoyoshi Nozaki, Tokyo, Japan). This construct was verified by sequencing. G3 *Eh* were harvested during mid-log growth and transfected with a silencing plasmid (pSAP2-gunma-cox) using the Lipofectamine (Life technologies) and OPTIMEMI medium (Life Technologies) supplemented with 5 mg/ml L-cysteine and 1 mg/ml ascorbic acid (transfection medium) and pH 6.8 as previously described (Fisher et al., 2006) Transfected *Eh* were selected with G418 (Sigma) over a 3-week period, starting with 6 µg/ml and ending with 24 µg/ml. Silencing was assessed in these strains using quantitative reverse transcription-PCR (qRT-PCR) and western blot analysis. Once gene silencing was confirmed, the G418 selection was removed, and then silencing was again confirmed and quantified.

Preparation of *E. histolytica* Nuclear Proteins (*Eh*NP)

Eh were washed twice in PBS and suspended in lysis buffer [100 mM Tris (pH 7.4), 1 µg/ml E-64 (Sigma), 2 µg/ml leupeptin, 7.4 µg/ml aprotinin and 0.5% Nonidet P-40 detergent] on ice for 15 min. Nuclei were pelleted by centrifugation at 2,000 × g for 15 min, washed with lysis buffer, and suspended in 0.1 M sodium phosphate buffer (pH 7.0). The protein concentration was determined by the bicinchoninic acid method using bovine serum albumin as protein standard (Thermo Scientific).

TABLE 1 | Primers used in this study.

	Name	Sequence 5′-3′	Annealing temp (°C)
E. histolytica	*Eh*Cox	Fwd:5′ stu1: AGGCCTATGACTGGAAATAAAGAAT	55
		Fwd: 3′ sac1: GAGCTCGAAACTGCTTCTGTTA	
	*Eh*Cox RT	Fwd: TGACTGGAAATAAAGAATGGGA	59
		Rev: CCATAAGACTAATCAAAATATCTGACT	
	CP5 RT	Fwd: AATTCATGGGGAACTATTTGG	59
		Rev: CATCAGCAACCCCAACTGG	
	CP4 RT	Fwd: GTTAACCATGGTGTTGCCGCTGTA	59
		Rev: GCATCATGAGCACCAGTTGGGAAA	
	CP1 RT	Fwd: ATAAACACTTCACAGCAGTTGA	59
		Rev: TTCTTCATTTGTCATAGCAGC	
	CP2 RT	Fwd: ATCCAAGCACCAGAATCAGT	59
		Rev: TTCCTTCAAGAGCTGCAAGT	
	rDNA RT	Fwd: TCAAAAAGCAACGTCGCTA	59
		Rev: AGCCCGTAAGGTGATTTCT	
Murine	IL-1β	Fwd: GCCTCGTGCTGTCGGACCCA	58
		Rev: CTGCAGGGTGGGTGTGCCGT	
	TNF-α	Fwd: ATGAGCACAGAAAGCATGATC	60
		Rev: TACAGGCTTGTCACTCGAATT	
	IFN-γ	Fwd: TCAAGTGGCATAGATGTGGAAGAA	58
		Rev: TGGCTCTGCAGGATTTTCATG	
	Actin	Fwd: CTACAATGAGCTGCGTGTG	58
		Rev: TGGGGTGTTGAAGGTCTC	
	KC	Fwd: ACCCAAACCGAAGTCATAGC	60
		Rev: TCTCCGTTACTTGGGGACAC	

Quantitative Real-Time (qRT) PCR-Based Analysis of Gene Expression

Total RNA was extracted from logarithmic-growth-phase *Eh* using a Trizol reagent method (Invitrogen; Life Technologies, Burlington, ON) and the yield and purity determined by the ratio of absorbance at 260/280 nm (NanoDrop, Thermo Scientific). DNase I-treated total RNA was used in the RT reaction using qScript cDNA Synthesis kit and PerfeCTa SYBR Green Supermix (Quantabio). Real-time qPCR was performed using a Rotor Gene 3000 real-time PCR system (Corbett Research). The PCR reaction mix (20 μl) comprised 1x SYBR Green, 25 ng cDNA and 1 μM of primers. A complete list of the primer sequences and conditions used are listed in **Table 1**. Results were analyzed using the 2-ΔΔCT methods and expressed as fold changes.

Sample Preparation for Proteomics

Eh lysates were prepared as described before. After proteins precipitation with TCA, the supernatant was discarded and proteins were air dried and suspended in 200 μL of urea/HCl. The sample was then treated with 10 mM of dithiothreitol and incubated at 37°C for 30 min and transferred into Microcon YM-30 (Millipore) and centrifuge at 14,000 × g at 20°C for 15 min. The eluates were discarded, 200 μL of UA was pipetted into the filtration unit, and the units were centrifuged again. Then 100 μL of 0.05 M iodoacetamide in Urea/Tris was added to the filters, and samples were incubated in darkness for 20 min. Filters were washed twice with 100 μL of Urea/Tris and, with 100 μL of 0.05 M ammonium bicarbonate at 14,000 × g for 15 min. Proteins were digested in 40 μL of trypsin in 0.05 M ammonium bicarbonate at 37°C overnight. The released peptides were collected by centrifugation at 14,000 × g for 10 min followed by two washes with 0.05 M, 40 μL ammonium bicarbonate and with 40 μL of 0.05 M NaCl. After isolation of the peptides, samples were transferred into new Eppendorf tube.

LC-MS/MS Analysis

Total protein and peptides content were analyzed on an Orbitrap Fusion Lumos Tribrid mass spectrometer (Thermo Scientific) operated with Xcalibur (version 4.0.21.10) and coupled to a Thermo Scientific Easy-nLC (nanoflow Liquid Chromatography) 1,200 system. Isolated trypsin treated peptides (2 μL) were loaded onto an Easy Spray Column (ES803) at a maximum of 700 bars (2 μm particle column). Further, peptides were eluted using a 120 min gradient from 5 to 40% (5 to 28% in 105 min followed by an increase to 40% B in 15 min) of 0.1% formic acid in 80% LC-MS grade acetonitrile at a flow rate of 0.3 μL/min and separated on a C18 analytical column (ES803). Then, peptides were electrosprayed using 2.0 kV voltages into the ion transfer tube (300°C) of the Orbitrap Lumos operating in positive mode. A full MS scan was performed by Orbitrap at a resolution of 12,0000 FWHM to detect the precursor ion having a *m*/*z* between 375 and 1575 and a +2 to +7 charge. The Orbitrap AGC (Auto Gain control) and the maximum injection time were set at 4e5 and 50 ms, respectively. The Orbitrap was working with a 3 s cycle time for precursor selection and most intense precursor ions presenting a peptidic isotopic profile, having an intensity threshold of at least 5,000 were isolated using the quadrupole and fragmented with HCD (30% collision energy) in the ion routing multipole. The fragment ions (MS^2) were analyzed in the ion trap at a rapid scan rate. The AGC and the maximum injection time were set at 1e4 and 35 ms, respectively, for the ion trap. Dynamic exclusion was enabled for 45 s to avoid of the acquisition of same precursor ion having a similar m/z (plus or minus 10 ppm).

Database Search

With the help Raw Converter (v1.1.0.18; The Scripps Research Institute), raw data files (*.raw) were converted into Mascot Generic Format (MGF). Monoisotopic precursors having a charge state of +2 to +7 were selected for conversion. The mgf file was used to search a database by using Mascot algorithm (Matrix Sciences; version 2.4). Search parameters for MS data included trypsin as enzyme, a maximum number of missed cleavage of 1, a peptide charge equal to 2 or higher, cysteine carbamidomethylation as fixed modification, methionine oxidation as variable modification and a mass error tolerance of 10 ppm. A mass error tolerance of 0.6 Da was selected for the fragment ions. Only peptides identified with a score having a confidence higher than 95% were kept for further analysis. The Mascot dat files were imported into Scaffold (v4.3.4, Proteome Software Inc.) for comparison of different samples based on their mass spectral counting.

Western Blots

Proteins (30 μg) were loaded on 12% SDS-PAGE gel followed by transfer onto polyvinylidene fluoride (PVDF) membrane and blocking in 5% skim milk. Blots were then probed with 1:5,000 *Eh*Cox antibody or 1:1,000 *Eh*CP5 antibody/1:500 *Eh*CP4 antibody/1:1,000 Actin antibody for 16 h at 4°C. After incubation with one of the previously described primary antibodies, the blots were incubated with appropriate HRP-conjugated secondary antibody for 1 h at RT, and then developed using ChemiLucent ECL detection (EMD Millipore).

*Eh*Cox Activity Assay

*Eh*COX activity assay was performed on nuclear fractions of *Eh* (*Eh*NP). *Eh*NP (100 μg) was incubated for 30 min with 1 mM aspirin (ASA) followed by 100 μM arachidonic acid (AA) or vehicle for 1 h at 37°C in sodium phosphate buffer containing 200 μM tryptophan and 2 μM hematin (Sigma) in 500 μl volume. After centrifugation, PGE_2 in the supernatant was extracted with Amprep C2 ethyl columns (Amersham Biosciences) following manufacturer's protocol. PGE_2 was quantified by using an enzyme immunoassay kit (Cayman Chemical, Ann Arbor, MI).

Eh Cysteine Proteinase Activity

*Eh*CP5 and *Eh*CP4 activity in lysate and secretory protein was determined using known chromophoric substrate benzyloxycarbonyl-L-arginyl-L-arginine p-nitroanilide (Z-Arg-Arg-pNA) and fluorogenic substrate benzyloxycarbonyl-L-val-L-val- 7-amino-4-methylcoumarin (Z-VVR-AMC), respectively, as previously described (Leippe et al., 1995; He et al., 2010). Briefly, substrate was incubated for 0–20 min at 37°C with either *Eh* lysate/secretory proteins (50 μg) alone or pretreated with CP inhibitor-E64 [L-trans-epoxysuccinyl-leucyl-amido-(4-guanidino) butane]/CP-1(WRR483) and CP-4 (WRR605) inhibitors. Cleavage of the chromophoric (Z-Arg-Arg-pNA) and fluorogenic (Z-VVR-AMC) substrate were detected at the 405 and 460 nm wavelength, respectively.

Gelatinase Gel Substrate Gel Electrophoresis

For analysis of protease activity by gelatinase substrate gel electrophoresis, 12% SDS polyacrylamide was copolymerized with 0.1% gelatin as described previously (Hellberg et al., 2000). Briefly, *Eh* lysate were prepared by three freeze-thaw cycles in HBSS and centrifuged for 10 min at 10,000 × g. Supernatant was separated on 0.1% gelatin copolymerized 12% SDS PAGE. After separation of proteins, SDS was removed by two washings in 2.5% Triton X-100 for 1 h at room temperature. Gel was then incubated in developing buffer (20 mM DTT, 100 mM sodium acetate, pH 4.2, and 1% Triton X-100) at 37°C for 3 h. The gel was stained with Coomassie blue. Clear band represent cysteine protease activity.

Eh Erythrophagocytosis Assay

Fresh human erythrocytes were obtained in DPBS and stained with Phicoerythrin by using PKH26 Red Fluorescent cell linker kit (PKH26, Sigma-Aldrich). The erythrocytes were counted and used in 1:100 (*Eh:* erythrocyte) ratio. *Eh* and erythrocytes were incubated for 20 min at 37°C in DPBS. After interaction, cells were washed twice with DPBS and centrifuged at 3,000 × g for 5 min at 4°C. Lysis buffer (RBC lysis buffer, Sigma-Aldrich) was added for 1 min at RT followed by 0.5 ml addition of FBS and washed again with DPBS. The cells were fixed with 4% p-formaldehyde for 20 min at RT and washed with DPBS. To each sample a drop of fluoresave reagent was used for the slide preparation. The slides were observed under confocal microscope and fluorescent intensity was quantified by selecting region of interest (ROI) containing phagocytose erythrocyte and measuring the fluorescent intensity by using Image J software. The data was plotted as mean fluorescent intensity.

Eh Cytopathic Assay

Caco-2 human colonic adenocarcinoma cells (ATCC, Manassas, VA) were grown to obtain confluent monolayers in DMEM medium (Invitrogen-Gibco) supplemented with 5% fetal bovine serum and 5 mg/ml penicillin-streptomycin under 5% CO_2 at 37°C (Sigma-Aldrich). *Eh* disruption of a Caco-2 cell monolayer was determined using a previously described protocol (Belley et al., 1996). Briefly, *Eh* (10^5/well) were incubated with Caco-2 cell monolayers in 24-wells tissue culture plates at 37°C. The incubation was stopped by placing the plates on ice and *Eh* were removed by washing with cold PBS. The Caco-2 cells that remained attached to the plates were stained with methylene blue (0.1% in 0.1 M borate buffer, pH 8.7). The dye was extracted from stained cells with 0.1 M HCl and color intensity of the extracted dye was measured spectrophotometrically at OD 660.

Stability of *Eh*CP-A4 and *Eh*CP-A5 Protein

Eh and *EhCoxgs* were inoculated at 2.5×10^5 and grown in TYI-S-33 media for 48 h before treatment with the protein synthesis inhibitor, cycloheximide at 100 μg/ml for 6, 12, and 24 h. After treatment *Eh* were harvested, wash in PBS and cell lysates were prepared in RIPA buffer 100 mM Tris-HCl, 150 mM NaCl, 2 mM EDTA, 0.1% sodium dexycholate pH 7.4 containing a protease inhibitor cocktail and 2 nM PMSF (Cruz-Vera et al., 2003). *Eh*CP protein remaining after treatment with cycloheximide was calculated as percentage protein remaining of levels at time zero (0 h). Protein half-life ($t_{1/2}$) was calculated by linear regression analysis.

Mice Colonic Loop Studies

$Math1^{GFP}$ mice were purchased from Jackson laboratory and bred in-house. Colonic loops studies were done by inoculating live *Eh* suspended in 100 μL PBS (1×10^6) into closed colonic loops as described previously (Belley and Chadee, 1999) This is a short-term infection model (3 h after infection). After 3 h, the colons were excised and tissue pro-inflammatory gene expression and myeloperoxidase activity was analyzed.

Colonic Myeloperoxidase Activity Assay (MPO)

MPO activity was assayed in mouse colon samples as described previously (Kumar et al., 2017). Briefly, fresh frozen tissues were homogenized in 0.5% hexadecyltri-methylammonium bromide. Homogenized tissue was freeze-thawed three times, sonicated, and centrifuged at 10,000 g for 10 min at 4°C. Clear supernatant was collected and the reaction was initiated by addition of 1 mg/ml dianisidine dihydrochloride (Sigma, St. Louis, MO) and 1% H_2O_2, and change in optical density was measured at 450 nm.

Math1 Expression via Non-invasive Whole-Body Imaging *ex vivo*

After 3 h of *Eh* infection, colons of $Math1^{GFP}$ mice were surgically removed, imaged *ex vivo* using an *in vivo* Xtreme 4MP-imaging platform (Bruker, Billerica, MA, USA) to detect GFP expression. The imaging was performed in two steps. The first one is reflectance imaging (2 s exposure time) and the second one was with excitation at 470 nm and emission at 535 nm (5 s exposure time) i.e., fluorescent imaging. Images were acquired and analyzed from the *in vivo* Xtreme using Bruker molecular imaging software MI SE (version 7.1.3.20550). GFP expression in the colon was quantified by measuring the mean fluorescence (after background subtraction) in a constant ROI.

Ethics Statements

All studies were carried out with the approval of the University of Calgary Animal Care Committee. Animal care committee have approved experimental procedure proposed and certifies that animal care was in accordance with recent policies by the Canadian council on Animal care.

Statistical Analysis

Data was analyzed using Graphpad Prism 7 (Graph-Pad Software, San Diego, CA) for all statistical analysis. Student's *t*-test was used when two groups were compared. Statistical significance was assumed at $P < 0.05$.

RESULTS

Silencing of the *Eh* Cyclooxygenase Like Gene Responsible for PGE_2 Biosynthesis

Eh-derived PGE_2 not only induces pro-inflammatory IL-8 production but also disrupts colonic epithelial cell tight junction by coupling through EP4 receptors (Dey et al., 2003; Dey and Chadee, 2008; Lejeune et al., 2011). To analyze the biological functions of endogenous *Eh*Cox and *Eh*PGE_2 mediated pro-inflammatory responses, we silenced the expression of the gene by small RNA-mediated transcriptional gene silencing in the G3 strain (Bracha et al., 2006). The specific gene repression was confirmed by reverse transcription PCR of corresponding cDNA and immunoblot analysis of proteins by using *Eh*Cox specific antibody. Complete silencing of *Eh*Cox was achieved in comparison to the *Eh* control (**Figures 1A,B, Supplementary Figure 1**). Immunoblot analysis detected the 72 and 66 Kda protein band in the lysate of control *Eh* as previously described (Dey et al., 2003). As predicted, *Eh*Cox enzymatic assay using nuclear fractions isolated from log-phase *Eh* showed almost no aspirin (ASA) inhibited PGE_2 release (Dey et al., 2003) by *EhCoxgs* in comparison to control *Eh* incubated with arachidonic acid (AA) substrate (**Figure 1C**). We used ASA inhibited PGE_2 release to accurately quantify PGE_2 levels as *EhCoxgs* showed modest non-specific binding by enzyme immunoassay (EIA) that was not inhibited with ASA.

Growth Kinetics of *EhCoxgs*

To determine whether *EhCoxgs* had an effect on cell proliferation, the growth kinetics of *EhCoxgs* and control *Eh* were compared. We analyzed the growth of *Eh* over time and showed that during the first 24 h growth kinetics were similar, however at 48 and 72 h *EhCoxgs* proliferation was significantly slower than control *Eh* (**Figure 1D**). These results suggest that *Eh*Cox might be essential for cell growth and proliferation.

*Eh*Cox Gene Silencing Caused Limited Proteome Change

To determine if *EhCoxgs* also affected the expression of other proteins, we took a proteomic approach and analyzed the proteome from *EhCoxgs* and control *Eh*. Only a limited number of proteins showed three-fold or higher expression (**Supplementary Table 1**). In *EhCoxgs*, 23 proteins were up regulated and 19 proteins were down regulated compared to control *Eh* (**Table 2**). *Eh*Cox protein (Q9U3Z8_ENTHI) was not detected in *EhCoxgs* proteome that confirms complete absence of the *Eh*Cox protein and gene specific silencing. Among the proteins that were up regulated included those encoding for several uncharacterized proteins (M7X297_ENTHI, A0A175JHX8_ENTHI, A0A175JJQ8_ENTHI, A0a175JU71_ENTHI, A0A175JQL9_ENTHI, A0A175LQ0_ENTHI, A0A175JJP8_ENTHI) and Rab family GTPase proteins (A0A175JL18_ENTHI, A0A175JT01_ENTHI, A0A175JSR0_ENTHI), UDP-glucose:glycoproteine glucosyltransferase (C4M0W6_ENTHI), WD domain containing protein

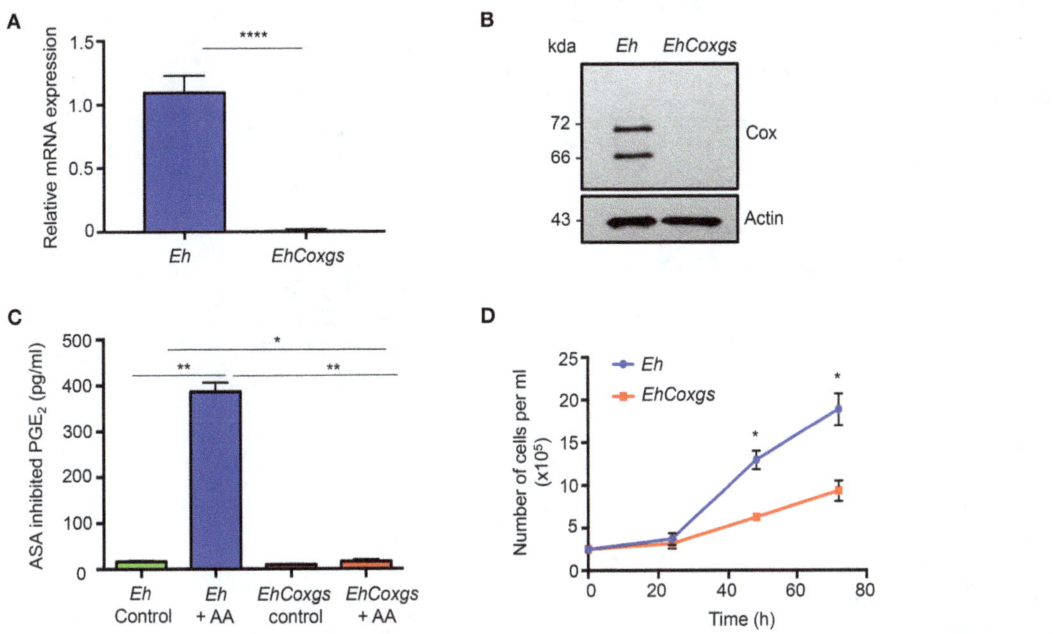

FIGURE 1 | Silencing of the Cox-like protein in *E. histolytica*. **(A)** qPCR was used to monitor cox expression using cDNA from *E. histolytica*. The data indicate the changes in mRNA expression compared with controls. **(B)** Immunoblot blot analysis was performed on lysate prepared from control *Eh* and *EhCoxgs*. The proteins were separated on 8% SDS PAGE gels and analyzed with a polyclonal cox antibody or actin antibody. **(C)** PGE_2 production was quantified using enzyme-linked immunosorbent assay kits following treatment of *Eh*NP with or without AA or aspirin (ASA) for 1 h at 37°C. The bars indicate the means and the error bars indicate the standard errors of the means for three different experiments. **(D)** Approximately 2.5×10^5 control *Eh* and *EhCoxgs* in the logarithmic growth phase were inoculated into 14 mL fresh culture medium and *Eh* were counted every 24 h. Data shown are the means and the error bars indicate the standard errors of the means for three different experiments. The asterisks indicate the results of comparisons with the controls. $^*P < 0.05$, $^{**}P < 0.01$, $^{****}P < 0.001$. *Eh, E. histolytica*.

(A0A175JMP8_ENTHI), Galactose specific adhesin light subunit (A0A175JFH2_ENTHI) and cysteine protease (A0A175JGF5_ENTHI) suggesting that increased expression of these genes particularly Rab family GTAPase and WD domain containing proteins that regulate vesicular trafficking of cysteine protease, may be involved in EhCox-mediated cysteine protease upregulation. The proteomics data showed a slightly increase in other cysteine proteases including CP1 and CP2 (**Table 3**). However, we did not detect *Eh*CP-A4 or *Eh*CP-A5 specifically in the dataset (**Table 2**, **Supplementary Table 1**). These observations led us to hypothesize that the increased expression and activity of CP5 and CP4 was not limited to a specific protease but rather, all the major CPs were regulated by *Eh*Cox. Similar to up regulated proteins we found several down regulated uncharacterized proteins (A0A175JKF9_ENTHI, C4LZW1_ENTHI, A0A175JJ73_ENTHI, A0A175JJ95_ENTHI). Other down regulated proteins were DNAj family protein (A0A175JFG6_ENTHI), Ras guanine nucleotide exchange factor (A0A175JYJ4_ENTHI), Ph domain containing protein (A0A175JQH4_ENTHI), and V-type proton ATPase subunit (A0A175JK72_ENTHI).

Gene Silencing of *Eh*Cox Increases Cysteine Protease Expression and Activity

Cysteine proteases play major roles in the pathogenesis of *Eh*. Specifically, *Eh*CP-A5 has been shown to be involved in tissue invasion by disrupting the protective mucus layer and stimulating pro-inflammatory response in colonic cells (Moncada et al., 2003; Hou et al., 2010). To determine the functional significance of *Eh*Cox derived PGE_2 in *Eh* virulence, we analyzed the expression of *Eh*CPs protein and mRNA in *EhCoxgs*. Cell lysates from *EhCoxgs* and control *Eh* were assayed for CP expression by western blotting using *Eh*CP-A5 and *Eh*CP-A4 specific antibodies. These proteases are highly expressed and released extracellular basally and during infection (He et al., 2010; Kissoon-Singh et al., 2011). An unexpected finding was that *EhCoxgs* showed a slight increased in *Eh*CP-A5 and significantly up regulated *Eh*CP-A4 protein expression compared to control *Eh* (**Figure 2A**, **Supplementary Figure 2**). Surprisingly, we did not detect a corresponding increase in CPs transcripts by qPCR (**Figure 2B**) using primer specific for *CP1, CP2, CP4*, and *CP5* (**Table 1**). These results suggest that *Eh*Cox was regulating CPs at the translational level independent of transcription. To assess whether the increase in *Eh*CPs protein expression resulted in a corresponding increase in *Eh*CPs enzymatic activity, gelatin substrate gel electrophoresis was performed with *Eh* lysates that showed prominent bands of CPs activity in *EhCoxgs* as compared to control *Eh* lysate which was not present in E64 (CP inhibitor) treated *Eh* lysate (**Figure 2C**). To verify increased enzymatic activity, *EhCoxgs* and control *Eh* lysates were incubated with known substrates and proteinase activity was quantified by the liberation of chromogenic leaving group p-nitroanilide

TABLE 2 | List of genes that are up or down regulated ≥3-fold upon *Eh*Cox gene silencing.

Protein name	Accession no.	Regulation
Uncharacterized protein	M7X297_ENTHI	Up
Uncharacterized protein	A0A175JHX8_ENTHI	Up
UDP-glucose:glycoprotein glucosyltransferase	C4M0W6_ENTHI	Up
Uncharacterized protein	A0A175JJQ8_ENTHI	Up
tRNA cytosine 5 methyltransferase putative	A0A175JGM4_ENTHI	Up
Leucine-rich repeat containing protein	A0A175JM48_ENTHI	Up
Uncharacterized protein	A0A175JU71_ENTHI	Up
Uncharacterized protein	A0A175JQL9_ENTHI	Up
Uncharacterized protein	A0A175JLQ0_ENTHI	Up
Alpha-soluble nsf attachment protein putative	A0A175JLV9_ENTHI	Up
Serine-rich protein	A0A060N047_ENTHI	Up
Uncharacterized protein	A0A175JJP8_ENTHI	Up
Uncharacterized protein	A0A175JFS2_ENTHI	Up
Rab family GTPase	A0A175JLI8_ENTHI	Up
Uncharacterized protein	A0A175JRL0_ENTHI	Up
Uncharacterized protein	A0A175JV24_ENTHI	Up
LIM zinc finger domain containing protein	A0A060N6K9_ENTHI	Up
WD domain containing protein	A0A175JMP8_ENTHI	Up
Galactose-specific adhesin light subunit	A0A175JFH2_ENTHI	Up
Rab family GTPase	A0A175JT01_ENTHI	Up
Uncharacterized protein	A0A175JYV1_ENTHI	Up
tRNA (guanine-N(7)-)-methyltransferase non-catalytic subunit	A0A175K0F2_ENTHI	Up
Rab family GTPase	A0A175JSR0_ENTHI	Up
Cysteine protease	A0A175JGF5_ENTHI	Up
Uncharacterized protein	A0A175JKF9_ENTHI	Down
Uncharacterized protein	C4LZW1_ENTHI	Down
Uncharacterized protein	A0A175JJ73_ENTHI	Down
Uncharacterized protein	A0A175JJ95_ENTHI	Down
DNAj family protein	A0A175JFG6_ENTHI	Down
Ras guanine nucleotide exchange factor putative	A0A175JYJ4_ENTHI	Down
Uncharacterized protein	A0A175JL03_ENTHI	Down
Uncharacterized protein	A0A175K128_ENTHI	Down
Ph domain containing protein	A0A175JQH4_ENTHI	Down
V-type proton ATPase subunit	A0A175JK72_ENTHI	Down
70kDa heat shock protein	M2RGX4_ENTHI	Down
Spry domain protein	A0A175JUJ4_ENTHI	Down
Mov34 mpn pad 1 family protein	A0A175JY43_ENTHI	Down
Uncharacterized protein	A0A060N091_ENTHI	Down
Uncharacterized protein	A0A175JLR6_ENTHI	Down
Rho guanine nucleotide exchange factor putative	A0A175JXR9_ENTHI	Down
Casein kinase putative	A0A175JLP4_ENTHI	Down
Uncharacterized protein	A0A175JN68_ENTHI	Down
Type a flavoprotein putative	A0A175JLL6_ENTHI	Down

and the fluorescent leaving group 7-amino-4-methylcoumarin (AMC) from *Eh*CP5 and *Eh*CP4 peptide substrates, Z-Arg-Arg-pNA and Z-VVR-AMC, respectively. Degradation of *Eh*CPs substrate occurred in linear mode over time (**Figures 2D,E**) with significantly higher enzymatic activity in *EhCoxgs* as compared to control *Eh* lysates. Specificity for CPs enzymatic activity was confirmed using specific *Eh*CP-A5 and *Eh*CP-A4 inhibitors, WRR483 and WRR605, respectively (**Figures 2D,E**). *Eh*CP-A5 and *Eh*CP-A1 are unique as they both cleave the common substrate Z-Arg-Arg-pNA and here we used the *Eh*CP-A1 specific inhibitor WRR483 to show that *Eh*CP-A5 enzyme activity was specifically increased (St-Pierre et al., 2017). E64 inhibits all CPs in *Eh*. As *Eh*CPs are secreted extracellular we also found significantly increased *Eh*CP5/4 enzyme activity in *EhCoxgs*

TABLE 3 | Analyzed cysteine protease expression in *EhCoxgs* compared to control *Eh* by using total spectral counts.

Identified proteins	Accession no.	Fold change
Cysteine protease putative	A0A175JGF5_ENTHI	3.0
Cysteine proteinase 1	A0A060N046_ENTHI	1.3
Cysteine proteinase 2	A0A060N5V8_ENTHI	1.2
Cysteine proteinase 1	S0AV91_ENTHI	1.3

compared to control *Eh* (**Figures 2F,G**). These results clearly show that *EhCoxgs* expressed higher levels and activity of CPs, which was regulated by *Eh*Cox protein.

Effect of Arachidonic Acid (AA), Aspirin and Prostaglandin E_2 on Cysteine Protease Activity

From the studies above it was unclear if inhibition of *Eh* PGE_2 biosynthesis and/or Cox enzyme activity was regulating CP expression and enzyme activity in *EhCoxgs*. In live *Eh*, PGE_2 is produced in a time-dependent manner in the presence of AA substrate (Dey et al., 2003). AA is the most important rate-limiting step in *Eh*Cox driven biosynthesis of PGE_2 and aspirin is the only inhibitor known to inhibit *Eh*Cox enzymatic activity (Dey et al., 2003). To evaluate if PGE_2 played a role in regulating *Eh*CP5 activity, control *Eh* was incubated with exogenous AA or aspirin and they had no effect on enzyme activity (**Figures 3A,B**). Similarly, the addition of exogenously prostaglandin (PGE_2) to *EhCoxgs* showed no difference in *Eh*CP5 activity (**Figure 3C**). These results strongly suggest that the increase in *Eh*CP5/4 activity was not dependent on Cox enzymatic activity but rather appear to be a direct effect of the Cox protein on *Eh*CP expression and activity.

EhCoxgs Stabilizes *Eh*CP-A5 Protein Degradation

To address the mechanism whereby *EhCoxgs* increased protein expression and enzymatic activity, we hypothesize that the CPs in *EhCoxgs* were not degraded based on increased protein expression (**Figure 2A**). As several proteins were up/down regulated in *EhCoxgs* (**Table 2**), we were surprised that more proteins were ubiquitinated and destine for 26S proteasome degradation in *EhCoxgs* as compared to *Eh* (**Figure 4A**). Based on these findings we theorize that proteins critical in regulating the stability of *Eh*CPs maybe degraded and quantified the half-lives of both *Eh*CP-A4/5. To do this, *Eh* and *EhCoxgs* were treated with cycloheximide and the percentage protein remaining over 24 h determined. Surprisingly, *Eh*CP-A4 protein was not degraded whereas the half-life for *Eh*CP-A5 was 19.3 h in *EhCoxgs* as compared to 12.2 h for control *Eh* (**Figures 4B,C**). The increase in *Eh*CP-A5 protein stability in *EhCoxgs* may account for increase protein accumulation and increase enzyme activity. In contrast, *Eh*CP-A4 protein was very stable and turnover rate low. We did not treat *Eh* longer than 24 h with cyclohexamide (95% viable by trypan blue exclusion) as cells became rounded and detached from the glass tubes and we were concern about cell death.

Increased Cysteine Protease Expression Results in Increased Erythrophagocytosis and Cytopathic Activity

Experimental evidence suggests a direct correlation between *Eh* virulence and the rate of phagocytosis and protease activity (Ankri et al., 1998, 1999; Okada et al., 2005; Hirata et al., 2007). Erythrophagocytosis is considered as one of the prominent marker of *Eh* virulence (Trissl et al., 1978; Orozco et al., 1983; Bhattacharya et al., 2002). Accordingly, we assayed the ability of *EhCoxgs* to phagocytose fluorescently labeled RBCs and measured the fluorescence intensity by confocal microscopy. *EhCoxgs* showed significantly higher RBCs uptake in comparison to control *Eh* (**Figure 5A**). *EhCoxgs* also significantly destroyed 27% of a Caco-2 monolayer after 2 h incubation compared to control *Eh* that destroyed 11% (**Figure 5B**). These results show that *EhCoxgs* is highly phagocytic with increased cytopathic activity.

Differential Math1 Transcriptional Activity in Math1^{GFP} Mice Exposed to *EhCoxgs*

Based on the results above, we then determined if there was a similar increase in *EhCoxgs* virulence using closed colonic loops in mice (Kissoon-Singh et al., 2013). We have previously shown that *Eh* induces hyper secretion of mucus by goblet cells and elicits an acute pro-inflammatory response in colonic loops (Dharmani et al., 2009). In particular, *Eh*CP5 RGD motif has been shown to bind $\alpha v\beta 3$ integrin on goblet cells to elicit mucin hyper secretion (Cornick et al., 2016). We hypothesized that increase CPs activity would result in a differential response toward mucin biosynthesis and secretion to *EhCoxgs* as compared to control *Eh*. To interrogate this, we used Math1^{GFP} mice containing the green fluorescent protein (GFP) reporter for Math1-expressing goblet cells. In the colon, Math1 is expressed in epithelial cells to differentiate into Muc2-producing goblet cells lineage. Basally, Math1^{GFP} activity was higher in the proximal colon in control mice. However, following *Eh* infection, Math1 activity was significantly decreased in the proximal colon, which was decreased further when mice were infected with *EhCoxgs* (**Figure 6**). We have previously shown that decrease in Math1^{GFP} activity correlates with increase pro-inflammatory activity in response to DSS-induced colitis (Tawiah et al., 2018).

Pro-inflammatory Responses Are Exacerbated in Math1 Mice Exposed to *EhCoxgs* Compared Control *Eh*

It is well-known that *Eh* infection in the gut elicits an acute pro-inflammatory response with the production of pro-inflammatory cytokines IL-1β, IL-8, IFN-γ, and TNF-α (Bansal et al., 2009; Galván-Moroyoqui et al., 2011). Based on the results above showing a marked decrease in Math1^{GFP} activity in the proximal

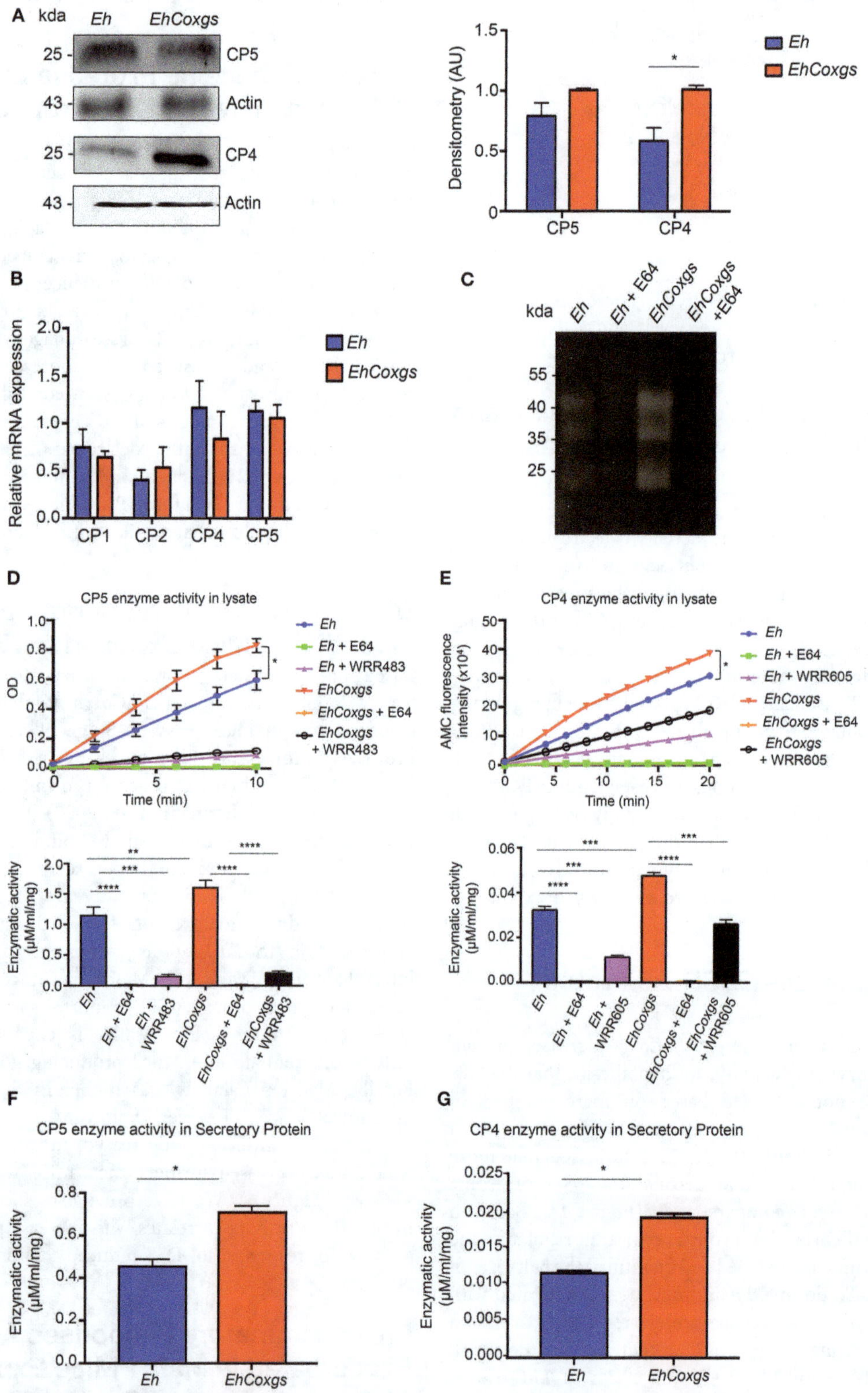

FIGURE 2 | Gene silencing of *Eh*Cox increases cysteine protease expression and activity. **(A)** Immunoblot blot analysis was performed on lysate prepared from control *Eh* and *EhCoxgs*. The proteins were separated on 12% SDS PAGE gels and analyzed with CP5, CP4 or actin antibody. Quantifications of CP5/4 were performed by densitometric analysis from three independent experiments shown in right panel. **(B)** qPCR was used to monitor CPs expression using cDNA from *Eh* and *EhCoxgs*. Data indicate changes in mRNA expression compared with controls. **(C)** Gelatin substrate gel electrophoresis of lysate from control *Eh* and *EhCoxgs* treated/untreated

(Continued)

FIGURE 2 | with E64. **(D,E)** CPs enzymatic activity was evaluated by incubating inhibitor-treated/non-treated *Eh* with *Eh*CP-A5 or *Eh*CP-A4 substrates for 10 and 20 min, respectively and calculated in μM/min/mg, shown in the bottom panel. **(D)** *Eh*CP-A5 enzymatic activity in lysate with known substrates (Z-RR) and 20 μM of inhibitor WRR483. **(E)** *Eh*CP-A4 enzymatic activity in lysate with known substrates (Z-VVR) and 20 μM of inhibitor WRR605 and 100 μM E64. **(F)** *Eh*CP-A5 and **(G)** *Eh*CP-A4 enzymatic activity in secreted protein. The bars indicate the means and the error bars indicate the standard errors of the means for three different experiments. The asterisks indicate the results of comparisons with the controls. $^{*}P < 0.05$, $^{**}P < 0.01$, $^{***}P < 0.002$, $^{****}P < 0.001$.

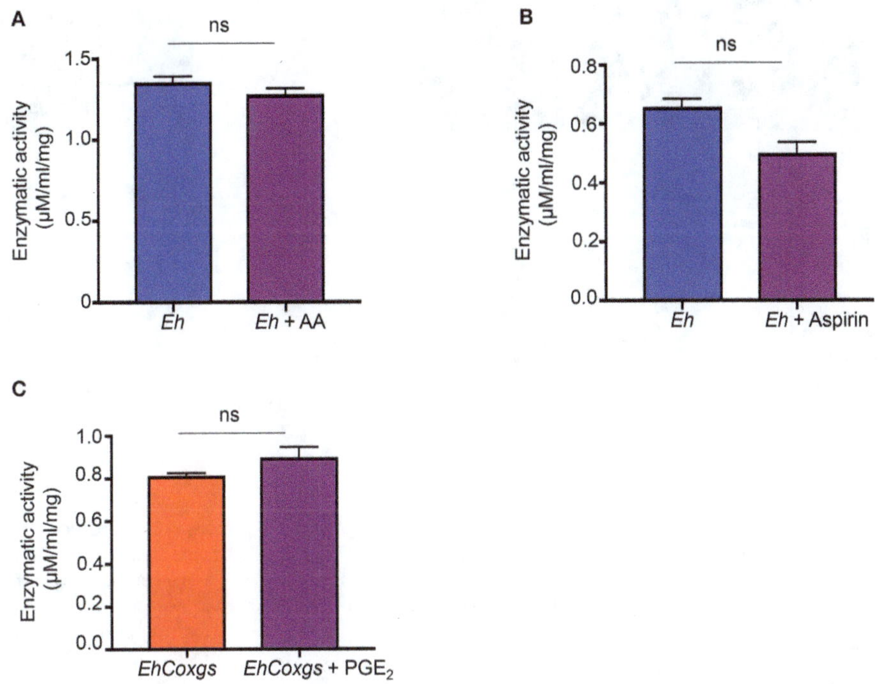

FIGURE 3 | Effect of arachidonic acid, aspirin and prostaglandin on *Eh*CP-A5 cysteine protease activity. Live control *Eh* were pretreated with drugs for 16 h at 37°C. **(A)** Arachidonic acid (100 μM), **(B)** aspirin (1 mM) and **(C)** PGE_2 (1 μM) for 16 h at 37°C. Lysates were prepared from drug treated/non-treated *Eh* using three cycles of freeze-thaw lysis. The bars indicate the means and the error bars indicate the standard errors of the means for three different experiments.

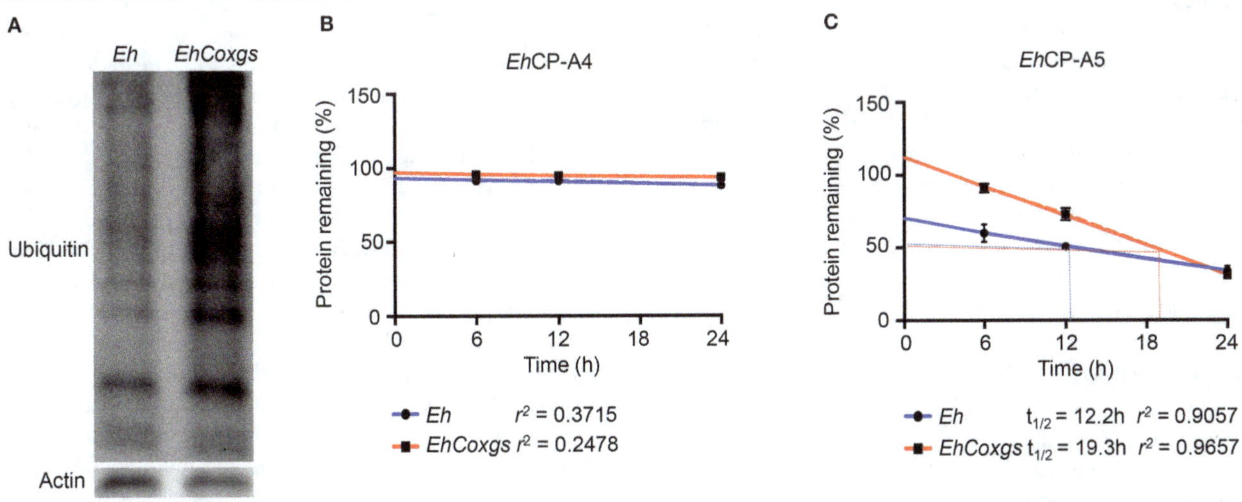

FIGURE 4 | *EhCoxgs* stabilizes *Eh*CP-A5 protein degradation. **(A)** Log phase *Eh* and *EhCoxgs* proteins (30 μg) were loaded on a 12% SDS-PAGE gel and immunoblotted with an ubiquitin antibody (P4D1). Actin was used as a loading control. **(B,C)** The half-life of *Eh*CP-A4 and *Eh*CP-A5 protein was determined by treating *Eh* with cyclohexamide (see details in Materials and Methods) and the remaining CPs quantified by Western blot over 24 h. Protein half-life ($t_{1/2}$) was calculated using regression analysis.

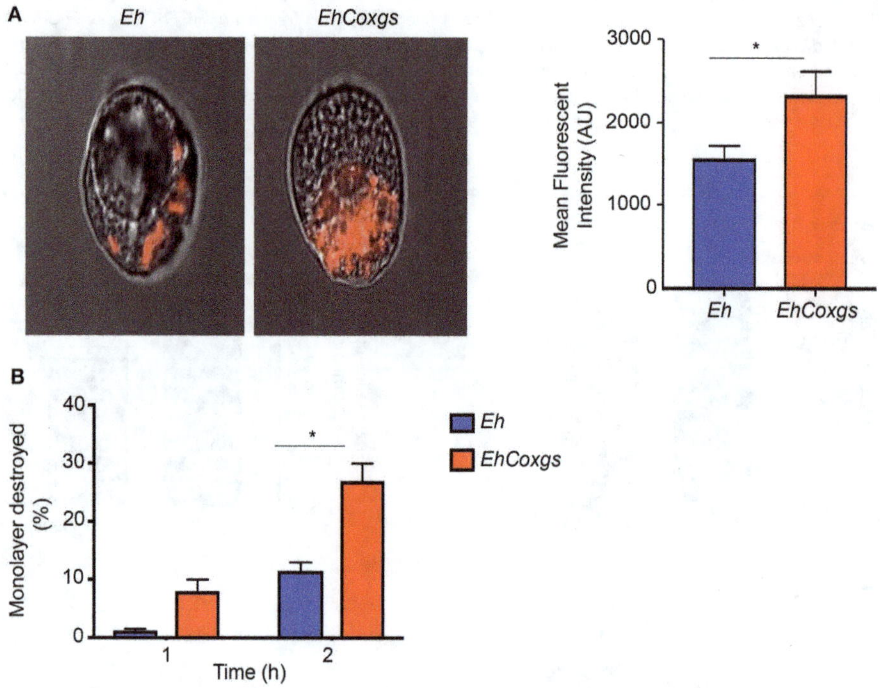

FIGURE 5 | Effect of *EhCox* gene silencing on erythrophagocytosis and cytopathic activity. **(A)** Confocal microscopy of Eh after 20 min incubation with Phicoerythrin labeled RBC at 37°C. Quantitation of erythrophagocytosis was performed with mean florescent intensity (MFI) analysis from three independent experiments, AU, arbitrary units. **(B)** *EhCoxgs* showed increase Caco-2 cells monolayer destruction in comparison to control *Eh* in a time-dependent manner. The bars indicate the means and the error bars indicate the standard errors of the means for different experiments. The asterisks indicate the results of comparisons with the controls. $^{*}P < 0.05$.

colon, we hypothesize that enhanced pro-inflammatory cytokines were suppressing Math1 activity. Indeed, pro-inflammatory cytokines expression in colonic tissues after 3 h exposure with *EhCoxgs* showed increased expression of IL-1β and KC (human IL-8 homolog) but not TNF-α and IFN-γ as compared to *Eh*-inoculated loops (**Figure 7**). Both IL-1β and KC are released by epithelial and immune cells recruited to the site of infection that can exacerbate tissue injury (Mortimer and Chadee, 2010). Specifically, KC is a potent neutrophil chemo attractant that recruits neutrophils to the site of infection but is ineffective in clearing the parasite. Pro-inflammatory cytokine expression correlated with increased myeloperoxidase (MPO) activity in response to *EhCoxgs* as compared to control *Eh* (**Figure 7**). These results reveal that *EhCoxgs* with increased CP enzyme expression and activity enhanced virulence in the mouse colon to elicit increased pro-inflammatory responses.

DISCUSSION

In this study, we describe how *Eh* cysteine protease expression and activity is regulated by another enzyme, cyclooxygenase (Cox). Cox is the critical rate limiting step in the biosynthesis of PGE_2 (Smith and Marnett, 1991; Vane et al., 1998). Cox was identified in *Eh* that showed little homology to known Cox1/2 enzyme across different species with absence of conserved arachidonic acid binding domain and catalytic site that are present in other species. However, endogenous and recombinant *Eh*Cox showed Cox like enzymatic activity by using arachidonic acid as substrate that was inhibited only by aspirin but not by another Cox-1/2 inhibitors (Dey et al., 2003). In a later study, Cox like protein (Acc No. AF208390) was characterized as an actinin like protein in *Eh* as it has actin- and calcium-binding domains. The actin binding domain of *Eh* actinin like protein share only 30% identity with other actin binding proteins however, the protein showed 28% sequence identity to *D. discoideum* actinin protein. Based on some of the unusual domain architecture feature of *Eh* actinin like proteins it was proposed that this unusual protein might differ in function from known actinin proteins (Heike et al., 2005). Beside actin bundling, multiple cellular functions of the actinin protein have been proposed with putative interacting partners (Otey and Carpen, 2004; Cabello et al., 2007). For example, mammalian actinin regulates several receptor activity by linking the cytoskeleton to a variety of trans membrane proteins (Cabello et al., 2007). From these studies and our findings, we proposed that besides Cox like activity and actin polymerization function, this protein might have multifunctional roles in the regulation of several other proteins in *Eh*. Based on its molecular structure and proposed multiple functions we developed *EhCoxgs* to determine its biological function in the pathogenesis of amebiasis.

Cysteine proteases (CPs) are ubiquitous and are differentially regulated in virulent and non-virulent strains of *Eh*. Previous studies have showed that CPs are key virulent factors in the pathogenesis of *Eh* that are released during tissue invasion and

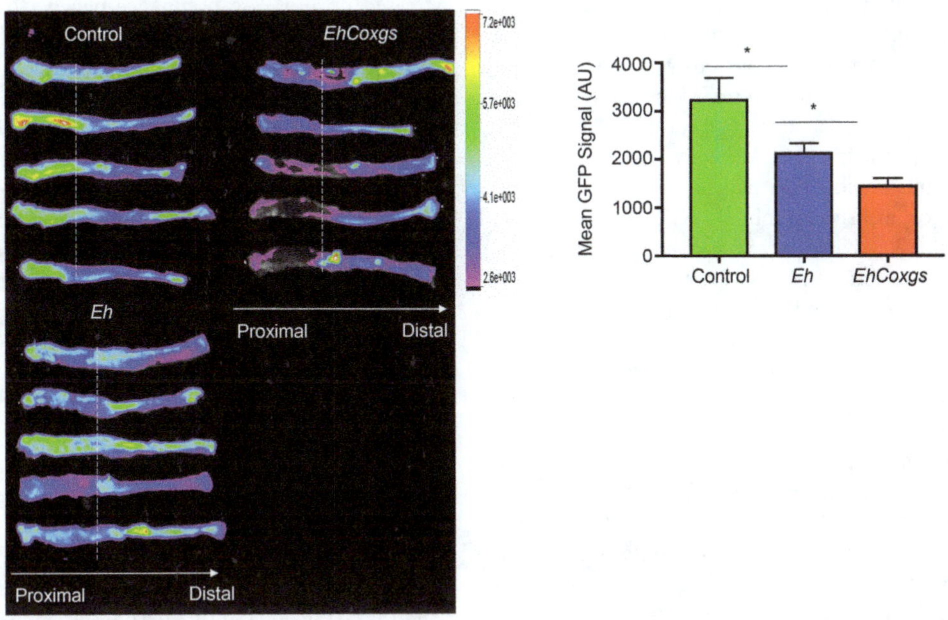

FIGURE 6 | Differential Math1 transcriptional activity in Math1 GFP mice exposed to *EhCoxgs* due to increased cysteine proteases activity. **(A)** Math1 expression heatmap in Math1^{GFP} mice colons, dotted line indicates the colonic loop ligation. **(B)** GFP signal quantification in the proximal colon. GFP, green fluorescent protein; AU, arbitrary units. $^*P < 0.05$.

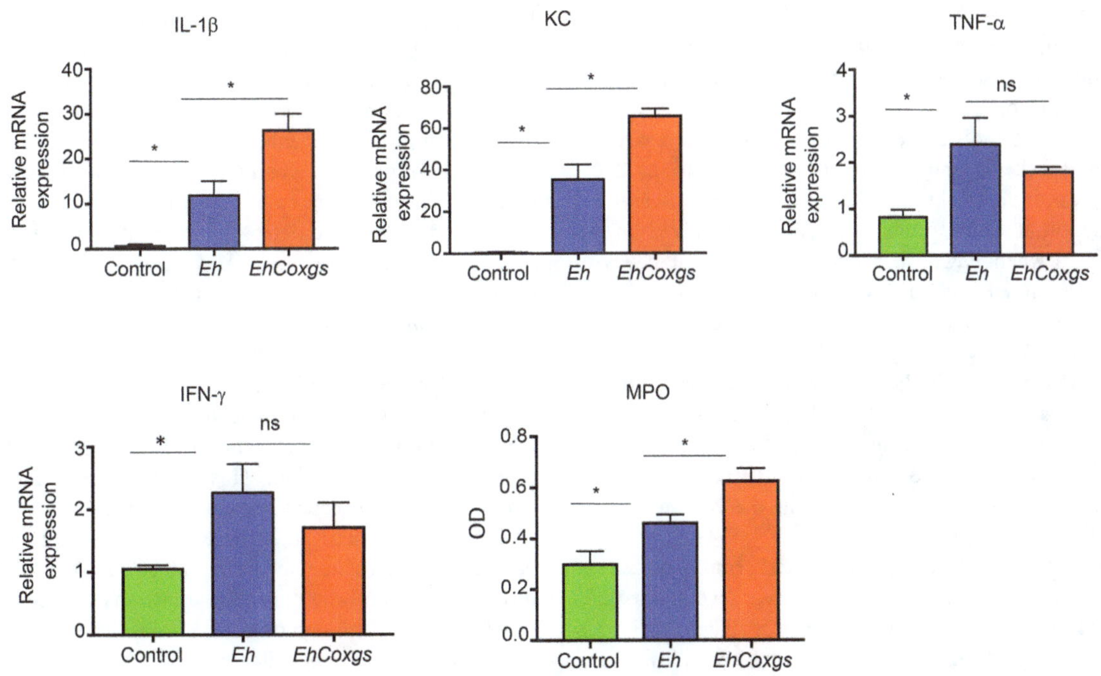

FIGURE 7 | Pro-inflammatory responses are exacerbated in Math1 mice exposed to *EhCoxgs* compared control *Eh*. Math1^{GFP} mice were infected with control *Eh* or *EhCoxgs* for 3 h. Gene expression of IL-1β, KC, TNF-α, and IFN-γ was examined from excised tissues from the proximal colon. Myeloperoxidase activity in the proximal colons of mice inoculated with control *Eh* or *EhCoxgs*. The bars indicate the means and the error bars indicate the standard errors of the means for different experiments. $^*P < 0.05$.

one of the most important protein involved in phagocytosis (Okada et al., 2005; Hirata et al., 2007). In the present study, we have shown that silencing the Cox gene increased cysteine protease expression and activity endogenously and extracellular without affecting CPs transcript. Increased cysteine protease activity led us to hypothesize that Cox derived PGE_2 was negatively regulating cysteine protease activity. However, the addition of exogenous arachidonic acid to live *Eh* to increase PGE_2 production or aspirin to inhibit PGE_2 or exogenous PGE_2 did not affect CP activity. These observations suggest that increase in CPs expression and activity was not the effect of Cox enzymatic activity/end product of biosynthesis but rather was regulated by the Cox protein itself. The *Eh*Cox protein acted as a negative regulator of CPs. Since expression of CPs was not regulated at the transcriptional level, there is the possibility of post-translational modification of CPs up regulating its expression and enzymatic activity. In support of this we have shown increased *Eh*CP-A5 protein stability in *EhCoxgs* as compared to control *Eh*. While the mechanism of this post-translational regulation is not known, our results suggest that proteins critically involved in regulating *Eh*CP-A5 turnover were degraded in *EhCoxgs* by the appearance of more ubiquitinated proteins. In contrast, *Eh*CP-A4 protein was stable and turnover rate low over 24 h that suggest different regulatory mechanisms between the CPs. No doubt uncovering the post-translational regulation of CPs enzyme will provide the basis to understand the mechanism of Cox mediated regulation and promote the development of more efficient therapeutic strategies of indirectly targeting CPs enzyme.

Proteomic analysis of the *EhCoxgs* revealed high expression of Rab family GTAPase and WD domain containing proteins as compared to control *Eh*. These proteins are involved in various cellular process including membrane trafficking, cytoskeletal assembly and cell proliferation (Saito-Nakano et al., 2005; Nakada-Tsukui and Nozaki, 2015). Based on this observation, we proposed that these proteins might be involved in up regulating CPs when *Eh*Cox is silenced. However, it needs to be further determined what functional advantages or constraints drive CPs up regulation. We also found iron-sulfur falvoprotein (A0A175JR31, M7W6A3; **Supplementary Table 1**) among the down regulated proteins in *EhCoxgs* which supports reduced growth of *EhCoxgs* as these proteins have been shown to be essential for the growth and survival of *Eh* under different condition (Nozaki et al., 1998; Shahi et al., 2016). However, the question that remains to be answered is the mechanism of how *Eh*Cox regulates *Eh* growth.

Phagocytosis is an active process in *Eh* and prominent marker of parasite pathogenicity. Phagocytosis involves several steps and activation of signaling pathways (Orozco et al., 1983; Hirata et al., 2007). A proteomic study of phagosome showed the involvement of several proteins in this process including cysteine protease and vesicular transport proteins (Okada et al., 2005). Since more cysteine protease (activity assay and expression) and several vesicular trafficking proteins (proteomics analysis) were observed in *EhCoxgs*, we analyzed the phagocytosis capacity of *EhCoxgs* as compared to control *Eh*. Unexpectedly, we found increased erythrophagocytosis and cytopathic activity in *EhCoxgs* as compared to control *Eh*. While it is difficult to explain how increased in *Eh* CPs can enhance phagocytosis, these data are consistent with previous studies that showed CPs are directly involved in destruction of colonic epithelial cells, tissue invasion, phagocytosis and degrade host antibodies and complement in immune evasion and disease pathogenesis (Hirata et al., 2007; Mortimer and Chadee, 2010; Nakada-Tsukui and Nozaki, 2016).

Several *in vivo* and *ex vivo* assays reported the recruitment of inflammatory cell in *Eh*-induced infection/lesion as a consequence of localized expression of chemokines and cytokines at the site of infection, leading to an inflammatory response (Bansal et al., 2009; Kissoon-Singh et al., 2013; Nakada-Tsukui and Nozaki, 2016). To address whether *EhCoxgs* were more virulent, we used closed colonic loop as short infection model to quantify acute inflammatory responses. Our study revealed that the Cox protein played a major role in *Eh*- induced fluid secretions and pro-inflammatory cytokine responses by regulating CPs activity. In particular, *EhCoxgs* elicited high levels of IL-1β and KC expression demonstrating cysteine protease dependent induction of IL-1β and IL-8 expression as observed in *Eh* infected SCID mouse-human intestinal xenograft (Seydel et al., 1997). Previous studies have shown CP5 to be important in enhancing mucosal inflammation by cleaving the released pro-IL-1β into its active form and inducing IL-8 expression in mast cell (Zhang et al., 2000; Lee et al., 2014). Both TNF-α and IFN-γ were up regulated in response to *Eh* and was not enhanced further by *EhCoxgs*. In *EhCoxgs* inoculated colonic loops we also found elevated MPO activity, a marker for increased flux of neutrophils that are responsible for exacerbating tissue injury.

Increased CP expression and virulence in *EhCoxgs* is intriguing which led us to propose the following hypotheses. First, *Eh*Cox is as endogenous inhibitor of cysteine proteases. While examples of identified cysteine proteinase inhibitors produced by parasites are rare they can be targeted to treat disease related to increased protease activity. For example, papain inhibitors were detected in parasitic protozoa including *Leishmania, Trichomonas,* and *Trypanosoma*, suggesting existence of these inhibitors are widespread (Irvine et al., 1992). In *Schistosoma mansoni*, a gene was identified which encode papain inhibitors (Cao et al., 1993). In *Eh*, few CP inhibitors have been characterized that negatively regulates CP secretion and thus, virulence of the parasite (Sato et al., 2006). Second, CP regulation by Cox is a negative feedback mechanism to reduce host inflammation. This negative feedback regulation may counteract excessive cysteine protease function at site of inflammation and thus, decrease the likelihood of tissue damage that led to amebic lesion/colitis. This phenomenon may furthered explain why most *Eh* infections are asymptomatic. Consistent with this hypothesis, a study in mice showed that ribosomal protein S19 interact with macrophage migration inhibitory factor and function as an extracellular inhibitory factor by attenuating its pro-inflammatory function (Filip et al., 2009). Another study in *Arabidopsis thaliana* proposed the formation of a complex network of cysteine protease-Serpin1 interaction controlling innate immunity during plant development (Rustgi et al., 2017). Based on these findings it would be interesting to determine whether these proteins can interact together; it is likely these interactions could regulate CPs activity either as a result of conformational changes of the enzyme or by impacting subcellular localization of CPs and thus affecting its interactions with Cox, to further modulate its activity. Furthermore, the effect of this interaction on activity and expression of cysteine protease or vice versa can be analyzed. This information can be used to develop chemotherapeutic target against *Eh* infection. Clearly further studies are needed to understand the underlying molecular mechanisms by which *EhCoxgs* increases CPs expression and activity.

AUTHOR CONTRIBUTIONS

PS and KC conceived and design the experiments and wrote the manuscript. PS and FM performed the experiments. PS analyzed the data.

FUNDING

This work was supported by an operating grant from the Canadian Institutes of Health Research (KC; MOP-142776).

ACKNOWLEDGMENTS

We thank the staff of the SAMS Center at the University of Calgary for help with proteomic analysis of the data. We also thank Dr. Björn Petri from the Snyder Mouse Phenomics Resources Laboratory for acquiring the non-invasive whole-body imaging *ex vivo* and the Snyder Live Cell Imaging facility for technical support. PS was supported by an Eyes High Postdoctoral Scholar award from the University of Calgary.

SUPPLEMENTARY MATERIAL

Supplementary Table 1 | Entire proteomics profile of control *Eh* and *EhCoxgs* with mass spectrometry counts, accession number and protein ID.

Supplementary Figure 1 | Full scan of blots for Cox protein shown in **Figure 1B.**

Supplementary Figure 2 | Full scan blots of CP5/4/actin shown in **Figure 2A.**

REFERENCES

Ahrenstedt, O., Hällgren, R., and Knutson, L. (1994). Jejunal release of prostaglandin E2 in Crohn's disease: relation to disease activity and first-degree relatives. *J. Gastroenterol. Hepatol.* 9, 539–43.

Alcantara, C., Stenson, W. F., Steiner, T. S., and Guerrant, R. L. (2001). Role of inducible cyclooxygenase and prostaglandins in *Clostridium difficile* toxin a-induced secretion and inflammation in an animal model. *J. Infect. Dis.* 184, 648–652. doi: 10.1086/322799

Ankri, S., Stolarsky, T., Bracha, R., Padilla-Vaca, F., and Mirelman, D. (1999). Antisense inhibition of expression of cysteine proteinases affects *Entamoeba histolytica*-induced formation of liver abscess in hamsters. *Infect. Immun.* 67, 421–422.

Ankri, S., Stolarsky, T., and Mirelman, D. (1998). Antisense inhibition of expression of cysteine proteinases does not affect *Entamoeba histolytica* cytopathic or haemolytic activity but inhibits phagocytosis. *Mol. Microbiol.* 28, 777–785. doi: 10.1046/j.1365-2958.1998.00837.x

Bansal, D., Ave, P., Kerneis, S., Frileux, P., Boche, O., Baglin, A. C., et al. (2009). An *ex-vivo* human intestinal model to study *Entamoeba histolytica* pathogenesis. *PLoS Negl. Trop. Dis.* 3:e551. doi: 10.1371/journal.pntd.0000551

Belley, A., and Chadee, K. (1999). Prostaglandin E(2) stimulates rat and human colonic mucin exocytosis via the EP(4) receptor. *Gastroenterology* 117, 1352–1362.

Belley, A., and Chadee, K. (2000). Production of prostaglandin E2 by *Entamoeba histolytica* via a novel cyclooxygenase. *Arch. Med. Res.* 31, 74–75. doi: 10.1016/S0188-4409(00)00226-5

Belley, A., Keller, K., Grove, J., and Chadee, K. (1996). Interaction of LS174T human colon cancer cell mucins with *Entamoeba histolytica*: an *in vitro* model for colonic disease. *Gastroenterology* 111, 1484–1492.

Bhattacharya, S., Bhattacharya, A., and Petri, W. A. (2002). Examining *Entamoeba*. *Trends Parasitol.* 18, 196–197. doi: 10.1016/S1471-4922(02)02279-1

Bracha, R., Nuchamowitz, Y., Anbar, M., and Mirelman, D. (2006). Transcriptional silencing of multiple genes in trophozoites of *Entamoeba histolytica*. *PLoS Pathog.* 2:e48. doi: 10.1371/journal.ppat.0020048

Cabello, N., Remelli, R., Canela, L., Soriguera, A., Mallol, J., Canela, E. I., et al. (2007). Actin-binding protein α-actinin-1 interacts with the metabotropic glutamate receptor type 5b and modulates the cell surface expression and function of the receptor. *J. Biol. Chem.* 282, 12143–12153. doi: 10.1074/jbc.M608880200

Cao, M., Chao, H., and Doughty, B. L. (1993). A cDNA from Schistosoma mansoni eggs sharing sequence features of mammalian cystatin. *Mol. Biochem. Parasitol.* 57, 175–176.

Cornick, S., Moreau, F., and Chadee, K. (2016). *Entamoeba histolytica* cysteine proteinase 5 evokes mucin exocytosis from colonic goblet cells via αvβ3 integrin. *PLoS. Pathog.* 12:e1005579. doi: 10.1371/journal.ppat.1005579

Cruz-Vera, J., Clara, L., Hernandez-Kelly, R., Alfredo Mendez, J., Perez-Salazar, E., and Ortaga, A. (2003). Collagen-induces STAT family members activation in *Entamoeba histolytica* trophozoites. *FEMS Microbiol. Lett.* 229 203–209. doi: 10.1016/S0378-1097(03)00822-X

Dey, I., and Chadee, K. (2008). Prostaglandin E2 produced by *Entamoeba histolytica* binds to EP4 receptors and stimulates interleukin-8 production in human colonic cells. *Infect. Immun.* 76, 5158–5163. doi: 10.1128/IAI.00645-08

Dey, I., Keller, K., Belley, A., and Chadee, K. (2003). Identification and characterization of a cyclooxygenase-like enzyme from *Entamoeba histolytica*. *Proc. Natl. Acad. Sci. U.S.A.* 100, 13561–13566. doi: 10.1073/pnas.1835863100

Dharmani, P., Srivastava, V., Kissoon-Singh, V., and Chadee, K. (2009). Role of intestinal mucins in innate host defense mechanisms against pathogens. *J. Innate Immun.* 1, 123–135. doi: 10.1159/000163037

Faust, D. M., and Guillen, N. (2012). Virulence and virulence factors in *Entamoeba histolytica*, the agent of human amoebiasis. *Microbes Infect.* 14, 1428–1441. doi: 10.1016/j.micinf.2012.05.013

Filip, A.-M., Klug, J., Cayli, S., Fröhlich, S., Henke, T., Lacher, P., et al. (2009). Ribosomal protein S19 interacts with macrophage migration inhibitory factor and attenuates Its pro-inflammatory function. *J. Biol. Chem.* 284, 7977–7985. doi: 10.1074/jbc.M808620200

Fisher, O., Siman-Tov, R., and Ankri, S. (2006). Pleiotropic phenotype in *Entamoeba histolytica* overexpressing DNA methyltransferase (Ehmeth). *Mol. Biochem. Parasitol.* 147, 48–54. doi: 10.1016/j.molbiopara.2006.01.007

Galván-Moroyoqui, J. M., del Carmen Domínguez-Robles, M., and Meza, I. (2011). Pathogenic bacteria prime the induction of toll-like receptor signalling in human colonic cells by the Gal/GalNAc lectin carbohydrate recognition domain of *Entamoeba histolytica*. *Int. J. Parasitol.* 41, 1101–1112. doi: 10.1016/j.ijpara.2011.06.003

He, C., Nora, G. P., Schneider, E. L., Kerr, I. D., Hansell, E., Hirata, K., et al. (2010). A novel *Entamoeba histolytica* cysteine proteinase, EhCP4, is key for invasive amebiasis and a therapeutic target. *J. Biol. Chem.* 285, 18516–18527. doi: 10.1074/jbc.M109.086181

Heike, B., Thomas, J., Britta, U., and Matthias, L. (2005). An exceptionally short a-actinin-like protein from the protozoan parasite *Entamoeba histolytica*. *J. Biol. Sci.* 5, 76–81. doi: 10.3923/jbs.2005.76.81

Hellberg, A., Leippe, M., and Bruchhaus, I. (2000). Two major "higher molecular mass proteinases" of *Entamoeba histolytica* are identified as cysteine proteinases 1 and 2. *Mol. Biochem. Parasitol.* 105, 305–309. doi: 10.1016/S0166-6851(99)00194-2

Hirata, K. K., Que, X., Melendez-Lopez, S. G., Debnath, A., Myers, S., Herdman, D. S., et al. (2007). A phagocytosis mutant of *Entamoeba histolytica* is less virulent due to deficient proteinase expression and release. *Exp. Parasitol.* 115, 192–199. doi: 10.1016/j.exppara.2006.08.004

Hou, Y., Mortimer, L., and Chadee, K. (2010). *Entamoeba histolytica* cysteine proteinase 5 binds integrin on colonic cells and stimulates NFkappaB-mediated pro-inflammatory responses. *J. Biol. Chem.* 285, 35497–35504. doi: 10.1074/jbc.M109.066035

Irvine, J. W., Coombs, G. H., and North, M. J. (1992). Cystatin-like cysteine proteinase inhibitors of parasitic protozoa. *FEMS Microbiol. Lett.* 75, 67–72.

Kissoon-Singh, V., Moreau, F., Trusevych, E., and Chadee, K. (2013). *Entamoeba histolytica* exacerbates epithelial tight junction permeability and proinflammatory responses in muc2$^{-/-}$ mice. *Am. J. Pathol.* 182, 852–865. doi: 10.1016/j.ajpath.2012.11.035

Kissoon-Singh, V., Mortimer, L., and Chadee, K. (2011). *Entamoeba histolytica* cathepsin-like enzymes: interactions with the host gut. *Adv. Exp. Med. Biol.* 712, 62–83. doi: 10.1007/978-1-4419-8414-2_5

Kumar, M., Kissoon-Singh, V., Coria, A. L., Moreau, F., and Chadee, K. (2017). Probiotic mixture VSL#3 reduces colonic inflammation and improves intestinal barrier function in Muc2 mucin-deficient mice. *Am. J. Physiol. Liver Physiol.* 312, G34–G45. doi: 10.1152/ajpgi.00298.2016

Lee, Y. A., Nam, Y. H., Min, A., Kim, K. A., Nozaki, T., Saito-Nakano, Y., et al. (2014). *Entamoeba histolytica*-secreted cysteine proteases induce IL-8 production in human mast cells via a PAR2-independent mechanism. *Parasite* 21:1. doi: 10.1051/parasite/2014001

Leippe, M., Sievertsen, H. J., Tannich, E., and Horstmann, R. D. (1995). Spontaneous release of cysteine proteinases but not of pore-forming peptides by viable *Entamoeba histolytica*. *Parasitology* 111, 569–574.

Lejeune, M., Moreau, F., and Chadee, K. (2011). Prostaglandin E2 produced by *Entamoeba histolytica* signals via EP4 receptor and alters claudin-4 to increase ion permeability of tight junctions. *Am. J. Pathol.* 179, 807–818. doi: 10.1016/j.ajpath.2011.05.001

Lidell, M. E., Moncada, D. M., Chadee, K., and Hansson, G. C. (2006). *Entamoeba histolytica* cysteine proteases cleave the MUC2 mucin in its C-terminal domain and dissolve the protective colonic mucus gel. *Proc. Natl. Acad. Sci. U.S.A.* 103, 9298–9303. doi: 10.1073/pnas.0600623103

Marie, C., and Petri, W. Jr. (2014). Regulation of virulence of *Entamoeba histolytica*. *Annu. Rev. Microbiol.* 493–520. doi: 10.1146/annurev-micro-091313-103550

Moncada, D., Keller, K., and Chadee, K. (2003). *Entamoeba histolytica* cysteine proteinases disrupt the polymeric structure of colonic mucin and alter its protective function. *Infect. Immun.* 71, 838–844. doi: 10.1128/IAI.71.2.838-844.2003

Moonah, S. N., Jiang, N. M., and Petri, W. A. (2013). Host immune response to intestinal amebiasis. *PLoS Pathog.* 9:e1003489. doi: 10.1371/journal.ppat.1003489

Mortimer, L., and Chadee, K. (2010). The immunopathogenesis of *Entamoeba histolytica*. *Exp. Parasitol.* 126, 366–380. doi: 10.1016/j.exppara.2010.03.005

Nakada-Tsukui, K., and Nozaki, T. (2015). "Molecular basis of the trafficking of cysteine proteases and other soluble lysosomal proteins in *Entamoeba histolytica*," in *Amebiasis*, eds T. Nozaki and A. Bhattacharya (Tokyo: Springer), 279–304.

Nakada-Tsukui, K., and Nozaki, T. (2016). Immune response of amebiasis and immune evasion by *Entamoeba histolytica*. *Front. Immunol.* 7:175. doi: 10.3389/fimmu.2016.00175

Nozaki, T., Asai, T., Kobayashi, S., Ikegami, F., Noji, M., Saito, K., et al. (1998). Molecular cloning and characterization of the genes encoding two isoforms of cysteine synthase in the enteric protozoan parasite *Entamoeba histolytica*. *Mol. Biochem. Parasitol.* 97, 33–44. doi: 10.1016/S0166-6851(98)00129-7

Nozaki, T., and Bhattacharya, A. (2015). *Amebiasis: Biology and Pathogenesis of Entamoeba*. Tokyo: Springer.

Okada, M., Huston, C. D., Mann, B. J., Petri, W. A., Kita, K., Nozaki, T., et al. (2005). Proteomic analysis of phagocytosis in the enteric protozoan parasite *Entamoeba histolytica*. *Eukaryot. Cell* 4, 827–831. doi: 10.1128/EC.4.4.827-831.2005

Orozco, E., Guarneros, G., Martinez-Palomo, A., and Sánchez, T. (1983). *Entamoeba histolytica*. Phagocytosis as a virulence factor. *J. Exp. Med.* 158, 1511–1521. doi: 10.1084/jem.158.5.1511

Otey, C. A., and Carpen, O. (2004). Alpha-actinin revisited: a fresh look at an old player. *Cell Motil. Cytoskeleton* 58, 104–111. doi: 10.1002/cm.20007

Resta-Lenert, S., and Barrett, K. E. (2002). Enteroinvasive bacteria alter barrier and transport properties of human intestinal epithelium: role of iNOS and COX-2. *Gastroenterology* 122, 1070–1087. doi: 10.1053/gast.2002.32372

Rustgi, S., Boex-Fontvieille, E., Reinbothe, C., von Wettstein, D., and Reinbothe, S. (2017). Serpin1 and WSCP differentially regulate the activity of the cysteine protease RD21 during plant development in *Arabidopsis thaliana*. *Proc. Natl. Acad. Sci. U.S.A.* 114, 2212–2217. doi: 10.1073/pnas.1621496114

Saito-Nakano, Y., Loftus, B. J., Hall, N., and Nozaki, T. (2005). The diversity of Rab GTPases in *Entamoeba histolytica*. *Exp. Parasitol.* 110, 244–252. doi: 10.1016/j.exppara.2005.02.021

Sanchez-Ramirez, B., Ramirez-Gil, M., Vazquez-Moctezuma, I., Ramos-Martinez, E., and Talamas-Rohana, P. (2004). *Entamoeba histolytica*: induction of cyclooxygenase-2 expression during amoebic liver abscess formation in hamsters (*Mesocricetus auratus*). *Exp Parasitol* 106, 119–125. doi: 10.1016/j.exppara.2004.03.004

Sato, D., Nakada-Tsukui, K., Okada, M., and Nozaki, T. (2006). Two cysteine protease inhibitors, EhICP1 and 2, localized in distinct compartments, negatively regulate secretion in *Entamoeba histolytica*. *FEBS Lett.* 580, 5306–5312. doi: 10.1016/j.febslet.2006.08.081

Seydel, K. B., Li, E., Swanson, P. E., and Stanley, S. L. (1997). Human intestinal epithelial cells produce proinflammatory cytokines in response to infection in a SCID mouse-human intestinal xenograft model of amebiasis. *Infect. Immun.* 65, 1631–1639.

Shahi, P., Trebicz-Geffen, M., Nagaraja, S., Hertz, R., Alterzon-Baumel, S., Methling, K., et al. (2016). N-acetyl ornithine deacetylase is a moonlighting protein and is involved in the adaptation of *Entamoeba histolytica* to nitrosative stress. *Sci. Rep.* 6:36323. doi: 10.1038/srep36323

Smith, W. L., and Marnett, L. J. (1991). Prostaglandin endoperoxide synthase: structure and catalysis. *Biochim. Biophys. Acta* 1083, 1–17.

Stanley, S. L. (2003). Amoebiasis. *Lancet*, 361, 1025–1034. doi: 10.1016/S0140-6736(03)12830-9

Stenson, W. F., Zhang, Z., Riehl, T., and Stanley, J. (2001). Amebic infection in the human colon induces cyclooxygenase-2. *Infect. Immun.* 69, 3382–3388. doi: 10.1128/IAI.69.5.3382-3388.2001

St-Pierre, J., Moreau, F., Cornick, S., Quach, J., Begum, s., Fernandez, L., et al. (2017). The macrophage cytoskeleton acts as a contact sensor upon interaction with *Entamoeba histolytica* to trigger IL-1β secretion. *PLoS Pathog.* 13:e1006592. doi: 10.1371/journal.ppat.1006592.

Tawiah, A., Moreau, F., Kumar, M., Tiwari, S., Falguera, J., and Chadee, K. (2018). High MUC2 mucin biosynthesis in goblet cells impedes restitution and wound healing by elevating endoplasmic reticulum stress and altered production of growth factors. *Am. J. Pathol.* 188, 2025–2041. doi: 10.1016/J.AJPATH.2018.05.013

Trissl, D., Martinez-Palomo, A., de la Torre, M., de la Hoz, R., and Perez de Suárez, E. (1978). Phagocytosis of human erythrocytes by *Entamoeba histolytica*. *Quant. Study. Arch. Investig. Méd.* 9(Suppl. 1), 219–222.

Vane, J. R., Bakhle, Y. S., and Botting, R. M. (1998). Cyclooxygenase 1 and 2. *Annu. Rev. Pharmacol. Toxicol.* 38, 97–120. doi: 10.1146/annurev.pharmtox.38.1.97

Verkerke, H. P., Petri, W. A., and Marie, C. S. (2012). The dynamic interdependence of amebiasis, innate immunity, and undernutrition. *Semin. Immunopathol.* 34, 771–785. doi: 10.1007/s00281-012-0349-1

World Health Organization (1997). Amoebiasis. *Wkly. Epidemiol. Rec.* 72, 97–100.

World Health Organization (1998). *The World Health Report 1998: Life in the 21st Century A Vision for All.* World Heal. Organ. 226.

Zhang, Z., Yan, L., Wang, L., Seydel, K. B., Li, E., Ankri, S., et al. (2000). *Entamoeba histolytica* cysteine proteinases with interleukin-1 beta converting enzyme (ICE) activity cause intetinal inflammation and tissue damage in amoebiasis. *Mol. Microbiol.* 37, 542–548. doi: 10.1046/j.1365-2958.2000.02037.x

7

The *Entamoeba histolytica* Syf1 Homolog is Involved in the Splicing of AG-Dependent and AG-Independent Transcripts

Diana M. Torres-Cifuentes [1], José M. Galindo-Rosales [1], Odila Saucedo-Cárdenas [2,3] and Jesús Valdés [1]*

[1] RNA Laboratory, Department of Biochemistry, Centro de Investigación y de Estudios Avanzados del Instituto Politécnico Nacional, Mexico City, Mexico, [2] Departamento de Histología, Facultad de Medicina, Universidad Autónoma de Nuevo León, Monterrey, Mexico, [3] División de Genética, Centro de Investigación Biomédica del Noreste, Instituto Mexicano del Seguro Social, Monterrey, Mexico

Correspondence:
Jesús Valdés
jvaldes@cinvestav.mx

Syf1 is a tetratricopeptide repeat (TPR) protein implicated in transcription elongation, spliceosome conformation, mRNA nuclear-cytoplasmic export and transcription-coupled DNA repair. Recently, we identified the spliceosomal components of the human parasite *Entamoeba histolytica*, among them is EhSyf. Molecular predictions confirmed that EhSyf contains 15 type 1 TPR tandem α-antiparallel array motifs. Amoeba transformants carrying plasmids overexpressing HA-tagged or EhSyf silencing plasmids were established to monitor the impact of EhSyf on the splicing of several test Entamoeba transcripts. EhSyf Entamoeba transformants efficiently silenced or overexpressed the proteins in the nucleus. The overexpression or absence of EhSyf notably enhanced or blocked splicing of transcripts irrespective of the strength of their 3′ splice site. Finally, the absence of EhSyf negatively affected the transcription of an intron-less transcript. Altogether our data suggest that EhSyf is a bona fide Syf1 ortholog involved in transcription and splicing.

Keywords: Xab2, Prp19C, splice sites, transcription, nuclear, CTD, human parasite

INTRODUCTION

The spliceosome carries out co-transcriptional pre-mRNA (pre-messenger RNA) splicing (Wahl et al., 2009) with dynamical and sequential assembly of subunits on the pre-mRNA substrate for every splicing episode (Wahl and Lührmann, 2015) by, identifying conserved intronic elements. Whereas the U1 snRNP (small nuclear ribonucleoprotein) first binds to the 5′ss (splice site), SF1 (splicing factor 1) and U2AF65/35 (U2 snRNP auxiliary factors of 65 and 35 kDa) bind the BS (branch point sequence), the pY (polypyrimidine tract) and the 3′ss, respectively, thus forming complex A. Next, the small RNA molecule of U2 snRNP replaces SF1 forming a double stranded RNA hybrid with the BS, bulging the conserved A of the branch necessary for the first of the two transesterification reactions involved in the elimination of the intron-lariat and splicing of exons. Upon entry of the U4/U6.U5 tri-snRNP complex B is formed, which becomes an active spliceosome (B^{ACT}) when U4/U6 basepairing is unwound allowing U6 snRNA to form two mutually exclusive interactions with the 5′ss and U2 snRNA, destabilizing U1 and U4 snRNPs. The first transesterification reaction occurs when U6/U2 and U2/BS RNA/RNA interactions position the bulged BS adenosine to attack the 5′ss, producing 5′ exon and intron lariat-3′ exon intermediates. The active spliceosome undergoes various rearrangements to form complex C that carries out the second transesterification reactions, ligating the exons and removing the intron-lariat (Wahl et al., 2009).

Other non-snRNPs factors are major players in the splicing process (Wahl et al., 2009), among them the components of the Prp19 complex or NTC in yeast: Prp19, Cefl, Syfl, Syf2, Syf3, Snt309, Isy1, and Ntc20 (Fabrizio et al., 2009). Prp19 is the scaffold for NTC formation, and it is essential for splicing but does not constitute any of the individual spliceosomal snRNPs (Tarn et al., 1993a,b, 1994). The NTC joins the spliceosome before, or during, U4/U6 unwinding and remain associated with the spliceosome during the two steps of splicing, marking the change from the inactive B to the active B^{ACT} spliceosome (Chan et al., 2003). Recent evidence shows that NTC regulates spliceosome conformations and fidelity (Hogg et al., 2010), and as part of the intron lariat complex participates in spliceosome disassembly (Fourmann et al., 2013).

It has been shown that U2AF65 and NTC interact both *in vitro* and *in vivo*, and this interaction is required for activation of splicing (David et al., 2011). U2AF65 binds directly to the Ser2 phosphorylated carboxy terminus domain of RNA Pol II (CTD), strengthening U2AF65 and NTC recruitment to the pre-mRNA (David et al., 2011). Thus U2AF65/NTC tether the spliceosome and pre-mRNA to the CTD of elongating Pol II. By this mechanism the CTD enhances splicing, and describes interactions important for splicing and its coupling to transcription (David et al., 2011). In addition, such mechanism links Syfl to transcription elongation, mRNA export, and to the nuclear excision DNA repair machinery in a transcription-coupled manner.

The human-to-yeast conserved TREX (TRanscription /EXport) complex shuttles mRNA from the nucleus to the cytoplasm. TREX is formed by the THO complex along with mRNA export proteins UAP56/Sub2 and Aly/Yra1. Strong evidence links TREX to transcription elongation in yeast. Strains carrying mutations in any of the four THO members fail to export mRNA and are defective in transcription elongation accumulating transcripts in or near their transcription start sites (Carmody and Wente, 2009). Furthermore, it has been shown that Syfl acts as a novel transcription elongation factor required for TREX occupancy at transcribed genes (Chanarat et al., 2011). In mammals, TREX binds the mRNA co-transcriptionally suggesting that TREX is associated with the late stages of splicing. Whereas HPR1, a member of the THO complex, directly interacts with UAP56/Sub2 and is essential for UAP56/Sub2 and Aly/Yra1 recruiting to the mRNA (Zenklusen et al., 2002), in humans all THO components co-purify with spliceosomes (Jurica and Moore, 2003; Reed and Cheng, 2005).

Additionally, damage/alterations in DNA structure can interfere with DNA and RNA polymerases or compromise replication and transcription fidelity. Damaged DNA is restored by nuclear excision repair (NER). Two major NER pathways exist: global genome repair (GGR) and transcription-coupled repair (TCR). In the former, damage recognition is carried out by a DDB heterodimer which binds to the XPC-RAD23B-CEN2 complex (Hamann et al., 1995). In the later, proteins CSA and CSB together with Syfl recognize DNA damage and recruit the DNA repairing machinery (Venema et al., 1990; Nakatsu et al., 2000). Both pathways converge in the following steps of DNA damage repair (Hanawalt and Spivak, 2008).

The protozoan parasite *Entamoeba histolytica* is the causative agent of amebiasis. *E. histolytica* infects approximately 1% of the human population, resulting in approximately 100,000 deaths annually (Nakada-Tsukui and Nozaki, 2016). Because pre-mRNA splicing mechanisms are almost unknown in this parasite, despite the limited amount of data, significant advances have been made to identify the Entamoeba splicing machinery and particular machineries (Miranda et al., 1996; Hernández-Rivas et al., 2000; Davis et al., 2007; Dávila López et al., 2008; Marchat et al., 2008; Hon et al., 2013; Valdés et al., 2014). Previous work using molecular biology and bioinformatic approaches revealed: splicing factor Prp6 (Hernández-Rivas et al., 2000), U2, U4, U5, and U6 snRNAs (Miranda et al., 1996; Davis et al., 2007), the possible lack of U1 snRNA in *E. histolytica* (Dávila López et al., 2008), the DExH/D RNA helicases involved in the proofreading of the sequential steps of spliceosome assembly and catalysis (Marchat et al., 2008), the preferred route of alternative splicing and the wide variety of alternative splice sites utilized by the Entamoeba spliceosome (Hon et al., 2013). Other proteins involved in pre-mRNA processing and maturation such as cleavage and specificity factors (CPSF160, 100, 73, and 30), cleavage stimulating factors (CstF77, 64, and 50), the cleavage factor Im of 25 kDa, both subunits of CFIIm (C1P1 and PCF11), FIP1, poly(A) polymerase, poly(A) binding protein, RBBP6 (Mpe1 in yeast), WDR33, PNAS-120, and PC4 (López-Camarillo et al., 2005, 2014). We have cloned HA-tagged snRNP component U1A and immunoprecipitated *in vivo* assembled pre-mRNA splicing complexes (Valdés et al., 2014). Among the nearly forty splicing factors identified by mass spectrometry were members of every splicing event, including factors involved in the formation of the aforementioned complexes A, B, and B^{ACT}, as well as catalytic, post-catalytic, intron lariat and disassembly complexes (reviewed by Valdés et al., this issue). Of note is the E. histolytica putative ortholog of U2AF65, which participates in spliceosome/pre-mRNA (at the 3′ss of the intron)/CTD of Pol II. Factors of the *Entamoeba histolytica* NTC, Prp19 (EHI_13870), Cwc2 (EHI_126150), Cefl (EHI_000550) and Syf (EHI_073300) were also identified. Furthermore, microarray data showed that EhSyf transcripts were overexpressed in amoebas transformed with HA-U1A (not shown) and splicing factor 1 (SF1). Trying to understand EhSyf participation in fundamental biological processes and to provide evidence about a key molecule that links transcription and splicing in a deep branched eukaryote, we cloned and characterized the general impact of EhSyf on splicing irrespective of 3′ss strength of Entamoeba virulence-related and virulence-unrelated introns.

MATERIALS AND METHODS

Entamoeba Cultures

Axenic cultures of *E. histolytica* trophozoites strain HM-1:IMSS Cl-6 were incubated at 37°C in 13 × 100 mm screw-capped Pyrex glass tubes or plastic culture flasks in BI-S-33 medium as described (Diamond et al., 1972, 1978, 1995).

Plasmid Constructs and Amoeba Transfectants

The *EhSyf* gene was amplified by PCR using oligonucleotides containing appropriate restriction sites. PCR products were cloned in plasmids pEhExHA (Saito-Nakano et al., 2004) and pKT3M 04-trigger (Morf et al., 2013). To facilitate EhSyf cloning, a Sma I site was inserted in the pKT3M 04-trigger plasmid by site-directed mutagenesis. Constructs were verified by sequencing. Trophozoites were transformed with plasmids by liposome-mediated transfection as previously described (Nozaki et al., 1999). Transformants were selected with 5 or 10 μg/ml of Geneticin.

Western Blot and Immunofluorescence

Protein extracts (60 μg) of amoeba transformants were separated by 10% SDS-PAGE and analyzed by western blotting using mouse anti-αSyf (human XAB2; Thermo Scientific), goat anti-Pol II (Santa Cruz Biotechnology), mouse anti-Actin, and secondary horseradish peroxidase-conjugated anti-IgG antibody (Sigma-Aldrich). The human anti-αSyf antibody target in EhSyf was validated by CLUSTALW alignment (Figure S1A). Enhanced chemiluminescent reagent (Perkin Elmer) was used to detect the proteins. To immunolocalize HA-EhSyf in amoeba transformants, cells were fixed and permeabilized in methanol at −20°C using anti-HA Alexa Fluor Labeled for viewing in a Zeiss LSM700 confocal microscope. All experiments were conducted in experimental and biological triplicates.

RT-PCR

For overexpression, silencing and *in vivo* splicing assays EhSyf, Sam50, RabX13, MybS6, ClcB1, Cdc2, actin, and RNA polymerase II expression was monitored by RT-PCR. Total RNA of amoeba transformants was extracted with Trizol (Invitrogen) and the synthesis of cDNA was performed using the SuperScript III First Strand Synthesis System (Invitrogen) according to the manufacturer's instructions. Unspliced pre-mRNA/intron retained (IR) and mRNA molecules were detected with their respective primers (Table S1). Three biological replicates were done for each experiment. PCR products were resolved by electrophoresis and images of the gels were acquired in color inversion mode.

Statistical and Bioinformatics Analyses

Phylogenetic trees were constructed with MEGA 7.0 (http://www.megasoftware.net/) using the neighbor-joining method; the significance of nodes was assessed using a bootstrap test with 1,000 (Tamura et al., 2013). To identify the type of TPR repeat consensus of EhSyf, CLUSTALW and CTREE alignments of the C-terminus of EhSyf (EHI_073300), *Homo sapiens XAB2* (accession number NP_064581), *Saccharomyces cerevisiae* (NP_010704), *Drosophila melanogaster* ORF de CG6197 accession number NP_610891, *Caenorhabditis elegans* ORF C50F2.3, accession number NP_491250, *Schizosaccharomyces pombe* ORF SPBC211.02c, accession number NP_596612 were carried out. EhSyf modeling was carried out with I-Tasser. For RT-PCR and western blots, differences between means were determined by *t*-test with GraphPad Prism 5.0. *p*-values were calculated comparing all pairs of the expression percentages obtained from the normalized IntDen values of densitometries using ImageJ. To eliminate plasmid transfection-effect, differences of transcript-expression values were normalized with respect to 18S rRNA (EhSyf) or RNA polymerase II (monitor transcripts) and were expressed as percent of the total expression (unspliced plus spliced gene products) as previously reported (Goren et al., 2006; de la Mata et al., 2010). Comparisons were carried out between empty vector and EhSyf constructs, prior verification of comparable copy number of plasmids by RT-PCR.

RESULTS

We first performed phylogenetic inference of EhSyf. All EhSyf hits in the BLAST analysis were used to construct the rooted phylogeny tree (**Figure 1A**). As expected for E. histolytica proteins, the identity values of its relatives ranged from 20 to 30% (Table S2). The node of EhSyf relatives include the angiosperm *Phalaenopsis equestris*, the aphid *Myzus persicae*, the calanoid copepod *Eurytemora affinis*, the animal pathogen *Basidiobolus meristosporus*, *E. nuttalli*, *E. invadens*, *E. dispar*, other *E. histolytica* strains. Most importantly such node includes a representative of the deepest branching clade of fungi *Rozella allomycis*, and the only extant representative of basal metazoans *Trichoplax adhaerens* suggesting an early origin of EhSyf. This node appears somewhat distant from the rest of EhSyf relatives, however no other tetratricopeptide repeats (TPR) proteins were identified in the initial BLAST.

TPR proteins participate in a wide variety of functions involving protein-protein interactions (Das et al., 1998; Blatch and Lässle, 1999; Makiuchi et al., 2013). As deduced from the last six TPR motifs alignment with human, yeasts, insects and worms (**Figure 1B**), and *in silico* structural models, EhSyf contains 15 TPR class I (Sikorski et al., 1991) motifs in antiparallel α-helix arrays (**Figures 1C,D**). Interestingly, the C-terminus domain of EhSyf keeps low identity (I) but significant similarity (S) percentages with human (I 16.6%; S 36.4%), *S. cerevisiae* (I 19.3%; S 36.8%), *S. pombe* (I 25.2%; S 42.8%), *D. melanogaster* (I 16.9%; S 33.7%), and *C. elegans* (I 17.6%; S 35.2%).

To partially understand EhSyf functions, pKT3M plasmid-based silencing (Morf et al., 2013) and HA-tagged over

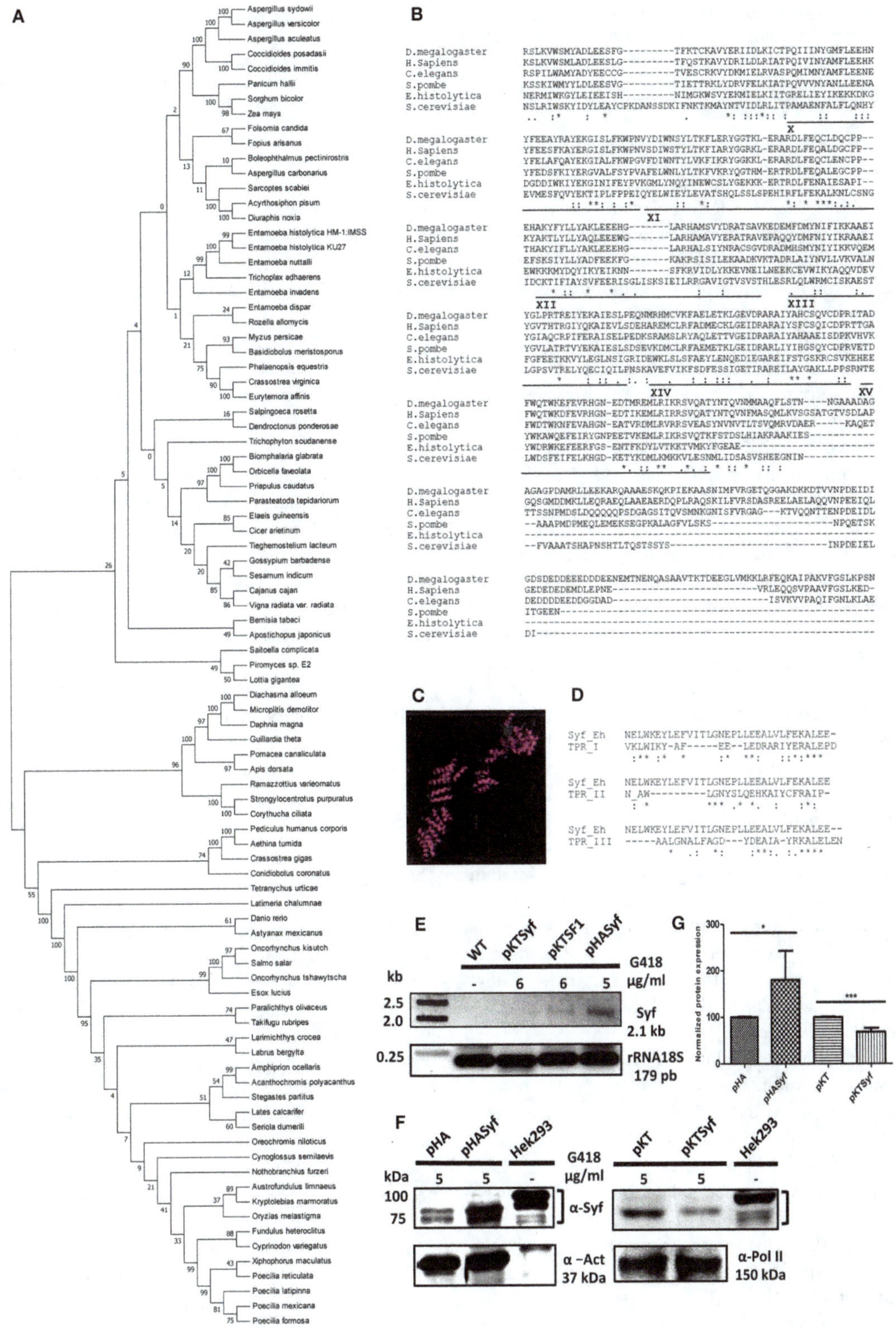

FIGURE 1 | *In silico* and expression analysis of the *EhSyf* gene in amoeba transformants. **(A)** Evolutionary relationships of *EhSyf*. 89 protein sequences retrieved from EhSyf protein BLAST were used to construct the phylogenetic tree using MEGA 5.05 by the neighbor-joining method with 1,000 bootstrap replicates. **(B)** CLUSTALW alignments of the last 6 TPR motifs of EhSyf with Syf proteins from *Drosophila melanogaster, Homo sapiens, Caenorhabditis elegans, Schizosaccharomyces pombe* and *Saccharomyces cerevisiae*. **(C)** I-Tasser structure model of the 699 amino acids of EhSyf. **(D)** CTREE alignments of human TPR Types I-III motifs consensus sequences with EhSyf TPRs, showing that EhSyf possess Type I TPRs (Sikorski et al., 1991). **(E)** EhSyf silenced (pKTSyf) and over expressed (pHASyf) amoeba

(Continued)

FIGURE 1 | transformants were established by selection with the indicated amounts of G418 and Syf transcripts were monitored by RT-PCR. Basal post-transfection expression was compared to the Splicing Factor 1 silenced (pKTSF1) transfectants, and 18S rRNA was used for normalization. **(F)** Western blots were carried out with anti-αSyf (human) antibodies to assess protein overexpression and silencing of EhSyf in amoeba transformants, compared to the human Hek293 cell extracts. For normalization, actin and RNA polymerase II proteins were used. **(G)** Plot of normalized EhSyf protein overexpression (80%) and silencing (32%) in amoeba transformants. Error bars indicate the SD of three independent experiments, asterisks show statistically significant differences (t-Student P * < 0.05 *** < 0.001) compared to empty vectors.

expression plasmid pEhExHA (Saito-Nakano et al., 2004) Syf Entamoeba transformants were established by selection with different amounts of geneticin, and their respective transcription and protein expression were monitored by RT-PCR and western blot. Contrary to transcriptomic analyses reported in AmoebaDB, we were not able to detect wild type EhSyf mRNA (**Figure 1E**), suggesting that Entamoeba expresses very low amounts of EhSyf. This is consistent with our previous findings in which EhSyf was not detected in MS2 aptamer-tagged RabX13 intron immunoprecipitates, which contained components of splicing B and C complexes, although other members of U2 snRNP and NTC were detected (Valdés et al., 2014; Valdes et al. this issue), reflecting NTC rearrangements within the spliceosome during pre-spliceosome to pre-catalytic complex transition. In spite of our observations, and because we expect constitutive EhSyf expression, we ensured the lack of EhSyf by means of pKTSyf-mediated silencing. To eliminate off-target effect another splicing-related protein SF1 (pKTSF1) was silenced, and we observed that EhSyf mRNA expression was enhanced, instead of reduced. Conversely, more EhSyf mRNA was detected in pHASyf overexpression transformants. In agreement with this, whereas the ≈ 84 kDa EhSyf was robustly expressed in mock-transfected amoebae (pHA), pHASyf transformants expressed 80% more, nearly as abundant as that of Hek293 human cells (**Figure 1F**, Figures S1A–D). Although we cannot ascertain EhSyf mRNA reduction, only 32% reduction of EhSyf protein expression was achieved in pKTSyf amoeba transformants (**Figure 1G**). Finally, anti-HA confocal microscopy immunofluorescence experiments showed that EhSyf localized to the nucleus similar to the HA-U1A splicing factor control (**Figure 2A** and Figure S1E).

To determine its role in splicing, we reasoned that slight changes of EhSyf expression, being part of the NTC, would imbalance wild type pre-mRNA/mRNA ratios in a general manner. Despite the capacity of U1 snRNP components to define the 5′ss and of the U2AF dimer to define the 3′ss. These protein/RNA interactions must be taken into consideration since most 5′ss (GUUUGUUU) are strong and conserved in Entamoeba (Hon et al., 2013), in the absence of U1 snRNA RNA (Dávila López et al., 2008). Therefore 5′ss definition must be carried out by U1 snRNP components and splicing auxiliary factors as described for other systems (Förch et al., 2002; Huang et al., 2012). For 3'ss definition, whereas strong (AG-independent) poly-pyrimidine tracts do not always require U2AF35, both U2AF35/65 are required to define AG-dependent 3'ss with weak poly-pyrimidine tracts (Wu et al., 1999). A collection of introns was analyzed with respect to their AG-dependency (**Figure 2B**) and several were chosen to test our hypothesis. AG-dependent introns of *Sam50* and *Cdc2*, and AG-independent introns of *RabX13*, *MybS6* and intron 1 of *ClcB*. As a control the intron-less Actin transcript was analyzed. These introns were also selected because they represent both virulence-related [*Sam50*, *MybS6*, and *ClcB* are downregulated after trophozoites recuperated from hamster liver abscesses (Weber et al., 2016)] and virulence-unrelated transcripts. Furthermore, in steady state conditions, they always produce unspliced pre-mRNA/intron retained (IR) and mRNA variants facilitating the monitoring of splicing variats. *In vivo* splicing assays were carried out using RNA extracts from the EhSyf expresser and silenced transformants. Compared to the HA control, spliced mRNA increased in all HASyf expresser transformants at the expense of pre-mRNA/IR variants. Correspondingly, EHSyf silencing resulted in pre-mRNA/IR accumulation at the expense of mRNA, compared to the pKT silencing controls (**Figure 2C**). Statistically different transcription levels are shown (**Figure 2D**). Unexpectedly this approach allowed us to detect that high selective pressure EhSyf silencing affected Actin gene expression too. This change was not observed in U2AF-silenced ameba transformants (psU2AF) selected with the same amount of G418 (**Figures 2B,C**), indicating that low amounts of EhSyf impact transcription of intron-less genes too.

DISCUSSION

EhSyf gene encodes a tetratricopeptide repeats protein involved in several nuclear functions. The Entamoeba *Syf* gene products appear to have low copy number that can be boosted during transfection of unrelated genes. This might reflect the direct/indirect participation of EhSyf in transcription, or it might reflect that the introduction of plasmid DNA evokes general transcription/DNA-repair mechanisms, increasing in turn *EhSyf* transcripts. The impact of plasmid transfection on endogenous genes has been documented since the pioneering works attempting heterologous expression of proteins in *E. histolytica* (Hamann et al., 1995).

EhSyf expression directly impacts splicing in a general manner. This reflects its relationship with the large subunit of U2AF which binds to poly-pyrimidine tracts in front of the 3′ss, and tethers the pre-mRNA/spliceosome to the CTD. Interestingly, EhSyf silencing but not overexpression, negatively affected transcription even of intron-less genes indicating its role in transcription elongation.

Together, our data suggest the coordinated functions of EhSyf in transcription and splicing in this early branched protist.

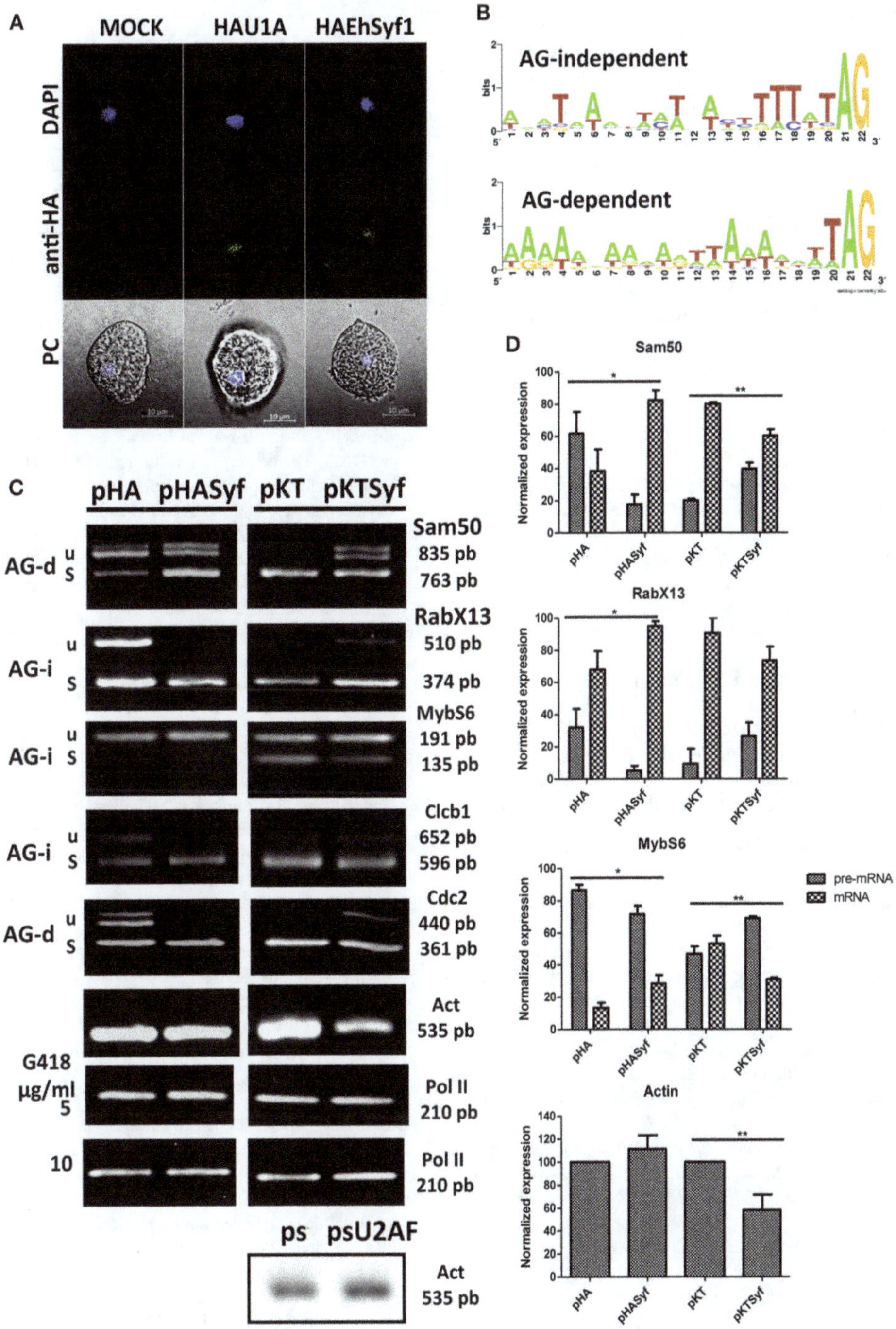

FIGURE 2 | pre-mRNA splicing is favored in amoebae overexpressing EhSyf and defective with the knockdown. **(A)** *Entamoeba histolytica* HA-Syf transformants were plated onto microscopy slides, incubated with FITC-coupled anti-HA antibodies to detect appropriate nuclear localization of *EhSyf* protein by confocal microscopy. Nuclei were stained with DAPI. **(B)** WebLogos of the 3′ss of *E. histolytica* AG-independent (AG-i) and AG-dependent (AG-d) introns (Wu et al., 1999).
(C) Representative semi-quantitative RT-PCR assays with specific primers to amplify Sam50, RabX13, MybS6, Clcb1, Cdc2 and the intron-less Actin gene products in 5 or 10 µg/ml G418 selected amoeba transformants. RNA polymerase II transcript was used to normalize the expression levels. For comparison, Actin gene expression was also monitored in U2AF splicing silenced amoebae (psU2AF). **(D)** Error bars indicate the SD of three independent experiments. The asterisks show significant differences (t-Student $P^{*} < 0.05$ $^{**} < 0.01$) compared to empty vector transfectants. Whereas for Sam50, RabX13 and Actin the results shown correspond to HASyf expresser and knockdown transformants selected with 5 and 10 µg/ml G418, respectively; MybS6 gene selection of HASyf expression and knockdown figures show the data of transformants selected with 10 and 5 µg/ml G418, respectively. Clcb1 and Cdc2 gene products showed no significant differences in any selection (shown 5 µg/ml G418).

Although the impact of EhSyf in transcription termination and mRNA export still remains to be tested. We conclude that EhSyf is a *bona fide Entamoeba histolytica* Syf1 ortholog that participates in splicing and transcription elongation. To our knowledge this is the first evidence of the molecular link between transcription and splicing in *Entamoeba histolytica*.

ACKNOWLEDGMENTS

The authors are grateful to Tomoyoshi Nozaki and Upinder Singh for plasmids. Funding was provided by CONACYT (Grants 127557-M and 236104 to JV; Scholarship 141030016 to DT-C).

AUTHOR CONTRIBUTIONS

JV, DT-C conception, experimental design, manuscript preparation; DT-C, JG-R, OS-C, and JV data acquisition and interpretation.

REFERENCES

Blatch, G. L., and Lässle, M. (1999). The tetratricopeptide repeat: a structural motif mediating protein-protein interactions. *Bioessays* 21, 932–939. doi: 10.1002/(SICI)1521-1878(199911)21:11<932::AID-BIES5>3.0.CO;2-N

Carmody, S. R., and Wente, S. R. (2009). mRNA nuclear export at a glance. *J. Cell Sci.* 122, 1933–1937. doi: 10.1242/jcs.041236

Chan, S. P., Kao, D. I., Tsai, W. Y., and Cheng, S. C. (2003). The Prp19p-associated complex in spliceosome activation. *Science* 302, 279–282. doi: 10.1126/science.1086602

Chanarat, S., Seizl, M., and Strässer, K. (2011). The Prp19 complex is a novel transcription elongation factor required for TREX occupancy at transcribed genes. *Genes Dev.* 25, 1147–1158. doi: 10.1101/gad.623411

Das, A. K., Cohen, P. W., and Barford, D. (1998). The structure of the tetratricopeptide repeats of protein phosphatase 5: implications for TPR-mediated protein-protein interactions. *EMBO J.* 17, 1192–1199. doi: 10.1093/emboj/17.5.1192

David, C. J., Boyne, A. R., Millhouse, S. R., and Manley, J. L. (2011). The RNA polymerase II C-terminal domain promotes splicing activation through recruitment of a U2AF65-Prp19 complex. *Genes Dev.* 25, 972–983. doi: 10.1101/gad.2038011

Dávila López, M., Rosenblad, M. A., and Samuelsson, T. (2008). Computational screen for spliceosomal RNA genes aids in defining the phylogenetic distribution of major and minor spliceosomal components. *Nucleic Acids Res.* 36, 3001–3010. doi: 10.1093/nar/gkn142

Davis, C. A., Brown, M. P., and Singh, U. (2007). Functional characterization of spliceosomal introns and identification of U2, U4, and U5 snRNAs in the deep-branching eukaryote *Entamoeba histolytica*. *Eukaryotic Cell* 6, 940–948. doi: 10.1128/EC.00059-07

de la Mata, M., Lafaille, C., and Kornblihtt, A. R. (2010). First come, first served revisited: factors affecting the same alternative splicing event have different effects on the relative rates of intron removal. *RNA* 16, 904–912. doi: 10.1261/rna.1993510

Diamond, L. S., Clark, C. G., and Cunnick, C. C. (1995). YI-S, a casein-free medium for axenic cultivation of *Entamoeba histolytica*, related Entamoeba, Giardia intestinalis and *Trichomonas vaginalis*. *J. Eukaryot. Microbiol.* 42, 277–278. doi: 10.1111/j.1550-7408.1995.tb01579.x

Diamond, L. S., Harlow, D. R., and Cunnick, C. C. (1978). A new medium for the axenic cultivation of *Entamoeba histolytica* and other Entamoeba. *Trans. R. Soc. Trop. Med. Hyg.* 72, 431–432. doi: 10.1016/0035-9203(78)90144-X

Diamond, L. S., Mattern, C. F., and Bartgis, I. L. (1972). Viruses of *Entamoeba histolytica*. I. Identification of transmissible virus-like agents. *J. Virol.* 9, 326–341.

Fabrizio, P., Dannenberg, J., Dube, P., Kastner, B., Stark, H., Urlaub, H., et al. (2009). The evolutionarily conserved core design of the catalytic activation step of the yeast spliceosome. *Mol. Cell* 36, 593–608. doi: 10.1016/j.molcel.2009.09.040

Förch, P., Puig, O., Martínez, C., Séraphin, B., and Valcárcel, J. (2002). The splicing regulator TIA-1 interacts with U1-C to promote U1 snRNP recruitment to 5' splice sites. *EMBO J.* 21, 6882–6892. doi: 10.1093/emboj/cdf668

Fourmann, J. B., Schmitzová, J., Christian, H., Urlaub, H., Ficner, R., Boon, K. L., et al. (2013). Dissection of the factor requirements for spliceosome disassembly and the elucidation of its dissociation products using a purified splicing system. *Genes Dev.* 27, 413–428. doi: 10.1101/gad.207779.112

Goren, A., Ram, O., Amit, M., Keren, H., Lev-Maor, G., Vig, I., et al. (2006). Comparative analysis identifies exonic splicing regulatory sequences–The complex definition of enhancers and silencers. *Mol. Cell* 22, 769–781. doi: 10.1016/j.molcel.2006.05.008

Hamann, L., Nickel, R., and Tannich, E. (1995). Transfection and continuous expression of heterologous genes in the protozoan parasite *Entamoeba histolytica*. *Proc. Natl. Acad. Sci. U.S.A.* 92, 8975–8979. doi: 10.1073/pnas.92.19.8975

Hanawalt, P.C., and Spivak, G. (2008). Transcription-coupled DNA repair: two decades of progress and surprises. *Nat. Rev. Mol. Cell Biol.* 9, 958–970. doi: 10.1038/nrm2549

Hernández-Rivas, R., Ramírez, C., Guillén, N., and Vargas, M. (2000). DNA cloning of the *Entamoeba histolytica* PRP6 gene: a putative U4/U6 small nuclear ribonucleoprotein particle (snRNP). *Arch. Med. Res.* 31, S294–295. doi: 10.1016/S0188-4409(00)00119-3

Hogg, R., McGrail, J. C., and O'Keefe, R. T. (2010). The function of the NineTeen Complex (NTC) in regulating spliceosome conformations and fidelity during pre-mRNA splicing. *Biochem. Soc. Trans.* 38, 1110–1115. doi: 10.1042/BST0381110

Hon, C. C., Weber, C., Sismeiro, O., Proux, C., Koutero, M., Deloger, M., et al. (2013). Quantification of stochastic noise of splicing and polyadenylation in *Entamoeba histolytica*. *Nucleic Acids Res.* 41, 1936–1952. doi: 10.1093/nar/gks1271

Huang, S. C., Ou, A. C., Park, J., Yu, F., Yu, B., Lee, A., et al. (2012). RBFOX2 promotes protein 4.1R exon 16 selection via U1 snRNP recruitment. *Mol. Cell. Biol.* 32, 513–526. doi: 10.1128/MCB.06423-11

Jurica, M. S., and Moore, M. J. (2003). Pre-mRNA splicing: awash in a sea of proteins. *Mol. Cell* 12, 5–14. doi: 10.1016/S1097-2765(03)00270-3

López-Camarillo, C., López-Rosas, I., Ospina-Villa, J. D., and Marchat, L. A. (2014). Deciphering molecular mechanisms of mRNA metabolism in the deep-branching eukaryote *Entamoeba histolytica*. *Wiley Interdiscip. Rev. RNA* 5, 247–262. doi: 10.1002/wrna.1205

López-Camarillo, C., Orozco, E., and Marchat, L. A. (2005). *Entamoeba histolytica*: comparative genomics of the pre-mRNA 3' end processing machinery. *Exp. Parasitol.* 110, 184–190. doi: 10.1016/j.exppara.2005.02.024

Makiuchi, T., Mi-ichi, F., Nakada-Tsukui, K., and Nozaki, T. (2013). Novel TPR-containing subunit of TOM complex functions as cytosolic receptor for Entamoeba mitosomal transport. *Sci. Rep.* 3:1129. doi: 10.1038/srep01129

Marchat, L. A., Orozco, E., Guillen, N., Weber, C., and López-Camarillo, C. (2008). Putative DEAD and DExH-box RNA helicases families in *Entamoeba histolytica*. *Gene* 424, 1–10. doi: 10.1016/j.gene.2008.07.042

Miranda, R., Salgado, L. M., Sánchez-López, R., Alagon, A., and Lizardi, P. M. (1996). Identification and analysis of the u6 small nuclear RNA gene from *Entamoeba histolytica*. *Gene* 180, 37–42. doi: 10.1016/S0378-1119(96)00397-6

Morf, L., Pearson, R. J., Wang, A. S., and Singh, U. (2013). Robust gene silencing mediated by antisense small RNAs in the pathogenic protist *Entamoeba histolytica*. *Nucleic Acids Res.* 41, 9424–9437. doi: 10.1093/nar/gkt717

Nakada-Tsukui, K., and Nozaki, T. (2016). Immune response of amebiasis and immune evasion by *Entamoeba histolytica*. *Front. Immunol.* 7:175. doi: 10.3389/fimmu.2016.00175

Nakatsu, Y., Asahina, H., Citterio, E., Rademakers, S., Vermeulen, W., Kamiuchi, S., et al. (2000). XAB2, a novel tetratricopeptide repeat protein involved in transcription-coupled DNA repair and transcription. *J. Biol. Chem.* 275, 34931–34937. doi: 10.1074/jbc.M004936200

Nozaki, T., Asai, T., Sanchez, L. B., Kobayashi, S., Nakazawa, M., and Takeuchi, T. (1999). Characterization of the gene encoding serine acetyltransferase, a regulated enzyme of cysteine biosynthesis from the protist parasites *Entamoeba histolytica* and Entamoeba dispar. Regulation and possible function of the cysteine biosynthetic pathway in Entamoeba. *J. Biol. Chem.* 274, 32445–32452. doi: 10.1074/jbc.274.45.32445

Reed, R., and Cheng, H. (2005). TREX, SR proteins and export of mRNA. *Curr. Opin. Cell Biol.* 17, 269–273. doi: 10.1016/j.ceb.2005.04.011

Saito-Nakano, Y., Yasuda, T., Nakada-Tsukui, K., Leippe, M., and Nozaki, T. (2004). Rab5-associated vacuoles play a unique role in phagocytosis of the enteric protozoan parasite *Entamoeba histolytica*. *J. Biol. Chem.* 279, 49497–49507. doi: 10.1074/jbc.M403987200

Sikorski, R. S., Michaud, W. A., Wootton, J. C., Boguski, M. S., Connelly, C., and Hieter, P. (1991). TPR proteins as essential components of the yeast cell cycle. *Cold Spring Harb. Symp. Quant. Biol.* 56, 663–673. doi: 10.1101/SQB.1991.056.01.075

Tamura, K., Stecher, G., Peterson, D., Filipski, A., and Kumar, S. (2013). MEGA6: Molecular Evolutionary Genetics Analysis version 6.0. *Mol. Biol. Evol.* 30, 2725–2729. doi: 10.1093/molbev/mst197

Tarn, W. Y., Hsu, C. H., Huang, K. T., Chen, H. R., Kao, H. Y., Lee, K. R., et al. (1994). Functional association of essential splicing factor(s) with PRP19 in a protein complex. *EMBO J.* 13, 2421–2431.

Tarn, W. Y., Lee, K. R., and Cheng, S. C. (1993a). Yeast precursor mRNA processing protein PRP19 associates with the spliceosome concomitant with or just after dissociation of U4 small nuclear RNA. *Proc. Natl. Acad. Sci. U.S.A.* 90, 10821–10825. doi: 10.1073/pnas.90.22.10821

Tarn, W. Y., Lee, K. R., and Cheng, S. C. (1993b). The yeast PRP19 protein is not tightly associated with small nuclear RNAs, but appears to associate with the spliceosome after binding of U2 to the pre-mRNA and prior to formation of the functional spliceosome. *Mol. Cell. Biol.* 13, 1883–1891. doi: 10.1128/MCB.13.3.1883

Valdés, J., Nozaki, T., Sato, E., Chiba, Y., Nakada-Tsukui, K., Villegas-Sepúlveda, N., et al. (2014). Proteomic analysis of *Entamoeba histolytica in vivo* assembled pre-mRNA splicing complexes. *J. Proteomics* 111, 30–45. doi: 10.1016/j.jprot.2014.07.027

Venema, J., Mullenders, L. H., Natarajan, A. T., van Zeeland, A. A., and Mayne, L. V. (1990). The genetic defect in Cockayne syndrome is associated with a defect in repair of UV-induced DNA damage in transcriptionally active DNA. *Proc. Natl. Acad. Sci. U.S.A.* 87, 4707–4711. doi: 10.1073/pnas.87.12.4707

Wahl, M. C., and Lührmann, R. (2015). SnapShot: spliceosome Dynamics, I. *Cell* 161, 1474–e1471. doi: 10.1016/j.cell.2015.05.050

Wahl, M. C., Will, C. L., and Lührmann, R. (2009). The spliceosome: design principles of a dynamic RNP machine. *Cell* 136, 701–718. doi: 10.1016/j.cell.2009.02.009

Weber, C., Koutero, M., Dillies, M. A., Varet, H., Lopez-Camarillo, C., Coppeé, J. Y., et al. (2016). Extensive transcriptome analysis correlates the plasticity of *Entamoeba histolytica* pathogenesis to rapid phenotype changes depending on the environment. *Sci. Rep.* 6:35852. doi: 10.1038/srep 35852

Wu, S., Romfo, C. M., Nilsen, T. W., and Green, M. R. (1999). Functional recognition of the 3' splice site AG by the splicing factor U2AF35. *Nature* 402, 832–835. doi: 10.1038/45590

Zenklusen, D., Vinciguerra, P., Wyss, J. C., and Stutz, F. (2002). Stable mRNP formation and export require cotranscriptional recruitment of the mRNA export factors Yra1p and Sub2p by Hpr1p. *Mol. Cell. Biol.* 22, 8241–8253. doi: 10.1128/MCB.22.23.8241-8253.2002

8

Postsplicing-Derived Full-Length Intron Circles in the Protozoan Parasite *Entamoeba histolytica*

María S. Mendoza-Figueroa[1], *Eddy E. Alfonso-Maqueira*[1], *Cristina Vélez*[2], *Elisa I. Azuara-Liceaga*[3], *Selene Zárate*[3], *Nicolás Villegas-Sepúlveda*[4], *Odila Saucedo-Cárdenas*[5,6] *and Jesús Valdés*[1*]

[1] Departamento de Bioquímica, Centro de Investigación y de Estudios Avanzados del Instituto Politécnico Nacional, Mexico City, Mexico, [2] Departamento de Biología Celular, Centro de Investigación y de Estudios Avanzados del Instituto Politécnico Nacional, Mexico City, Mexico, [3] Posgrado en Ciencias Genómicas, Universidad Autónoma de la Ciudad de Mexico, Mexico City, Mexico, [4] Departamento de Biomedicina Molecular, Centro de Investigación y de Estudios Avanzados del Instituto Politécnico Nacional, Mexico City, Mexico, [5] Departamento de Histología, Facultad de Medicina, Universidad Autónoma de Nuevo León, Monterrey, Mexico, [6] División de Genética, Centro de Investigación Biomédica del Noreste, Instituto Mexicano del Seguro Social, Monterrey, Mexico

Correspondence:
Jesús Valdés
jvaldes@cinvestav.mx

Noncoding circular RNAs are widespread in the tree of life. Particularly, intron-containing circular RNAs which apparently upregulate their parental gene expression. *Entamoeba histolytica*, the causative agent of dysentery and liver abscesses in humans, codes for several noncoding RNAs, including circular ribosomal RNAs, but no intron containing circular RNAs have been described to date. Divergent RT-PCR and diverse molecular approaches, allowed us to detect bona fide full-length intronic circular RNA (flicRNA) molecules. Self-splicing reactions, RNA polymerase II inhibition with Actinomycin D, and second step of splicing-inhibition with boric acid showed that the production of flicRX13 (one of the flicRNAs found in this work, and our test model) depends on mRNA synthesis and pre-mRNA processing instead of self-splicing. To explore the cues and factors involved in flicRX13 biogenesis *in vivo*, splicing assays were carried out in amoeba transformants where splicing factors and Dbr1 (intron lariat debranching enzyme 1) were silenced or overexpressed, or where Rabx13 wild-type and mutant 5′ss (splice site) and branch site minigene constructs were overexpressed. Whereas SF1 (splicing factor 1) is not involved, the U2 auxiliary splicing factor, Dbr1, and the GU-rich 5′ss are involved in postsplicing flicRX13 biogenesis, probably by Dbr1 stalling, in a similar fashion to the formation of ciRNAs (circular intronic RNAs), but with distinctive 5′-3′ss ligation points. Different from the reported functions of ciRNAs, the 5′ss GU-rich element of flicRX13 possibly interacts with transcription machinery to silence its own gene in *cis*. Furthermore, introns of *E. histolytica* virulence-related genes are also processed as flicRNAs.

Keywords: ncRNA, circular RNA, Dbr1, virulence, splicing, 5′ss, branch point sequence

INTRODUCTION

Circular RNAs (circRNAs) are a group of noncoding RNAs (ncRNAs) that originated from protein coding genes. They were described nearly 40 years ago through electron microscopy studies (Hsu and Coca-Prados, 1979); however, their prevalence in different cellular conditions, biogenesis and possible functions have been explored only recently with the advent of massive sequencing of the transcriptomes.

Most of them still lack a specific function but it has been described that some may act as postranscriptional regulators in the cytoplasm or may act as cotranscriptional regulators in the nucleus (Hansen et al., 2013; Memczak et al., 2013; Ashwal-Fluss et al., 2014; Li et al., 2015), suggesting that circRNAs have important functions in modifying gene expression.

The best studied circRNAs are exon-coded cytoplasmic microRNA sponges (Hansen et al., 2013; Memczak et al., 2013), while others consist of exons that include full intronic sequences, named ElciRNAs, which compete with splicing to control their parental gene expression in *cis* via their interaction with RNA Pol II and the U1 small nuclear RNA at their respective promoter regions (Ashwal-Fluss et al., 2014; Li et al., 2015). The biogenesis of circRNAs and ElciRNAs involves backsplicing or is mediated by an exon-containing lariat precursor, pathways favored by complementary sequences, such as ALU repeats, in the introns bracketing the circularized exons and in some cases mediated by the splicing factors *muscleblind* or *quaking* (Jeck et al., 2013; Memczak et al., 2013; Ashwal-Fluss et al., 2014; Barrett et al., 2015; Conn et al., 2015; Ivanov et al., 2015).

Cytoplasmic (and some nuclear) stable intronic sequence RNAs (sisRNAs) and ciRNAs conform an additional type of splicing-related circular RNA molecules that escape debranching reaction of intron lariats (Zhang et al., 2013; Talhouarne and Gall, 2014). Cytoplasmic sisRNAs are lariats lacking the 3′ terminal tail (approximately 30 nt upstream the 3′ss) and are present during early embryogenesis in the cytoplasm of *Xenopus tropicalis*. It has been proposed that they avoid debranching before leaving the nucleus since they are opened by nuclear, but not cytoplasmic, extracts of *Xenopus laevis* (Talhouarne and Gall, 2014). Conversely, ciRNA production in human cells depends on the presence of a GU rich sequence element close to the 5′ss and a C-rich element near to the branch site (BP). These elements are not present in introns that are not circularized, and more importantly they enable the lariats that contain such elements to escape debranching. Therefore, Dbr1 appears to be involved in the biogenesis of sisRNAs and ciRNAs through particular mechanisms not yet described. The ciRNAs interact with the phosphorylated RNA Pol II to activate the transcription of its parental genes (Zhang et al., 2013).

To date, the best characterized circular RNA molecules have been described in multicellular eukaryotes, yeasts, *Plasmodium falciparum* and *Dictyostelium discoideum* (Wang et al., 2014), but not in other protists of clinical relevance, such as *Entamoeba histolytica,* the etiologic agent of amoebiasis which still causes over 55,000 annual deaths worldwide, and 2.2 million disability-adjusted life years (Lozano et al., 2012; Murray et al., 2012). However, *E. histolytica* is not devoid of regulatory ncRNAs which include stressed-induced self-circularized 5′-external transcribed spacer rRNAs (Gupta et al., 2012), and microRNAs (De et al., 2006; Mar-Aguilar et al., 2013).

Entamoeba histolytica possess small introns of ≈75 nt in length with extremely conserved 5′ and 3′ss, GUUUGUU and UAG, respectively (Wilihoeft et al., 2001; Davis et al., 2007; Lorenzi et al., 2010; Hon et al., 2013). The BP sequence (YNYYRAY) of amoebic introns has been identified only *in silico* and lacks the conservation maintained in other protozoans (Wilihoeft et al., 2001; Vanácová et al., 2005; Davis et al., 2007).

Here, we explored the existence of *E. histolytica* splicing products similar to the vertebrate circRNAs, ElcircRNAs, or ciRNAs. For the first time we report circular ncRNA molecules from different amoeba gene products, including some overexpressed in virulence. Different from their vertebrate counterparts, these are conformed by full-length intronic circular RNAs (flicRNAs). Characterization of the intron circle of *RabX13* (flicRX13) showed that it originates from transcription/splicing of its parental gene and is more stable than the IR (intron retained), spliced and lariat variants that originated thereof. FlicRX13 biogenesis can be attributed to the intronic 5′ss GU-rich element and possibly to Dbr1 activity, which we are still investigating. Due to their distinctive 5′-3′ss ligation points, we propose that flicRNAs might arise from stalled Dbr1 with the aid of additional factors. Different from the reported functions of ciRNA, minigene intron constructs carrying 5′ss GU-rich element mutants evidenced a *cis*-regulatory role of flicRX13 silencing its parental gene, possibly via interaction with factors of the transcription machinery.

MATERIALS AND METHODS

E. histolytica Cultures and Drug Treatments

Trophozoites of the *E. histolytica* strain HM1:IMSS were axenically cultured in Trypticase-yeast extract-iron serum (TYI-S-33) medium at 37°C and harvested as described (Diamond et al., 1995). For *in vivo* assays (splicing, inhibition of second step of splicing or Dbr1 inhibition), 10^6 log phase (48 h) wild type or transfectant trophozoites per experimental point, either alone or treated with 1.3 μM Actinomycin D (Sigma Aldrich) as described (López-Camarillo et al., 2003), or with different concentrations of boric acid (pH 7.9) (Shomron and Ast, 2003) during 1.5 h. After treatments, cells were harvested, and total RNA was isolated and analyzed by reverse transcription (RT) followed by polymerase chain reaction (PCR) amplification of the DNA.

RNA and DNA Isolation

Genomic DNA (gDNA) and total RNA were isolated using the TRIzol Reagent as specified by the manufacturer (Invitrogen). For RNA isolation, preparations were treated with RQ1 DNase (Promega) or with RNase R (Epicentre), when specified. For gDNA purification, preparations were treated with RNases T1 and A.

Retro Transcription and Polymerase Chain Reactions

All primers and PCR conditions are listed in **Table S1**. *RabX13* (EHI_065790), *U6 snRNA* (U43841), *18S rRNA* (AB426549), *RNA Pol II* (EHI_087360), and *EhActin* (EHI_107290) gene expression were monitored by RT-PCR using specific primer pairs, M-MLV retro transcriptase, and Taq DNA Polymerase, as specified by the manufacturer (Invitrogen). All PCR products were cloned into the pCR2.1 plasmid vector (Invitrogen) and sequenced.

To detect circular RNA molecules, specific outward facing primer pairs targeted to the introns of the *E. histolytica* genes *RabX13*, *rpL12* (EHI_191750), *rpS14* (EHI_074090), *Cdc2* (L03810), and intron 2 of *ClcB* (EHI_186860), respectively, were designed as described (Vogel et al., 1997). The primers were used in circular RT-PCR using the aforementioned conditions. In some cases, PCR reactions were carried out with the 5′-end radiolabeled Rab2BSs oligonucleotide. Radiolabeling was carried out with the T4 PNK enzyme (New England BioLabs) as suggested by the manufacturer. Where indicated, RT reactions were carried out in the presence of 5 μM Actinomycin D (Sigma-Aldrich), adding the drug immediately after the denaturing step (Houseley and Tollervey, 2010). PCR products were resolved in 8% urea-polyacrylamide gels. The Kappa Syber Fast Universal One-Step qRT-PCR kit (Sigma Aldrich) was used for quantitative RT-PCR with 10 ng of cDNA input in 10 μL.

SF1, U2AF, and DBR1 Plasmid Constructs and Entamoeba Transformants

Using *E. histolytica* gDNA as a template and the respective primer pairs in which the SmaI and XhoI restriction sites were included, the full-length and C-terminus deleted (ΔC) U2AF and Dbr1ΔC, were amplified by PCR and ligated into the SmaI/XhoI-digested pEhExHA expression plasmid able to express N-terminal hemagglutinin (HA)-tagged fusion protein (Saito-Nakano et al., 2007). The wild type and mutant *RabX13* minigenes were purchased to GeneScript (**Table S2**) and subcloned into pEhExHA. The full-length *EhSF1* gene was amplified by PCR and ligated in inverted orientation into the SmaI/XhoI-digested silencing pKT3M plasmid (Morf et al., 2013). Plasmids were transfected into *E. histolytica* HM1:IMSS trophozoites as described (Nozaki et al., 1999). To avoid lethality, 24 h after transfection the expression of HA-Dbr1ΔC fusion proteins in transient transfectants was induced by the addition of 1.5 μg/mL during 48 h. Stable HA-U2AF, HA-U2AFΔC, and pK-SF1 transfectants were established by culturing in 3, 6, or 10 μg/mL G418 as above. *In vivo* splicing assays were carried out with purified RNA from log phase cultures of transformants to detect *RabX13* unspliced, spliced, lariats and circular RNA variants.

Western Blots

HA-Dbr1, HA-U2AFΔC proteins as well as histone H3 were detected by western blot assays using the anti-HA (Covance) and anti-histone H3 (Cell Signaling) antibodies diluted 1:25,000 and 1:1,000, respectively. SF1 was detected with anti-human SF1 antibodies (Santa Cruz) diluted 1:1,000.

Statistical Analyses

The intensity of each splice isoform was measured using NIH ImageJ software from at least three RT-PCR experiments and analyzed using Student's *t*-test and One-Way ANOVA with SigmaPlot software. For reference, the mean value of each isoform in the absence of Boric acid or at the zero time points was set to 1. qRT-PCR data was analyzed using the $2^{-\Delta\Delta C_T}$ method (Livak and Schmittgen, 2001).

RESULTS

Identification and Validation of Full-Length Intron Circular RNAs

To detect circular intronic noncoding RNAs, outward facing primers (**Figure 1A** and **Table S1**) targeted to five genes of different functions and intron sizes were used in circular RT-PCR (Vogel et al., 1997): the Rab GTPase family member *RabX13* (136 nt intron); the ribosomal protein S14 gene *rpS14* (73 nt intron); the ribosomal protein L12 gene *rpL12* (106 nt intron); the yeast homolog *p34^cdc2^ Cdc2* (79 nt intron); and the chloride anion channel *ClcB* (57 nt intron 1 and 81 nt intron 2) (Salas-Casas et al., 2006). These genes were selected because their intron size is larger than the mean of *E. histolytica* introns, therefore facilitating their study. Like intron 1 of *ClcB*, the majority of introns initially chosen for this study were too small and/or were A-T rich and were left out because were not amenable to such analyses.

Surprisingly no sequence reads of the introns analyzed corresponded to branched molecules showing a typical miss-incorporation of an A for T at the lariat's BP (Vogel et al., 1997; Barrett et al., 2015). Instead, the sequences corresponded to full-length intronic circularized RNAs (flicRNAs), with ligated G residues of the ends of the introns, 6–15 nt larger than the products expected from the lariat amplicons (**Figures 1B,C**, black arrowheads). No 3′ tail-less lariat structures such as those observed in vertebrates or other types of branched lariats (Li-Pook-Than and Bonen, 2006; Gao et al., 2008; Taggart et al., 2012, 2017; Zhang et al., 2013) were detected. The remaining amplicons (white asterisks) did not match their respective intronic sequences. None of the *Cdc2* reads were informative; therefore, this intron was not analyzed further. Since the *Rabx13* flicRNA (flicRX13) is readily detected in different Entamoeba strains, it was chosen for further characterization and analyses.

Experiments were carried out to discard any given condition that could render artifactual 5′-3′ss joined amplicons. First, to rule out intron tandem genomic templates, we compared the products obtained in circular RT-PCR experiments using DNase I-treated total RNA, with and without RT, and RNase A+T1-treated gDNA without RT reactions. FlicRX13 was detected only in plus RT DNase I-treated total RNA samples (**Figure 2A**). Second, to eliminate the possible inter-molecular trans-splicing origin of flicRNAs, cDNA synthesis was carried out with the primer EhActR or Rab2BSas, targeted to the *EhActin* gene and to the *RabX13* intron, respectively. Then, independent PCR reactions were carried out with each cDNA, using the respective reverse primers employed in the RT reaction (EhActR or Rab2BSas) and the forward primers targeted to different transcripts (e.g., *rpS14*) as shown in **Figure 2B**. Except for the *EhActin* controls (lane 1), no PCR products were detected. Third, to discard possible self-ligation events due to diluted RNA samples, we used increasing amounts of total RNA input in the circular RT-PCR experiments and observed a proportional increase in flicRX13 amplification (**Figure 2C**). To eliminate artifactual inter- and intra-molecular RT jumps, cDNA was synthesized in the presence of Actinomycin D (Houseley and Tollervey, 2010) with increasing amounts of total RNA inputs. As expected, Actinomycin D increased flicRX13 specific

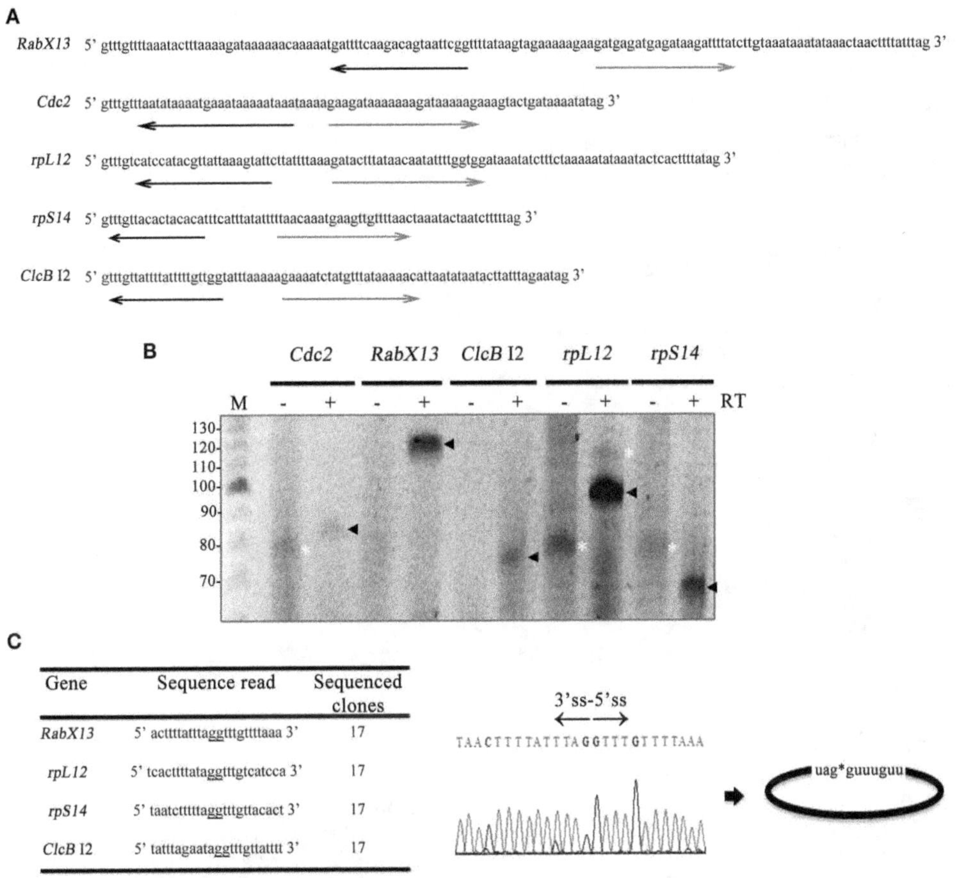

FIGURE 1 | *E. histolytica* full-length intronic circular RNAs. **(A)** Sequences of the introns analyzed in this work. Antisense (black) and sense (gray) outward-facing primers used in circular RT-PCRs. **(B)** 8% urea-polyacrylamide gels showing the amplicons obtained in the circular RT-PCRs alongside a 10 bp ladder (M). Black arrowheads indicate products ~5–10 nt larger than the tailed lariats, e.g., flicRNAs. White asterisks indicate products that do not correspond to their respective intron sequences. PCRs with (+) and without (−) RT reactions are indicated. **(C)** Sequence reads of amplicon clones showing ligation points between the 5′ss and the 3′ss (underlined gg residues; also denoted by an asterisk), suggesting full-length intronic circular RNA molecules (right). The electropherogram corresponds to flicRX13.

amplification as a function of the RNA input (**Figure 2D**). Together these experiments suggest that at least flicRX13 does not result from noncanonical trans-splicing events.

To verify the circularity of the intronic RNA molecules, additional criteria were considered. First, stringent northern blot hybridization was performed with a probe spanning the 3′ss G-5′ss G ligation point of flicRX13 (dashed arrow in **Figure 2E**). Next, total RNA was treated with RNAse R to degrade linear RNA (Suzuki et al., 2006; Burd et al., 2010; Salzman et al., 2012; Jeck et al., 2013; Ashwal-Fluss et al., 2014) and was used to perform circular RT-PCR using primer Rab2BSas (black arrow in **Figure 2F**) for cDNA synthesis. Only a specific PCR product corresponding to flicRX13 was amplified with the probe and sense primer (dashed and gray arrows respectively). Furthermore, as expected for intronic circular ncRNA (Zhang et al., 2013) we were able to amplify flicRNAs from nuclear RNA and from RNA extracted with miRNA isolation kits. Altogether, our results support the notion that *E. histolytica* flicRNAs are *bona fide* circular intronic RNA molecules.

Postsplicing Origin of flicRNAs

Circular RNA molecules are more stable than their corresponding splicing variants (Jeck et al., 2013). This is also true for flicRX13, since this product appears early in the growth phase and is maintained throughout a 72-h standard growth culture (not shown) incubated in the presence of Actinomycin D at different time points. After 3 h of transcription inhibition, *RabX13* pre-mRNA and spliced variants nearly disappear while the flicRNA population remained up to 6 h of treatment (**Figures 3A,B**). As previously observed (López-Camarillo et al., 2003), the expression of *EhActin* remained unchanged. U6 snRNA and 18S rRNA were also not affected, indicating that RNA polymerases III (Miranda et al., 1996) and I (Oakes et al., 1993), respectively, were not affected (**Figure 3C**). These results show the different stability between pre-mRNA, mRNA and flicRX13, and that the half-life of flicRX13 is greater than that of its parental mRNA.

To explore the splicing or postsplicing origin of flicRNAs we first silenced the E complex factor SF1 (Loftus et al., 2005; Valdés et al., 2014) and analyzed flicRX13 abundance

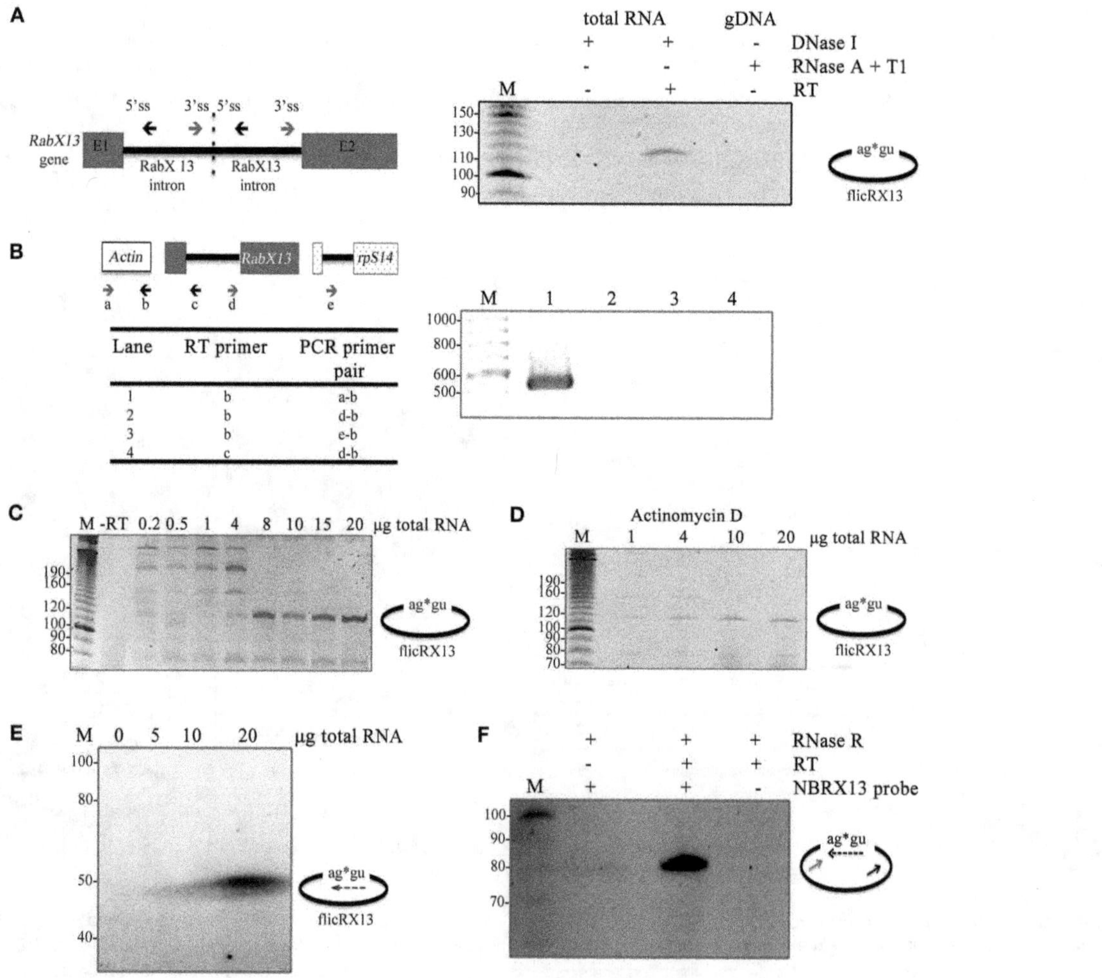

FIGURE 2 | flicRX13 is not a product of intron duplication, trans-splicing, or self-circularization events. **(A)** A diagram of the theoretical intron duplication event is depicted to the left showing the 5′ss, the 3′ss, and the outward facing primers. flicRX13 was detected only in plus RT DNase I-treated total RNA samples suggesting that no tandem templates exist in the genome. E1, exon 1; E2, exon 2. **(B)** Analysis of the possible intermolecular noncanonical trans-splicing events. Details are described in the text. Except for *EhActin* controls (lane 1), no PCR products were detected suggesting that flicRX13 is not a product of either intermolecular trans-splicing nor RT jumps. **(C)** Increasing amounts of total RNA input in the circular RT-PCR experiments proportionally increased flicRX13 amplification, ruling out possible self-ligation events due to dilute RNA samples. **(D)** Addition of Actinomycin D to the RT reaction increased flicRX13 specific amplification as a function of RNA input. **(E)** Different amounts of total trophozoite RNAs were blotted onto nylon membrane and hybridized at full stringency with a radiolabeled probe spanning the splice site ligation points. **(F)** RNase R treated RNA samples were used as input for cDNA synthesis with the antisense primer of **Figure 1** in the presence (+) or absence (−) of RT. Circular PCR was carried out with the sense primer and the probe used in **(E)**. Numbers to the left of the gel images indicate the bp ladder (M).

in the transfected amoebas. After confirming SF1 mRNA depletion by RT-PCR, we observed that reduced levels of SF1 moderately increased intron retained/spliced precursor and RabX13 spliced variants but not flicRX13, demonstrating its role in splicing, but not in flicRNA production (**Figure 4A**). We next overexpressed the E complex U2 auxiliary splicing factor, U2AF. Full-length U2AF slightly increased flicRNA formation in response to increased overall synthesis of unspliced and spliced RabX13 transcripts; however, overexpression of the C-terminus deleted U2AF strongly increased both splicing and flicRNA production (**Figure 4B**), suggesting that flicRNAs are byproducts of splicing after complex E has been assembled.

To seek whether flicRNA formation occurs during or after the first step of splicing, we compared the abundance of unspliced pre-mRNA/intron retained, spliced mRNA, lariats and flicRNAs in RNA extracts from Entamoeba cultured in boric acid, an inhibitor of the second step of splicing (Shomron and Ast, 2003). By circular RT-PCR using a radioactive primer, we detected *RabX13* and *rpS14* lariats with the predicted BP (**Figure S1** and **Figure 4C**) and with the expected 6–11 nt size, which is smaller compared to flicRNAs. As expected, 5 mM boric acid significantly affected the amplification of all splicing products (ANOVA $P \leq 0.001$), particularly flicRX13. However, with 10 mM boric acid, a slight recovery of flicRX13 and lariat molecules (including actual

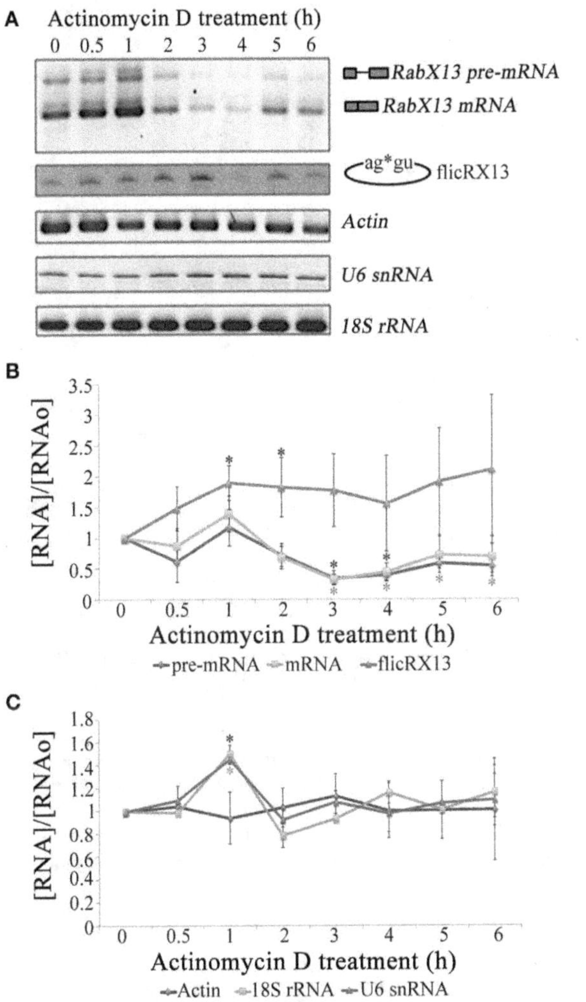

FIGURE 3 | flicRX13 is an RNA processing byproduct and is more stable than its corresponding splicing linear variants. **(A)** *RabX13* gene expression after RNA Pol II inhibition by Actinomycin D. As the loading control *EhActin* gene expression was analyzed. Pol I (18S rRNA) and Pol III (U6 snRNA) inhibition by Actinomycin D was also monitored. **(B)** Quantitative analysis of RabX13 gene expression after RNA Pol II inhibition by Actinomycin D shown in **(A)**. The increase of flicRX13 expression at 1 and 2 h posttreatment is significantly different (t-Student $P < 0.0061$; $P < 0.0041$, respectively) as well as the decrease in pre-mRNA and mRNA (t-Student $P < 0.001$ at 3 h; black and gray asterisks, respectively). **(C)** Quantitative analysis of 18S rRNA, U6 snRNA and *EhActin* gene expression after RNA Pol II inhibition by Actinomycin D shown in **(A)**. The increases in 18S rRNA and U6 snRNA (black and gray asterisks, respectively) are statistically significative (t-Student $P < 0.001$).

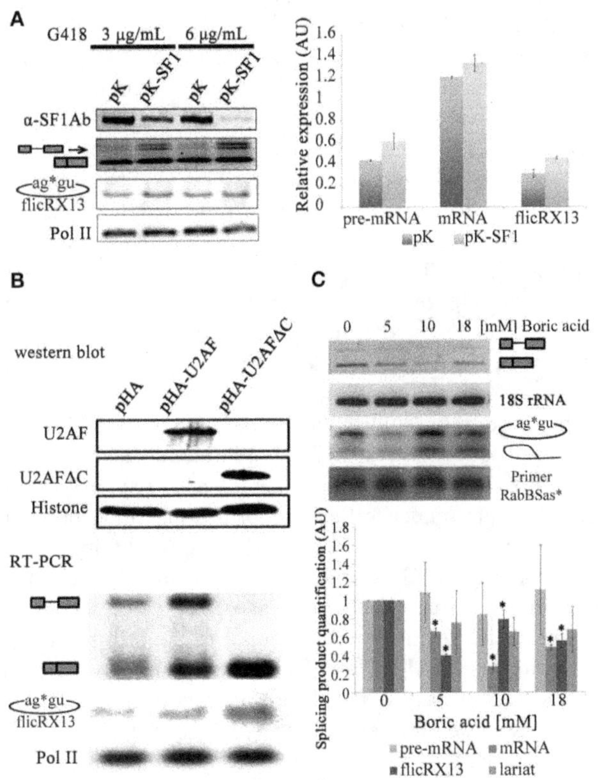

FIGURE 4 | Inhibition of the second step of splicing alters flicRNA production. **(A)** Stable SF1-silencing (pK-SF1) and empty pKT3M vector (pK) transfectants were established at 3 and 6 μg/mL G418. Silencing was assessed by western blot (top) achieving 40–90% efficiency. Absence of SF1 slightly increased pre-mRNA/unspliced and mRNA *Rabx13* transcripts (middle), and flicRX13 production (bottom); however, such increments were not statistically significant (right plot). **(B)** Amoeba transformants overexpressing wt (HA-U2AF) and carboxy-terminal deleted (HA-U2AFΔC) U2 auxiliary splicing factor were established. Appropriate expression of the hemagglutinin-U2AF fusion proteins were monitored and compared to histone H3 expression by western blot (top). Compared to the empty Entamoeba HA expression plasmid (pHA) pHA-U2AF increased the overall expression of all *RabX13* transcription products. However, HA-U2AFΔC substantially increased mRNA (spliced) products and flicRX13. RNA polymerase II expression was equivalent between the transformants. **(C)** Expression of the *RabX13* gene transcript variants (unspliced, spliced, flicRX13 and intron lariat) after incubation of *E. histolytica* trophozoites with different concentrations of boric acid, an inhibitor of the second step of splicing. 18S rRNA expression was used for normalization purposes. To detect intron lariats, circular RT-PCR was carried out with the ^{32}P-labeled Rab2BSas primer (Rab2BSas*), which was used as the loading control. Bottom panel, products in the upper panel were quantitated and statistically analyzed. Decrease of spliced *RabX13* variant and flicRX13 were statistically significant (ANOVA $P \leq 0.001$, asterisks in bold). Values are the average of three independent experiments.

and cryptic BP lariats, and lariat-3′ exon intermediaries) was observed at the expense of the spliced products (**Figure 4C**). These results suggest that flicRX13 is another final product of splicing, most likely originated by the circularization of lariats. Because *in vivo* boric acid treatment is a novel experimental approach, the accumulation of lariats in boric acid treated mammalian cell cultures was validated as well. Lariats of the HPV16 proximal 3′ss accumulated in infected HeLa cells only (**Figure S1**).

Elements and Factors Involved in flicRNAs Biogenesis

Structurally, flicRNAs resemble circular group I and group II introns. We did not explore the possible origin of flicRNAs by self-splicing reactions homologous to group I introns because *E. histolytica* introns have no discernible internal guide sequences that facilitate self-splicing (Winter et al., 1990), and we did not observe circle ligation points containing guanine triplets, that would result by the attack of an exogenous αG to the 5′ss, followed by the 5′ exon attack to the 3′ss as previously reported (Hausner et al., 2014). To explore whether flicRNAs are self-spliced such as group II introns, synthetic radio-labeled RabX13 and ai5γ group II intron transcripts were incubated in the appropriate buffers. Whereas the intron-3′ exon intermediate and mRNA were produced from the ai5γ intron transcript, only intact RabX13 transcripts were observed suggesting that flicRNAs might not originate through this mechanism (**Figure S2**). However, since RabX13 intron does not have the RNA elements required for auto excision (data not shown), we cannot completely discard this route of intron circularization in *E. histolytica*.

To escape from the debranching reaction, ciRNA biogenesis requires a GU-rich 5′ss and a C-rich element upstream of the BP (Zhang et al., 2013). Therefore, to explore whether these elements influence flicRNA formation, minigene intron Entamoeba transfectants were established harboring the wt intron, a minus GU-rich 5′ss (ΔGU) intron, an intron containing a C-rich element 11 nt upstream of the BP (C; uncommon in the Entamoeba genome), and an intron with both modifications (ΔGU-C), all of which are flanked with partial exon sequences tagged with plasmid-specific sequences. The different RNA species transcribed from the transfected plasmids were monitored by qRT-PCR with primers CS+116 and Rab-REx2. The elimination of the GU-rich element at the 5′ss affected flicRNA formation even in the presence of the synthetic C-rich element. The C-rich element alone has a similar effect but not as strong as the 5′ss-GU element indicating that the GU-rich element is sufficient to promote intron circularization (**Figure 5A**).

Dbr1 participates in sisRNAs and ciRNAs biogenesis (Zhang et al., 2013; Talhouarne and Gall, 2014). To explore the possible *E. histolytica* Dbr1 involvement in flicRNAs biogenesis, we attempted siRNA-mediated Dbr1 silencing without success. Also, the establishment of the catalytically deficient Dbr1 (Dbr1ΔC) overexpressor amoebas was unsuccessful. Therefore, *in vivo* splicing assays were conducted using Dbr1ΔC transiently transfected trophozoites under low selection pressure (1.5 μg/mL G418). After assessing Dbr1ΔC expression by western blot, the different *RabX13* splicing products were monitored (**Figure 6**). Surprisingly, compared to the control Dbr1ΔC overexpression increased flicRNA levels. Taken together, our data indicate that *E. histolytica* flicRNAs originate from lariat molecules after the second step of splicing has taken place, and that the GU-rich 5′ss and Dbr1 are implicated in their biogenesis. However, the implication of Dbr1 in this process might be indirect or require additional factors.

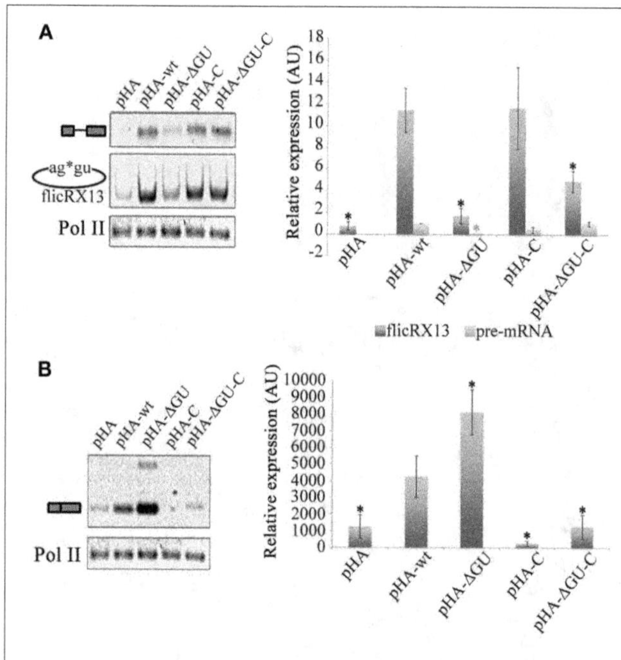

FIGURE 5 | The GU-rich 5′ss element of the intron is involved in flicRNA biogenesis and function. Amoeba transformants expressing wt, 5′ss mutant (GUUUGUUU to GUAAGAA), C-enriched BP mutant (AACTAACTTTT**A** to ACCTCCCTCTT**A**; A in bold corresponds to the BP mapped in **Figure S1**), and double mutant *RabX13* minigene constructs were established, and the impact on unspliced, spliced, and flicRX13 *RabX13* variant expression was assessed by qRT-PCR using primers CS+116 and Rab-REx2 targeted to plasmid sequences **(A)** and endogenous *RabX13* mRNA **(B)**. Decreases of plasmid-derived unspliced *RabX13* variants and flicRX13 were statistically significant; likewise, the increase of endogenous mRNA was statistically significant (ANOVA black asterisk $P \leq 0.0001$, gray asterisk $P \leq 0.01$, respectively). Values are the average of three independent experiments.

Insights Into flicRNAs Possible Functions

circRNAs bound to the U1 snRNA promote the transcription of their parental genes, which interact with the RNA polymerase II at the promoter or during elongation (Zhang et al., 2013; Li et al., 2015). Our experimental design with the minigene constructs allowed us to explore the possible function of Entamoeba flicRNAs irrespective of the snRNA involved. Again, *in vivo* splicing assays were performed using RNA from minigenes transformed amoebas and the different endogenous RNA species were monitored. Unexpectedly, mutations in the 5′ss-GU element resulted in an increase of endogenous *RabX13* expression (**Figure 5B**), indicating that such elements of flicRX13 silences the expression of its parental gene in *cis*.

Finally, to explore the general nature of flicRNAs in the Entamoeba ncRNA repertoire, we sought additional flicRNAs, particularly those involved in liver abscess formation (Meyer et al., 2016). We detected flicRNAs from the gene products in the loci EHI_014170 (intron 1), EHI_169670 (both introns), and the mono-intronic EHI_192510 (**Figure 7**), suggesting that flicRNAs are common ncRNA species in *E. histolytica* involved in gene expression regulation.

DISCUSSION

Here, we identified full-length intronic circular RNAs or flicRNAs, whose 5′ss is ligated to the 3′ss, in the protozoan parasite *E. histolytica*, which differs from other parasitic or mammalian circular RNAs. For example, *D. discoideum* and *P. falciparum* circular RNAs contain exons and some, are related to exon-skipping splicing events (Wang et al., 2014), indicating that in protozoa there might exist a wide repertoire of circular noncoding RNAs that originated by distinct mechanisms in protozoa.

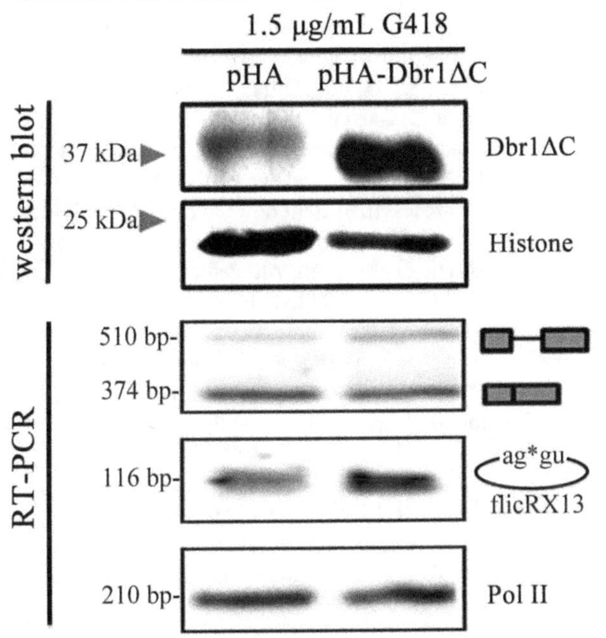

FIGURE 6 | flicRX13 is a postsplicing product: Dbr1 is involved in Entamoeba flicRNA production. *E. histolytica* trophozoites were transiently transfected with the empty vector pEhExHA (pHA), or with the C-terminus deleted Dbr1 (pHA-Dbr1ΔC) plasmids and 24 h latter were tested under low selection pressure (1.5 μg/mL G418). Overexpression of Dbr1 (wt or ΔC) was monitored by western blot using anti-HA antibody compared to anti-histone H3 (loading control). The effect of Dbr1 (wt or ΔC) overexpression on flicRX13, *RabX13* mRNA, and RNA Pol II (loading control) gene expression was analyzed by RT-PCRs.

flicRNAs Biogenesis in *E. histolytica*

Exon-intron-containing circular RNAs are generated by backsplicing, mainly favored by protein-mediated or sequence-mediated approximation of intronic repetitive sequences that flank nonconsecutive circularized exons (Ashwal-Fluss et al., 2014; Jeck and Sharpless, 2014; Conn et al., 2015; Ivanov et al., 2015). The molecular mechanisms involved are not fully understood, but it is clear that circRNA formation competes with splicing (Ashwal-Fluss et al., 2014) and, in spite of the lack of direct biochemical evidence (Barrett et al., 2015), the occurrence of some circular RNAs have been correlated to exon-skipping splicing events (Zaphiropoulos, 1996; Surono et al., 1999; Zhang et al., 2014), as reported for the exon-derived circular RNAs found in *D. discoideum* and *P. falciparum* (Wang et al., 2014). The biogenesis of *E. histolytica* flicRNAs characterized here does not depend on complex E splicing formation, possibly due to the strong (Larson and Hoskins, 2017) and most frequent Entamoeba 5′ss (GUUUGUU) (Davis et al., 2007; Hon et al., 2013) since SF1 is not related to splice site definition nor to flicRNA formation. The impact of the U2 auxiliary factor in flicRNA formation indicates a closer relationship between complex A factors and the requirements for intron circularization, particularly those recruited with the entrance of the U2 snRNP, facilitated by U2AF, that not only defines the 3′ss (Shepard et al., 2002; Förch and Valcarcel, 2003), but also contacts both RNA polymerase II and the nineteen complex (David et al., 2011), which is part of the spliceosomal intron lariat complex, along with other components of the U2 snRNP, and remain attached to the lariat after spliceosomal disassembly (Yoshimoto et al., 2009; Fourmann et al., 2013). Likewise, such impact of U2AF on flicRX13 formation supports the notion that flicRNAs originate by postsplicing events, ruling out the autosplicing route of flicRNA biogenesis.

The circular RNAs in *E. histolytica* are similar to some human ncRNAs. They are full-length intronic circles with joined 5′ and 3′ss and are, thus flicRNAs. Although functionally related, mammalian EIcircRNAs are dissimilar to flicRNAs since they contain both intronic and exonic sequences (Li et al., 2015).

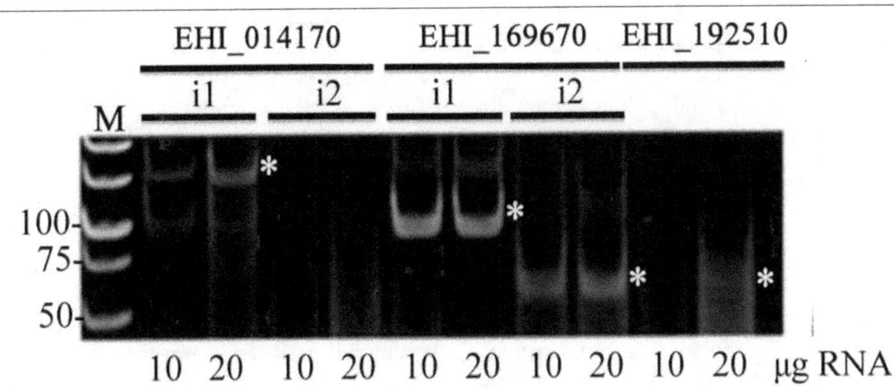

FIGURE 7 | Introns of some virulence-related genes also render flicRNAs. Appropriate sets of outward-facing primers were designed to amplify virulence-related flicRNAs (white asterisks) by circular RT-PCR as in **Figure 2F**. Different amounts of small RNA input isolated with the miRNA isolation kit were used. Gene accession numbers are indicated; i1, intron 1; i2, intron 2. Numbers to the left indicate the bp ladder (M).

Circular ncRNAs are structurally similar to flicRNAs, which are 1) the tail-less ciRNAs consisting of circular intron lariats derived from splicing, which escape lariat-debranching enzyme activity, due to a 7 nt GU-rich element at the 5′ss and a C-rich element 11 nt upstream of the BP (Zhang et al., 2013), and 2) the senescence-related and translation-inhibiting human intron-originated circular RNAs, similar to cirRNAs and flicRNAs, whose biogenesis remains unknown (Taggart et al., 2012, 2017; Abdelmohsen et al., 2017; Panda et al., 2017).

C-rich elements are absent in the genome and the BP environment of Entamoeba introns explaining why even the addition of synthetic C elements fails to elicit flicRNA production. The closest resemblances of such elements are the NYYUAY pyrimidine-rich elements in the vicinity of the BP (Wilihoeft et al., 2001), suggesting that other cis elements are necessary for their biogenesis. The GUUUGUU 5′ss consensus sequence of *E. histolytica* introns resembles the GU-rich element of ciRNAs. Here, we showed that nucleotide substitutions of this 5′ss for a vertebrate 5′ss consensus (GUAAGAA) almost abolishes the formation of flicRNAs, suggesting that such GU-rich elements are essential for splicing and flicRNA biogenesis, probably by allowing escape from the debranching reaction. Interestingly, the artificial introduction of a C-rich BP element had no ostensible effect in flicRNA formation indicating that the Entamoeba genome adapted to a C-poor environment to carry out flicRNA biogenesis using only strong 5′ss GU-rich elements. During splicing complex E formation, U1 snRNA binds to the 5′ss (Larson and Hoskins, 2017). In *E. histolytica*, the U1 snRNP proteins U1A, U1C, and U170k are able to recruit the pre-mRNA processing machinery (Valdés et al., 2014) even in the absence of the U1 snRNA (Dávila López et al., 2008). However, as reported in yeast and *in vitro* systems (Kandels-Lewis and Seraphin, 1993; Rhode et al., 2006), it is possible that the Entamoeba U6 snRNA activates the 5′ss and splicing due to their high degree of base complementarity. Therefore, compared to the wild type 5′ss the changes introduced in the ΔGU mutant elicited a different splicing response due to impaired 5′ss activation. The link of the GU-rich element to debranching reaction escape is still under investigation.

Taggart and coworkers detected the first intron-derived circular molecules similar to flicRNAs by deep sequencing (Taggart et al., 2012, 2017). They observed that approximately 3% of the BP corresponded to the 3′ss of the respective transcripts, thus circular 5′-3′ss ligated molecules, and, although they did not characterize such molecules further, they proposed their postsplicing origin either by a third nucleophilic attack or by a debranching-ligation event. Our results using boric acid as the second step of splicing inhibitor (Shomron and Ast, 2003) suggest a postsplicing origin of flicRX13. We cannot discard that flicRNAs may originate via a third nucleophilic attack as proposed for Group II introns (Murray et al., 2001). However, a more complex debranching-ligation reactions scenario is more likely to occur since it must involve additional factors. Whereas in situations where 2′-5′ phosphodiester bond hydrolysis is impaired, such as in human and yeast Dbr1-deficient cells, intron lariats accumulate (Montemayor et al., 2014; Han et al., 2017), overexpression of an equally impaired Dbr1 in amoeba transformants, unexpectedly increased flicRX13 formation, strengthening the notion that flicRNAs originate from accumulated lariats and that other factors might participate in circularization of Entamoeba introns.

BP conformation is essential for stable recognition and catalysis by Dbr1 CTD and lariat recognition loop (LRL) domains; therefore it is possible that CTD-less Dbr1 might have hydrolyzed the BP and, due to the unstable LRL-BP interaction and the 5′ss GU-rich element, the intron was now exposed to yet to be identified circularization factors, RNA ligase for example, in addition to the intron lariat large complex (U2, U5 and U6 snRNPs, Ntr1, Prp43, and Dnr1) (Yoshimoto et al., 2009; Fourmann et al., 2013; Garrey et al., 2014). Finally, removal of the 3′ tail of the lariat precedes debranching (Chapman and Boeke, 1991; Salem et al., 2003), and we detected that the 3′ss of RabX13 and rps14 lariats are less than 10 nt downstream of the BP, placing them within the LRL-BP recognition groove and protecting them from exonucleolytic degradation. Altogether, these observations support the role of Dbr1 in flicRNA biogenesis and suggest that debranching limits access/competes with other necessary factors for intron circularization. We cannot rule out the possibility that flicRNAs arise from a third nucleophilic attack even though such reaction has not been reported in postsplicing events.

flicRNAs Possible Functions

Cytoplasmic exon-containing circRNAs function as miRNA sponges (Jeck and Sharpless, 2014; Chen, 2016). Conversely, the small (thus without space to accommodate miRNA target sites), and nuclear *E. histolytica* flicRNAs most likely have different functions. It is currently accepted that intron containing linear and circular RNAs are retained in the nuclei by a similar mechanism (Chen, 2016). Although by mechanisms not fully understood, intronic circular RNAs participate in gene transcription regulation (Chen, 2016). CLIP-Seq experiments identified intronic circular RNAs associated with Pol II (Li et al., 2015), and the depletion of the abundantly expressed ciRNAs such as ci-ankrd52 and ci-sirt7 results in lower transcription of their parental genes (ANKRD52 y SIRT7) indicating that they promote their transcription by interacting with the Pol II elongation complex (Zhang et al., 2013). Other nuclear circRNAs interact with the U1 snRNP and Pol II on the promoter of their parental genes, stimulating their transcription. Both knockdown of these circRNAs as well as disruption of U1 snRNA-circRNA binding with morpholinos anti-U1 diminishes transcription of their parental genes (Li et al., 2015). In contrast, expression of ΔGU minigenes showed that Entamoeba flicRX13 apparently inhibits transcription of its parental gene, in which the 5′ss GU-rich element again seems to be actively involved. Although direct evidence of flicRNA-RNA Pol II interaction still lacks, our findings suggest an inhibitory role of flicRNAs on transcription. Recently, it has been shown that small regulatory RNAs inhibit RNA polymerase during elongation in the nematode *C. elegans* (Guang et al., 2010). Interestingly the addition of a C-rich BP element positively affected transcription in *cis* probably due to poly C binding hnRNPs (Chaudhury et al., 2010; Han et al., 2010), which are able to bind to such elements in the transcripts, favoring their expression and transcription over other genes (Kim et al., 2005; Meng et al., 2007).

Current experiments are directed to support our present models in which silencing of *Rabx13* transcription might occur via flicRX13-U6 snRNA binding or flicRNA-U1A/TIA-1/TIAR binding prior interaction with Pol II at the promoter or during elongation. In conclusion flicRNAs are common ncRNA species in *E. histolytica* that are involved in gene expression regulation of different regulatory processes including virulence traits.

AUTHOR CONTRIBUTIONS

MM-F, EA-M, NV-S, and JV conception and experimental design. MM-F, EA-M, CV, EA-L, SZ, NV-S, OS-C, and JV data acquisition and interpretation. MM-F and JV manuscript preparation.

FUNDING

The authors are grateful to Tomoyoshi Nozaki and Upinder Singh for plasmids. Funding was provided by CONACYT (Grants 127557-M and 236104).

REFERENCES

Abdelmohsen, K., Panda, A. C., Munk, R., Grammatikakis, I., Dudekula, D. B., De, S., et al., (2017). Identification of HuR target circular RNAs uncovers suppression of PABPN1 translation by CircPABPN1. *RNA Biol.* 14, 361–369. doi: 10.1080/15476286.2017.1279788

Ashwal-Fluss, R., Meyer, M., Pamudurti, N. R., Ivanov, A., Bartok, O., Hanan, M., et al. (2014). CircRNA biogenesis competes with pre-mRNA splicing. *Mol. Cell* 56, 55–66. doi: 10.1016/j.molcel.2014.08.019

Barrett, S. P., Wang, P. L., and Salzman, J. (2015). Circular RNA biogenesis can proceed through an exon-containing lariat precursor. *Elife* 4:e07540. doi: 10.7554/eLife.07540

Burd, C. E., Jeck, W. R., Liu, Y., Sanoff, H. K., Wang, Z., and Sharpless, N. E. (2010). Expression of linear and novel circular forms of an INK4/ARF-associated non-coding RNA correlates with atherosclerosis risk. *PLoS Genet.* 6:e1001233. doi: 10.1371/journal.pgen.1001233

Chapman, K. B., and Boeke, J. D. (1991). Isolation and characterization of the gene encoding yeast debranching enzyme. *Cell* 65, 483–492. doi: 10.1016/0092-8674(91)90466-C

Chaudhury, A., Chander, P., and Howe, P. H. (2010). Heterogeneous nuclear ribonucleoproteins (hnRNPs) in cellular processes: focus on hnRNP E1's multifunctional regulatory roles. *RNA* 16, 1449–1462. doi: 10.1261/rna.2 254110

Chen, L. L. (2016). The biogenesis and emerging roles of circular RNAs. *Nat. Rev. Mol. Cell Biol.* 17, 205–211. doi: 10.1038/nrm.2015.32

Conn, S. J., Pillman, K. A., Toubia, J., Conn, V. M., Salmanidis, M., Phillips, C. A., et al. (2015). The RNA binding protein quaking regulates formation of circRNAs. *Cell* 160, 1125–1134. doi: 10.1016/j.cell.2015.02.014

David, C. J., Boyne, A. R., Millhouse, S. R., and Manley, J. L. (2011). The RNA polymerase II C-terminal domain promotes splicing activation through recruitment of a U2AF65-Prp19 complex. *Genes Dev.* 25, 972–983. doi: 10.1101/gad.2038011

Dávila López, M., Rosenblad, M. A., and Samuelsson, T. (2008). Computational screen for spliceosomal RNA genes aids in defining the phylogenetic distribution of major and minor spliceosomal components. *Nucleic Acids Res.* 36, 3001–3010. doi: 10.1093/nar/gkn142

Davis, C. A., Brown, M. P., and Singh, U. (2007). Functional characterization of spliceosomal introns and identification of U2, U4, and U5 snRNAs in the deep-branching eukaryote *Entamoeba histolytica*. *Eukaryot. Cell* 6, 940–948. doi: 10.1128/EC.00059-07

De, S., Pal, D., and Ghosh, S. K. (2006). *Entamoeba histolytica*: computational identification of putative microRNA candidates. *Exp. Parasitol.* 113, 239–243. doi: 10.1016/j.exppara.2006.01.009

Diamond, L. S., Clark, C. G., and Cunnick, C. C. (1995). YI-S, a casein-free medium for axenic cultivation of *Entamoeba histolytica*, related Entamoeba, *Giardia Intestinalis* and *Trichomonas vaginalis*. *J. Eukaryot. Microbiol.* 42, 277–278. doi: 10.1111/j.1550-7408.1995.tb01579.x

Förch, P., and Valcarcel, J. (2003). Splicing regulation in Drosophila sex determination. *Prog. Mol. Subcell. Biol.* 31, 127–151. doi: 10.1007/978-3-662-09728-1_5

Fourmann, J. B., Schmitzova, J., Christian, H., Urlaub, H., Ficner, R., Boon, K. L., et al. (2013). Dissection of the factor requirements for spliceosome disassembly and the elucidation of its dissociation products using a purified splicing system. *Genes Dev.* 27, 413–428. doi: 10.1101/gad.207779.112

Gao, K., Masuda, A., Matsuura, T., and Ohno, K. (2008). Human branch point consensus sequence is yUnAy. *Nucleic Acids Res.* 36, 2257–2267. doi: 10.1093/nar/gkn073

Garrey, S. M., Katolik, A., Prekeris, M., Li, X., York, K., Bernards, S., et al. (2014). A homolog of lariat-debranching enzyme modulates turnover of branched RNA. *RNA* 20, 1337–1348. doi: 10.1261/rna.044602.114

Guang, S., Bochner, A. F., Burkhart, K. B., Burton, N., Pavelec, D. M., and Kennedy, S. (2010). Small regulatory RNAs inhibit RNA polymerase II during the elongation phase of transcription. *Nature* 465, 1097–1101. doi: 10.1038/nature09095

Gupta, A. K., Panigrahi, S. K., Bhattacharya, A., and Bhattacharya, S. (2012). Self-circularizing 5'-ETS RNAs accumulate along with unprocessed pre ribosomal RNAs in growth-stressed *Entamoeba histolytica*. *Sci. Rep.* 2:303. doi: 10.1038/srep00303

Han, B., Park, H. K., Ching, T., Panneerselvam, J., Wang, H., Shen, Y., et al. (2017). Human DBR1 modulates the recycling of snRNPs to affect alternative RNA splicing and contributes to the suppression of cancer development. *Oncogene* 36, 5382–5391. doi: 10.1038/onc.2017.150

Han, S. P., Tang, Y. H., and Smith, R. (2010). Functional diversity of the hnRNPs: past, present and perspectives. *Biochem. J.* 430, 379–392. doi: 10.1042/BJ20100396

Hansen, T. B., Kjems, J., and Damgaard, C. K. (2013). Circular RNA and miR-7 in cancer. *Cancer Res.* 73, 5609–5612. doi: 10.1158/0008-5472.CAN-13-1568

Hausner, G., Hafez, M., and Edgell, D. R. (2014). Bacterial group I introns: mobile RNA catalysts. *Mob. DNA* 5:8. doi: 10.1186/1759-8753-5-8

Hon, C. C., Weber, C., Sismeiro, O., Proux, C., Koutero, M., Deloger, M., et al. (2013). Quantification of stochastic noise of splicing and polyadenylation in *Entamoeba histolytica*. *Nucleic Acids Res.* 41, 1936–1952. doi: 10.1093/nar/gks1271

Houseley, J., and Tollervey, D. (2010). Apparent non-canonical trans-splicing is generated by reverse transcriptase *in vitro*. *PLoS ONE* 5:e12271. doi: 10.1371/journal.pone.0012271

Hsu, M. T., and Coca-Prados, M. (1979). Electron microscopic evidence for the circular form of RNA in the cytoplasm of eukaryotic cells. *Nature* 280, 339–340. doi: 10.1038/280339a0

Ivanov, A., Memczak, S., Wyler, E., Torti, F., Porath, H. T., Orejuela, M. R., et al. (2015). Analysis of intron sequences reveals hallmarks of circular RNA biogenesis in animals. *Cell Rep.* 10, 170–177. doi: 10.1016/j.celrep.2014.12.019

Jeck, W. R., and Sharpless, N. E. (2014). Detecting and characterizing circular RNAs. *Nat. Biotechnol.* 32, 453–461. doi: 10.1038/nbt.2890

Jeck, W. R., Sorrentino, J. A., Wang, K., Slevin, M. K., Burd, C. E., Liu, J., et al. (2013). Circular RNAs are abundant, conserved, and associated with ALU repeats. *RNA* 19, 141–157. doi: 10.1261/rna.035667.112

Kandels-Lewis, S., and Seraphin, B. (1993). Involvement of U6 snRNA in 5' splice site selection. *Science* 262, 2035–2039. doi: 10.1126/science.8266100

Kim, S. S., Pandey, K. K., Choi, H. S., Kim, S. Y., Law, P. Y., Wei, L. N., et al. (2005). Poly(C) binding protein family is a transcription factor in mu-opioid receptor gene expression. *Mol. Pharmacol.* 68, 729–736. doi: 10.1124/mol.105.012245

Larson, J. D., and Hoskins, A. A. (2017). Dynamics and consequences of spliceosome E complex formation. *Elife* 6:e27592. doi: 10.7554/eLife.27592

Li, Z., Huang, C., Bao, C., Chen, L., Lin, M., Wang, X., et al. (2015). Exon-intron circular RNAs regulate transcription in the nucleus. *Nat. Struct. Mol. Biol.* 22, 256–264. doi: 10.1038/nsmb.2959

Li-Pook-Than, J., and Bonen, L. (2006). Multiple physical forms of excised group II intron RNAs in wheat mitochondria. *Nucleic Acids Res.* 34, 2782–2790. doi: 10.1093/nar/gkl328

Livak, K. J., and Schmittgen, T. D. (2001). Analysis of relative gene expression data using real-time quantitative PCR and the $2^{-\Delta\Delta C_T}$ method. *Methods* 25, 402–408. doi: 10.1006/meth.2001.1262

Loftus, B., Anderson, I., Davies, R., Alsmark, U. C., Samuelson, J., Amedeo, P., et al. (2005). The genome of the protist parasite *Entamoeba histolytica*. *Nature* 433, 865–868. doi: 10.1038/nature03291

López-Camarillo, C., Luna-Arias, J. P., Marchat, L. A., and Orozco, E. (2003). EhPgp5 mRNA stability is a regulatory event in the *Entamoeba histolytica* multidrug resistance phenotype. *J. Biol. Chem.* 278, 11273–11280. doi: 10.1074/jbc.M211757200

Lorenzi, H. A., Puiu, D., Miller, J. R., Brinkac, L. M., Amedeo, P., Hall, N., et al. (2010). New assembly, reannotation and analysis of the *Entamoeba histolytica* genome reveal new genomic features and protein content information. *PLoS Negl. Trop. Dis.* 4:e716. doi: 10.1371/journal.pntd.0000716

Lozano, R., Naghavi, M., Foreman, K., Lim, S., Shibuya, K., Aboyans, V., et al. (2012). Global and regional mortality from 235 causes of death for 20 age groups in 1990 and 2010: a systematic analysis for the global burden of disease study 2010. *Lancet* 380, 2095–2128. doi: 10.1016/S0140-6736(12)61728-0

Mar-Aguilar, F., Trevino, V., Salinas-Hernandez, J. E., Tamez-Guerrero, M. M., Barron-Gonzalez, M. P., Morales-Rubio, E., et al. (2013). Identification and characterization of microRNAs from *Entamoeba histolytica* HM1-IMSS. *PLoS ONE* 8:e68202. doi: 10.1371/journal.pone.0068202

Memczak, S., Jens, M., Elefsinioti, A., Torti, F., Krueger, J., Rybak, A., et al. (2013). Circular RNAs are a large class of animal RNAs with regulatory potency. *Nature* 495, 333–338. doi: 10.1038/nature11928

Meng, Q., Rayala, S. K., Gururaj, A. E., Talukder, A. H., O'Malley, B. W., and Kumar, R. (2007). Signaling-dependent and coordinated regulation of transcription, splicing, and translation resides in a single coregulator, PCBP1. *Proc. Natl. Acad. Sci. U.S.A.* 104, 5866–5871. doi: 10.1073/pnas.0701065104

Meyer, M., Fehling, H., Matthiesen, J., Lorenzen, S., Schuldt, K., Bernin, H., et al. (2016). Overexpression of differentially expressed genes identified in non-pathogenic and pathogenic *Entamoeba histolytica* clones allow identification of new pathogenicity factors involved in amoebic liver abscess formation. *PLoS Pathog* 12:e1005853. doi: 10.1371/journal.ppat.1005853

Miranda, R., Salgado, L. M., Sanchez-Lopez, R., Alagon, A., and Lizardi, P. M. (1996). Identification and analysis of the u6 small nuclear RNA gene from *Entamoeba histolytica*. *Gene* 180, 37–42. doi: 10.1016/S0378-1119(96)00397-6

Montemayor, E. J., Katolik, A., Clark, N. E., Taylor, A. B., Schuermann, J. P., Combs, D. J., et al. (2014). Structural basis of lariat RNA recognition by the intron debranching enzyme Dbr1. *Nucleic Acids Res.* 42, 10845–10855. doi: 10.1093/nar/gku725

Morf, L., Pearson, R. J., Wang, A. S., and Singh, U. (2013). Robust gene silencing mediated by antisense small RNAs in the pathogenic protist *Entamoeba histolytica*. *Nucleic Acids Res.* 41, 9424–9437. doi: 10.1093/nar/gkt717

Murray, C. J., Vos, T., Lozano, R., Naghavi, M., Flaxman, A. D., Michaud, C., et al. (2012). Disability-adjusted life years (DALYs) for 291 diseases and injuries in 21 regions, 1990-2010: a systematic analysis for the global burden of disease study 2010. *Lancet* 380, 2197–2223. doi: 10.1016/S0140-6736(12)61689-4

Murray, H. L., Mikheeva, S., Coljee, V. W., Turczyk, B. M., Donahue, W. F., Bar-Shalom, A., et al. (2001). Excision of group II introns as circles. *Mol. Cell* 8, 201–211. doi: 10.1016/S1097-2765(01)00300-8

Nozaki, T., Asai, T., Sanchez, L. B., Kobayashi, S., Nakazawa, M., and Takeuchi, T. (1999). Characterization of the gene encoding serine acetyltransferase, a regulated enzyme of cysteine biosynthesis from the protist parasites *Entamoeba histolytica* and *Entamoeba dispar*. Regulation and possible function of the cysteine biosynthetic pathway in Entamoeba. *J. Biol. Chem.* 274, 32445–32452. doi: 10.1074/jbc.274.45.32445

Oakes, M., Nogi, Y., Clark, M. W., and Nomura, M. (1993). Structural alterations of the nucleolus in mutants of *Saccharomyces cerevisiae* defective in RNA polymerase I. *Mol. Cell. Biol.* 13, 2441–2455. doi: 10.1128/MCB.13.4.2441

Panda, A. C., Abdelmohsen, K., and Gorospe, M. (2017). RT-qPCR Detection of senescence-associated circular RNAs. *Methods Mol. Biol.* 1534, 79–87. doi: 10.1007/978-1-4939-6670-7_7

Rhode, B. M., Hartmuth, K., Westhof, E., and Luhrmann, R. (2006). Proximity of conserved U6 and U2 snRNA elements to the 5' splice site region in activated spliceosomes. *EMBO J.* 25, 2475–2486. doi: 10.1038/sj.emboj.7601134

Saito-Nakano, Y., Mitra, B. N., Nakada-Tsukui, K., Sato, D., and Nozaki, T. (2007). Two Rab7 isotypes, EhRab7A and EhRab7B, play distinct roles in biogenesis of lysosomes and phagosomes in the enteric protozoan parasite *Entamoeba histolytica*. *Cell Microbiol.* 9, 1796–1808. doi: 10.1111/j.1462-5822.2007.00915.x

Salas-Casas, A., Ponce-Balderas, A., Garcia-Perez, R. M., Cortes-Reynosa, P., Gamba, G., Orozco, E., et al. (2006). Identification and functional characterization of EhClC-A, an *Entamoeba histolytica* ClC chloride channel located at plasma membrane. *Mol. Microbiol.* 59, 1249–1261. doi: 10.1111/j.1365-2958.2006.05023.x

Salem, L. A., Boucher, C. L., and Menees, T. M. (2003). Relationship between RNA lariat debranching and Ty1 element retrotransposition. *J. Virol.* 77, 12795–12806. doi: 10.1128/JVI.77.23.12795-12806.2003

Salzman, J., Gawad, C., Wang, P. L., Lacayo, N., and Brown, P. O. (2012). Circular RNAs are the predominant transcript isoform from hundreds of human genes in diverse cell types. *PLoS ONE* 7:e30733. doi: 10.1371/journal.pone.0030733

Shepard, J., Reick, M., Olson, S., and Graveley, B. R. (2002). Characterization of U2AF(6), a splicing factor related to U2AF(35). *Mol. Cell. Biol.* 22, 221–230. doi: 10.1128/MCB.22.1.221-230.2002

Shomron, N., and Ast, G. (2003). Boric acid reversibly inhibits the second step of pre-mRNA splicing. *FEBS Lett.* 552, 219–224. doi: 10.1016/S0014-5793(03)00928-1

Surono, A., Takeshima, Y., Wibawa, T., Ikezawa, M., Nonaka, I., and Matsuo, M. (1999). Circular dystrophin RNAs consisting of exons that were skipped by alternative splicing. *Hum. Mol. Genet.* 8, 493–500. doi: 10.1093/hmg/8.3.493

Suzuki, H., Zuo, Y., Wang, J., Zhang, M. Q., Malhotra, A., and Mayeda, A. (2006). Characterization of RNase R-digested cellular RNA source that consists of lariat and circular RNAs from pre-mRNA splicing. *Nucleic Acids Res.* 34:e63. doi: 10.1093/nar/gkl151

Taggart, A. J., DeSimone, A. M., Shih, J. S., Filloux, M. E., and Fairbrother, W. G. (2012). Large-scale mapping of branchpoints in human pre-mRNA transcripts *in vivo*. *Nat. Struct. Mol. Biol.* 19, 719–721. doi: 10.1038/nsmb.2327

Taggart, A. J., Lin, C. L., Shrestha, B., Heintzelman, C., Kim, S., and Fairbrother, W. G. (2017). Large-scale analysis of branchpoint usage across species and cell lines. *Genome Res.* 27, 639–649. doi: 10.1101/gr.202820.115

Talhouarne, G. J., and Gall, J. G. (2014). Lariat intronic RNAs in the cytoplasm of *Xenopus tropicalis* oocytes. *RNA* 20, 1476–1487. doi: 10.1261/rna.045781.114

Valdés, J., Nozaki, T., Sato, E., Chiba, Y., Nakada-Tsukui, K., Villegas-Sepulveda, N., et al. (2014). Proteomic analysis of *Entamoeba histolytica in vivo* assembled pre-mRNA splicing complexes. *J. Proteomics* 111, 30–45. doi: 10.1016/j.jprot.2014.07.027

Vanácová, S., Yan, W., Carlton, J. M., and Johnson, P. J. (2005). Spliceosomal introns in the deep-branching eukaryote *Trichomonas vaginalis*. *Proc. Natl. Acad. Sci. U.S.A.* 102, 4430–4435. doi: 10.1073/pnas.0407500102

Vogel, J., Hess, W. R., and Borner, T. (1997). Precise branch point mapping and quantification of splicing intermediates. *Nucleic Acids Res.* 25, 2030–2031. doi: 10.1093/nar/25.10.2030

Wang, P. L., Bao, Y., Yee, M. C., Barrett, S. P., Hogan, G. J., Olsen, M. N., et al. (2014). Circular RNA is expressed across the eukaryotic tree of life. *PLoS* ONE 9:e90859. doi: 10.1371/journal.pone.0090859

Wilihoeft, U., Campos-Gongora, E., Touzni, S., Bruchhaus, I., and Tannich, E. (2001). Introns of *Entamoeba histolytica* and *Entamoeba dispar*. *Protist* 152, 149–156. doi: 10.1078/1434-4610-00053

Winter, A. J., Groot Koerkamp, M. J., and Tabak, H. F. (1990). The mechanism of group I self-splicing: an internal guide sequence can be provided in trans. *EMBO J.* 9, 1923–1928.

Yoshimoto, R., Kataoka, N., Okawa, K., and Ohno, M. (2009). Isolation and characterization of post-splicing lariat-intron complexes. *Nucleic Acids Res.* 37, 891–902. doi: 10.1093/nar/gkn1002

Zaphiropoulos, P. G. (1996). Circular RNAs from transcripts of the rat cytochrome P450 2C24 gene: correlation with exon skipping. *Proc. Natl. Acad. Sci. U.S.A.* 93, 6536–6541. doi: 10.1073/pnas.93.13.6536

Zhang, X. O., Wang, H. B., Zhang, Y., Lu, X., Chen, L. L., and Yang, L. (2014). Complementary sequence-mediated exon circularization. *Cell* 159, 134–147. doi: 10.1016/j.cell.2014.09.001

Zhang, Y., Zhang, X. O., Chen, T., Xiang, J. F., Yin, Q. F., Xing, Y. H., et al. (2013). Circular intronic long noncoding RNAs. *Mol. Cell* 51, 792–806. doi: 10.1016/j.molcel.2013.08.017

9

Entamoeba histolytica Trophozoites Induce a Rapid Non-Classical NETosis Mechanism Independent of NOX2-Derived Reactive Oxygen Species and PAD4 Activity

César Díaz-Godínez [1], Zayda Fonseca [1], Mario Néquiz [2], Juan P. Laclette [1], Carlos Rosales [1] and Julio C. Carrero [1]**

[1] Laboratory of Immunology, Department of Immunology, Instituto de Investigaciones Biomédicas, Universidad Nacional Autónoma de México, Mexico City, Mexico, [2] Laboratory of Immunopathology, Department of Experimental Medicine, Hospital General de México, Facultad de Medicina, Universidad Nacional Autónoma de México, Mexico City, Mexico

***Correspondence:**
Carlos Rosales
carosal@biomedicas.unam.mx
Julio C. Carrero
carrero@biomedicas.unam.mx

Neutrophil extracellular traps (NETs) are DNA fibers decorated with histones and antimicrobial proteins from cytoplasmic granules released into the extracellular space in a process denominated NETosis. The molecular pathways involved in NETosis have not been completely understood. Classical NETosis mechanisms involve the neutrophil elastase (NE) translocation to nucleus due to the generation of reactive oxygen species (ROS) by NADPH oxidase (NOX2) or the peptidyl arginine deiminase 4 (PAD4) activation in response to an increase in extracellular calcium influx; both mechanisms result in DNA decondensation. Previously, we reported that trophozoites and lipopeptidophosphoglycan from *Entamoeba histolytica* trigger NET release in human neutrophils. Here, we demonstrated in a quantitative manner that NETs were rapidly form upon treatment with amoebic trophozoites and involved both nuclear and mitochondrial DNA (mtDNA). NETs formation depended on amoeba viability as heat-inactivated or paraformaldehyde-fixed amoebas were not able to induce NETs. Interestingly, ROS were not detected in neutrophils during their interaction with amoebas, which could explain why NOX2 inhibition using apocynin did not affect this NETosis. Surprisingly, whereas calcium chelation reduced NET release induced by amoebas, PAD4 inhibition by GSK484 failed to block DNA extrusion but, as expected, abolished NETosis induced by the calcium ionophore A23187. Additionally, NE translocation to the nucleus and serine-protease activity were necessary for NET release caused by amoeba. These data support the idea that *E. histolytica* trophozoites trigger NETosis by a rapid non-classical mechanism and that different mechanisms of NETs release exist depending on the stimuli used.

Keywords: ***Entamoeba Histolytica*, neutrophils, NETosis, NETs, ROS, NOX2, PAD4**

INTRODUCTION

Neutrophils are the most abundant leucocytes in the mammal peripheral blood. Neutrophils have different strategies to combat pathogens including phagocytosis, degranulation and production of neutrophil extracellular traps (NETs). NETs are DNA fibers decorated with histones and antimicrobial proteins from cytoplasmic granules (Papayannopoulos and Zychlinsky, 2009) that are combined in the cytosol and released into the extracellular space in a process denominated NETosis (Steinberg and Grinstein, 2007). NETosis has been described as a cellular death process different from apoptosis and necrosis as it is independent of caspase pathway and there is no phosphatidylserine exposition on cell surface. In addition, NETosis is culminated with DNA extrusion (Fuchs et al., 2007).

The molecular pathways involved in NETosis has not been completely understood. During phorbol miristate acetate (PMA) stimulation, NADPH oxidase (NOX2) assemble take place to produce reactive oxygen species (ROS) (Fuchs et al., 2007). ROS promote the translocation of neutrophil elastase (NE) from the cytoplasmic granules to the nucleus where this enzyme cleaves histones to promote DNA decondensation (Papayannopoulos et al., 2010). Nevertheless, calcium ionophores ionomycin and A23187 appear to induce NETosis independently of NOX2-derived ROS; however, they depend on peptidyl arginine deiminase 4 (PAD4) activity to promote DNA decondensation by changing positive charged arginine residues to none charged citrulline residues in histones (Wang et al., 2009). This mechanism occurs due to an increase in extracellular calcium influx that activates PAD4 (which has four sites for calcium binding), and theoretically any molecule with the capacity to form pores in the cytoplasmic membrane of neutrophils (e.g., bacterial toxins or complement) are able to induce NETosis through this pathway (Konig and Andrade, 2016). Additionally, mitochondrial DNA (mtDNA) NETosis (Yousefi et al., 2009) has been reported in neutrophils which were primed with granulocyte/macrophage-colony stimulatory factor (GM-CSF) and stimulated with lipopolysaccharide (LPS) or complement fraction C5a; this form of NETs release was named vital NETosis because only mtDNA is extruded without compromise cell viability of neutrophils, in contrast with the lethal nuclear NETosis.

Entamoeba histolytica is an intestinal parasite with high prevalence in developing countries (Tellevik et al., 2015; Ghenghesh et al., 2016). Neutrophils have been implicated in defense against this parasite playing a crucial protective role (Asgharpour et al., 2005); nevertheless, involvement of neutrophils and other leukocytes in tissue damage has also been reported (Olivos-García et al., 2007). Oxidative (ROS production) and non-oxidative mechanisms are proposed to be used by neutrophils to kill amoeba (Ghosh et al., 2010; Pacheco-Yépez et al., 2011; Campos-Rodríguez et al., 2016). Mechanisms triggering neutrophils by amoebas are unknown but they could involve innate immune receptors such as TLRs. In this sense, human monocytes TLR2 and TLR4 recognition of lipopeptidophosphoglycan (LPPG) present on cell surface of amoebic trophozoites results in IL-6 and TNF-α release, suggesting that at least amoebic LPPG can activate immune cells trough PRRs (Maldonado-Bernal et al., 2005). Previously, *in vitro* NETs production in response to *E. histolytica* trophozoites or the LPPG from this parasite was demonstrated by our group (Ávila et al., 2016). Interestingly, non-viable amoebas failed to induce NETosis and trophozoites treated with PMA-derived NETs did not decreased neither their viability nor the capacity to develop amoebic liver abscess in a hamster model (Ávila et al., 2016). The mechanism of NET induction by *E. histolytica* is still unknown and its characterization could contribute to our understanding of the still controversial role of neutrophils in amoebiasis.

Here, we demonstrated that *E. histolytica* trophozoites rapidly induced NETosis by a mechanism independent of NOX2-derived ROS and PAD4 activity; however, this mechanism was dependent on the presence of extracellular calcium and serine-protease activity. These data support the notion of the existence of different NETosis processes that are triggered depending on the stimuli used, the study of which may add to the understanding of the role of these innate immunity mechanisms in parasitic infections.

MATERIALS AND METHODS

Entamoeba histolytica Trophozoites

Entamoeba histolytica trophozoites (strain HM1:IMSS) were cultured axenically at 37°C in TYIS-33 medium supplemented with 15% heat-inactivated adult bovine serum and Diamond vitamin tween solution (Sigma). The cultures were incubated for 72 h and trophozoites were harvested by chilling on ice for 5 min and centrifugation at 1,500 rpm for 5 min at 4°C. The pelleted amoebas were resuspended in PBS pH 7.4 and counted. For some experiments, trophozoites were washed with PBS and formaldehyde-fixed or heat-inactivated at 56°C during 10 and 30 min, respectively.

Neutrophil Isolation

Neutrophils were isolated from peripheral blood of healthy volunteers using Ficoll-Paque gradient (GE Healthcare) and hypertonic shock to lyse erythrocytes, as previously described (García-García et al., 2013). Cells were resuspended in RPMI medium supplemented with 5% fetal bovine serum and kept until use at 4°C. This study was carried out in accordance with the recommendations and approval of the Ethical Committee for Studies on Humans of the Instituto de Investigaciones Biomédicas, UNAM. All subjects gave written informed consent in accordance with the Declaration of Helsinki.

NET Quantification Assay

Neutrophils (3×10^5 cells) were stimulated by co-culturing with viable or fixed or heat-inactivated non-viable *E. histolytica* trophozoites (1.5×10^4 cells) in 500 μL of RPMI during 4 h at 37°C under 5% CO_2 atmosphere; 20 nM PMA was used as positive control of NETosis instead of trophozoites. In selected experiments 10 μM of the calcium ionophore A23187 was used as NETosis inducer. After stimulation, supernatants were collected by centrifugation at 4,000 rpm for 2 min to eliminate cells and

50 μL of the supernatants were added to the wells of a 96 well-plate containing 50 μL of PBS pH 7.4 with 500 nM SYTOX Green (Thermo-Fisher). Fluorescence was read from the bottom of wells in a spectrofluorometer using 485 nm excitation and 528 nm emission filters.

To obtain fluorescence values during the first 1 h of stimulation, neutrophils (1×10^5) were co-cultured with viable *E. histolytica* trophozoites (5×10^3) in 100 μL RPMI added with 500 nM SYTOX Green. Fluorescence values were measured each 5 min during 1 h with the 485 nm excitation and 528 nm emission filters as above.

In parallel experiments, neutrophils were pre-incubated before each stimulation with either DMSO-dissolved inhibitors apocynin (200 μM), PMSF (1 mM), or GSK484 (10 μM) at 4°C during 30 min. In the experiments with EGTA (20 mM), it was added 20 min before stimulation.

NET Visualization

Single DNA Staining

NETs staining was performed by co-culturing 2×10^5 neutrophils with 1×10^4 *E. histolytica* trophozoites (20:1 ratio) in 200 μL RPMI medium using Chamber Slide™ System (Lab-Tek) for the respective time-points at 37°C under 5% CO_2 atmosphere. After indicated time-periods, cultures were fixed with 4% formaldehyde for 10 min, washed three times with PBS and stained with 5 μg/mL DAPI. The coverslips were mounted with Fluoroshield (Sigma) before observation in a fluorescence microscope (Olympus BX51).

Immunofluorescence

NETs were induced with *E. histolytica* trophozoites on the Chamber Slide™ System as described above, and the cells were fixed with 4% paraformaldehyde for 10 min. The fixed cells were then permeabilized by adding 0.2% Triton X-100 in PBS for 5 min. Detergent was washed out three times with cold PBS and unspecific protein binding was blocked with a solution of 1% BSA, 0.3 M glycine, 0.1% Tween 20 in PBS for 30 min at 37°C. The samples were incubated with primary anti-NE (Santa Cruz Biotechnology), anti-myeloperoxidase (Abcam), anti-histone H4 (Abcam), or anti-citrulline (Abcam) antibodies diluted 1:100 in 1% BSA, 0.1%Tween 20 in PBS during 1 h at room temperature. The cells were gently washed with cold PBS and incubated with secondary anti-mouse IgG-FITC (Sigma) or anti-rabit IgG-TRITC (Zymax) antibodies diluted 1:50 in the same solution that primary antibody for 1 h at room temperature in darkness. The cells were then washed with PBS and stained with 5 μg/mL DAPI. The coverslips were mounted with Fluoroshield (Sigma) before observation in a fluorescence microscope (Olympus BX51).

Scanning Electron Microscopy

For scanning electron microscopy, neutrophils (3×10^5) were co-cultured with *E. histolytica* trophozoites (1.5×10^4) in RPMI medium on cover glass previously coated with poly-lysine. After 4 h of incubation, samples were fixed with 2.5% glutaraldehyde, washed with PBS and dehydrated by increasing concentrations of ethanol. Samples were air dried and coated with gold using Fine Coat Ion Sputter before analysis in an electron microscope Jeol JSM-7600F.

Apoptosis and Necrosis Detection

DNA Fragmentation Assay

DNA integrity assay was performed by incubating neutrophils under different conditions. Neutrophils were stimulated with 20 nM PMA or 10 μM A23187 or *E. histolytica* trophozoites at 37°C for 1 h to induce NETosis. Necrosis, and in a lesser extent apoptosis, were induced by culturing neutrophils at 56°C for 1 h. The samples were centrifuged at 7,000 rpm during 5 min, the pellets were resuspended in 20 μL of lysis buffer (2 mM EDTA, 100 mM Tris-HCl, 0.8% SDS, pH 8.0) and 10 μL of 20 mg/mL proteinase K was added. Samples were incubated during 1.5 h at 56°C and mixed with DNA loading buffer. Finally, the samples were run in 1.5% agarose gel and stained with ethidium bromide for visualization.

Annexin V Assay

Phosphatidylserine exposure was tested by FITC Annexin V Apoptosis Detection Kit I (Beckton Dickinson). In brief, necrotic cells (and in a lesser extent apoptotic cells) obtained after heat-treatment or NETotic cells obtained with PMA, A23187 or amoebas, as described above, were washed with PBS and then resuspended in binding buffer at a concentration of 1×10^7 cells/mL. A total of 100 μL from the cell suspension were transferred to a new tube, and added with 5 μL of FITC annexin V. After gently vortexing, samples were incubated in darkness for 15 min at room temperature and observed by fluorescence microscopy. A total of 300 cells were counted to determine the percentage of apoptotic cells in the samples.

ROS Measurement

ROS generation was determined by flow cytometry using 2′,7′-dichlorodihydrofluorescein (H_2DCFDA). In brief, 1×10^6 neutrophils were pre-incubated with 10 μM H_2DCFDA (Sigma) for 30 min at 37°C and washed three times with PBS. Cells were resuspended in 1 mL of PBS, stimulated with 5×10^4 *E. histolytica* trophozoites or 20 nM PMA (positive control for ROS production) and incubated at 37°C. Cultures were fixed with 4% formaldehyde at 0 or 1 h. Finally, the 2′7′-dichlorofluorescein (DCF) fluorescence was measured using a FACScalibur cytometer. At least 1×10^4 gated events of each sample were analyzed. Not stained and stained but not-stimulated cells were used as autofluorescence and negative controls, respectively.

Amplification of Nuclear and Mitochondrial Genes From NETs

Obtaining of NET Solution

To obtain NETs solution, neutrophils (1×10^6) were co-cultured with *E. histolytica* trophozoites (5×10^5) in serum-free RPMI for 15 min. Supernatants were collected after centrifugation at 4,000 rpm for 2 min three times to eliminate residual cells. DNA concentration was measured with NanoDrop 2000.

Neutrophil DNA Isolation

Neutrophils (4×10^6) were lysed in 400 μl lysis buffer containing 1% SDS, 50 mM Tris–HCl at pH 8, 100 mM EDTA and 200 μg/ml proteinase K at 56 °C for 2 h. After addition of 125 μl of 5M NaCl solution, DNA was precipitated adding ice-cold isopropanol, re-suspended in 100 μL nuclease-free water, and extracted with phenol-chloroform-isoamyl alcohol (25:24:1). DNA was precipitated from aqueous fraction adding 0.25 M sodium acetate (pH 5.2) and absolute ethanol. After a final wash with ice-cold 70% ethanol, DNA was resuspended in water (Cotter and Muruve, 2006) and the concentration determined in NanoDrop 2000 (Thermo-Fisher).

Trophozoite DNA Isolation

DNA from *E. histolytica* trophozoites was obtained as described elsewhere (Bhattacharya et al., 1988). Trophozoites from 72 h cultures were harvested by centrifugation and resuspended in 5 mL of NET Buffer containing 100 mM NaCl, 10 mM EDTA, 10 mM Tris, pH 8, and lysed with 0.2% SDS. DNA from suspension was extracted with phenol–chloroform (25:24) and precipitated with absolute ethanol. The precipitated DNA was dissolved in TNE Buffer containing 10 mM NaC1, 1 mM EDTA, 10 mM Tris, pH 8, treated with proteinase K at 37°C for 45 min, and extracted again with phenol-chloroform. After ethanol precipitation, the DNA was dissolved in TNE Buffer and its concentration was measured in NanoDrop 2000.

PCR Conditions

PCR was perform using HotStarTaq® Plus Master Mix Kit (Qiagen) according to the manufacturer instruction. The primers used were as previously designed by Yousefi et al. (2009). For (I) amplification of mitochondrial genes: ATP synthase subunit 6 (*atp6*) (5′-ATACACAACACTAAA GGACGAACCT-3′ and 5′-GAGGCTTACTAGAAGTGT GAAAACG-3′), cytochrome oxidase c subunit 1 (*co1*) (5′-GGAGTCCTAGGCACAGCTCTAA-3′ and 5′-GGAGGGTAG ACTGTTCAACCTG-3′), NADH dehydrogenase subunit 1 (*nd1*) (5′-GCATTCCTAATGCTTACCGAAC-3′ and 5′-AAG GGTGGAGAGGTTAAAGGAG-3′), cytochrome oxidase b (*cyb*) (5′-CTAGCAGCACTCCACCTCCTAT-3′ and 5′-GTTGTCCTC CGATTCAGGTTAG-3′); (II) amplification of nuclear genes: glyceraldehyde phosphate dehydrogenase (*gapdh*) (5′-CCCCTT CATTGACCTCAACTAC-3′ and 5′-GAGTCCTTCCACGAT ACCAAAG-3′), β-actine (*actb*) (5′-ATCTGGCACCACACC TTCTACAATGAGCTGCG-3′ and 5′-CGTCATACTCCTGCT TGCTGATCCACATCTGC-3′), and FAS receptor (*fas*) (5′-TCA CCACTATTGCTGGAGTCAT-3′ and 5′-TAAACATCCTTG GAGGCAGAAT-3′). PCR protocol included 30 cycles with an alignment temperature of 55°C for all primer pairs used. The PCR products were run in 1% agarose gels and stained with ethidium bromide for visualization.

Statistics

Statistical significance was tested with paired two-tailed Student's t-test. Data are reported as mean ± SD. A p-value ≤ 0.05 was considered statistically significant.

RESULTS

Characterization of NETs Induced by *E. histolytica* Trophozoites

Detection of NETs Components

DNA release during neutrophil/amoeba co-culturing has been reported previously (Ávila et al., 2016). Here, these structures were characterized to determine that they were effectively NETs. Neutrophils and amoebas were co-cultured in a proportion of 20:1, respectively, in RPMI medium supplemented with FBS 5% during 4 h. After this period, unstimulated neutrophils showed a cytoplasmic localization of NE and MPO, meanwhile, histone H4 co-localized with DNA as expected (**Figure 1A**). In contrast, in the neutrophil/amoeba co-culture, DNA extracellular fiber were detected by DAPI staining and these structures co-localized with proteins associated with NETs such as NE, MPO and histone H4 (**Figure 1B**). Similar structures were appreciated in neutrophils stimulated with 20 nM PMA, a well-characterized NETosis inductor (**Figure 1C**). Interestingly, while histone H4 showed a regular distribution along DNA filaments, NE and MPO were detected as immunostained spots only partially co-localized with DNA. Trophozoites were not stained with anti-NE or anti-MPO antibodies and the anti-histone H4 antibody showed a nuclear localization as expected (data not shown).

Scanning Electron Microscopy of NETs

NETs were analyzed by scanning electron microscopy to observe interaction of trophozoites with extracellular DNA. Non-stimulated neutrophils were visualized as adherent spherical cells with an irregular surface (**Figure 2A**), while trophozoites were detected as pleomorphic cells (**Figure 2B**). After neutrophil–amoeba interaction, trophozoites appeared embedded in the extracellular material (NETs) forming clusters and surrounded by fiber-like structures in close contact with amoebas (**Figures 2C–D**). None-intact neutrophils were visualized in this condition suggesting that all neutrophils undergo NETosis.

Trophozoites Induce NETosis and no Other Forms of Cell Death

In order to discard other forms of cell death during neutrophil–amoeba interaction, the nuclear morphology at the moments before DNA extrusion was analyzed. Non-stimulated neutrophils showed characteristic condensed-multilobular nuclei (**Figure 3A**), while PMA-treated neutrophils presented decondensed chromatin with loss of multilobular morphology associated to the NETosis process. During neutrophil–amoeba interaction, neutrophils also presented decondensed nuclei before DNA release suggesting NETosis process (**Figure 3A**). To confirm these observations, DNA from neutrophils treated with PMA, A23187, exposed to amoebas or subject to heat was run in agarose gels to verify its integrity. DNA from control neutrophils as well as neutrophils treated with PMA, A23187 or amoebas showed no fragmented DNA (**Figure 3B**), whereas smeared DNA was seen with heat-treated neutrophils. PMA-treated neutrophils, but above all, heat-treated neutrophils showed an increase in phosphatidylserine exposition respect to control

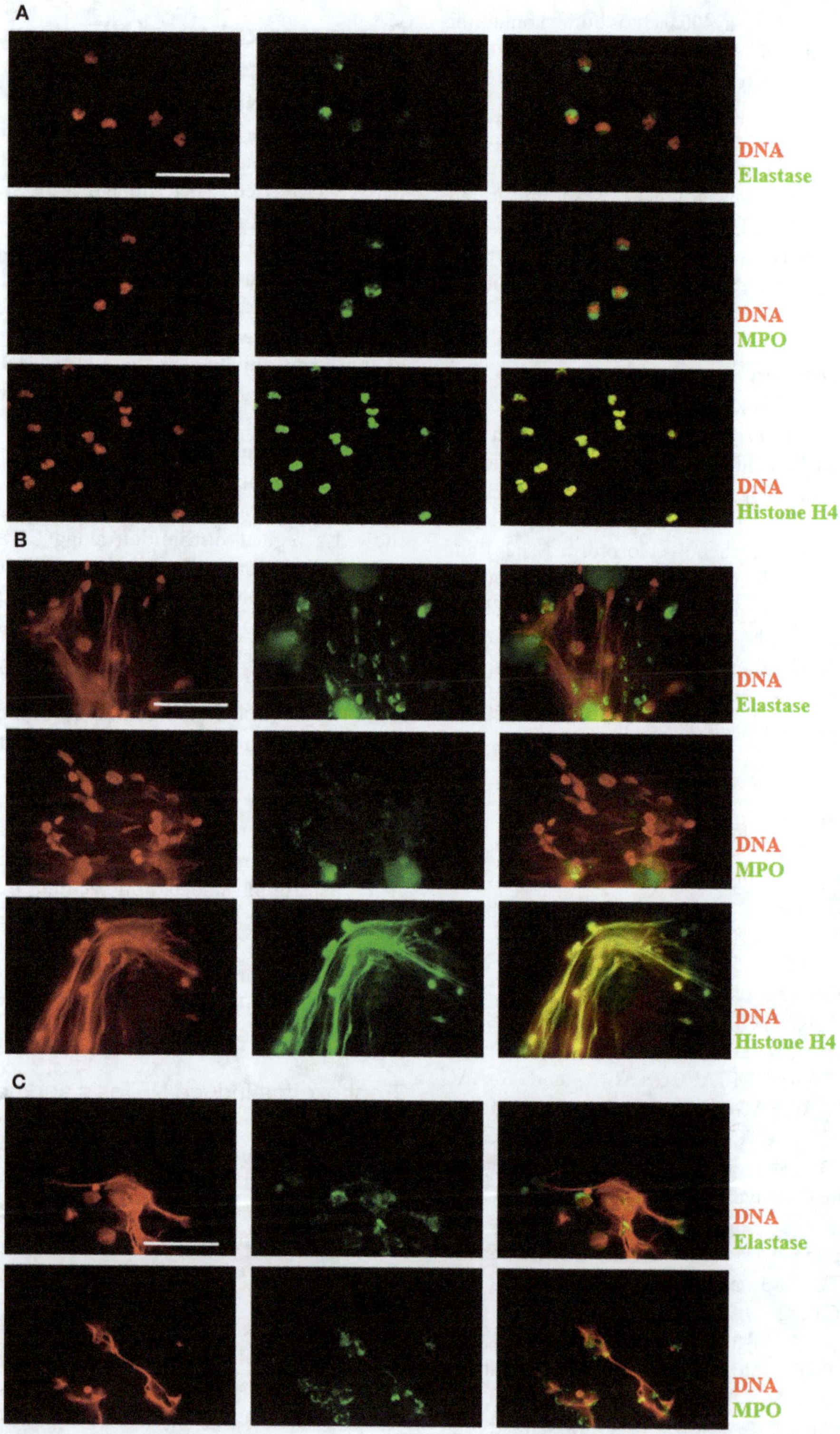

FIGURE 1 | Characterization of components in NETs induced by *E. histolytica* trophozoites. Human neutrophils (2×10^5) were cultured in absence of stimuli **(A)** or stimulated with 1×10^4 trophozoites **(B)** or 20 nM PMA **(C)** in RPMI medium during 4 h at 37°C. Cells were fixed and immunofluorescence was performed using anti-neutrophil elastase (NE), anti-myeloperoxidase (MPO) or anti-histone H4 antibodies followed by anti-mouse IgG conjugated to FITC (for NE and MPO) or anti-rabbit IgG conjugated to TRITC (for histone H4). DNA was stained with DAPI. Images were taken at 100x magnification. Scale bar 50 μm.

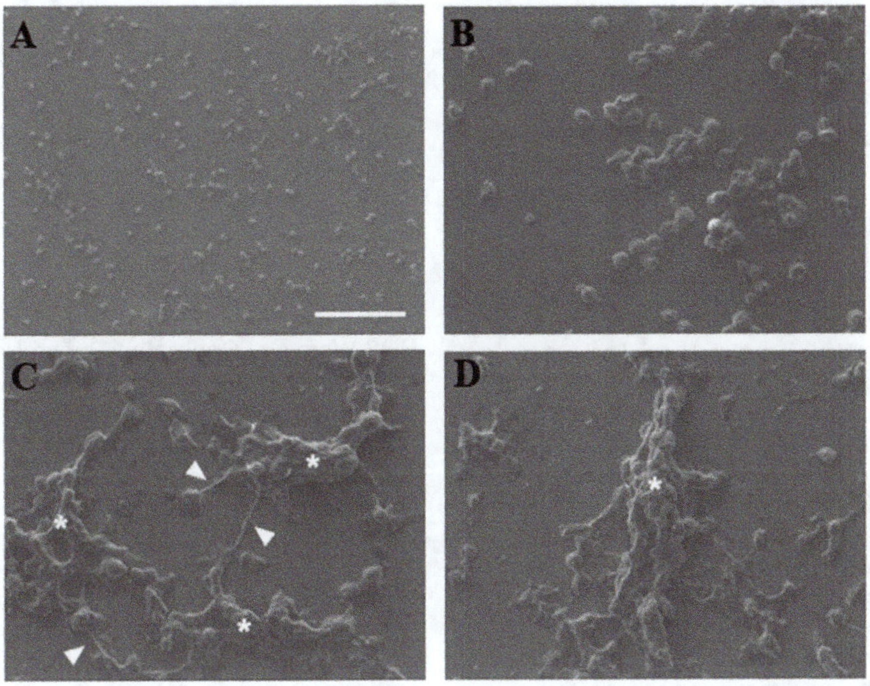

FIGURE 2 | Scanning electron microscopy of NETs induced by amoebas. **(A)** Neutrophils, **(B)** trophozoites, or **(C,D)** co-cultured neutrophils-amoebas (ratio 20:1) were incubated during 4 h at 37°C. Posteriorly, cells were fixed, dehydrated, air dried, and coated with gold. Fibrillar structures (arrowhead) and clusters of amoebas trapped in the fibrillar material (asterisks) are shown. Images were taken at 250x magnification. Scale bar 100 μm.

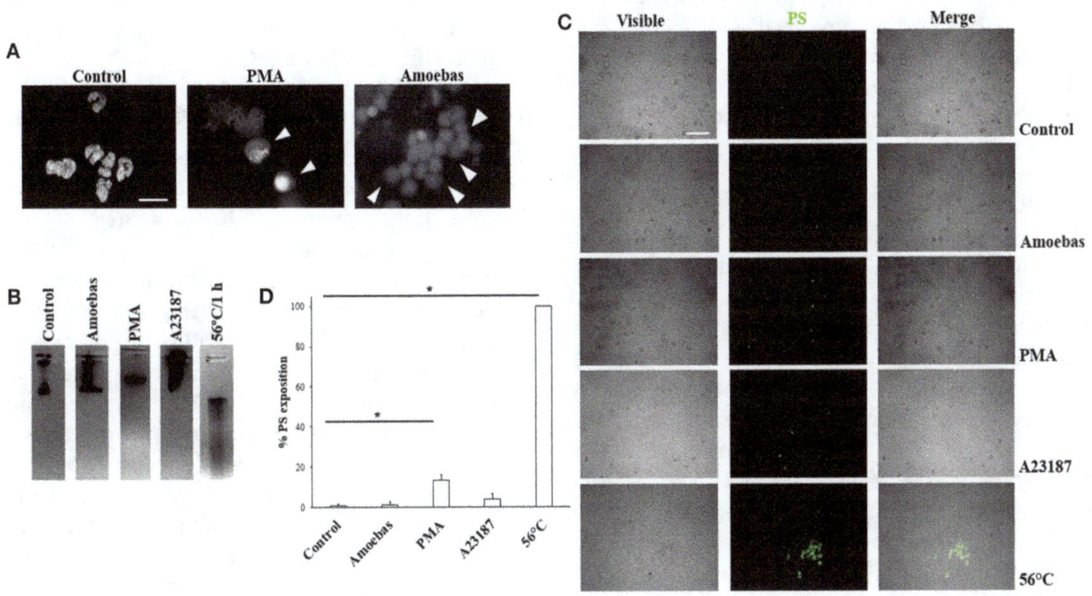

FIGURE 3 | Trophozoites induces NETosis without evidence of apoptosis or necrosis. **(A)** Neutrophils were incubated with 20 nM PMA or trophozoites (ratio 20:1). After 4 h of incubation, cells were fixed and stained with DAPI. Decondensed chromatin is shown (arrowheads). Images were taken at 100x magnification. Scale bar 10 μm. **(B)** DNA from neutrophils (1×10^6) treated for 1 h with trophozoites (5×10^4) or 20 nM PMA or 10 μM A23187 or heat (50°C) were extracted and run in 1.8% agarose gel and the bands visualized by staining with ethidium bromide. **(C)** Phosphatidylserine (PS) exposition was assessed by fluorescence microscopy using FITC-annexin V. **(D)** Percentage of cells positive to PS was determined in a total of 300 stained neutrophils. Values are means ± SD of three independent experiments. $^*p < 0.001$.

(**Figures 3C,D**); meanwhile, A23187 and amoebas did not show phosphatidylserine exposition.

NETosis Occurs Rapidly and Depends on the Viability of Amoebas

Previously, we demonstrated in a qualitative manner that *E. histolytica* trophozoites induce a rapid NETs release (Ávila et al., 2016); here, these results were verified quantitatively. We show that neutrophils extruded DNA evidently after 25 min of interaction with amoebas (**Figure 4A**) and the amounts of expelled DNA increased in the time-course of following 4 h (**Figure 4B**). PMA-treated neutrophils underwent NETosis after 1 h of stimulation and control-neutrophils did not release DNA in our experiments. These data were confirmed by fluorescence microscopy: control neutrophils were observed with multilobular and condensed nuclei (**Figure 4C**, panel i), PMA-treated neutrophils showed decondensed chromatin and extracellular DNA fibers (**Figure 4C**, panel ii), whereas in neutrophil-amoebas co-cultures, scarce intact neutrophils were observed and the trophozoites appeared surrounded by extracellular DNA fibers (**Figure 4C**, panels iii–vi).

Fixed amoebas have been reported to be unable to induce NETosis after 1 h of interaction with neutrophils (Ávila et al., 2016). Because some stimuli take more than 1 h to induce this phenomenon, NETs amounts were determined after 4 h of stimulation with either PMA, viable trophozoites or formaldehyde-fixed or heat-inactivated amoebas. As described before, PMA-treated neutrophils and neutrophils co-cultured with viable trophozoites extruded DNA (**Figures 5A,B**, panels iii and iv), but heat-inactivated or formaldehyde-fixed trophozoites failed to induce NETs after the same incubation period even when they were in close contact with neutrophils (**Figures 5A,B**, panels v and vi). These data suggest that the surface molecules present on the trophozoites are not the unique stimuli necessary to induce NETosis.

NETs Contain Both Nuclear and Mitochondrial DNA

Previous studies show that DNA from NETs can have either nuclear or mitochondrial origin, or both, depending on stimuli used (Yousefi et al., 2009). Here, we assessed the origin of DNA from NETs amplifying three nuclear and four mitochondrial neutrophil genes. As expected, all amplicons were obtained from neutrophil DNA while no amplicons were obtained from purified *E. histolytica* DNA (**Figure 6A**) indicating that trophozoite DNA co-purified from NETs does not contribute to the amplification. The presence of both nuclear and mtDNA was detected from supernatant of amoebas-neutrophils co-cultured for 15 min (**Figure 6B**). No amplification was obtained using supernatant from PMN cultured alone for 4 h (**Figure 6C**).

Dependence of NETosis Process of ROS Generation

NETs Were Generated Independently of NOX2-Derived ROS

To establish the mechanisms involved in the induction of NETs by amoebas, we determined the dependency of this process on NOX2-derived ROS production using apocynin as inhibitor of NOX2 activity (the widely used NOX2 inhibitor DPI caused amoebas death; data not shown). As expected, apocynin (200 μM) inhibited NETosis pretended with PMA treatment for 4 h showing that the mechanism of PMA-induced NETosis depends on ROS production. However, apocynin treatment did not decrease DNA release induced by trophozoites indicating that trophozoite-induced NETosis is independent of ROS production by NOX2 (**Figure 7A**). Apocynin treatment did not lead to morphological alterations in control neutrophils as well as did not affect NETs amount visualized by microscopy in neutrophils stimulated with trophozoites (**Figure 7B**).

ROS Were Not Generated During Neutrophil–Amoeba Interaction

ROS generation has been previously linked to the defense against *E. histolytica* (Denis and Chadee, 1989). For this reason, assuming that NETosis induced by this parasite was independent of NOX2-derived ROS, the production of ROS from this source was investigated during neutrophil–amoeba interaction by flow cytometry. Population corresponded to neutrophils was selected by flow cytometry according to size and granularity features (**Figure 8A**). Negative region M1 was defined as covering the 98% events in the absence of stimuli; positive region M2 was defined as all values superior to M1.

Basal DCF fluorescence levels were detected in PMA-stimulated neutrophils at 0 h but these increased significantly after 1 h of stimulation indicating ROS generation (**Figures 8B,D**). On the other hand, no significant differences were observed in neutrophils co-cultured with trophozoites after 1 h as compared to the starting time point suggesting that ROS production did not take place during interaction of neutrophils with the parasite (**Figures 8C,D**).

Requirements for Neutrophil Elastase During NET Formation

NE Is Translocated to Nucleus During NETosis

Nuclear translocation of NE is a step of NETosis that has been proposed to require ROS production by NOX2 (Papayannopoulos et al., 2010). This concept was explored in our model even though amoeba-induced NETosis resulted independent of NOX2-derived ROS. By immunofluorescence, control neutrophils showed multilobular nuclei and NE was localized to cytoplasm, as expected (**Figure 9**), while 20 nM PMA treatment caused NE migration to nucleus after 1 h of stimulation and before DNA decondensation (**Figure 9**). In both cases, a NE remnant was also detected in cytoplasm. Surprisingly, neutrophils co-cultured with trophozoites also presented co-localization of the enzyme with chromatin with patterns of irregular distribution in pre-NETotic nuclei after 15 min of interaction (**Figure 9**). These results indicate that NE translocation to the nucleus can take place independently of ROS generation by NOX2 during NETosis induced by trophozoites.

Serine-Protease Inhibition Results in Reduction of NET Release

NE is a serine-protease that decondense chromatin after its translocation to nucleus in the process of NETosis

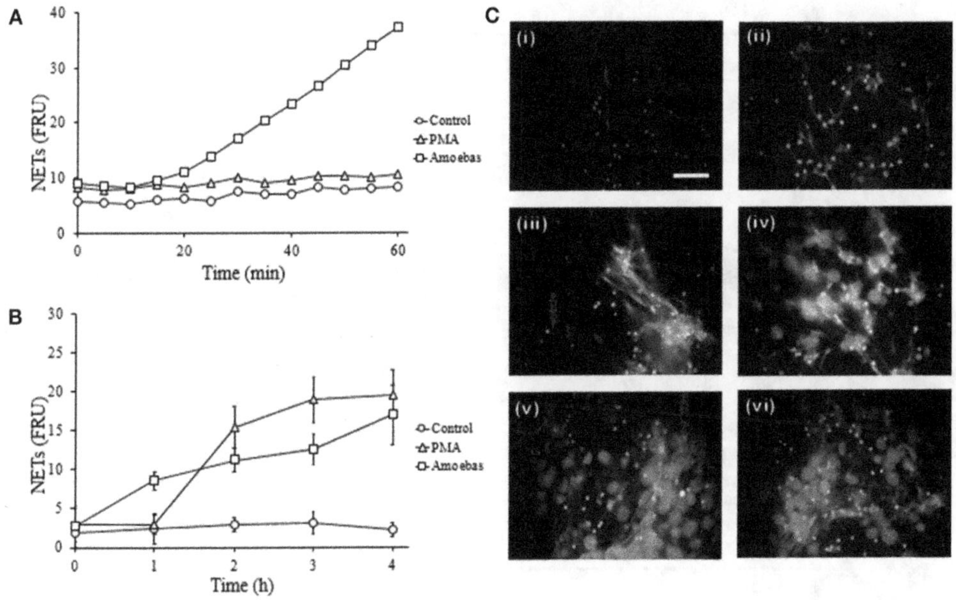

FIGURE 4 | *E. histolytica* trophozoites induces a rapid NETosis process. **(A)** Neutrophils (1×10^5) were co-culture with trophozoites (5×10^3) in RPMI medium added with 500 nM SYTOX Green and fluorescence values were measured every 5 min during 1 h. **(B)** Neutrophils (3×10^5) were co-cultured with trophozoites (1.5×10^4) in RPMI medium for the indicated times; supernatants were collected, mixed 1:1 with 500 nM SYTOX Green and the fluorescence measured. In **(A,B)** 20 nM PMA was used as positive control of NETosis, NETs amount is expressed in fluorescence relative units (FRU) and values are means ± SD of three independent experiments in triplicate. **(C)** Neutrophils were stimulated with 20 nM PMA (4 h) or amoebas (ratio 20:1) during 1, 2, 3, and 4 h and the cells fixed and stained with DAPI. Control neutrophils (i), neutrophils treated with PMA (ii), neutrophils co-cultured with amoebas for 1 h (iii), 2 h (iv), 3 h (v), and 4 h (vi). Images were taken at 60x magnification. Scale bar 50 μm.

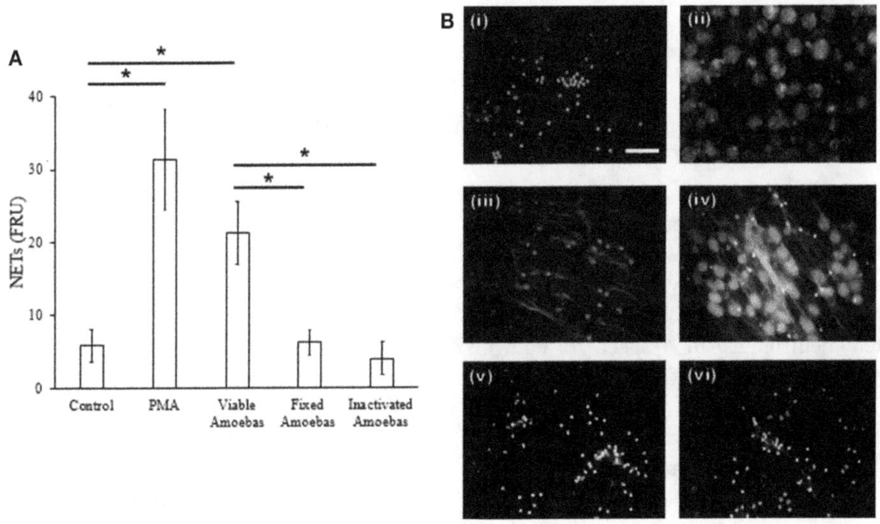

FIGURE 5 | NET release depends on amoeba viability. **(A)** Neutrophils (3×10^5) were co-cultured with viable, formaldehyde-fixed or heat-inactivated trophozoites (1.5×10^4) in RPMI medium for 4 h. PMA at 20 nM was used as positive control of NETosis. Supernatants were collected, mixed 1:1 with SYTOX Green (500 nM) and fluorescence was measured. NETs amount is expressed in fluorescence relative units (FRU). Values are means ± SD of three independent experiments in triplicate. $^*p < 0.001$. **(B)** Neutrophils were stimulated with 20 nM PMA or viable or non-viable amoebas (ratio 20:1) during 4 h; cells were fixed and staining with DAPI. Control neutrophils (i), control amoebas (ii), neutrophils treated with PMA (iii), neutrophils co-cultured with viable (iv), fixed (v), or heat-inactivated amoebas (vi). Images were taken at 60x magnification. Scale bar 50 μm.

(Papayannopoulos et al., 2010). To study the role of NE in NETosis induced by *E. histolytica* trophozoites, 1 mM phenylmethylsulfonyl fluoride (PMSF) was used to inhibit its activity in neutrophils. Serine protease inhibition caused a statistically significant decrease in NET amounts released by neutrophils stimulated with 20 nM PMA or *E. histolytica*

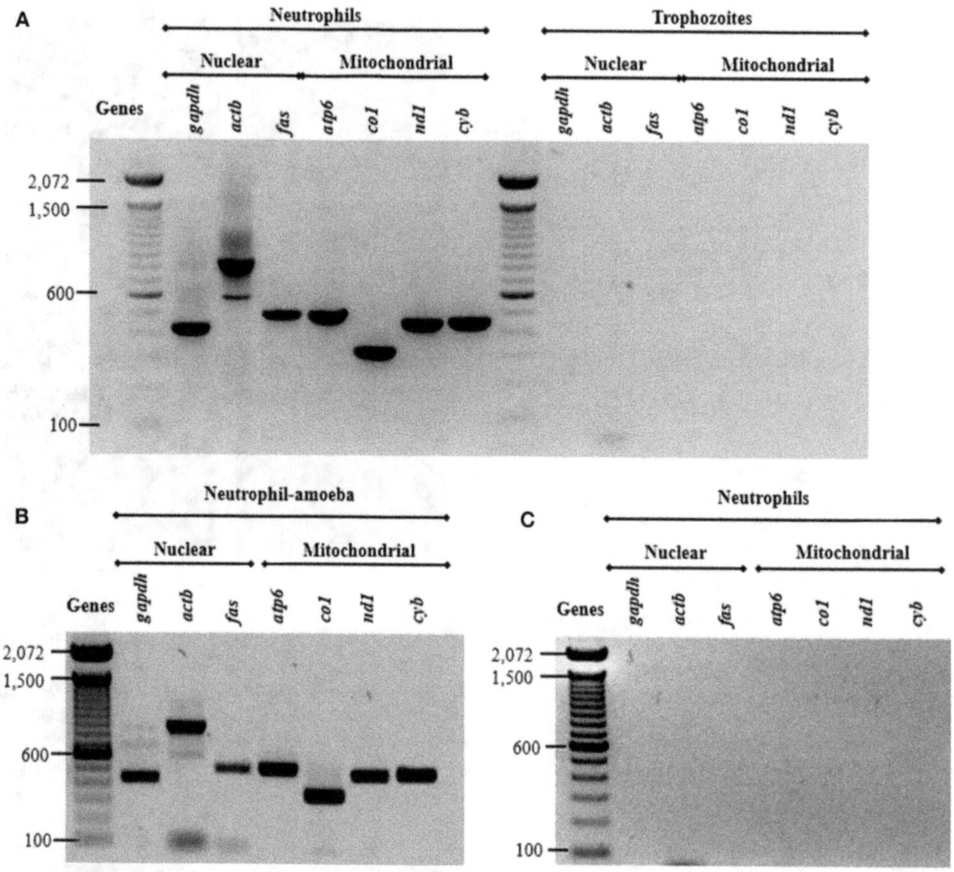

FIGURE 6 | Both nuclear and mitochondrial DNA composes NETs induced by *E. histolytica* trophozoites. **(A)** DNA from neutrophils and trophozoites were extracted and PCR was performed to amplify three nuclear (*gapdh, actb,* and *fas*) and four mitochondrial (*atp6, co1, nd1,* and *cyb*) genes. Supernatant from **(B)** neutrophil (1×10^6)-trophozoites (5×10^4) co-cultures or **(C)** from neutrophils without any stimulus were directly used as template for PCR reactions to amplify the nuclear and mitochondrial genes. PCR amplicons were run 1% agarose gels and stained with ethidium bromide for visualization.

trophozoites (**Figure 10A**). In these experiments, PMSF did not affect cell viability (data not shown). The result was confirmed under fluorescence microscopy showing that PMSF reduced the numbers of extracellular DNA fibers in PMA- or trophozoites-treated neutrophils in respect to controls. Additionally, major numbers of non-NETotic cells were noted when neutrophils were pre-treated with PMSF (**Figure 10B**). These results suggest that a serine-protease, probably NE, is required to induce NET release in neutrophils co-cultured with trophozoites.

Role of PAD4 in Netosis Induced by Amoebas

Extracellular Calcium Is Required for NETosis

Extracellular calcium influx required for PAD4 activation was considered to be linked to NETosis processes independent of NOX2-derived ROS (Konig and Andrade, 2016). Therefore, herein calcium was chelated from the medium by adding 20 mM EGTA before neutrophil stimulation with 20 nM PMA or trophozoites. EGTA treatment did not affect cell viability of both neutrophils and amoebas (data not shown). EGTA addition reduced significantly DNA extrusion by neutrophils after stimulation with *E. histolytica* trophozoites; however, NETosis induced by PMA was also reduced (**Figure 11A**). This result was corroborated by fluorescence microscopy showing that extracellular DNA fibers were less abundant with respect to controls in PMA- or amoeba-treated neutrophils when calcium was previously chelated (**Figure 11B**). These data suggest that NETosis induced by amoeba is dependent on extracellular calcium, which appears to be required for NETosis process independently of requirements for PAD4 activity as PMA-induced NETosis do not depend on PAD4.

PAD4 Inhibition Do Not Affect NET Release

Extracellular calcium dependent-NETosis has been associated to DNA decondensation by PAD4 activity (Douda et al., 2015). In order to explore the participation of PAD4 in NETosis induced by *E. histolytica* trophozoites, GSK484 was used to inhibit its activity. Neutrophils treated with 10 μM GSK484 were able to form NETs after stimulation with PMA; on the other hand, neutrophils stimulated with the calcium ionophore A23187, a known

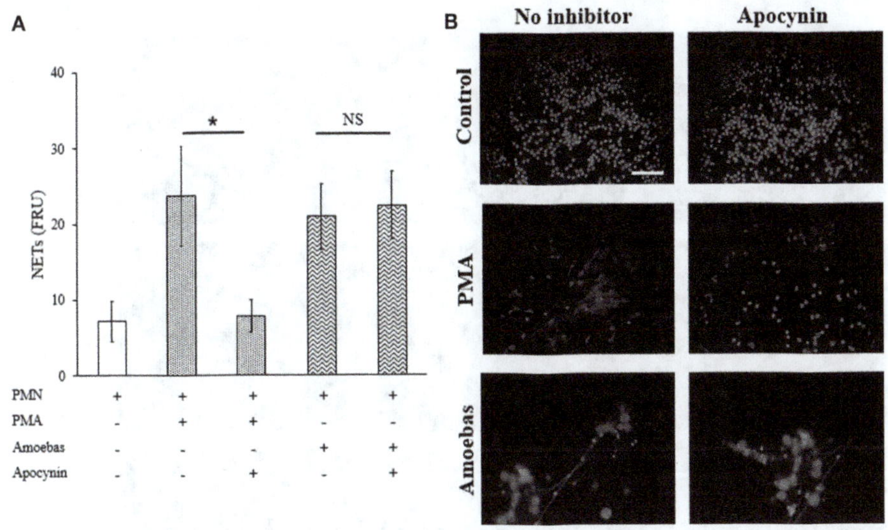

FIGURE 7 | NETosis induced by trophozoites is independent of NOX2-derived ROS. **(A)** Neutrophils (3×10^5) were pre-incubated with 200 μM apocynin or DMSO for 30 min and then stimulated with 20 nM PMA or co-cultured with trophozoites (1.5×10^4) during 4 h. Supernatants were collected, mixed 1:1 with SYTOX Green (500 nM) and fluorescence was measured. NETs amount is expressed in fluorescence relative units (FRU). Values are means ± SD of three independent experiments in triplicate. *$p < 0.001$; NS: statistically non-significant. **(B)** Neutrophils were treated as describe previously, cells were fixed and stained with DAPI. Images were taken at 60x magnification. Scale bar 50 μm.

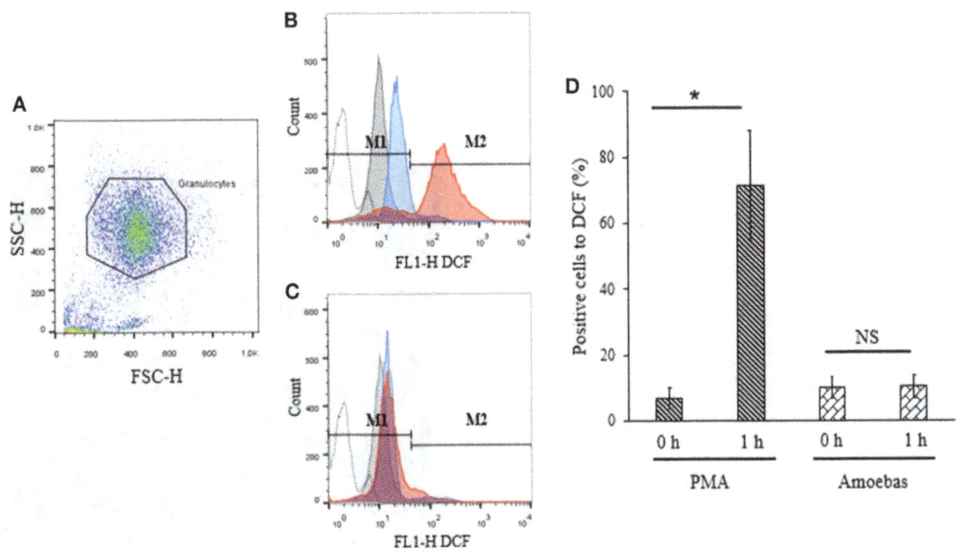

FIGURE 8 | ROS were not detected during neutrophil–amoeba interaction. Neutrophils (1×10^6) were pre-incubated with 10 μM H_2DCFDA for 30 min and stimulated with 5×10^4 trophozoites or 20 nM PMA for 1 h. DCF fluorescence was measured using a FACScalibur cytometer. **(A)** Neutrophils population selected for analysis. **(B)** Histogram of neutrophils stimulated with PMA. **(C)** Histogram of neutrophils co-cultured with trophozoites. M1 negative region (cells with low fluorescence); M2 positive region (cells with high fluorescence). Histograms: dotted, autofluorescence; gray, non-stimulated; blue, stimulated 0 h; red, stimulated 1 h. **(D)** Percentage of positive cells to DCF respect to the control. Values are means ± SD of three independent experiments. *$p < 0.001$. NS, statistically non-significant.

inducer of PAD4-dependent NETosis, decreased NET release when neutrophils were pre-treated with GSK484 (**Figure 12A**). Surprisingly, neutrophils pre-treated with PAD4 inhibitor and co-cultured with amoebas retained their capacity to form NETs (**Figure 12A**). As seen by fluorescence microscopy, GSK484 did not affect the morphology of neutrophils in respect to controls, and no differences were detected in the release of NETs between neutrophils treated or not with the inhibitor after stimulation with PMA (**Figure 12B**). In a similar way, PAD4 inhibition did not affect NET release in neutrophils co-cultured with trophozoites; however, neutrophils pre-treated with GSK484 formed less NETs upon stimulation with A23187 (**Figure 12B**).

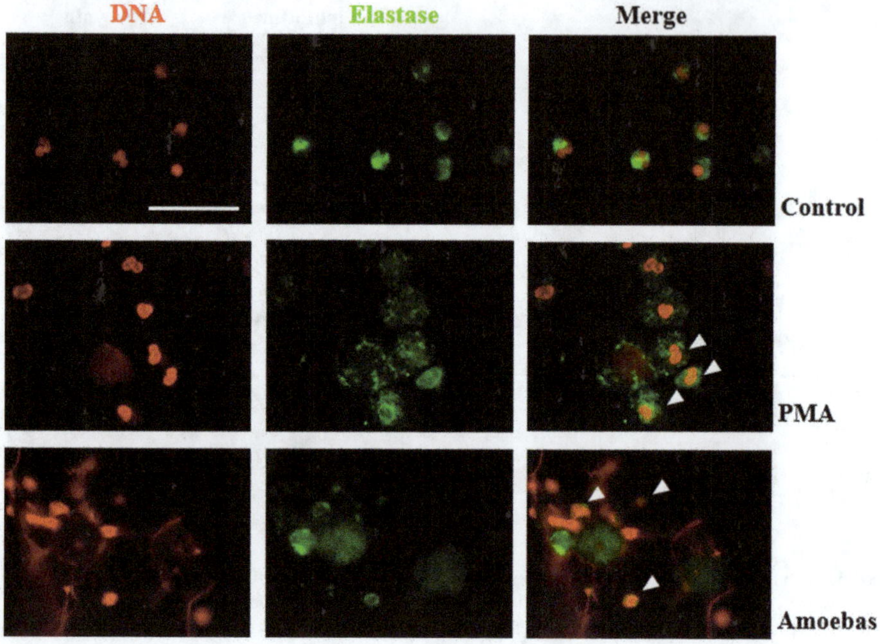

FIGURE 9 | Neutrophil elastase (NE) translocation to the nucleus take place during NETosis induced by trophozoites. Non-stimulated neutrophil (2×10^5) and neutrophils stimulated by 20 nM PMA or co-culture with 1×10^4 trophozoites during 4 h were fixed and immunofluorescence performed using anti-NE antibody and anti-mouse IgG conjugated to FITC. DNA was staining with DAPI. Arrowheads indicate nuclear localization of NE. Images were taken at 100x magnification. Scale bar 50 μm.

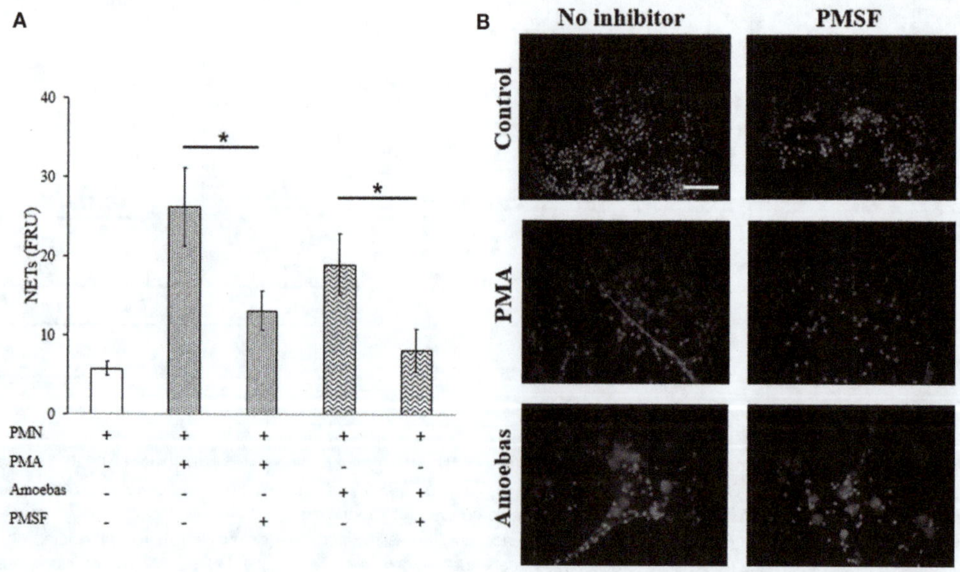

FIGURE 10 | Serine protease activity is required for NETosis induce by *E. histolytica* trophozoites. **(A)** Neutrophils (3×10^5) were pre-incubated with 1 mM PMSF or DMSO for 30 min and then stimulated with 20 nM PMA or co-cultured with trophozoites (1.5×10^4) during 4 h. Supernatants were collected, mixed 1:1 with SYTOX Green (500 nM) and fluorescence was measured. NETs amount is expressed in fluorescence relative units (FRU). Values are means ±SD of three independent experiments in triplicate. $^*p < 0.001$. **(B)** Neutrophils were treated as describe previously, fixed and stained with DAPI. Images were taken at 60x magnification. Scale bar 50 μm.

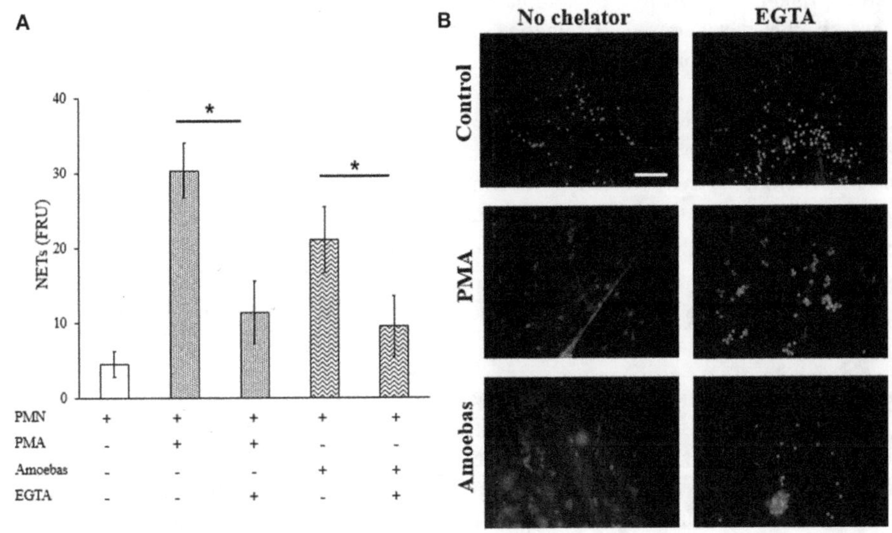

FIGURE 11 | NETosis induced by *E. histolytica* trophozoites require the presence of extracellular calcium. **(A)** Neutrophils (3×10^5) were culture in the presence or absence of 20 mM EGTA. EGTA-treated neutrophils were stimulated with 20 nM PMA or co-cultured with trophozoites (1.5×10^4) during 4 h. Supernatants were collected, mixed 1:1 with SYTOX Green (500 nM) and fluorescence was measured. NETs amount is expressed in fluorescence relative units (FRU). Values are means ± SD of three independent experiments in triplicate. $^*p < 0.001$. **(B)** Neutrophils were treated as describe previously, fixed and stained with DAPI. Images were taken at 60x magnification. Scale bar 50 μm.

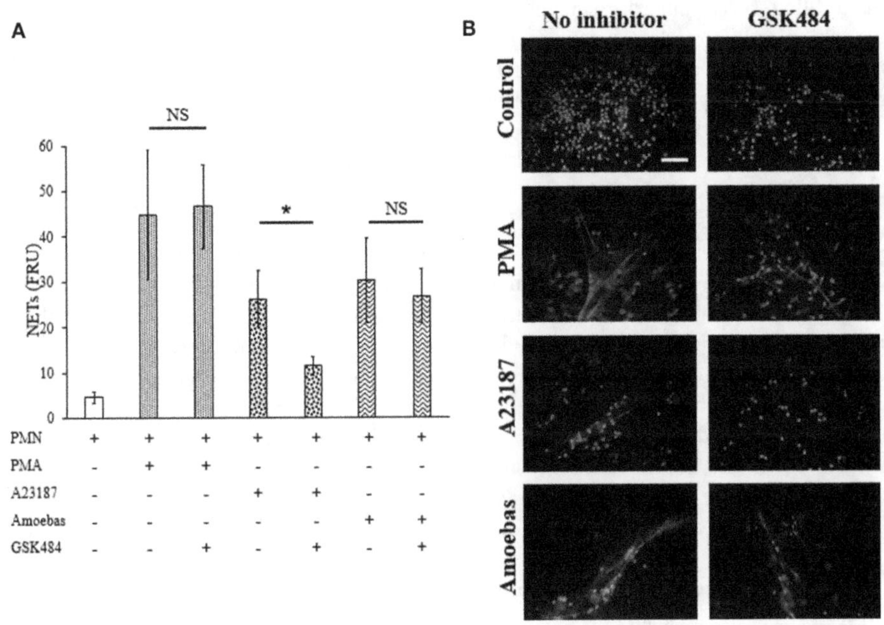

FIGURE 12 | NETosis induced by *E. histolytica* trophozoites is independent of PAD4 activity. **(A)** Neutrophils (3×10^5) were pre-incubated with 10 μM GSK484 or DMSO for 30 min and then stimulated with 20 nM PMA, 10 μM A23187, or co-cultured with trophozoites (1.5×10^4) during 4 h. Supernatants were collected, mixed 1:1 with SYTOX Green (500 nM) and fluorescence was measured. NETs amount is expressed in fluorescence relative units (FRU). Values are means ±SD of three independent experiments in triplicate. $^*p < 0.001$. NS: statistically non-significant. **(B)** Neutrophils were treated as describe previously, fixed and stained with DAPI. Images were taken at 60x magnification. Scale bar 50 μm.

Detection of Citrullinated Proteins

Citrullinated proteins are considered as markers of PAD4-mediated NETosis (Wang et al., 2009). Here we assayed if NETosis induced by trophozoites generated citrullination of neutrophil proteins even though PAD4 activity was not required for NETosis process. Control and PMA-treated neutrophils showed few citrullinated proteins, principally in cytoplasm, and were less frequent in the decondensed chromatin of PMA-induced neutrophils (**Figure 13**). Conversely, citrullinated proteins were abundant in NETs induced by A23187 or *E. histolytica* trophozoites, co-localizing with extruded DNA in both cases. Interestingly, citrullinated proteins were detected in a spot pattern similar to the observed during the detection of NE in NETs induced by trophozoites. These results suggest that protein citrullination take place in the NETosis triggered by amoeba.

DISCUSSION

NETosis is a relatively new mechanism of innate immunity that has been linked to the defense against different pathogens including bacteria, fungi and protozoa by killing or inhibiting their growth, preventing their spread and contributing to the establishment of a protective immune response against pathogens (Brinkmann et al., 2004; Urban et al., 2006; Guimarães-Costa et al., 2009; Röhm et al., 2014; Halverson et al., 2015; Sousa-Rocha et al., 2015). However, contradictory reports have emerged since the formation of NET seems to depend on the pathogen size, with the large pathogens or aggregates of the small ones being responsible for triggering NETosis, while the small non-aggregated pathogens are targeted by phagocytosis (Branzk et al., 2014). In addition, several microorganisms evade the action of NETs by inhibiting their release, degrading the DNA with nucleases or resisting the anti-microbial effect of the NET-associated proteins through encapsulation (reviewed in Storisteanu et al., 2017). On the other hand, the excessive development of NETs has recently begun to be associated with autoimmune and vasculitic diseases, contributing in general to the pathology of some diseases associated with microbial infections (Yipp and Kubes, 2013). Therefore, the role of NETs in the outcome of most infectious diseases is still unknown and is a matter of intensive studies. Nevertheless, the mechanisms underlying the formation of NETs remain poorly understood.

E. histolytica is a parasite that causes intestinal amoebiasis and, in some cases, amoebic liver abscesses. Very early in both pathologies, neutrophils are rapidly recruited to the site of infection becoming the cell of the innate immunity more prevalent in the lesions. However, the role of neutrophils in the amoebic infection is still not well understood. Studies on the outcome of the interaction of neutrophils with amoeba *in vitro* have shown that priming of these cells with recombinant cytokines IFN-γ and TNF-α make them capable to kill 97% of *E. histolytica* trophozoites in a H_2O_2-dependent manner (Denis and Chadee, 1989). In contrast, non-primed neutrophils suffer apoptosis and/or are highly phagocyted when exposed to virulent *E. histolytica* trophozoites (Sim et al., 2004; Ávila et al., 2016). Likewise, *in vivo*, while some reports confer to neutrophils a protective activity during the infection (Asgharpour et al., 2005), evidence exists that immune cells, including neutrophils, are implicated in tissue damage (Olivos-García et al., 2007). More recently, we have reported that *E. histolytica* trophozoites were capable of inducing NETosis in human neutrophils (Ávila et al., 2016), but the role of this process in amoebiasis and the molecular mechanisms implicated in its formation were not clarified. Herein we study some important characteristics associated to the NETosis process induced by neutrophil–trophozoite interaction.

First, to verify the NETosis occurrence in neutrophils co-cultures with amoebas, the presence of NETs components was tested. Like other reports, NE, MPO and histone H4 (Brinkmann et al., 2004; Kaplan and Radic, 2012) were found co-localized with extracellular DNA released by neutrophils after their interaction with trophozoites. By scanning electron microscopy, NETs were observed as extracellular fibers trapping clusters of amoebas in a similar way observed with other pathogens (Guimarães-Costa et al., 2009; Brinkmann and Zychlinsky, 2012; Della Coletta et al., 2015). Afterwards, we determined that during neutrophil–amoeba interaction the NETosis process took place and no other forms of cell death. As expected, the NETosis inducer PMA caused nuclear decondensation on neutrophils without affecting DNA integrity; however, an increase in the exposition of phosphatidylserine occurred in <20% of the treated neutrophils, which agrees with a report showing that PMA induces phosphatidylserine exposition in neutrophils (Saito et al., 2005). Necrotic and at lesser extent apoptotic neutrophils induced by treatment with heat showed DNA degradation and phosphatidylserine exposition as it has been reported in other cells (Krysko et al., 2004; Li and Zhou, 2016). Different reports indicate that *E. histolytica* trophozoites induce apoptosis in diverse cell types including neutrophils (Seydel and Stanley, 1998; Huston et al., 2000; Sim et al., 2004). However, we show that under our conditions, the interaction of trophozoites with human neutrophils resulted in rapid decondensation of the neutrophil nuclei without phosphatidylserine exposition in their external surfaces or genomic DNA breakdown, followed by DNA release to the extracellular space, indicating that neutrophils undergo NETosis and discarding both apoptosis and necrosis in the presence of amoebas. The result was similar to the effect obtained with the calcium ionophore A23187, another NETosis inductor, which did not affect the integrity of the neutrophils DNA and prevented phosphatidylserine exposition in the external surface. Together, the results suggest at this point that amoebas and the calcium ionophore could share similar NETosis pathways which are different to those of PMA.

The most important component of NETs is the DNA released from the neutrophils. Early studies of NETosis showed that traps were exclusively generated from nuclear DNA (nDNA) (Fuchs et al., 2007). Posteriorly, it was observed that under specific conditions, neutrophils were able to form NETs exclusively from mtDNA without compromise the cell viability (Yousefi et al., 2009). Here, we showed that NETs triggered by *E. histolytica* trophozoites contain both nDNA and mtDNA, as it has been reported using other stimuli as PMA and the nitric oxide donor DETA-NONOate (Keshari et al., 2012). The release of mtDNA during NETosis has been linked to autoimmune pathologies such as eritematous systemic lupus due to its pro-inflammatory properties (Lood et al., 2016). Thus, mtDNA of NETs could cause a positive feedback through TLR9 propitiating that more neutrophils enter to NETosis (Itagaki et al., 2015). In this regard, we can speculate that mtDNA of NETs induced by trophozoites could contribute to the pathogenesis of the

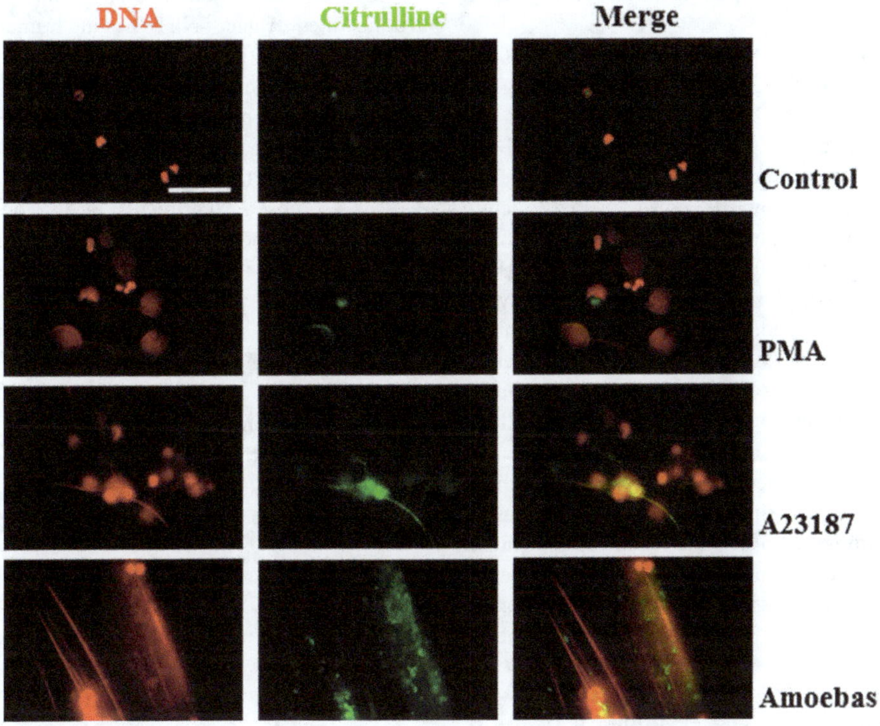

FIGURE 13 | Protein citrullination occurs during NET release induce by *E. histolytica* trophozoites. Non-stimulated neutrophil (2×10^5) and neutrophils stimulated with 20 nM PMA, 10 μM A23187 or co-cultured with 1×10^4 trophozoites during 4 h were fixed and immunofluorescence performed using anti-citrulline antibody and anti-rabbit IgG conjugated to TRITC. DNA was staining with DAPI. Images were taken at 100x magnification. Scale bar 50 μm.

disease promoting inflammation, a well-known feature of the tissular damage caused by *E. histolytica*. However, we cannot rule out that mtDNA could come from neutrophils lysed during the interaction with amoebas. Therefore, further studies using specific mtDNA markers are necessary to confirm that NETs induced by amoebas effectively contain this type of DNA.

Initially, NETosis process was described as a slow mechanism when compared with phagocytosis and degranulation (Fuchs et al., 2007), taking ~2 h since addition of stimulus until DNA release. In contrast, *E. histolytica* trophozoites induced NET release on few minutes after the contact with neutrophils, similarly to other stimuli as ionomicyn, *Staphylococcus aureus* or *Leishmania amanzonensis* promastigotes (Pilsczek et al., 2010; Douda et al., 2015; Rochael et al., 2015). It is worth to mention that these rapid stimuli were shown to induce NETosis through a distinct mechanism compared to PMA and recent evidence effectively suggest that the NETosis process varies depending on the stimuli used (Muth et al., 2017). In this regard, the mechanism underlying the formation of NETs induced by amoebas seems to be non-classical. Thus, ROS production was not detected when human neutrophils were co-cultured with *E. histolytica* trophozoites in our study and apocynin, a NOX2 inhibitor, failed to inhibit amoeba-induced NETosis. Since generation of ROS has been reported during the interaction of neutrophils with *E. histolytica* trophozoites at higher ratio of trophozoites that the ratio we used here (10:1 vs. 20:1; Sim et al., 2004, 2005), our results suggest that the mechanism of NETosis induced by amoebas is independent of high concentration of ROS, or at least, of ROS generated from NOX2. Like amoebas, different stimuli induce NETosis independently of NOX2 activity including calcium ionophores, uric acid or immune complexes (Parker et al., 2012; Arai et al., 2014; Kraaij et al., 2016). Nevertheless, we detected that amoebas induced NE translocation to nucleus of neutrophils, an important step during NOX2-dependent NETosis that requires ROS formation (Papayannopoulos et al., 2010; Metzler et al., 2014). Since ROS-independent NE translocation has not been described and evidence suggests that histone cleavage takes place in NOX2-independent NETosis (Muth et al., 2017), we speculate that NOX2-independent ROS could be participating in the NETosis triggered by amoebas promoting NE translocation to the nucleus. Recently, other sources of ROS such as the mitochondrial respiratory chain or exogenous hydrogen peroxide produced by microorganisms have been considered necessary for NETosis induced by calcium ionophores and *Candida albicans* hypha, respectively (Douda et al., 2015; Muth et al., 2017). Therefore, we cannot discard that another ROS source, producing amounts that might not be detected with the methodology we used here, play a crucial role in the amoeba-induced NETosis. On the other hand, the translocation of NE to the nucleus in combination with our result showing that the inhibition of its serine protease activity with PMSF reduced the amount of NETs induced by amoeba, confirms that NE translocation is an important step in this mechanism.

PAD4 is a peptidyl arginine deiminase that catalyzes the conversion of arginine into citrulline residues in histones and requires calcium for activation (Jones et al., 2009; Bicker and Thompson, 2013). PAD4 activity is relevant to decondense DNA in some NETosis processes independent of NOX2-derived ROS and in the NETosis induced by the non-regulated calcium influx caused by calcium ionophores or calcium channel-forming proteins (Wang et al., 2009; Li et al., 2010; Konig and Andrade, 2016). Since *E. histolytica* possess amoebapores (Lynch et al., 1982), pore-forming peptides implicated in pathogenicity (Bracha et al., 2002; Zhang et al., 2004), we tested in our model the role of PAD4 in amoebic NETosis. Noteworthy, PAD4 inhibition did not affect amoebic NETosis but chelation of extracellular calcium does. This controversy can be explained by the fact that calcium is required for neutrophil adhesion, which in turn, is important for NETosis since neutrophils in suspension produce less NETs compared to adherent neutrophils (Fuchs et al., 2007). Is worth to mention that in contrast to amoebas, PAD4 inhibition reduced NETosis induced by calcium ionophore A23187, suggesting that at this point of nuclear decondensation, the NETosis processes triggered by amoebas and A23187 are different.

Because of its activity, the presence of citrullinated proteins, principally histones, is considered as a marker of PAD4-mediated NETosis (Brinkmann et al., 2016; Li et al., 2017). In accordance to other reports, our results showed that citrullinated proteins were scarce in control and PMA-treated neutrophils (Neeli and Radic, 2013; Konig and Andrade, 2016; Muth et al., 2017); however, abundant citrullinated proteins were seen in neutrophils treated with A23187 and amoebas. Considering that inhibition of PAD4 using GSK484 failed to inhibit NET release induced by amoebas, the results together suggest that protein citrullination take place but it could be no necessary in the NETosis induced by trophozoites. Further experiments are being carried out to elucidate the participation of citrullination in the process. In this regard, it was recently suggested that protein citrullination can be a mechanism that microorganisms employ to evade the immune response by inactivating the antimicrobial action of NETs proteins (Konig and Andrade, 2016). This notion may explain our previous observation that NETs failed to kill trophozoites *in vitro* and did not ever reduced their capacity to cause amoebic liver abscesses in hamsters (Ávila et al., 2016).

In conclusion, our results show that *E. histolytica* trophozoites trigger NETosis in human neutrophils by a non-classical pathway independent of NOX2-derived ROS and PAD4 activity but dependent of extracellular calcium and the serine protease activity of NE translocated to the nucleus. Our data contribute to understand how NETs are formed in the presence of *E. histolytica* trophozoites. However, more experiments are required to completely elucidate the mechanism of NETs formation triggered by this parasite and its role in protection or pathogenesis of amoebiasis.

AUTHOR CONTRIBUTIONS

JC and CD-G conceived and designed the experiments. CD-G, ZF, and MN performed the experiments. CD-G, JC, and CR analyzed the data. JC, JL, and CR contributed reagents, materials, and analysis tools. JC and CD-G wrote the paper.

FUNDING

This work was supported in part by Grant 284830 (to JC) and Grant 254434 (to CR) from Consejo Nacional de Ciencia y Tecnología (CONACyT), Mexico (http://conacyt.mx), by Grant IN206316 (to JC) from Dirección General de Asuntos del Personal Académico, Universidad Nacional autónoma de México (http://dgapa.unam.mx), and by a special Grant for encouragement of medical research (to JC) from the Miguel Alemán Valdés Foundation, Mexico (https://www.miguelaleman.org). Funding agencies had no role in study design, data collection and analysis, decision to publish, or preparation of the manuscript.

ACKNOWLEDGMENTS

CD-G is a Ph.D. student of the Programa de Maestría y Doctorado en Ciencias Bioquímicas, UNAM, and is recipient of a scholarship from Consejo Nacional de Ciencia y Tecnología (CONACyT), Mexico (432205/596731). We thank Patricia de la Torre for help in PCR standardization; Carlos Castellanos-Barba for flow cytometry assistance; Omar Rafael Alemán and Nancy Mora for technical assistance and Pavel Petrosyan for critical reading of the manuscript.

REFERENCES

Arai, Y., Nishinaka, Y., Arai, T., Morita, M., Mizugishi, K., Adachi, S., et al. (2014). Uric acid induces NADPH oxidase-independent neutrophil extracellular trap formation. *Biochem. Biophys. Res. Commun.* 443, 556–561. doi: 10.1016/j.bbrc.2013.12.007

Asgharpour, A., Gilchrist, C., Baba, D., Hamano, S., and Houpt, E. (2005). Resistance to intestinal *Entamoeba histolytica* infection is conferred by innate immunity and Gr-1+ cells. *Infect. Immun.* 73, 4522–4529. doi: 10.1128/IAI.73.8.4522-4529.2005

Bhattacharya, S., Bhattacharya, A., and Diamond, L. S. (1988). Comparision of repeated DNA from stains of *Entamoeba histolytica* and other *Entamoeba* 27, 257–262.

Bicker, K. L., and Thompson, P. R. (2013). The protein arginine deiminases: structure, function, inhibition, and disease. *Biopolymers* 99, 155–163. doi: 10.1002/bip.22127

Bracha, R., Nuchamowitz, Y., and Mirelman, D. (2002). Amoebapore is an important virulence factor of *Entamoeba histolytica. J. Biosci.* 27, 579–587. doi: 10.1007/BF02704851

Branzk, N., Lubojemska, A., Hardison, S. E., Wang, Q., Gutierrez, M. G., Brown, G. D., et al. (2014). Neutrophils sense microbe size and selectively release neutrophil extracellular traps in response to large pathogens. *Nat. Immunol.* 15, 1017–1025. doi: 10.1038/ni.2987

Brinkmann, V., Abed, U. A., Goosmann, C., and Zychlinsky, A. (2016). Immunodetection of NETs in paraffin-embedded tissue. *Front. Immunol.* 7:513. doi: 10.3389/fimmu.2016.00513

Brinkmann, V., Reichard, U., Goosmann, C., Fauler, B., Uhlemann, Y., Weiss, D. S., et al. (2004). Neutrophil extracellular traps kill bacteria. *Science* 303, 1532–1535. doi: 10.1126/science.1092385

Brinkmann, V., and Zychlinsky, A. (2012). Neutrophil extracellular traps: is immunity the second function of chromatin? *J. Cell Biol.* 198, 773–783. doi: 10.1083/jcb.201203170

Campos-Rodríguez, R., Gutiérrez-Meza, M., Jarillo-Luna, R. A., Drago-serrano, M. E., Abarca-rojano, E., Ventura-juárez, J., et al. (2016). A review of the proposed role of neutrophils in rodent amebic liver abscess models. *Parasite* 23:6. doi: 10.1051/parasite/2016006

Cotter, M. J., and Muruve, D. A. (2006). Isolation of neutrophils from mouse liver: a novel method to study effector leukocytes during inflammation. *J. Immunol. Methods* 312, 68–78. doi: 10.1016/j.jim.2006.02.019

Della Coletta, A. M., Bachiega, T. F., de Quaglia e Silva, J. C., Victoriano de Campos Soares, Â. M., De Faveri, J., Marques, S. A., et al. (2015). Neutrophil extracellular traps identification in tegumentary lesions of patients with paracoccidioidomycosis and different patterns of NETs generation *in vitro*. *PLoS Negl. Trop. Dis.* 9:e0004037. doi: 10.1371/journal.pntd.0004037

Denis, M., and Chadee, K. (1989). Human neutrophils activated by interferon-gamma and tumour necrosis factor-alpha kill *Entamoeba histolytica* trophozoites *in vitro*. *J. Leukoc. Biol.* 46, 270–274. doi: 10.1002/jlb.46.3.270

Douda, D. N., Khan, M. A., Grasemann, H., and Palaniyar, N. (2015). SK3 channel and mitochondrial ROS mediate NADPH oxidase-independent NETosis induced by calcium influx. *Proc. Natl. Acad. Sci. U.S.A.* 112, 2817–2822. doi: 10.1073/pnas.1414055112

Ávila, E. E., Salaiza, N., Pulido, J., Rodríguez, M. C., Díaz-Godínez, C., Laclette, J. P., et al. (2016). *Entamoeba histolytica* trophozoites and lipopeptidophosphoglycan trigger human neutrophil extracellular traps. *PLoS ONE* 11:e0158979. doi: 10.1371/journal.pone.0158979

Fuchs, T. A., Abed, U., Goosmann, C., Hurwitz, R., Schulze, I., Wahn, V., et al. (2007). Novel cell death program leads to neutrophil extracellular traps. *J. Cell Biol.* 176, 231–241. doi: 10.1083/jcb.200606027

García-García, E., Uribe-Querol, E., and Rosales, C. (2013). A simple and efficient method to detect nuclear factor activation in human neutrophils by flow cytometry. *J. Vis. Exp.* 74, 1–7. doi: 10.3791/50410

Ghenghesh, K. S., Ghanghish, K., BenDarif, E. T., Shembesh, K., and Franka, E. (2016). Prevalence of *Entamoeba histolytica*, *Giardia lamblia*, and *Cryptosporidium spp.*in Libya: 2000-2015. *Libyan J. Med.* 11, 1–6. doi: 10.3402/ljm.v11.32088

Ghosh, A. S., Dutta, S., and Raha, S. (2010). Hydrogen peroxide-induced apoptosis-like cell death in *Entamoeba histolytica*. *Parasitol. Int.* 59, 166–172. doi: 10.1016/j.parint.2010.01.001

Guimarães-Costa, A. B., Nascimento, M. T. C., Froment, G. S., Soares, R. P. P., Morgado, F. N., Conceição-Silva, F., et al. (2009). *Leishmania amazonensis* promastigotes induce and are killed by neutrophil extracellular traps. *Proc. Natl. Acad. Sci. U.S.A.* 106, 6748–6753. doi: 10.1073/pnas.0900226106

Halverson, T. W. R., Wilton, M., Poon, K. K. H., Petri, B., and Lewenza, S. (2015). DNA is an antimicrobial component of neutrophil extracellular traps. *PLoS Pathog.* 11:e1004593. doi: 10.1371/journal.ppat.1004593

Huston, C. D., Houpt, E. R., Mann, B. J., Hahn, C. S., and Petri, W. A. (2000). Caspase 3-dependent killing of host cells by the parasite *Entamoeba histolytica*. *Cell. Microbiol.* 2, 617–625. doi: 10.1046/j.1462-5822.2000.00085.x

Itagaki, K., Kaczmarek, E., Lee, Y. T., Tang, I. T., Isal, B., Adibnia, Y., et al. (2015). Mitochondrial DNA released by trauma induces neutrophil extracellular traps. *PLoS ONE* 10:e0120549. doi: 10.1371/journal.pone.0120549

Jones, J. E., Causey, C. P., Knuckley, B., Slack-Noyes, J. L., and Thompson, P. R. (2009). Protein arginine deiminase 4 (PAD4): current understanding and future therapeutic potential. *Curr. Opin. Drug Discov. Devel.* 12, 616–627.

Kaplan, M. J., and Radic, M. (2012). Neutrophil extracellular traps: double-edged swords of innate immunity. *J. Immunol.* 189, 2689–2695. doi: 10.4049/jimmunol.1201719

Keshari, R. S., Jyoti, A., Kumar, S., Dubey, M., Verma, A., Srinag, B. S., et al. (2012). Neutrophil extracellular traps contain mitochondrial as well as nuclear DNA and exhibit inflammatory potential. *Cytometry A* 81, 238–247. doi: 10.1002/cyto.a.21178

Konig, M. F., and Andrade, F. (2016). A critical reappraisal of neutrophil extracellular traps and NETosis mimics based on differential requirements for protein citrullination. *Front. Immunol.* 7:461. doi: 10.3389/fimmu.2016.00461

Kraaij, T., Tengström, F. C., Kamerling, S. W. A., Pusey, C. D., Scherer, H. U., Toes, R. E. M., et al. (2016). A novel method for high-throughput detection and quantification of neutrophil extracellular traps reveals ROS-independent NET release with immune complexes. *Autoimmun. Rev.* 15, 577–584. doi: 10.1016/j.autrev.2016.02.018

Krysko, O., De Ridder, L., and Cornelissen, M. (2004). Phosphatidylserine exposure during early primary necrosis (oncosis) in JB6 cells as evidenced by immunogold labeling technique. *Apoptosis* 9, 495–500. doi: 10.1023/B:APPT.0000031452.75162.75

Li, P., Li, M., Lindberg, M. R., Kennett, M. J., Xiong, N., and Wang, Y. (2010). PAD4 is essential for antibacterial innate immunity mediated by neutrophil extracellular traps. *J. Exp. Med.* 207, 1853–1862. doi: 10.1084/jem.20100239

Li, R. H. L., Ng, G., and Tablin, F. (2017). Lipopolysaccharide-induced neutrophil extracellular trap formation in canine neutrophils is dependent on histone H3 citrullination by peptidylarginine deiminase. *Vet. Immunol. Immunopathol.* 193–194, 29–37. doi: 10.1016/j.vetimm.2017.10.002

Li, Z., and Zhou, Z. (2016). How are necrotic cells recognized by their predators? *Worm* 5:e1120400. doi: 10.1080/21624054.2015.1120400

Lood, C., Blanco, L. P., Purmalek, M. M., Carmona-Rivera, C., De Ravin, S. S., Smith, C. K., et al. (2016). Neutrophil extracellular traps enriched in oxidized mitochondrial DNA are interferogenic and contribute to lupus-like disease. *Nat. Med.* 22, 146–153. doi: 10.1038/nm.4027

Lynch, E. C., Rosenberg, I. M., and Gitler, C. (1982). An ion-channel forming protein produced by *Entamoeba histolytica*. *EMBO J.* 1, 801–804.

Maldonado-Bernal, C., Kirschning, C. J., Rosenstein, Y., Rocha, L. M., Rios-Sarabia, N., Espinosa-Cantellano, M., et al. (2005). The innate immune response to *Entamoeba histolytica* lipopeptidophosphoglycan is mediated by toll-like receptors 2 and 4. *Parasite Immunol.* 27, 127–137. doi: 10.1111/j.1365-3024.2005.00754.x

Metzler, K. D., Goosmann, C., Lubojemska, A., Zychlinsky, A., and Papayannopoulos, V. (2014). Myeloperoxidase-containing complex regulates neutrophil elastase release and actin dynamics during NETosis. *Cell Rep.* 8, 883–896. doi: 10.1016/j.celrep.2014.06.044

Muth, A., Mondal, S., Kenny, E. F., Herzig, A., Kru, R., Thompson, P. R., et al. (2017). Diverse stimuli engage different neutrophil extracellular trap pathways. *Elife* 6:e24437. doi: 10.7554/eLife.24437

Neeli, I., and Radic, M. (2013). Opposition between PKC isoforms regulates histone deimination and neutrophil extracellular chromatin release. *Front. Immunol.* 4:38. doi: 10.3389/fimmu.2013.00038

Olivos-García, A., Carrero, J. C., Ramos, E., Nequiz, M., Tello, E., Montfort, I., et al. (2007). Late experimental amebic liver abscess in hamster is inhibited by cyclosporine and N-acetylcysteine. *Exp. Mol. Pathol.* 82, 310–315. doi: 10.1016/j.yexmp.2006.09.005

Pacheco-Yépez, J., Rivera-Aguilar, V., Barbosa-Cabrera, E., Rojas Hernández, S., Jarillo-Luna, R. A., and Campos-Rodríguez, R. (2011). Myeloperoxidase binds to and kills *Entamoeba histolytica* trophozoites. *Parasite Immunol.* 33, 255–264. doi: 10.1111/j.1365-3024.2010.01275.x

Papayannopoulos, V., Metzler, K. D., Hakkim, A., and Zychlinsky, A. (2010). Neutrophil elastase and myeloperoxidase regulate the formation of neutrophil extracellular traps. *J. Cell Biol.* 191, 677–691. doi: 10.1083/jcb.201006052

Papayannopoulos, V., and Zychlinsky, A. (2009). NETs: a new strategy for using old weapons. *Trends Immunol.* 30, 513–521. doi: 10.1016/j.it.2009.07.011

Parker, H., Dragunow, M., Hampton, M. B., Kettle, A. J., and Winterbourn, C. C. (2012). Requirements for NADPH oxidase and myeloperoxidase in neutrophil extracellular trap formation differ depending on the stimulus. *J. Leukoc. Biol.* 92, 841–849. doi: 10.1189/jlb.1211601

Pilsczek, F. H., Salina, D., Poon, K. K. H., Fahey, C., Yipp, B. G., Sibley, C. D., et al. (2010). A novel mechanism of rapid nuclear neutrophil extracellular trap formation in response to *Staphylococcus aureus*. *J. Immunol.* 185, 7413–7425. doi: 10.4049/jimmunol.1000675

Rochael, N. C., Guimarães-Costa, A. B., Nascimento, M. T. C., DeSouza-Vieira, T. S., Oliveira, M. P., Garcia e Souza, L. F., et al. (2015). Classical ROS-dependent and early/rapid ROS-independent release of Neutrophil Extracellular Traps triggered by Leishmania parasites. *Sci. Rep.* 5:18302. doi: 10.1038/srep18302

Röhm, M., Grimm, M. J., D'Auria, A. C., Almyroudis, N. G., Segal, B. H., and Urban, C. F. (2014). NADPH oxidase promotes neutrophil extracellular trap formation in pulmonary aspergillosis. *Infect. Immun.* 82, 1766–1777. doi: 10.1128/IAI.00096-14

Saito, T., Takahashi, H., Doken, H., Koyama, H., and Aratani, Y. (2005). Phorbol myristate acetate induces neutrophil death through activation of p38 mitogen-activated protein kinase that requires endogenous reactive oxygen species other than HOCl. *Biosci. Biotechnol. Biochem.* 69, 2207–2212. doi: 10.1271/bbb.69.2207

Seydel, K. B., and Stanley, S. L., J. (1998). *Entamoeba histolytica* induces host cell death in amebic liver abscess by a non-fas-dependent, non-tumor necrosis factor alpha-dependent pathway of apoptosis. *Infect. Immun.* 66, 2980–2983.

Sim, S., Kim, K. A., Yong, T. S., Park, S. J., Im, K. L, and Shin, M. H. (2004). Ultrastructural observation of human neutrophils during apoptotic cell death triggered by *Entamoeba histolytica*. *Korean J. Parasitol.* 42, 205–208. doi: 10.3347/kjp.2004.42.4.205

Sim, S., Yong, T.-S., Park, S.-J., Im, K.-I., Kong, Y., Ryu, J.-S., et al. (2005). NADPH oxidase-derived reactive oxygen species-mediated activation of ERK1/2 is required for apoptosis of human neutrophils induced by *Entamoeba histolytica*. *J. Immunol.* 174, 4279–4288. doi: 10.4049/jimmunol.174.7.4279

Sousa-Rocha, D., Thomaz-Tobias, M., Diniz, L. F. A., Souza, P. S. S., Pinge-Filho, P., and Toledo, K. A. (2015). *Trypanosoma cruzi* and its soluble antigens induce NET release by stimulating toll-like receptors. *PLoS ONE* 10:e0139569. doi: 10.1371/journal.pone.0139569

Steinberg, B. E., and Grinstein, S. (2007). Unconventional roles of the NADPH oxidase: signaling, ion homeostasis, and cell death. *Sci. STKE* 2007:pe11. doi: 10.1126/stke.3792007pe11

Storisteanu, D. M. L., Pocock, J. M., Cowburn, A. S., Juss, J. K., Nadesalingam, A., Nizet, V., et al. (2017). Evasion of neutrophil extracellular traps by respiratory pathogens. *Am. J. Respir. Cell Mol. Biol.* 56, 423–431. doi: 10.1165/rcmb.2016-0193PS

Tellevik, M. G., Moyo, S. J., Blomberg, B., Hjøllo, T., Maselle, S. Y., Langeland, N., et al. (2015). Prevalence of *Cryptosporidium parvum/hominis*, *Entamoeba histolytica* and *Giardia lamblia* among Young Children with and without Diarrhea in Dar es Salaam, Tanzania. *PLoS Negl. Trop. Dis.* 9:e0004125. doi: 10.1371/journal.pntd.0004125

Urban, C. F., Reichard, U., Brinkmann, V., and Zychlinsky, A. (2006). Neutrophil extracellular traps capture and kill *Candida albicans* and hyphal forms. *Cell. Microbiol.* 8, 668–676. doi: 10.1111/j.1462-5822.2005.00659.x

Wang, Y., Li, M., Stadler, S., Correll, S., Li, P., Wang, D., et al. (2009). Histone hypercitrullination mediates chromatin decondensation and neutrophil extracellular trap formation. *J. Cell Biol.* 184, 205–213. doi: 10.1083/jcb.200806072

Yipp, B. G., and Kubes, P. (2013). NETosis: how vital is it? *Blood* 122, 2784–2794. doi: 10.1182/blood-2013-04-457671

Yousefi, S., Mihalache, C., Kozlowski, E., Schmid, I., and Simon, H. U. (2009). Viable neutrophils release mitochondrial DNA to form neutrophil extracellular traps. *Cell Death Differ.* 16, 1438–1444. doi: 10.1038/cdd.2009.96

Zhang, X., Zhang, Z., Alexander, D., Bracha, R., Mirelman, D., and Stanley, S. L. (2004). Expression of amoebapores is required for full expression of *Entamoeba histolytica* virulence in amebic liver abscess but is not necessary for the induction of inflammation or tissue damage in amebic colitis. *Infect. Immun.* 72, 678–683. doi: 10.1128/IAI.72.2.678-683.2004

10

Entamoeba histolytica Up-Regulates MicroRNA-643 to Promote Apoptosis by Targeting XIAP in Human Epithelial Colon Cells

Itzel López-Rosas[1], César López-Camarillo[2], Yarely M. Salinas-Vera[2], Olga N. Hernández-de la Cruz[2], Carlos Palma-Flores[3], Bibiana Chávez-Munguía[4], Osbaldo Resendis-Antonio[5], Nancy Guillen[6], Carlos Pérez-Plasencia[7,8], María Elizbeth Álvarez-Sánchez[2], Esther Ramírez-Moreno[9] and Laurence A. Marchat[9*]*

[1] Catedrática CONACYT, Laboratorio de Genómica Funcional y Biología Molecular, Colegio de Postgraduados Campus Campeche, Campeche, Mexico, [2] Posgrado en Ciencias Genómicas, Universidad Autónoma de la Ciudad de Mexico, Mexico City, Mexico, [3] Catedrático CONACYT, Instituto Politécnico Nacional, Mexico City, Mexico, [4] Departamento de Infectómica y Patogénesis Molecular, Centro de Investigación y de Estudios Avanzados del Instituto Politécnico Nacional, Mexico City, Mexico, [5] Instituto Nacional de Medicina Genómica y Coordinación de la Investigación Científica, Red de Apoyo a la Investigación, Universidad Nacional Autónoma de Mexico, Mexico City, Mexico, [6] Unidad de Análisis Cuantitativo de Imágenes, Institute Pasteur, Paris, France, [7] Unidad de Biomedicina, Facultad de Estudios Superiores-Iztacala, Universidad Nacional Autónoma de México, Mexico City, Mexico, [8] Instituto Nacional de Cancerología, Mexico City, Mexico, [9] Programa en Biomedicina Molecular y Red de Biotecnología, Escuela Nacional de Medicina y Homeopatía, Instituto Politécnico Nacional, Mexico City, Mexico

***Correspondence:**
César López-Camarillo
genomicas@yahoo.com.mx
Laurence A. Marchat
lmarchat@gmail.com

MicroRNAs (miRNAs) are small non-coding RNAs that function as negative regulators of gene expression. Recent evidences suggested that host cells miRNAs are involved in the progression of infectious diseases, but its role in amoebiasis remains largely unknown. Here, we reported an unexplored role for miRNAs of human epithelial colon cells during the apoptosis induced by *Entamoeba histolytica*. We demonstrated for the first time that SW-480 colon cells change their miRNAs profile in response to parasite exposure. Our data showed that virulent *E. histolytica* trophozoites induced apoptosis of SW-480 colon cells after 45 min interaction, which was associated to caspases-3 and -9 activation. Comprehensive profiling of 667 miRNAs using Taqman Low-Density Arrays showed that 6 and 15 miRNAs were significantly ($FC > 1.5$; $p < 0.05$) modulated in SW-480 cells after 45 and 75 min interaction with parasites, respectively. Remarkably, no significant regulation of the 6-miRNAs signature (miR-526b-5p, miR-150, miR-643, miR-615-5p, miR-525, and miR-409-3p) was found when SW-480 cells were exposed to non-virulent *Entamoeba dispar*. Moreover, we confirmed that miR-150, miR-643, miR-615-5p, and miR-525 exhibited similar regulation in SW-480 and Caco2 colon cells after 45 min interaction with trophozoites. Exhaustive bioinformatic analysis of the six-miRNAs signature revealed intricate miRNAs-mRNAs co-regulation networks in which the anti-apoptotic XIAP, API5, BCL2, and AKT1 genes were the major targets of the set of six-miRNAs. Of these, we focused in the study of functional relationships between miR-643, upregulated at 45 min interaction, and its predicted target X-linked inhibitor of apoptosis protein (XIAP). Interestingly, interplay of amoeba with SW-480 cells resulted in downregulation of XIAP consistent with apoptosis activation. More importantly, loss of function studies using antagomiRs showed that forced inhibition of miR-643 leads to restoration of XIAP levels and suppression of both apoptosis and caspases-3 and -9 activation. Congruently, mechanistic studies using luciferase reporter assays confirmed that miR-643 exerts a postranscripcional negative regulation of XIAP by targeting its 3′-UTR indicating that it's a downstream effector. In summary, we provide novel lines of evidence suggesting that early-branched eukaryote *E. histolytica* may promote apoptosis of human colon cells by modulating, in part, the host microRNome which highlight an unexpected role for miRNA-643/XIAP axis in the host cellular response to parasites infection.

Keywords: *Entamoeba histolytica*, apoptosis, microRNAs, SW480, XIAP

INTRODUCTION

Entamoeba histolytica is the single-celled protozoan parasite causative of human amoebiasis that affects between 40 and 50 million people worldwide. About 10% of infected individuals are at risk for developing invasive amoebiasis, namely amoebic colitis and extra-intestinal disease, such as amoebic liver abscesses that can be fatal (Stanley, 2003). The parasite infection shown clinical variability associated to intestinal microbiota composition that may increase resistance to infection by decreasing the virulence properties and altering systemic immunity against parasites (Burgess et al., 2017). Indeed, specific gut microbiota patterns have been linked to colonization with parasitic protists. For instance, it was reported a differential fecal microbiota in subjects infected with *Giardia duodenalis* or *Entamoeba spp./Blastocystis hominis* (Iebba et al., 2016). Another study found that the *Entamoeba* is significantly correlated with microbiome composition and diversity, and that colonization can be predicted with 79% accuracy based on the composition of an individual's gut microbiota (Morton et al., 2015). Gilchrist et al. also reported that a high parasite burden coupled with increased levels of Prevotella copri was linked to symptomatic infection with *E. histolytica* in children (Gilchrist et al., 2016). In addition, dysbiosis induced by antibiotic treatment increased the severity of amebic colitis and delayed clearance of *E. histolytica* in an amoebic colitis mouse model (Watanabe et al., 2017). These data urge for a better understanding of the mechanisms underlying microbiota-mediated protection that may help explain clinical variability and help treat amoebiasis.

The main site of *E. histolytica* infection is the colon epithelium. Tissues damage resulting from adhesion, lysis, and phagocytosis of host cells is caused by the activity of several parasite proteins; however, the molecular mechanisms by which trophozoites cause epithelial damage are not fully understood. The activity of several parasite proteins including cysteine proteases (Sajid and McKerrow, 2002), the Gal/GalNAc lectin (Petri and Schnaar, 1995), and amoebapores (Leippe, 1997) among others, is important for disruption and invasion of colonic mucosa by *E. histolytica* trophozoites. Moreover, adherence of virulent amoebae to host cells results in cell death, mainly by apoptosis, both *in vitro* (Berninghausen and Leippe, 1997; Sim et al., 2007) and *in vivo* (Moncada et al., 2006), as well as in tissue inflammatory response (Seydel et al., 1997, 1998; Seydel and Stanley, 1998). These events are the result of the ability of parasites to alter gene expression in host cells. Several reports confirmed these assumptions, for instance genome-wide transcriptional analyses of mouse liver cells revealed the impact of *E. histolytica* on transcription of infected cells which contributes to the activation of apoptosis, regenerative and inflammatory cellular pathways in host cells (Pelosof et al., 2006). Also, transcriptional response to adhesion of virulent parasites to liver sinusoidal endothelial cells leads to death and actin cytoskeleton disorganization of host cells (Faust et al., 2011). These data highlights the impact of *E. histolytica* on the gene expression programs of human cells during infection.

Over the last decade, microRNAs (miRNAs) have emerged as a new prominent class of negative regulators of gene expression. MiRNAs are evolutionary conserved small non-coding single-stranded RNAs of 21–25 nt length which function as guide molecules in posttranscriptional gene silencing by binding to the 3′ untranslated region (3′UTR) of target genes resulting in mRNA degradation or translational repression in P-bodies (Bartel, 2004). Notably, aberrant expression of microRNAs may greatly contribute to development of diverse infectious diseases. Interestingly, miRNAs have been investigated in the host-pathogen interactions including viral, bacterial, fungus, and parasitic infections where they mainly mediate inflammatory response and apoptosis in response to inflection (Drury et al., 2017). For instance, *Toxoplasma gondii* inhibits the apoptotic response of infected host cells through upregulation of miR-17-92 expression and downregulation of pro-apoptotic Bim in human macrophages challenged with parasites (Cai et al., 2014). In addition, infection of cholangiocytes with *Cryptosporidium parvum*, a protist causing intestinal and biliary disease, decreased the expression of primary let-7i and mature let-7 which in turn regulate TLR4 expression and contributes to epithelial immune responses against parasite infection (Chen et al., 2007). These findings suggested that miRNAs mediate post-transcriptional regulation of cellular pathways critical to host-cell regulatory responses to parasite infection. Importantly, miRNAs may also represent *bonna fide* biomarkers of infections, mainly in virus and bacterial infections, as its levels significantly differs in patients relative to healthy individuals. For instance, it was reported that miR-18a, miR-21, miR-29, miR-106b, and miR-122 were downregulated in serum of patients with Hepatitis B virus infection and liver cirrhosis relative to patients with chronic hepatitis B without liver cirrhosis. This set of miRNAs was able to distinguish both groups of patient's sensitivity of 85 and specificity of 70% (Jin et al., 2015). These data highlighted the potential of miRNAs as novel diagnostic tools in infectious diseases. However, no studies on miRNAs as potential amoebiasis biomarkers, neither clinical data about the relevance of miRNAs in outcome of patients with intestinal diseases have been reported yet. One mechanism by which pathogens may survive and disseminate in host tissues is by inducing cell death and apoptosis of cells. The effects of parasites on host miRNAs expression have been described in a few protozoan and nematode species, but nothing is known in *E. histolytica*. Moreover, the exact role of miRNAs in cell death of host cells is largely unknown in the context of amoebiasis. In this study, we aimed to determine whether the modulation of host cellular miRNAs is involved in the pathophysiological responses of epithelial colon cells to amoeba interactions. Our results revealed for the first time a miRNAs signature of human SW-480 and Caco2 epithelial colon cells in response to exposure to virulent *E. histolytica* trophozoites. Also, we showed a functional role for miR-643/XIAP axis in the apoptosis activation of host cells.

MATERIALS AND METHODS

Parasite and Cell Cultures

Virulent *E. histolytica* trophozoites (strain HM1:IMSS) were grown under axenic conditions in Diamond's TYI-S-33 medium at 37°C (Diamond et al., 1978). Trophozoites in exponential phase of growth were used in all experiments. SW-480 (CCL-228) and Caco2 (HTB-37) human colorectal adenocarcinoma cell lines were purchased from ATCC collection and cultured in Dulbecco's modified Eagle's medium (DMEM; Invitrogen), supplemented with 10% fetal bovine serum, 100 U/ml penicillin and 100 mg/ml streptomycin. Cultures were maintained in a 5% CO_2 humidified atmosphere at 37°C. For interaction assays, SW-480 and Caco2 cells (250,000) were cultured overnight in 6-well plates until reach 100% confluence, then amoeba was incubated with monolayers at 10:1 ratio (SW-480:amoeba) during 0, 15, 30, 45 and 75 min for downstream analysis.

Transmission Electron Microscopy

After 15, 30, and 45 min interactions, SW-480/trophozoites co-cultures were washed twice with PBS to remove any unattached amoeba and fixed for 60 min with 2.5 % (v/v) glutaraldehyde in 0.1 M sodium cacodylate buffer, pH 7.2, and postfixed for 60 min with 1 % (w/v) osmium tetroxide in the same buffer. After dehydration, with increasing concentrations of ethanol and propylene oxide, samples were embedded in Polybed epoxy resins and polymerized at 60°C for 24 h. Thin sections (60 nm) were obtained and stained with uranyl acetate and lead citrate for its examination in a Philips Morgagni 268 D electron microscope.

miRNAs Profiling Using TaqMan Low Density Arrays

Profiling of microRNAs was performed as previously described with minor modifications (Flores-Pérez et al., 2016). Briefly, Total RNA was extracted from SW-480 cells, with or without interaction with *E. histolytica* trophozoites using the TRIzol reagent (Invitrogen). RNA integrity was assessed using capillary electrophoresis system Agilent 2100 Bioanalyzer with the eukaryotic nano-chip. Only samples with RNA integrity number (RIN) of six or higher were processed. Expression analysis of 667 human miRNAs was performed by reverse transcription and quantitative real-time polymerase chain reaction (RT-qPCR) using the Megaplex TaqMan Low-Density Arrays (TLDAs) v2.0 system (ThermoFisher), as described by the manufacturer. Briefly, 300 ng total RNA were retrotranscribed using stem-loop primers. In order to detect low abundant microRNAs, a pre-amplification step was included. The pre-amplified product was loaded into the TLDA and amplification signal detection was performed in the 7900 FAST real time thermal cycler (ABI). Data were exported to the DataAssist software version 2.0 (Life Technologies) and normalized using the small-nucleolar RNA RNU44. Mean relative quantity (RQ) was calculated and microRNAs differentially expressed between groups (SW-480 cells interacting with trophozoites vs. SW-480 cells alone) were defined as those with fold change >1.5- and p-value < 0.05.

Quantitative Real-Time Reverse Transcription-PCR (qRT-PCR)

The differential expression of six selected miRNAs (hsa-miR-409-3p, hsa-miR-526b-5p, hsa-miR-643, hsa-miR-150, hsa-miR-615-5p and hsa-miR-525) was verified using microRNA assays (Applied Biosystems, Foster City, CA, USA). Briefly, total RNA from SW-480 cells with and without interaction with *E. histolytica,* was reverse transcribed using a specific stem-loop RT primer for each miRNA and the MultiScribe™ reverse transcriptase. Then, diluted retro-transcription reaction (1:15) was independently mixed with Universal PCR Master Mix, No AmpErase® UNG (2X), in presence of individual PCR probes for miR-409-3p, miR-526b-5p, miR-150, miR-643, miR-615-5p, and miR-525. The PCR reactions were done in a GeneAmp® PCR System 9700 (Applied Biosystems), using the following program: 95°C for 10 min, and 40 cycles of 95°C for 15 s and 60°C for 1 min. The relative expression of microRNAs was measured by qRT-PCR using the comparative Ct ($2^{-\Delta\Delta CT}$) method. The snoRNA RNU44 was used as an internal control for data normalization.

Prediction of miRNAs Targets

MiRNA targets were predicted by using four microRNA target prediction programs: DIANA-microT (http://diana.imis.athena-innovation.gr/DianaTools/index.php?r=microT_CDS/index) [44], TargetScan (http://genes.mit.edu/targetscan) [45], miRanda (http://www.microrna.org) [46] and PicTar (http://pictar.mdc-berlin.de/). DIANA-microT identifies targets that are conserved in human and mouse; TargetScan reveals targets which are conserved in human, mouse, rat, chicken, and dog.

miRanda detects targets which are conserved among human, mouse, and rat; and PicTar finds targets which are conserved in human, chimpanzee, mouse, rat, and dog. We selected all target-genes miRNAs pairs that were predicted by at least three programs. Biological pathways of predicted target-genes microRNAs were identified using mirPath (http://diana.imis.athena-innovation.gr/DianaTools/index.php?r=mirpath/index), miRWalk (http://www.umm.uni-heidelberg.de/apps/zmf/mirwalk/predictedmirnapathway.php) and KEGG (http://www.genome.jp/kegg/pathway.html) databases.

Apoptosis Assays

Apoptosis of SW-480 cells after 15, 30, 45, and 75 min interaction with *E. histolytica* trophozoites was quantified by flow cytometry. Annexin-V/propidium iodide (PI) double assay was performed using the annexin V-EGFP apoptosis detection kit (Roche). For interaction assays, SW-480 cells (250,000) were cultured overnight in 6-well plates until reach 100% confluence, then amoeba was incubated with monolayers at 10:1 ratio (SW-480:amoeba) during 0, 15, 30, 45, and 75 min. Subsequently, cells were washed twice with cold 1X PBS to detach amoebas. Then monolayers were seeded and resuspended in 400 μl binding buffer and stained with 5 μl annexin V-EGFP according to the manufacturer's recommendations. Then, 10 μl PI were added and cells were incubated for 5 min at 4°C in the dark. Cells were analyzed in a FACS Calibur flow cytometer (BD Biosciences). The SW-480 cells cultured in DMEM or treated with 50 μM cisplatin for 24 h were used as controls. Assay was repeated three times in triplicate and data were expressed as mean ± standard deviation. Statistical analyses were performed using the Student's *t*-test and a *p*-value < 0.05 was set as significant.

Western Blots Assays

For interaction assays, SW-480 cells (250,000) were cultured overnight in 6-well plates until reach 100% confluence, then amoeba was incubated with monolayers at 10:1 ratio (SW-480:amoeba) during 0, 15, 30, and 45 min. Subsequently, cells were washed twice with cold 1X PBS to detach amoebas. Then remaining SW-480 cells were lysed in ice-cold cell lysis buffer (20 mM Tris, 250 mM NaCl, 2 mM EDTA, 1% Triton X-100, 0.4 mM PMSF), and 1X complete protease inhibitor cocktail (Roche). The protein concentration was determined with the Bradford protein assay kit (BioRad). Total protein extracts (30 μg) were separated through 15% SDS-PAGE and electrotransferred to a nitrocellulose membrane (BioRad) using standard protocols. After blocking with 5% dry skimmed milk, 0.2% Tween-20 in 1X PBS (pH 7.4), membranes were incubated with primary antibodies overnight at 4°C.Then, they were washed twice in 1X PBS with 0.1% Tween-20 for 5 min and incubated for 1 h at room temperature with secondary antibodies conjugated to horseradish peroxidase (HRP) (Jackson). Finally, membranes were washed four times for 10 min in 1X PBS- 0.1% Tween-20 and developed with the ECL Western Blotting substrate (Amersham), according to the manufacturer's instructions. Caspase-3 and caspase-9 antibodies (1:1000 dilution, Cell Signaling) and XIAP antibody (1:3000 dilution, Cell Signaling) were used as primary antibodies. Bands were analyzed by densitometry (myImage Analysis, Thermo), and actin expression was used to normalize data.

Inhibition of MIR-643 Expression Using Antagomirs

SW-480 cells were cultured in a 24-well plate (40,000 cells/well) and grown until reached a 100% confluence. Then cells were incubated with live *E. histolytica* trophozoites for 45 min. Subsequently, amoebas were removed by repeated washing of SW-480 monolayers with cold 1X PBS. Then, SW-480 cells were transfected with miR-643 inhibitor (at 30 and 50 nM) or scramble sequence (50 nM) using siPORT amine transfection agent (Ambion). Non-transfected SW-480 cells exposed to *E. histolytica* were used as control. After 24 h transfection, SW-480 cells were collected and total RNA was extracted using TRIzol reagent to evaluate miRNA-643 expression by stem-loop qRT-PCR and Western blot assays.

Luciferase Gene Reporter Assays

A DNA fragment corresponding to the XIAP 3′UTR (which contains a miR-643 biding site) was synthesized and cloned into the *Xba*I site, downstream from the stop codon of the luciferase gene, in the pGL3 vector (GenScript) to obtain the pGL3-XIAP-3′UTR construct. SW-480 cells (40,000 cells/well) were transfected with the pGL3-XIAP-3′UTR plasmid (1 μg) using lipofectamine 2000 (Invitrogen) according to the manufacturer's protocol. A pGL3-SIAH1-3′UTR construct that contains the 3′UTR of SIAH1 gene and lack of a miR-643 biding site was used as control. At 24 h postransfection SW-480 cells were incubated with *E. histolytica* trophozoites for 45 min, and then transfected with anti-miR-643 or scramble as described above. Luciferase activity was measured using the Dual-Luciferase Reporter Assay System (Promega) at 24 h post transfection. Data were normalized against values corresponding to SW-480 cells transfected with pGL3-XIAP without interaction with *E. histolytica*. Each assay was repeated three times in duplicate, and data were expressed as mean ± standard deviation.

Statistical Analysis

Statistical analyses were performed using the unpaired Student *t*-test to compare each condition with control cells and a p value$<$0.05 was considered as significant.

RESULTS

E. histolytica Alters miRNAs Expression During the Induced Apoptosis of Human SW-480 Colon Cells

Previous studies using *in vitro* and *in vivo* approaches demonstrated that *E. histolytica* induced apoptosis of human Caco2 and Jurkat cells (Seydel and Stanley, 1998; Huston et al., 2000, 2003; Kim et al., 2014; Lee et al., 2014). Here we asked about the contribution of non-coding miRNAs in apoptosis of SW-480 epithelial colon cells induced by *E. histolytica* live trophozoites as this issue remains completely understood. Firstly, we setup an interaction model of SW-480 cells with trophozoites and then evaluated the morphological changes induced during the

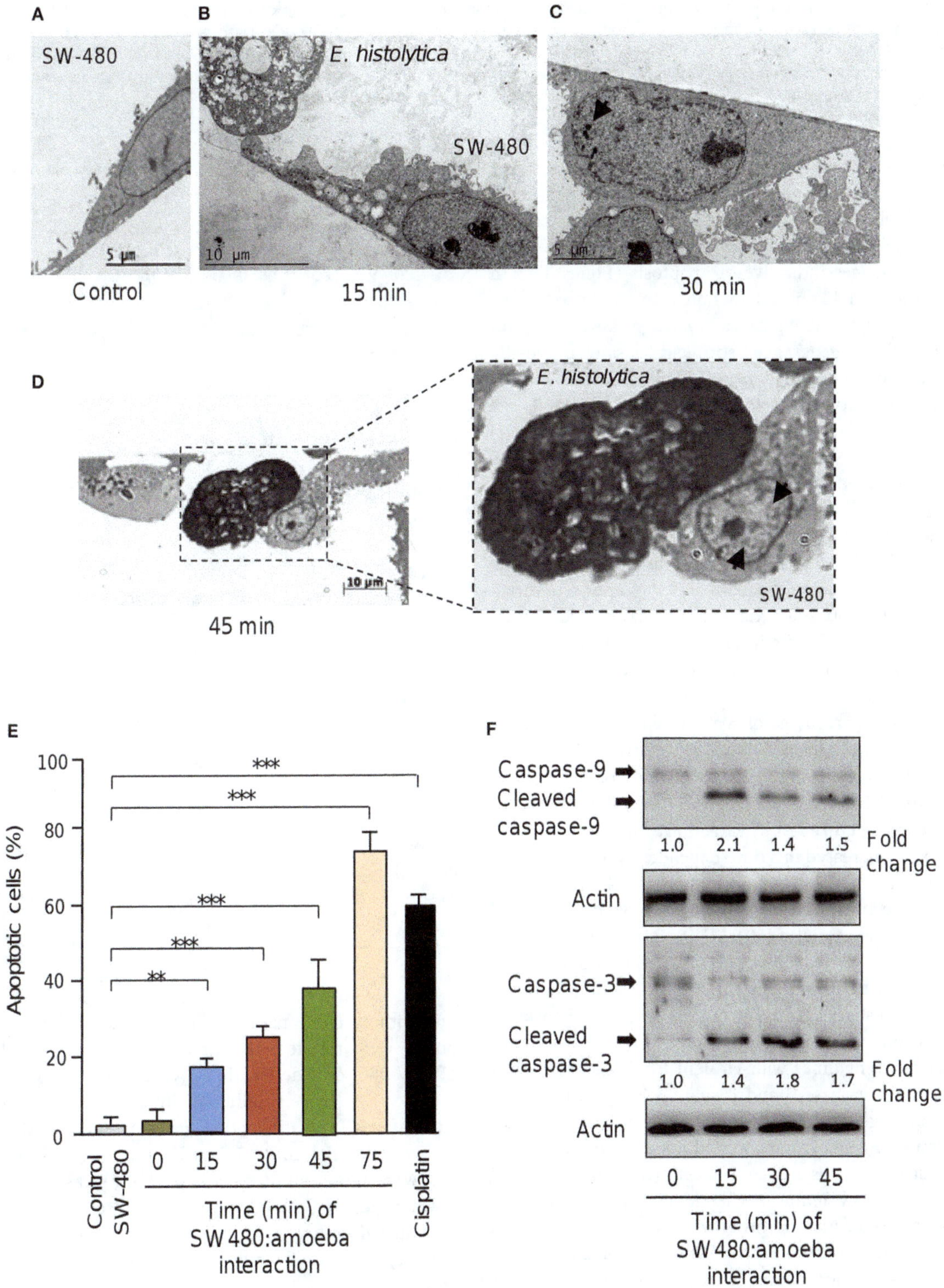

FIGURE 1 | *E. histolytica* induces apoptosis in SW-480 cells. **(A)** Representative transmission electron microscopy ultrastructure image of confluent SW-480 cells showing a well-spread cell with irregular microvilli, mitochondria distributed through the cytoplasm and enlarged nuclei. Scale bar 5 µM. **(B)** Image shows transmission electron microscopy ultrastructure images of trophozoites in contact with colon cells after 15, **(C)** 30 and **(D)** 45 min of co-culture. **(D)** SW-480 cells showing typical early changes associated with apoptosis including a general cell-shrinkage, loss of microvilli and nuclear chromatin condensation denoted by arrows (close up in **D**). Scale bar 10 µM. **(E)** Apoptosis assays. SW-480 cells after interaction with *E. histolytica* trophozoites for 0, 15, 30, 45, and 75 min were analyzed by flow cytometry using annexin V. SW-480 cells without exposure to trophozoites and cells treated with cisplatin (50 µM) for 24 h were used as controls. Data are representative

(Continued)

FIGURE 1 | of three independent experiments, performed in triplicate. Bars represent the mean of three independent experiments ± S.D. **$p < 0.01$. ***$p < 0.001$. **(F)** Western blot assays showing cropped images for immunodetection of caspase-9 and–3. Whole protein extracts were obtained from SW-480 cells after interaction with trophozoites for 0, 15, 30, and 45 min and submitted to Western blot assays using caspase-3 and caspase-9 antibodies. Actin antibodies were used as loading control. Immunodetected bands intensity was quantified by densitometry and normalized against actin. Numbers between panels represent the fold change values relative to control (time 0).

interaction. Data showed that control SW-480 cells incubated without parasites form monolayers of well-spread cells with irregular microvilli (**Figure 1A**). At early times of interaction between host cells and amoeba (15 min), we hardly observed morphological changes indicative of apoptosis (**Figure 1B**). In contrast, after 30 and 45 min interaction with trophozoites, the SW-480 cells exhibited the typical early changes associated with apoptosis including a general cell-shrinkage, loss of microvilli, and nuclear chromatin condensation (**Figures 1C,B,D**). Finally, after 75 min interaction we found extensive SW-480 cell death and monolayers destruction (**Supplementary Figures 1, 2**) representative of late stages of apoptosis and cell killing, thus we did not considered longer time for downstream molecular analysis. These data indicate that 45 min of amoeba-colon cells interaction was able to induce morphological changes associated with apoptosis in agreement with previous reports in other human cells including colonic Caco-2 and T lymphocyte Jurkat cells (Huston et al., 2000, 2003; Kim et al., 2014; Lee et al., 2014).

To confirm whether *E. histolytica* parasites induce apoptosis in SW-480 cells we performed flow cytometry analysis using annexin V method. Data showed that in the absence of trophozoites a low percentage of SW-480 control cells (3.7 ± 0.4%) were in apoptotic stage. A similar proportion of apoptotic cells (3.9 ± 0.6%) were found at time 0 interaction, which corresponds to initial time when trophozoites and SW-480 cells were co-incubated (**Figure 1E**). The fraction of apoptotic SW-480 cells significantly increased in a time-dependent way from 19.5% at 15 min co-cultures to 25.1, 40, and 78% at 30, 45, and 75 min interaction, respectively (**Figure 1E**). In SW-480 cells exposed to apoptosis-inducer cisplatin (50 μM) for 24 h, the proportion of apoptotic cells reached 59%. Next, we were wondering if apoptosis was related to intrinsic pathway activation, therefore we performed Western blot assays for caspase-3 and caspase-9 detection using whole protein extracts from SW-480 cells incubated at different times with virulent trophozoites. Results showed that both caspase-9 and caspase-3 were activated by proteolytic cleavage at 15, 30, and 45 min interaction with amoeba (**Figure 1F**). In contrast, we did not detected significant amounts of cleaved caspases in control cells (time 0). Actin used as control did not show significant changes during course of time. These data confirmed that *E. histolytica* trophozoites induced apoptosis via the intrinsic pathway in SW-480 colon cells.

MiRNAs are small non-coding RNAs that negatively regulate the expression of target genes involved in cell survival, migration, and apoptosis in diverse eukaryotic organisms (Bartel, 2004). We were asked whether apoptosis of SW-480 cells induced by trophozoites was mediated by changes in expression of miRNAs repertoire. To test this hypothesis, we performed a comprehensive profiling of 667 miRNAs using TaqMan Low Density Arrays (TLDAs) in SW-480 cells interacting or not with virulent parasites for 45 and 75 min. These time points were selected as represents the early and late stages of SW-480 cell destruction by trophozoites. Data showed that 6 miRNAs were differentially expressed ($FC > 1.5$; $p < 0.05$) after 45 min interaction. Particularly, 5 miRNAs denoted as miR-526b-5p, miR-150, miR-643, miR-615-5p, and miR-525 were significantly up-regulated, whereas miR-409-3p was down-regulated (**Table 1**). At 75 min interaction, we found 16 deregulated miRNAs (3 downregulated and 12 upregulated; **Table 1**). Intriguingly, none common miRNA was modulated at both times.

TABLE 1 | MicroRNAs modulated in human SW-480 epithelial colon cells after 45 and 75 min interaction with virulent *E. histolytica* trophozoites.

MicroRNAs	Fold change (log2 RQ)	*p*-value	*locus*
DOWNREGULATED AFTER 45 MIN INTERACTION			
hsa-miR-409-3p	−3.39	0.031	14q32.31
UPREGULATED AFTER 45 MIN INTERACTION			
hsa-miR-526b-5p	13.48	0.003	19q13.42
hsa-miR-643	3.41	0.019	19q13.41
hsa-miR-150	3.14	0.038	19q13.33
hsa-miR-615-5p	6.97	0.039	12q13.13
hsa-miR-525	8.67	0.044	19q13.42
DOWNREGULATED AFTER 75 MIN INTERACTION			
miR-10a	−5.33	0.0344	17q21.32
miR-642	−5.60	0.0487	19q13.32
miR-501	−7.61	0.0156	Xp11.23
UPREGULATED AFTER 75 MIN INTERACTION			
miR-100	2.02	0.0281	11q24.1
miR-452	3.02	0.0444	Xq28
miR-135a	3.07	0.0179	3p21.2
miR-26b	3.08	0.0047	2q35
miR-32	4.51	0.0387	9q31.3
miR-502-3p	4.53	0.0334	Xp11.23
miR-652	6.18	0.0220	Xq23
miR-101	4.49	0.0296	1p31.3
miR-221	4.14	0.0041	Xp11.3
miR-505*	4.97	0.0296	Xq27.1
miR-17	5.09	0.0344	13q31.3
miR-656	15.20	0.0334	14q32.31

To validate these findings, we selected the six-miRNAs signature deregulated at 45 min and reexamined its expression by stem-loop qRT-PCR using individual TaqMan probes. In agreement with TLDAs data, the expression of miR-526b-5p, miR-643, miR-150, miR-615-5p, and miR-525 was found increased, while the abundance of miR-409-3p was decreased in SW-480 colon cells after 45 min interaction with trophozoites

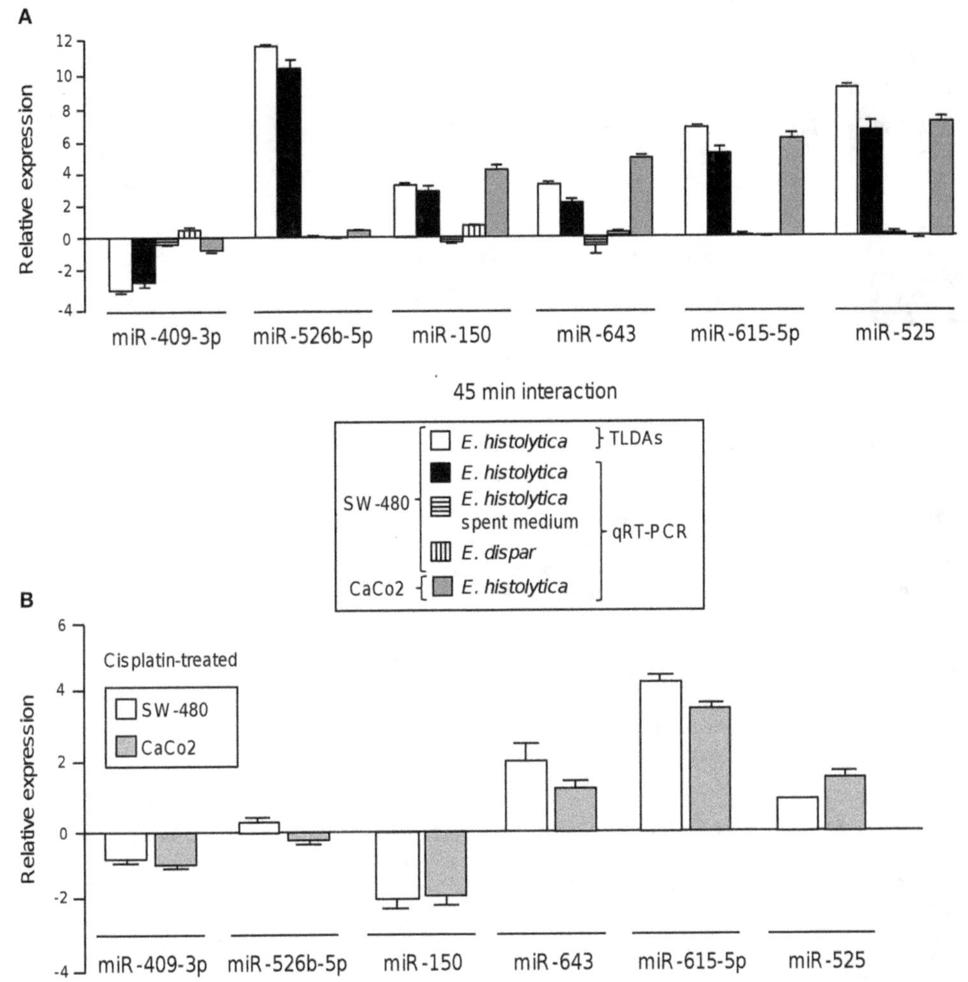

FIGURE 2 | Validation of differential expression of cellular miRNAs after interaction of colon cells with trophozoites. **(A)** Expression levels of the 6-miRNAs signature during the interplay of SW-480 cells with *E. histolytica* for 45 min using qRT-PCR assay (black bars) in comparison with data obtained using spent *E. histolytica* media, during interaction of *Entamoeba dispar* parasites with SW-480 cells and relative to TLDAs profiling (white bars). qRT-PCR assays of Caco2 cells interacting with trophozoites were carried out as an additional control (gray bars). Cell lines, treatments and experiments performed for the 6-miRNAs profiling are denoted in the box inset. **(B)** qRT-PCR assays of the 6-miRNAs in SW-480 and Caco2 colon cells treated with cisplatin as apoptosis control for 24 h. Data is representative of three independent experiments that were performed in duplicate, error bars represent S.D.

(**Figure 2A**). To distinguish the possibility that a soluble factor released by trophozoites could be contributing in the induction of changes in miRNAs abundance, we carried out qRT-PCR analysis of the six-miRNAs signature in the presence of spent medium obtained from parasite's culture media growing without colon cells and compared with the miRNAs levels found after 45 min contact of trophozoites with SW-480 cells. Data showed that the expression of the six miRNAs was very low in the presence of spent culture media in comparison to incubation with trophozoites, indicating no significant regulation of miRNAs (**Figure 2A**). In addition, we also ruled out the possibility that virulent-deficient parasites could be inducing changes in the miRNAs abundance. Results showed no significant expression on the six-miRNAs signature after interaction of SW-480 cells with non-virulent *Entamoeba dispar* trophozoites (**Figure 2A**). We further confirmed the changes of the six-miRNAs levels using an additional Caco2 epithelial colon cell line. Results showed that miR-150, miR-643, miR-615-5p, and miR-525 exhibited similar levels in SW-480 and Caco2 cells after 45 min incubation with virulent trophozoites (**Figure 2A**). In contrast, miR-409-3p and miR-526b-5p were expressed at very low levels in Caco2 cells in comparison to SW-480 cell line. Then, we analyzed the 6-miRNAs expression in SW-480 and Caco2 cells in the presence of cisplatin used as cell death inductor. Data showed that cisplatin modulated the expression of miR-409-3p, miR-643, miR-615-5p, and miR-525 in SW-480 and Caco2 cells in a similar way as observed after the 45 min interactions with virulent trophozoites (**Figure 2B**). Moreover, minimal differences in the 4-miRNAs levels in both cell types were observed after cisplatin treatment. In contrast, miR-526b-5p and miR-150 showed an inverse expression profile in cisplatin-treated SW-480 cells in

TABLE 2 | Validated targets for miRNAs regulated at 45 min in SW-480 cells after interaction with *E. histolytica* according to miRTarBase (http://mirtarbase.mbc.nctu.edu.tw/php/index.php).

miRNA	Validated target[a]	Protein name[b]	Biological context and disease
DOWNREGULATED MICRORNAs			
hsa-miR-409-3p	FGA	Fibrinogen alpha chain	Cardiovascular disease
	FGB	Fibrinogen beta chain	Cardiovascular disease
	FGG	Fibrinogen gamma chain	Cardiovascular disease
	PHF10	Phd finger protein 10	Gastric cancer
	ANG	Angiogenin, ribonuclease, rnase a family, 5	Fibrosarcoma
	IFNG	Interferon, gamma	Primary immune thrombocytopenia
UPREGULATED MICRORNAs			
hsa-miR-526b-5p	TRAF6	TNF receptor-associated factor 6	Colon cancer, esophageal squamous cell carcinoma, and human lung adenocarcinoma cell
	SLITRK4	SLIT and NTRK-like family, member 4	Breast carcinomas and brain tumor
	UBE2V2	Ubiquitin-conjugating enzyme E2 variant 2	Human colon carcinoma cells
	CREB1	Camp responsive element binding protein 1	Regulation of gonadotropin biosynthesis
	FGD4	FYVE, rhogef, and PH domain containing 4	Charcot-Marie-Tooth neuropathy
	PRMT2	Protein arginine methyltransferase 2	Breast cancer
	CBX5	Chromobox homolog 5	Chromodomains characterization in human
	EIF4E3	Eukaryotic translation initiation factor 4E family member 3	Tumor suppression
	RIMKLA	Ribosomal modification protein rimk-like family member A	Central nervous system function
	SCAMP1	Secretory carrier membrane protein 1	Organellar pH homeostasis
hsa-miR-643	TP53IN1	Tumor protein 53-induced nuclear protein 1	Lymphocytic leukemia
	CSF1	Colony stimulating factor 1 (macrophage)	Narcolepsy
	ZEB1	Zinc finger E-box binding homeobox 1	Breast cancer cells
	NR3C1	Nuclear receptor subfamily 3, group C, member 1	Cellular stress
	ER-alpha	Estrogen-related receptor alpha	Myeloma
hsa-miR-150	MYB	v-*myb* avian myeloblastosis viral oncogene homolog	Lymphocyte development
	EGR2	Early growth response 2	Gastric cancer
	VEGFA	Vascular endothelial growth factor a	Vascular diseases
	P2RX7	Purinergic receptor p2x, ligand-gated ion channel, 7	Cancer epithelial cells
	IGF2	Insulin-like growth factor 2 (somatomedin a)	Skeletal myogenesis
	CXCR4	Chemokine (c-x-c motif) receptor 4	Ischemic heart disease
	ZEB1	Zinc finger e-box binding homeobox 1	Esophageal squamous cell carcinoma
	NOTCH3	Notch 3	Thymocyte differentiation
	FLT3	Fms-related tyrosine kinase 3	Leukemia
	EP300	E1a binding protein p300	Gastric cancer
	TP53	Tumor protein p53	Lung cancer cells
hsa-miR-615-5p	IGF2	Insulin-Like Growth Factor 2 (Somatomedin A)	Cutaneous melanoma
hsa-miR-525	DOHH	Deoxyhypusine hydroxylase	Prostate cancer
	KLK4	Kallikrein-related peptidase	Lupus erythematosus
	E2F1	Transcription factor E2F1	Gastric cancer
	ERBB-2	Receptor tyrosine-protein kinase 2	Prostate cancer

[a]*Gene symbol.* [b]*Recommended protein name (UniProtKB).*

comparison to the observed after SW-480/amoeba interactions without cisplatin.

Modulated miRNAs Potentially Target Multiple Apoptosis-Related Genes

The identification of genes that could be targeted by miRNAs is a necessary step to understand its functions in host response to parasites. Several of the regulated miRNAs identified here have been previously described in various biological contexts and human diseases, and some gene targets have been functionally validated (**Table 2**). However, most of these studies have been performed in cancer cells from diverse types of human malignancies and until we know, there are no reports related to infectious diseases. To gain insights into the biological roles of cellular miRNAs that were modulated in SW-480 cells, we performed computational predictions to identify their gene targets using DIANA-microT, TargetScan, PicTar, and miRanda software's. We only focused in the bioinformatic analysis of potential gene targets of the set of miRNAs deregulated at 45 min as it represent the time in which apoptosis was clearly observed. Data showed that 120 predicted gene targets can be regulated by at least two miRNAs modulated at 45 min. In addition, DIANA-mirPath and miRWalk analyses revealed that 5 cellular pathways were mainly affected. These include mRNA surveillance pathway (16 genes), biosynthesis of unsaturated fatty acids (5 genes), ubiquitin mediated proteolysis (16 genes), PI3K/AKAT signaling pathway (5 genes), and apoptosis (8 genes). As others, here we also showed that incubation of amoebae with host cells resulted in apoptosis, therefore we decided to focus on this

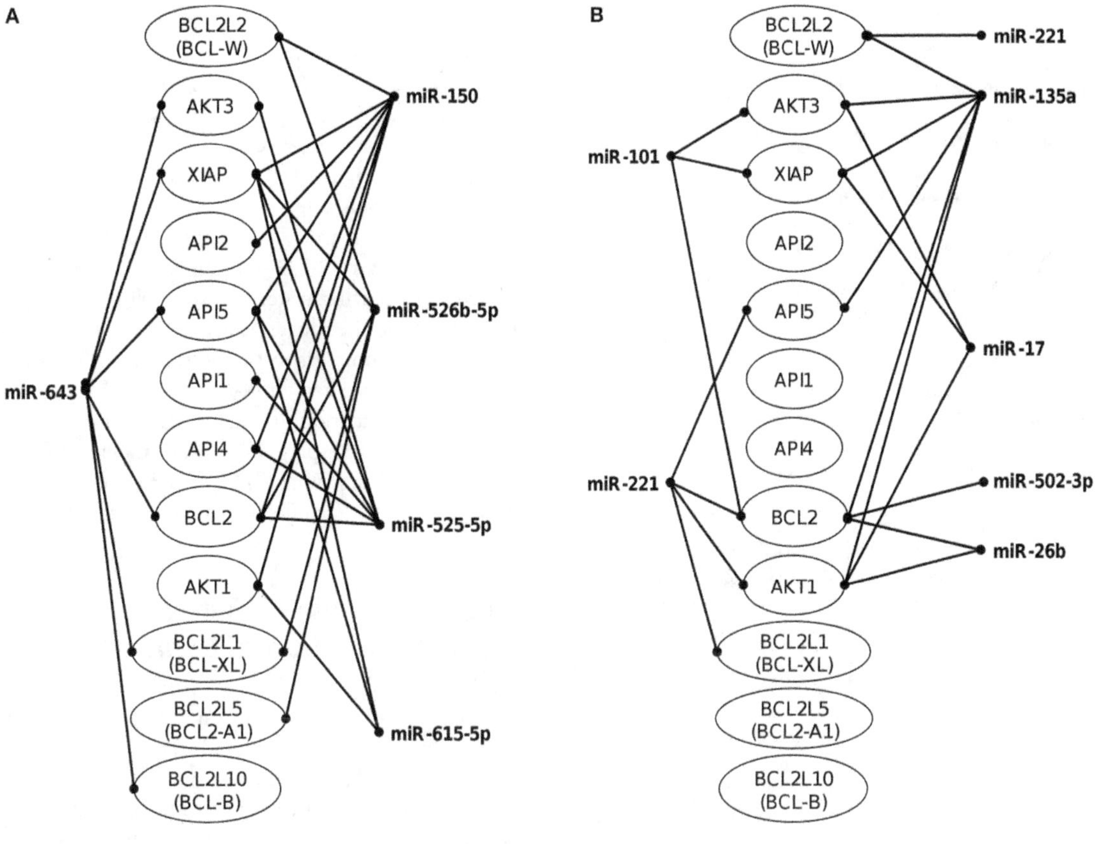

FIGURE 3 | Co-regulation networks of modulated miRNAs and predicted target mRNAs. Image depicts the interaction networks of miRNAs modulated at **(A)** 45 min and **(B)** 75 min after interaction of SW-480 cells with *E. histolytica*. Target mRNAs were predicted by at least two of the three programs used (DIANA-microT, TargetScan, and miRanda). Genes related to apoptosis were also included even if they were targeted by only one miRNA.

cellular process. Interestingly, *in silico* analyses revealed a complex miRNAs-mRNAs coregulation network in which the anti-apoptotic XIAP, API5, BCL2, AKT3, and AKT1 genes were the major targets of deregulated miRNAs at both 45 and 75 min (**Figure 3**; **Table 3**).

Apoptosis Inhibitor XIAP Is a Target of miR-643

To understand the biological role of cellular miRNAs in apoptosis during *E. histolytica* interplay, we initiated the functional characterization of miR-643 which was upregulated after 45 min interaction of trophozoites with SW-480 cells as it was predicted to modulate the expression of six genes related with apoptosis (**Table 1**, **Figure 3**). Bioinformatic analysis indicated that X-linked inhibitor of apoptosis protein XIAP (also known as inhibitor of apoptosis protein 3, IAP3 and baculoviral IAP repeat-containing protein 4, BIRC), a member of the inhibitor of apoptosis family of proteins (IAPs) (Deveraux et al., 1997), it's a predicted target of miR-643. To demonstrate the role of miR-643/XIAP axis in apoptosis, we first evaluated whether interaction of trophozoites with SW-480 cells have a negative effect on expression of XIAP. Western blot results showed that the amount of XIAP protein in SW-480 cells was decreased in a time-dependent way in response to exposition with trophozoites. At 30 and 45 min we found a 10 and 30% reduction in XIAP levels, respectively, in comparison to time 0 (**Figure 4A**). Actin used as control did not show significant changes during course of time.

Examination of the XIAP gene sequence allowed us to identify a miR-643 binding site at the 3′ UTR (1654 to 1660 nucleotide position) suggesting that it may be a direct target (**Figure 4B**). Thus to explore whether miR-643 may negatively regulate XIAP, we inhibited it's expression using a specific antagomiR. SW-480 cells were or not exposed to trophozoites for 45 min and transfected with miR-643 inhibitor (30 and 50 nM) or with scramble sequence (50 nM) as negative control. Results from qRT-PCR assays indicated that in control SW-480 cells grown without trophozoites, the relative expression of miR-643 was low (**Figure 4C**). Interestingly, miR-643 expression was induced six-fold in non-transfected SW-480 cells after interaction with trophozoites in agreement with original TLDAs data (**Table 1**; **Figure 4C**). Moreover, we found that miR-643 amount was dramatically reduced in cells transfected with anti-miR-643 when compared with non-transfected and scramble-transfected SW-480 control cells interacting with *E. histolytica*, indicating that

TABLE 3 | Modulated microRNAs in SW-480 cells interacting with *E. histolytica* for 45 min and predicted targets associated to apoptosis.

MicroRNAs	Predicted target[a]	Protein name[b]
Downregulated MICRORNAS		
miR-409-3p	BCL2	B-cell CLL/lymphoma 2
	BCL2L11	BCL2-like 11 (apoptosis facilitator)
	BCL2L15	BCL2-like 15 (apoptosis facilitator)
Upregulated MICRORNAS		
miR-526b-5p	XIAP	X-linked inhibitor of apoptosis
	BAK1	BCL2-antagonist/killer 1
	BNIP3L	BCL2/adenovirus E1B 19kDa interacting protein 3-like
miR-643	BCL2L1	BCL2-like 1
	BCL2L10	BCL2-like 10
	BCL2L11	BCL2-like 10
	BCL2L14	BCL2-like 14
	XIAP	X-linked inhibitor of apoptosis
	API5	Apoptosis inhibitor 5
miR-150	BCL2L2	BCL2-like 2
	NAIF1	Nuclear apoptosis inducing factor 1
	CASP7	Caspase 7, apoptosis-related cysteine peptidase
	CASP8	Caspase 8, apoptosis-related cysteine peptidase
	CFLAR	CASP8 and FADD-like apoptosis regulator
	AIFM3	Apoptosis-inducing factor, mitochondrion-associated, 3
	AIFM2	Apoptosis-inducing factor, mitochondrion-associated, 2
miR-615-5p	BCL2L1	BCL2-like 1
	BCLAF1	BCL2-associated transcription factor 1
	BMF	Bcl2 modifying factor
	AIFM3	Apoptosis-inducing factor, mitochondrion-associated, 3
	AATK	Apoptosis-associated tyrosine kinase
miR-525	BCL2L1	BCL2-like 1
	BCL2L13	BCL2-like 13
	BAG3	BCL2-associated athanogene 3
	BAG1	BCL2-associated athanogene
	XIAP	X-linked inhibitor of apoptosis
	CASP7	caspase 7, apoptosis-related cysteine peptidase
	BMF	Bcl2 modifying factor

[a]*Gene symbol,* [b]*Recommended protein name (UniProtKB).*

both antagomiR doses (30 and 50 nM) were effective to suppress the expression of endogenous miR-643 (**Figure 4C**).

To corroborate whether miR-643 can exerts posttranscriptional repression of XIAP, we performed luciferase reporter gene assays. A DNA fragment corresponding to the 3′UTR sequence of XIAP which contains the putative miR-643 binding site was cloned downstream of the luciferase coding region into pGL3 vector (**Figure 4B**). Recombinant pGL3-XIAP plasmid was transfected alone or together miR-643 inhibitor into SW-480 cells and luciferase activity was analyzed after 24 h. Data showed that SW-480 cells transfected with pGL3-XIAP construct alone showed a high luciferase activity which was taken as 100% (**Figure 4D**). Interestingly, transfection of pGL3-XIAP into SW-480 cells co-incubated with trophozoites for 45 min resulted in a substantial reduction of the relative luciferase activity in comparison with SW-480 monoculture used as control (**Figure 4D**). A similar reduction (81%) was observed when cells were co-transfected with scramble control. These data suggested that during interaction of amoeba with colon cells endogenous miR-643 levels were increased allowing the repression of pGL3-XIAP mRNA product and luciferase activity. Remarkably, luciferase enzyme activity was restored when expression of miR-643 was inhibited using two different doses of antagomiR (30 and 50 nM). Importantly, in SW-480 cells transfected with 50 nM, luciferase activity almost reached similar levels that observed in cells that were not exposed with amoebas (**Figure 4D**). This effect was counteracted when cells were co-transfected with anti-miR-643 and an unrelated pGL3-SIAH1 construct (containing the 3′UTR of SIAH1 gene lacking of miR-643 binding sites) used as control and (**Figure 4D**). Furthermore, Western blot assays corroborated that expression of endogenous XIAP protein was restored (fold change 1.4 in comparison to control) in SW-480 cells exposed to trophozoites when miR-643 was inhibited (**Figure 4E**), strengthening the notion that miRNA-643 targets the XIAP gene during the interplay of SW-480:amoeba. Taken altogether, these data suggested that XIAP is targeted by miR-643 during interaction of *E. histolytica* trophozoites with human colon cells.

Inhibition of miR-643 Impairs Apoptosis During Interaction of *E. histolytica* With Colon Cells

To obtain further evidence that upregulation of miR-643 is involved in apoptosis activation during the interplay of parasites with SW-480 cells, the expression of miR-643 was inhibited using antagomiRs and the effects in cell death were quantified using annexin-V assays. Again, results showed that in the absence of trophozoites a low percentage of SW-480 control cells were in apoptosis. In addition, data indicated that the fraction of apoptotic cells significantly decreased to 18% after 45 min interaction of miR-643-deficient SW-480 cells with parasites in comparison to cells transfected with scramble negative control and mock which display around 40% apoptosis (**Figure 5A**). In SW-480 cells exposed to cisplatin as control the proportion of apoptotic cells reached 61%. Then, we performed Western blot assays for the detection of caspases 3 and 9 using colon cells transfected with anti-miR-643 and controls. Results showed that activation of caspases 3 and 9 was decreased up to 47 and 49%, respectively, after 45 min interaction of antagomiR-643 transfected-SW-480 cells with amoeba (**Figures 5B,C**) in comparison to controls. Altogether these data suggested that *E. histolytica* induced apoptosis in SW-480 cells, at least in part, through induction of miR-643, which in turn downregulates XIAP.

DISCUSSION

It has been largely described that *E. histolytica* trophozoites produce important changes in genetic programs of host cells during the invasive process. In addition, the impact of host non-coding RNAs in the fine tuning regulation of genes involved in apoptosis is poorly understood. In the current study, we identified for the first time a specific miRNA-signature of SW-480 colon cells that may be involved in the pathophysiological responses to amoeba infection. Our data revealed that exposure

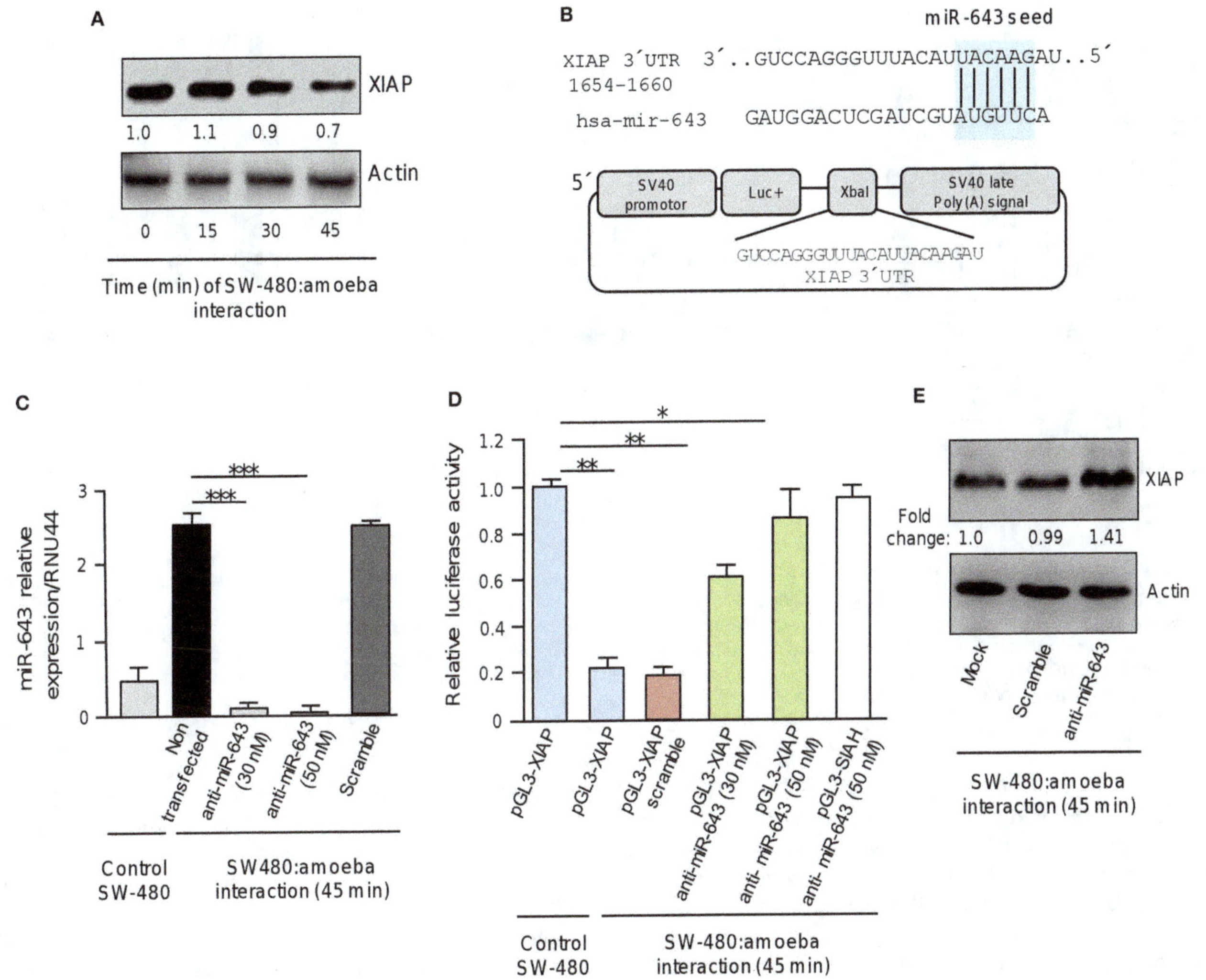

FIGURE 4 | XIAP 3′UTR is a target of miR-643. **(A)** Western blot assays for XIAP expression. SW-480 cells were incubated with trophozoites for 0, 15, 30, and 45 min. Total protein were extracted and XIAP expression was determined by Western blot assays using XIAP antibody (Cell signaling). Actin antibodies (Santa Cruz) were used as control. Numbers represents the fold change in XIAP expression quantified by densitometry and normalized against actin. Values are expressed relative to the control group (time 0 h). **(B)** Schematic representation of pGL3-XIAP construct containing the 3′UTR of XIAP gene cloned at the *Xba*I site downstream of firefly luciferase gene (Luc+) of pGL3 Luciferase Reporter Vector. The miR-643 seed sequence is indicated in the colored box. **(C)** qRT-PCR assays for expression analysis of miR643. SW-480 cells were incubated with trophozoites for 45 min and transfected with miR-643 inhibitor at 30 nM and 50 nM or with scramble sequence (50 nM). **(D)** Luciferase reporter gene assays. SW-480 cells transfected with the pGL3-XIAP were incubated with trophozoites for 45 min and co-transfected with anti-miR-643 (30 and 50 nm) or scramble (50 nM). Luciferase activity was measured after 24 h. SW-480 cells transfected with pGL3-XIAP but not exposed to parasites were used as control. **(E)** Western blot assays showing cropped images for XIAP expression. SW-480 cells transfected with anti-miR-643, scramble or not transfected were incubated with trophozoites for 45 min and then submitted to immunoblotting with XIAP and actin antibodies. Bands intensity was quantified by densitometry and normalized to actin. In all cases, data are representative of three independent experiments by duplicate. Error bars represent S.D. The unpaired Student *t*-test was used to compare each condition with control cells that were not exposed to *E. histolytica*. $^{*}p < 0.05$; $^{**}p < 0.01$; $^{***}p < 0.001$.

to virulent *E. histolytica* trophozoites resulted in a significant deregulation of miRNAs repertoire in epithelial colon cells, as illustrated by the up-regulation of miR-526b-5p, miR-643, miR-150, miR-615-5p, and miR-525, and the down-regulation of miR-409-3p after 45 min interaction. Of these, 4 miRNAs genes are located at the genomic locus 19q13 that is a chromosomal region frequently altered in many human cancers (Kontos, 2014). The small number of modulated miRNAs suggests that amoeba has a limited, but at the same important, impact on the post-transcriptional control of host gene expression mediated by miRNAs, at least at 45 min interaction. Notably, at longer time of cell-cell interactions (75 min) we found an increased number of modulated miRNAs, but none was common at both times. These intriguingly findings showed and suggested that: (i) the apoptosis process could be differentially regulated by miRNAs at 45 min and 75 min. These data is in agreement with the many differences at morphological and molecular level that we evidenced here using multiple approaches. At 45 min

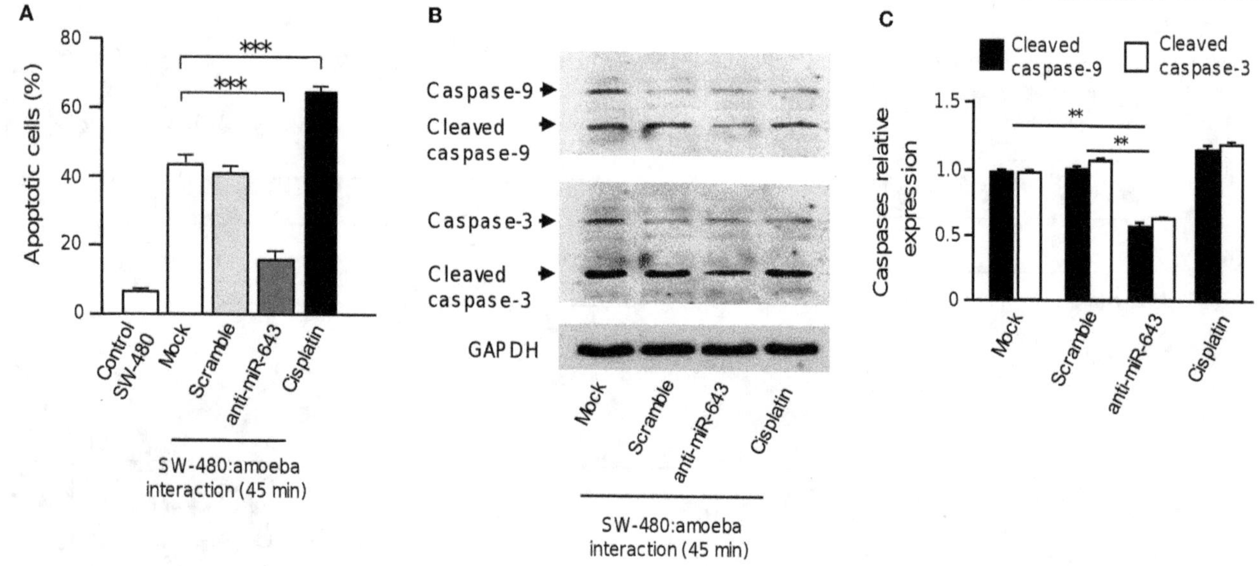

FIGURE 5 | Inhibition of miR-643 impairs apoptosis of SW-480 cells interacting with trophozoites. **(A)** SW-480 cells were or not transfected with miR-643 inhibitor or scramble and interacting with trophozoites for 45 min. Then apoptosis of SW-480 cells was quantified using annexin V assays. SW-480 cells without exposure to *E. histolytica* and cells treated with cisplatin (50 μM, during 12 h) were used as controls. **(B)** Protein extracts from miR-643 deficient SW-480 cells interacting with *E. histolytica* trophozoites for 45 min and controls were submitted to Western blot assays using caspase-3 and caspase-9 antibodies. GADPH antibodies were used as loading control. **(C)** Immunodetected bands intensity in panel B were quantified by densitometry and normalized to GAPDH. Values are expressed relative to the control group (0 h, interaction). $^{**}p < 0.01$; $^{***}p < 0.001$.

we observed about 40% apoptosis, whereas at 75 min most of colon cells showed apoptosis and presented severe damage and extensive cell death; thus is understood that differences at molecular level (miRNAs profile) also should be exist, (ii) our data also suggested that differential expression of miRNAs is not linear between 45 and 75 min, indicating that at late time of apoptosis a different set of miRNAs is needed to modulate the final stage of cell death, and; (iii) apoptosis is a complex event in which several gene regulation mechanisms are activated/deactivated at different stages of process. The different miRNAs modulated at both times revealed the different stages of apoptosis process and thus it's likely that they change during the time revealing a dynamic regulation of apoptosis by miRNAs. However, additional experimental evidences are needed to demonstrate these assumptions as well to understand the role of the deregulated miRNAs at late stage (75 min) of cell killing.

In related studies, the number of modulated miRNAs in response to parasite infection is variable, depending on the pathogen species and the use of an *in vivo* or *in vitro* model. For example, *Eimeria papillata*, another gastrointestinal protozoan, modulates only 4 miRNAs species in the mouse jejunum (Dkhil et al., 2011), while *Plasmodium*, *Cryptococus*, and *Leishmania* modulate a set of 19, 28, and 64 microRNAs in hepatocytes, cholangiocytes and fibroblasts, respectively (Chen et al., 2007; Delić et al., 2011; Lemaire et al., 2013). Thus our datasets size is in the range of regulated miRNAs observed in different pathogen-host cells studies. Importantly, one should keep on mind that a single miRNA can potentially regulate as many as 1,000 different genes (Krek et al., 2005). Indeed, the 6-modulated miRNAs at 45 min were individually predicted to regulate from 365 (miR-615) to 1057 (miR-525). Altogether, they can potentially affect the expression of genes participating in at least five important biochemical pathways in SW-480 cells, including mRNA surveillance pathways, biosynthesis of unsaturated fatty acids, ubiquitin mediated proteolysis, PI3K-AKT signaling pathway and apoptosis. These data indicate that trophozoites interaction represents a stress condition that induces a physiological and adaptive response in host cells. The modulation of proteins involved in mRNA surveillance and ubiquitin mediated proteolysis points out that host cells modify their gene expression after *E. histolytica* interaction. Importantly, bioactive lipid molecules promote apoptosis by modulating mitochondrial membrane permeability and activating different enzymes including caspases (Vanhaesebroeck et al., 2010; Huang and Freter, 2015). Amoeba may be inducing apoptosis in host cells by altering, in part, miRNAs regulating genes involved in lipid metabolism, PI3K-AKT signaling pathway and apoptosis. Notably, the six modulated microRNAs potentially target genes related to apoptosis. Thus, the expression of BCL2L11, XIAP, AIFM3, BCL2L1, and BMF can potentially be regulated by at least two of these miRNAs. SW-480 cells were induced to apoptosis and caspase-3 and-9 were processed following interaction with *E. histolytica* trophozoites, suggesting the activation of the apoptotic intrinsic pathway. Several of the miRNAs identified here have been previously described in cancer cells with a role in the regulation of cell proliferation and apoptosis. In addition, a few targets related to apoptosis have been validated. For instance, miR-409 promotes epithelial-to-mesenchymal transition and

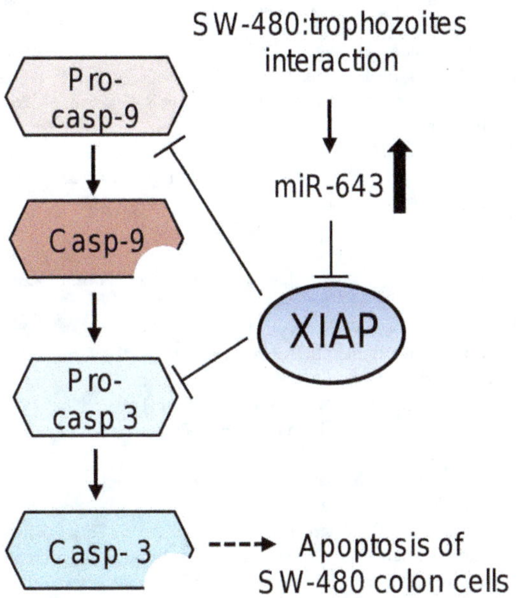

FIGURE 6 | Working model that describes the possible participation of miR-643 in apoptosis of SW-480 cells driven by *E. histolytica*. Upregulation of miR-643 occurs after contact of SW-480 cells with parasites. Then miR-643 may target the XIAP 3′UTR inducing the downregulation of XIAP protein levels, which release the inhibition of caspase-3 and -9. In consequence the executioner caspase-3 triggers degradation of cellular proteins inducing the apoptosis of SW-480 cells.

prostate tumorigenesis (Josson et al., 2015) while it suppresses tumor cell invasion and metastasis by directly targeting radixin in gastric cancer (Zheng et al., 2012). miR-150 promotes cell proliferation in gastric cancer and cancer epithelial cells (Zhou et al., 2008; Wu et al., 2010), while it functions as a tumor suppressor in human colorectal cancer by targeting c-Myb (Feng et al., 2014). miR-526b-5p induces cell cycle arrest and apoptosis in non-small cell lung cancer (Zhang et al., 2015). miR-615 functions as a tumor suppressor in pancreas and breast cancer (Bai et al., 2015; Sun et al., 2015).

Here we demonstrated that miR-643 target the anti-apoptotic XIAP gene in SW-480 cells. Previously, it was reported that miR-643 functions as a tumor suppressor gene in osteosarcoma cells. It was showed that miR-643 suppressed the cancer hallmarks and as a *bona fide* tumor suppressor it may also activates apoptosis (Wang et al., 2017). XIAP has a central regulatory role in programmed cell death by inhibiting the caspases cascade (Deveraux and Reed, 1999). In agreement, apoptosis of SW-480 cells was associated with XIAP repression mediated by upregulation of miR-643 in response to *E. histolytica* exposure. It is important to note that miR-643 and the other modulated miRNAs can also potentially regulate the expression of other target genes related to apoptosis, contributing to SW-480 cell death. Based on our results, we proposed a working model to describe the participation of cellular miRNAs in apoptosis driven by amoebas' interaction (**Figure 6**). In this model, after 45 min contact of SW-480 cells with parasites the miR-643 was upregulated. Then miR-643 target the XIAP 3′UTR inducing the downregulation of XIAP protein levels, which release the inhibition of caspase-3 and -9. In consequence the executioner caspase-3 triggers degradation of cellular components resulting in the apoptosis of SW-480 cells. Notably, miR-526-5p, miR-525, miR-150, and miR-615-5p could also contribute to XIAP inhibition, as they were upregulated during the SW480:amoeba interplay, and were also predicted to target XIAP, however additional experimental evidences are needed to support this assumption.

Limitations of the actual study include: (i) as in previous reports on apoptosis induced by *E. histolytica* in colonic Caco-2 and T lymphocyte Jurkat cells (Huston et al., 2000, 2003; Kim et al., 2014; Lee et al., 2014), the use of a particular cell line limits the extrapolation of findings to *in vivo* conditions; (ii) the miRNAs signature reported here are specific for SW-480 cell line; (iii) the parasite's processes that may trigger miRNAs changes during apoptosis of SW-480 cells remains unknown; (iv) the contribution of additional miRNAs in apoptosis and immune response evasion, and the mechanism by which amoeba contact regulates the transcription of selected host miRNAs remains to be elucidated. Our results showed that the knowledge of the impact of *E. histolytica* on host miRNAs may provide new insights into the relationships between this pathogen and human cells. This first miRNA profiling in SW-480 human colon cells exposed to amoeba revealed significant alterations in cellular miRNAs expression. The set of deregulated miRNAs represent a guide for further functional studies in apoptosis and immune response events. Thus, our findings represent novel data that contribute to our understanding of the cellular and molecular mechanisms activated by the host cells during *E. histolytica* contact.

AUTHOR CONTRIBUTIONS

IL-R, YS-V, OH, CP-F, and BC-M conducted all the experiments. BC-M performed the transmission electron microscopy of cells. MÁ-S, ER-M, and LM performed experiments with amoeba. OR-A performed the *in silico* analysis. CL-C, NG, CP-P and LM contributed to experimental design, intellectual input, and interpreting data. CL-C and LM wrote the manuscript.

ACKNOWLEDGMENTS

We thank Jacqueline Soto-Sanchez for helping with trophozoites cultures. We also acknowledge to Universidad Autónoma de la Ciudad de México and Instituto Politécnico Nacional for support.

REFERENCES

Bai, Y., Li, J., Li, J., Liu, Y., and Zhang, B. (2015). MiR-615 inhibited cell proliferation and cell cycle of human breast cancer cells by suppressing of AKT2 expression. *Int. J. Clin. Exp. Med.* 8, 3801–3808.

Bartel, D. P. (2004). MicroRNAs: genomics, biogenesis, mechanism, and function. *Cell* 116, 281–297. doi: 10.1016/S0092-8674(04)00045-5

Berninghausen, O., and Leippe, M. (1997). Necrosis versus apoptosis as the mechanism of target cell death induced by *Entamoeba histolytica. Infect. Immunity* 65, 3615–3621.

Burgess, S. L., Gilchrist, C. A., Lynn, T. C., and Petri, W. A. Jr. (2017). Parasitic protozoa and interactions with the host intestinal microbiota. *Infect Immun.* 19:85. doi: 10.1128/IAI.00101-17

Cai, Y., Chen, H., Mo, X., Tang, Y., Xu, X., Zhang, A., et al. (2014). *Toxoplasma gondii* inhibits apoptosis via a novel STAT3-miR-17-92-Bim pathway in macrophages. *Cell Signal.* 26, 1204–1212. doi: 10.1016/j.cellsig.2014.02.013

Chen, X. M., Splinter, P. L., O'Hara, S. P., and LaRusso, N. F. (2007). A cellular micro-RNA, let-7i, regulates Toll-like receptor 4 expression and contributes to cholangiocyte immune responses against *Cryptosporidium parvum* infection. *J. Biol. Chem.* 282, 28929–28938. doi: 10.1074/jbc.M702633200

Delić, D., Dkhil, M., Al-Quraishy, S., and Wunderlich, F. (2011). Hepatic miRNA expression reprogrammed by *Plasmodium chabaudi* malaria. *Parasit. Res.* 108, 1111–1121. doi: 10.1007/s00436-010-2152-z

Deveraux, Q. L., and Reed, J. C. (1999). IAP family proteins–suppressors of apoptosis. *Genes Dev.* 13, 239–252. doi: 10.1101/gad.13.3.239

Deveraux, Q. L., Takahashi, R., Salvesen, G. S., and Reed, J. C. (1997). X-linked IAP is a direct inhibitor of cell-death proteases. *Nature* 388, 300–304. doi: 10.1038/40901

Diamond, L. S., Harlow, D. R., and Cunnick, C. C. (1978). A new medium for the axenic cultivation of *Entamoeba histolytica* and other *Entamoeba. Trans. R. Soc. Trop. Med. Hyg.* 72, 431–432. doi: 10.1016/0035-9203(78)90144-X

Dkhil, M., Abdel-Baki, A. A., Delić, D., Wunderlich, F., Sies, H., and Al-Quraishy, S. (2011). *Eimeria papillata:* upregulation of specific miRNA-species in the mouse jejunum. *Exp. Parasitol.* 127, 581–586. doi: 10.1016/j.exppara.2010.11.002

Drury, R. E., O'Connor, D., and Pollard, A. J. (2017). The clinical application of microRNAs in infectious disease. *Front. Immunol.* 25:1182. doi: 10.3389/fimmu.2017.01182

Faust, D. M., Marquay-Markiewicz, J., Danckaert, A., Soubigou, G., and Guillen, N. (2011). Human liver sinusoidal endothelial cells respond to interaction with *Entamoeba histolytica* by changes in morphology, integrin signalling and cell death. *Cell Microbiol.* 13, 1091–1106. doi: 10.1111/j.1462-5822.2011.01604.x

Feng, J., Yang, Y., Zhang, P., Wang, F., Ma, Y., Qin, H., et al. (2014). miR−150 functions as a tumour suppressor in human colorectal cancer by targeting c-Myb. *J. Cell Mol. Med.* 18, 2125–2134. doi: 10.1111/jcmm.12398

Flores-Pérez, A., Marchat, L. A., Rodríguez-Cuevas, S., Bautista-Piña, V., Hidalgo-Miranda, A., et al. (2016). Dual targeting of ANGPT1 and TGFBR2 genes by miR-204 controls angiogenesis in breast cancer. *Sci. Rep.* 6:34504. doi: 10.1038/srep34504

Gilchrist, C. A., Petri, S. E., Schneider, B. N., Reichman, D. J., Jiang, N., Begum, S., et al. (2016). Role of the gut microbiota of children in diarrhea due to the protozoan parasite *Entamoeba histolytica. J. Infect. Dis.* 15, 1579–1585. doi: 10.1093/infdis/jiv772

Huang, C., and Freter, C. (2015). Lipid metabolism, apoptosis and cancer therapy. *Int. J. Mol. Sci.* 16, 924–949. doi: 10.3390/ijms16010924

Huston, C. D., Boettner, D. R., Miller-Sims, V., and Petri, W. A. Jr. (2003). Apoptotic killing and phagocytosis of host cells by the parasite Entamoeba histolytica. *Infect. Immunol.* 71, 964–972. doi: 10.1128/IAI.71.2.964-972.2003

Huston, C. D., Houpt, E. R., Mann, B. J., Hahn, C. S., and Petri, W. A. Jr. (2000). Caspase 3-dependent killing of host cells by the parasite *Entamoeba histolytica. Cell Microbiol.* 2, 617–625. doi: 10.1046/j.1462-5822.2000.00085.x

Iebba, V., Santangelo, F., Totino, V., Pantanella, F., Monsia, A., Di Cristanziano, V., et al. (2016). Gut microbiota related to *Giardia duodenalis, Entamoeba* spp. and *Blastocystis hominis* infections in humans from Côte d'Ivoire. *J. Infect. Dev. Ctries.* 30, 1035–1041. doi: 10.3855/jidc.8179

Jin, B. X., Zhang, Y. H., Jin, W. J., Sun, X. Y., Qiao, G. F., Li, N., et al. (2015). MicroRNA panels as disease biomarkers distinguishing hepatitis B virus infection caused hepatitis and liver cirrhosis. *Sci. Rep.* 12:15026. doi: 10.1038/srep15026

Josson, S., Gururajan, M., Sung, S. Y., Hu, P., Shao, C., Zhau, H. E., et al. (2015). Stromal fibroblast-derived miR-409 promotes epithelial-to-mesenchymal transition and prostate tumorigenesis. *Oncogene* 34, 2690–2699. doi: 10.1038/onc.2014.212

Kim, K. A., Min, A., Lee, Y. A., and Shin, M. H. (2014). Degradation of the transcription factors NF-κB, STAT3, and STAT5 is involved in *Entamoeba histolytica*-induced cell death in Caco-2 colonic epithelial cells. *Korean J. Parasitol.* 52, 459–469. doi: 10.3347/kjp.2014.52.5.459

Kontos, C. K. (2014). Protein-coding genes of the cancer-related genomic *locus* 19q13 and microRNAs as emerging tumor biomarkers. *Austin J. Cancer Clin. Res.* 1:1001.

Krek, A., Grün, D., Poy, M. N., Wolf, R., Rosemberg, L., Epstein, E. J., et al. (2005). Combinatorial microRNA target predictions. *Nat. Genet.* 37, 495–500. doi: 10.1038/ng1536

Lee, Y. A., Kim, K. A., Min, A., and Shin, M. H. (2014). Amoebic PI3K and PKC is required for Jurkat T cell death induced by *Entamoeba histolytica. Korean J. Parasitol.* 52, 355–365. doi: 10.3347/kjp.2014.52.4.355

Leippe, M. (1997). Amoebapores. *Parasitol. Today* 13, 178–183. doi: 10.1016/S0169-4758(97)01038-7

Lemaire, J., Mkannez, G., Guerfali, F., Gustin, C., Attia, H., Sghaier, R. M., et al. (2013). MicroRNA expression profile in human macrophages in response to Leishmania major infection. *PLoS Neglected Tropical Dis.* 7:e2478. doi: 10.1371/journal.pntd.0002478

Moncada, D., Keller, K., Ankri, S., Mirelman, D., and Chadee, K. (2006). Antisense inhibition of *Entamoeba histolytica* cysteine proteases inhibits colonic mucus degradation. *Gastroenterology* 130, 721–730. doi: 10.1053/j.gastro.2005.11.012

Morton, E. R., Lynch, J., Froment, A., Lafosse, S., Heyer, E., Przeworski, M., et al. (2015). Variation in rural african gut microbiota is strongly correlated with colonization by entamoeba and subsistence. *PLoS Genet.* 30:e1005658. doi: 10.1371/journal.pgen.1005658

Pelosof, L. C., Davis, P. H., Zhang, Z., Zhang, X., and Stanley, S. L. Jr. (2006). Co-ordinate but disproportionate activation of apoptotic, regenerative and inflammatory pathways characterizes the liver response to acute amebic infection. *Cell Microbiol.* 8, 508–522. doi: 10.1111/j.1462-5822.2005.00642.x

Petri, W. A. Jr., and Schnaar, R. L. (1995). Purification and characterization of galactose- and N-acetylgalactosamine-specific adhesin lectin of *Entamoeba histolytica. Methods Enzymol.* 253, 98–104. doi: 10.1016/S0076-6879(95)53011-8

Sajid, M., and McKerrow, J. H. (2002). Cysteine proteases of parasitic organisms. *Mol. Biochem. Parasitol.*121, 1–21. doi: 10.1016/S0166-6851(01)00438-8

Seydel, K. B., Li, E., Swanson, P. E., and Stanley S. L. Jr. (1997). Human intestinal epithelial cells produce proinflammatory cytokines in response to infection in a SCID mouse–human intestinal xenograft model of amoebiasis. *Infect. Immunity* 65, 1631–1639.

Seydel, K. B., Li, E., Zhang, Z., Stanley, S. L. Jr. (1998). Epithelial cell-initiated inflammation plays a crucial role in early tissue damage in amebic infection of human intestine. *Gastroenterology* 115, 1446–1453. doi: 10.1016/S0016-5085(98)70023-X

Seydel, K. B., and Stanley, S. L. Jr. (1998). *Entamoeba histolytica* induces host cell death in amebic liver abscess by a non-Fas-dependent, non-tumor necrosis factor alpha-dependent pathway of apoptosis. *Infect Immunity* 66, 2980–2983.

Sim, S., Park, S. J., Yong, T. S., Im, K. I., and Shin, M. H. (2007). Involvement of beta 2-integrin in ROS-mediated neutrophil apoptosis induced by *Entamoeba histolytica. Microbes Infect.* 9, 1368–1375. doi: 10.1016/j.micinf.2007.06.013

Stanley, S. L. Jr. (2003). Amoebiasis. *Lancet* 361, 1025–1034. doi: 10.1016/S0140-6736(03)12830-9

Sun, Y., Zhang, T., Wang, C., Jin, X., Jia, C., Yu, S., et al. (2015). MiRNA-615-5p functions as a tumor suppressor in pancreatic ductal adenocarcinoma by targeting AKT2. *PLoS ONE* 10:e0119783. doi: 10.1371/journal.pone.0119783

Vanhaesebroeck, B., Guillermet-Guibert, J., Graupera, M., and Bilanges, B. (2010). The emerging mechanisms of isoform-specific PI3K signalling. *Nat. Rev. Mol. Cell Biol.* 11, 329–341. doi: 10.1038/nrm2882

Wang, H., Xing, D., Ren, D., Feng, W., Chen, Y., Zhao, Z., et al. (2017). MicroRNA-643 regulates the expression of ZEB1 and inhibits tumorigenesis in osteosarcoma. *Mol. Med. Rep.* 16, 5157–5164. doi: 10.3892/mmr.2017.7273

Watanabe, K., Gilchrist, C. A., Uddin, M. J., Burgess, S. L., Abhyankar, M. M., Moonah, S. N. Jr., et al. (2017). Microbiome-mediated neutrophil recruitment via CXCR2 and protection from amebic colitis. *PLoS Pathog.* 17:e1006513. doi: 10.1371/journal.ppat.1006513

Wu, Q., Jin, H., Yang, Z., Luo, G., Lu, Y., Li, K., et al. (2010). MiR-150 promotes gastric cancer proliferation by negatively regulating the pro-apoptotic gene EGR2. *Biochem. Biophys. Res. Commun.* 392, 340–345. doi: 10.1016/j.bbrc.2009.12.182

Zhang, Z. Y., Fu, S. L., Xu, S. Q., Zhou, X., Liu, X. S., Xu, Y. J., et al. (2015). By downregulating Ku80, hsa-miR-526b suppresses non-small cell lung cancer. *Oncotarget* 6, 1462–1477. doi: 10.18632/oncotarget.2808

Zheng, B., Liang, L., Huang, S., Zha, R., Liu, L., Jia, D., et al. (2012). MicroRNA-409 suppresses tumour cell invasion and metastasis by directly targeting radixin in gastric cancers. *Oncogene* 31, 4509–4516. doi: 10.1038/onc.2011.581

Zhou, L., Qi, X., Potashkin, J. A., Abdul-Karim, F. W., and Gorodeski, G. I. (2008). MicroRNAs miR-186 and miR-150 down-regulate expression of the pro-apoptotic purinergic P2X7 receptor by activation of instability sites at the 3′-untranslated region of the gene that decrease steady-state levels of the transcript. *J. Biol. Chem.* 283, 28274–28286. doi: 10.1074/jbc.M802663200

11

Life and Death of mRNA Molecules in *Entamoeba histolytica*

Jesús Valdés-Flores[1]***, Itzel López-Rosas***[2]***, César López-Camarillo***[3]***, Esther Ramírez-Moreno***[4]***, Juan D. Ospina-Villa***[4†] ***and Laurence A. Marchat***[4*]

[1] Departamento de Bioquímica, CINVESTAV, Ciudad de Mexico, Mexico City, Mexico, [2] CONACyT Research Fellow – Colegio de Postgraduados Campus Campeche, Campeche, Mexico, [3] Posgrado en Ciencias Genómicas, Universidad Autónoma de la Ciudad de México, Ciudad de Mexico, Mexico City, Mexico, [4] Escuela Nacional de Medicina y Homeopatía, Instituto Politécnico Nacional, Ciudad de Mexico, Mexico City, Mexico

***Correspondence:**
Laurence A. Marchat
lmarchat@gmail.com;
lmarchat@ipn.mx

†Present Address:
Juan D. Ospina-Villa,
Grupo Biología y Control de Enfermedades Infecciosas, Universidad de Antioquia, Medellín, Colombia

In eukaryotic cells, the life cycle of mRNA molecules is modulated in response to environmental signals and cell-cell communication in order to support cellular homeostasis. Capping, splicing and polyadenylation in the nucleus lead to the formation of transcripts that are suitable for translation in cytoplasm, until mRNA decay occurs in P-bodies. Although pre-mRNA processing and degradation mechanisms have usually been studied separately, they occur simultaneously and in a coordinated manner through protein-protein interactions, maintaining the integrity of gene expression. In the past few years, the availability of the genome sequence of *Entamoeba histolytica*, the protozoan parasite responsible for human amoebiasis, coupled to the development of the so-called "omics" technologies provided new opportunities for the study of mRNA processing and turnover in this pathogen. Here, we review the current knowledge about the molecular basis for splicing, 3′ end formation and mRNA degradation in amoeba, which suggest the conservation of events related to mRNA life throughout evolution. We also present the functional characterization of some key proteins and describe some interactions that indicate the relevance of cooperative regulatory events for gene expression in this human parasite.

Keywords: *Entamoeba*, mRNA decay, mRNA processing, P-bodies, polyadenylation, protozoan parasite, splicing

INTRODUCTION

The metabolism of messenger RNA (mRNA) is a complex process that is essential for gene expression regulation and mRNA turnover in response to environmental signals and cell-cell communication in eukaryotic cells. During pre-mRNA synthesis by RNA polymerase II (RNA Pol II) in the nucleus, they are modified to generate mature transcripts that can be exported to the cytoplasm and translated to proteins. First, the 5′ end of nascent mRNA is capped by a 7-methyl guanosine linked by a 5′-5′ triphosphate bridge to the first nucleoside of the transcript (capping). These reactions are catalyzed by three enzymes: RNA triphosphatase, guanylyltransferase, and RNA (guanine-7-)-methyltransferase (RNMT) (Cowling, 2010). Then, introns are removed and exons are ligated by the catalytic activity of the spliceosome components that include five small nuclear RNA (snRNAs), namely U1, U2, U4, U5, and U6, and small nuclear ribonucleic proteins (snRNPs) (splicing) (Shi, 2017). Finally, a phosphodiester bond is hydrolyzed at the 3′ end of mRNA and a poly(A) tail is added by the coordinated activity of a large set of polyadenylation factors that recognize specific motifs in RNA 3′ untranslated region (3′UTR) (cleavage/polyadenylation)

(Xiang et al., 2014). After translation, the elimination of mRNA molecules is necessary to ensure proper course of gene expression and prevent the accumulation of transcripts (Christie et al., 2011). Pathways of mRNA decay depend on the formation of RNA-protein complexes in microscopically detectable cytoplasmic structures, called processing bodies (P-bodies) (Sheth and Parker, 2003), in which mRNAs are translationally repressed (silenced) or degraded; their re-incorporation into ribosomes is also possible (Eulalio et al., 2007). Transcript decay involves 3′ end deadenylation by CAF1 and CCR4/NOT1-5 complex (or by PARN, PAN2 and PAN3 deadenylases) followed by 5′ end decapping by DCP1-DCP2 complex and Lsm1-7 proteins, and 5′-3′ digestion by exonuclease XRN1; alternatively, deadenylated transcripts can be degraded from the 5′ end by the exosome complex, while the scavenger-decapping DCP enzyme hydrolyzes the remaining cap structure (Łabno et al., 2016). During translation, aberrant mRNAs with premature termination codons can be detected and eliminated through the nonsense-mediated decay (NMD) pathway (Rebbapragada and Lykke-Andersen, 2009).

Although pre-mRNA processing reactions have usually been studied separately, they occur co-transcriptionally, simultaneously and in a coordinated manner. Moreover, a large set of data has shown that they are interconnected with transcription, translation, and mRNA degradation; protein-protein interactions establish a functional link between the different molecular machineries and promote reciprocal regulation events to maintain the integrity of gene expression. Consequently, each of these processes plays a major role throughout the life cycle of mRNA. Thus, in addition to protect mRNA from 5′ to 3′ exonuclease cleavage, the m7G cap interacts with the cap-binding complex (CBC), which regulates spliceosome assembly, transcription termination, 3′ end processing, RNA export, and NMD in the nucleus. In the cytoplasm, CBC recruits eIF4G, RNA helicase eIF4A, and other proteins to promote translation initiation. Moreover, eIF4G interacts with poly(A) binding protein PABP1 bound to the poly(A) tail to create a mRNA pseudo-circularization and enhance the processivity of the ribosome. Furthermore, it has been recently demonstrated that 2′O methylated cap (cap 1) acts as a signature of self RNA molecules (Ramanathan et al., 2016). Several data indicate that U1 snRNP, the more abundant splicing factor, inhibits 3′ end processing. Notably, its interaction with PAP inhibits poly(A) tail synthesis and promotes degradation of U1A pre-mRNA (Gunderson et al., 1994, 1997). Moreover, its binding to the 5′ splice site (5′ss) of the terminal intron, avoids the use of premature cleavage and polyadenylation to protect the integrity of the transcriptome (Furth et al., 1994). Other data indicate that splicing and 3′ end processing factors may recruit each other and form a stabilized complex on the target pre-mRNA, resulting in reciprocal stimulation of efficiency. Thus, interactions between U2AF65 and CFIm59 (Millevoi et al., 2006), or U1A and CPSF160 (Lutz et al., 1996), enhance the polyadenylation reaction, while CPSF (Kyburz et al., 2006) and PAP (Vagner et al., 2000) stabilize U2AF65 to the terminal intron to stimulate splicing. On the other hand, exon–exon junction complexes (EJC) participate in mRNA degradation, as part of the CBC whose CBP80 component interacts directly with the NMD factor, up-frameshift 1 (UPF1), enhancing the efficiency of this process (Isken and Maquat, 2008). CFIm may bridge 3′ processing with capping through the binding of CFIm25 with CBP20 (Yang et al., 2011).

Until recently, little was known about mRNA metabolism in *Entamoeba histolytica*, the protozoan responsible for human amoebiasis. The availability of the *E. histolytica* genome sequence and the development of the so-called "omics" technologies have provided new opportunities for the study of mRNA processing and turnover in this parasite. To our knowledge, capping has not been described in *E. histolytica*, although preliminary searches in parasite genome database suggest the presence of genes that encode proteins with similarities to human capping enzymes. In this review, we focus on the current knowledge about the molecular basis for splicing, 3' end formation and mRNA degradation, and describe some interactions between these events.

WHAT IS KNOWN ABOUT SPLICING IN *E. HISTOLYTICA*

Splicing Factors

There are nearly four thousand introns in the 8333 annotated genes of *E. histolytica* (Weedall and Hall, 2011), most of them flanked by highly conserved 5′ and 3′ splice sites (ss), GUUUGU and UAG, respectively, but their branch point sequences (BS) lack such degree of conservation (Wilihoeft et al., 2001; Hon et al., 2013). Whereas, no minor U12 introns have been identified in amoeba and most likely neither in the eukaryotic ancestor (Collins and Penny, 2005; Bartschat and Samuelsson, 2010), the majority of the main spliceosome components have been predicted and identified.

Molecular evidence and cloning confirmed the presence of U2, U4, U5, and U6 snRNAs (Miranda et al., 1996; Davis et al., 2007), however no significant homology with eukaryotic U1 snRNAs has led to the conclusion that such small nuclear RNA is absent in *Entamoeba* (Dávila et al., 2008). Nonetheless bioinformatic analyses predicted the presence of the three U1 snRNP U1-A, U1-C, and U1-70k factors, suggesting that activation of the 5′ss might be due to direct interaction of snRNP proteins or by U6 snRNA-5′ss complementarity substitution as demonstrated in other systems (Kandels-Lewis and Seraphin, 1993; Förch et al., 2002; Rhode et al., 2006; Huang et al., 2012). *In vivo* expression of tag-cloned U1-A and cross-linking immunoprecipitation (CLIP) assays of nuclear proteins coupled to mass spectroscopy allowed the identification of at least 32 splicing factors in trophozoites (**Table 1**), namely U2, U4, and U5 snRNP, integral SmD1, SmD3, and SmF proteins; the U1 snRNP components and auxiliary factors U1-70k and TIA-1/TIAR; the U2 snRNP and related components U2-A′, SF3a120, SF3a60/Prp9, SF3b1, SF3b3, U2AF65, and U2AF35; the U5 snRNP components Prp8 and Prp6 [which was previously identified and cloned (Hernandez-Rivas et al., 2000)]; the U6 snRNP integral components LSm2 and LSm5; two alleles

TABLE 1 | Comparison of splicing factors in *Entamoeba histolytica* vs. human and yeast.

Particle/class	Splicing factor	Remodeling	*E. histolytica* protein	Locus[a]	UniProtKB
Sm/LSm snRNP	SmD1		snRNP Sm D1	EHI_052090	B1N466
	SmD3		snRNP	EHI_163710	*C4M3V1*
	SmF		snRNP F	EHI_060400	C4M6J5
	LSm2		U6 snRNA-associated Sm-like LSm2	EHI_068580	C4LU49
	LSm5		hypothetical protein	EHI_076840	B1N3I3
U1 snRNP U1-related No U1 snRNA	U1A, HA-tag		U1 snRNP-specific protein	EHI_050780	C4LTU8
	U1-70K		U1 snRNP subunit	EHI_153670	C4LSE9
	p68	A-B (U1-5'ss)	EhDEAD20	EHI_096390	C4LWF2
	TIA-1/TIAR		RNA-binding protein TIA-1	EHI_056660	C4M9T1
U2 snRNP U2-related U2 snRNA	U2A'		leucine rich repeat protein	EHI_167290	C4MAF8
	SF3a120		splicing factor	EHI_058680	C4LWT7
	SF3a60/Prp9^{PILC}		splicing factor 3A subunit 3	EHI_038600	C4LZP4
	SF3b1^{PILC}		splicing factor 3B subunit 1	EHI_049170	C4MAD8
	SF3b3^{PILC}		splicing factor 3b subunit 3	EHI_048160	C4M4A7
	U2AF65		U2 snRNP aux. fact. large subunit	EHI_098300	C4LXB3
	U2AF35		U2 snRNP auxiliary factor	EHI_192500	C4M1H0
	Prp43	ILS-disassembly	EhDExH9	EHI_184530	C4M6S9
	Prp43	ILS-disassembly	EhDExH13	EHI_090040	C4MA27
	Prp43	ILS-disassembly	EhDExH7	EHI_096230	C4LWD6
	Prp5	E-A (U2-3'ss)	EhDEAD3	EHI_013960	C4LXN8
U5 snRNP U5 snRNA	Snu114^{PILC}	B-B^{act}	U5 snRNP subunit	EHI_021380	B1N373
	Brr2^{PILC}	B-B^{act}; C-Post splicing	EhDExH10/U5 snRNP-specific 200kd	EHI_045170	C4LTD0
	Brr2^{PILC}	B-B^{act}; C-Post splicing	EhDExH1	EHI_131080	C4LXH6
	220K/Prp8^{PILC}		splicing factor Prp8	EHI_060350	C4M6K0
	102K/Prp6		pre-mRNA splicing factor	EHI_093960	C4LYI7
	Prp28	A-B	EhDEAD4	EHI_021440	C4M058
U4/U6 snRNP	CPR6		peptidyl-prolyl cis-trans isomerase	EHI_020340	C4M7U6
U4/U6 snRNA	CPR6		peptidyl-prolyl cis-trans isomerase	EHI_125840	O15729
U4/U6·U5 tri-snRNP	65K/SAD1		ubiquitin C-term hydrolase	EHI_152110	C4LSP9
	Prp38		PRP38 family protein	EHI_000490	C4LZA0
Prp19C/IBC	Prp19^{PILC}		WD domain containing protein	EHI_130870	C4LXF5
	CDC5^{PILC}		myb-like DNA-binding	EHI_000550	C4LZA6
	Aquarius		regulator of nonsense transcripts	EHI_193520	C4M4V4
	Syf1^{PILC}		Hypothetical protein	EHI_073300	C4LXJ5
	RBM22^{PILC}		pre-mRNA splicing factor cwc2	EHI_126150	C4LW00
EJC	CWC22$^{\#,PILC}$		cell cycle control protein	EHI_093720	C4LYG3
	Sub2p/UAP56	E-A (U2-3'ss)	EhDEAD18	EHI_151600	C4LSK1
RES complex	MGC13125^{PILC}		EF-hand calcium-binding	EHI_150550	C4M234
Complex B^{act}	Prp2	B^{act}-B*	EhDExH4	EHI_033720	C4M435
Complex C	Abstrakt		EhDEAD1	EHI_175030	C4LZM8
Step 2 factors	Prp22^{PILC}	Post splicing-ILS	EhDExH3	EHI_077640	C4M8N6
	Prp16	C-Post splicing	EhDExH5	EHI_122790	C4M5M5

[a]*AmoebaDB. E. histolytica splicing factors, U snRNAs and components of the post-catalytic/intron lariat spliceosome complexes (PILS in superscript) were described by Miranda et al. (1996), Hernandez-Rivas et al. (2000), Davis et al. (2007), Dávila et al. (2008), Fourmann et al. (2013), and Valdés et al. (2014). Previously undetected additional Entamoeba PILS components (shaded) were identified in the ProteomeXchange repository PXD001080. # indicates that CWC22 is also part of the Prp19C. Transitions of spliceosome complexes remodeling by the respective DExH/D-box helicases are indicated (Liu, 2002; Marchat et al., 2008; Hahn et al., 2012; Wahl and Luhrmann, 2015).*

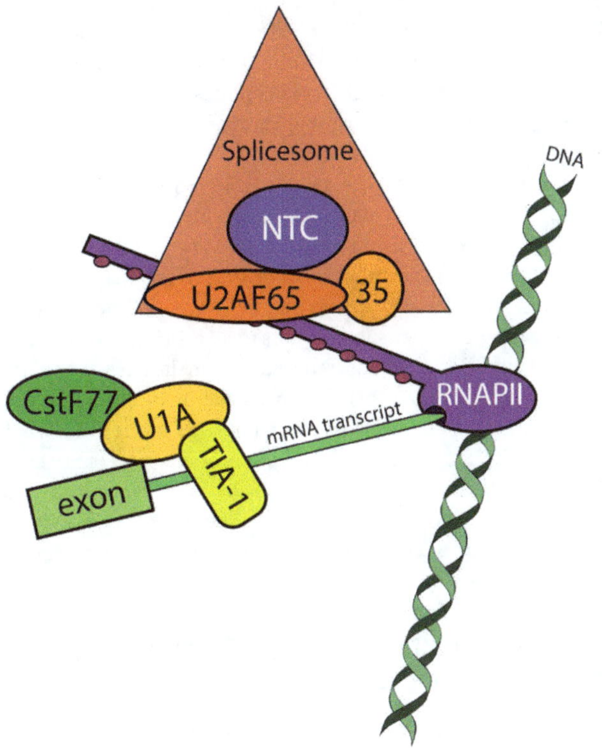

FIGURE 1 | Co-transcriptional pre-mRNA processing in *E. histolytica*: focus on splicing factors. The model summarizes the data available to date (Valdés et al., 2014). During transcript elongation by RNA polymerase II (RNAPII; purple), Ser2 residues of the few heptapeptide repeats of its carboxy-terminal domain become phosphorylated (PSer2-CTD; maroon circles) and apt to recruit the spliceosomal (salmon triangle) and polyadenylation machineries. The large subunit of the U2 Auxiliary Splicing Factor U2AF65 (of 84 kDa in *E. histolytica*; orange oval) is a major player in pre-mRNA processing by tethering the spliceosome and the pre-mRNA (light green boxes) to RNAPII. U2AF65 interacts with the RNAPII-PSer2-CTD and with splicing factors conforming the Prp19 Complex (NTC; blue circle). The NTC regulates the formation and progression of essential spliceosome conformations required for the two steps of spacing. Splicing complex E formation occurs when the snRNP U1-A (yellow oval) binds to the 5′ss (splice site) and the splicing factor TIA-1/TIAR (yellow box) binds to the U-rich sequence just downstream the 5′ss. Splicing complex E also involves the 3′ss definition (not shown). When RNAPII releases the 3′ss from the transcription site, splicing factor 1 binds the branch site at the same time that U2AF65 binds the intron's polypyrimidine tract located between the branch site and the 3′ss; also simultaneously, the small subunit of U2AF (U2AF35, of 29 kDa in *E. histolytica*; pale orange circle) recognizes the 3′ss. The interaction of U2AF65 with splicing factor 1 and U2AF65 at the 3′ss and with the CTD of RNAPII ensures that U2AF65 also tethers the pre-mRNA to RNAPII. Finally, in addition to the previously reported interactions of RNAPII with the polyadenylation complex (vide infra), U1-A directly or indirectly interacts with the splicing complexes B-C, and more importantly with CstF77 (dark green oval), a member of the polyadenylation machinery.

of the U4/U6 di-snRNP component CP6; the U4/U6.U5 tri-snRNP components SAD1 and Prp38; and the nineteen complex (NTC) components Prp19, KIAA0560/Aquarius intron-binding spliceosomal factor, DDX5, and Abstrakt/DDX41 (Valdés et al., 2014) (**Figure 1**).

Splicing E (early) complex formation involves 5′ss recognition by the U1 snRNP (Larson and Hoskins, 2017). However, the less conserved and poorly recognized (weak) 5′ss are activated by 5'ss-U1-C interactions or when TIA-1/TIAR binds to U-tracts localized in front of the 5′ss (Förch et al., 2002). Only U1-70k and TIA-1/TIAR were detected in the U1-A CLIP assays, therefore the most likely scenario for *Entamoeba* 5′ss activation involves direct interaction of U1-A/U1-70k with the 5′ss with the participation of TIA-1/TIAR bound to the U-rich most often spliced *Entamoeba* 5′ss (GUUUGUUU) (Hon et al., 2013) as described for weak 5′ss.

Because cross-linking was carried out with UV, the number of factors identified is limited but it represents all complexes formed during spliceosome assembly, first and second steps of splicing, disassembly, turnover, exon junction complex, and mRNA transport. Moreover, the presence of the core protein of the NTC, Prp19, and U2AF65, which interact with the PSer2 CTD of the large subunit of RNA pol II, ensure proper co-transcriptional activation of the spliceosome, splicing catalysis, termination factors recruitment, and extranuclear mRNA transport factors (David et al., 2011; Gu et al., 2013).

Also, DExH/D RNA helicases involved in the proofreading of the sequential steps of spliceosome assembly and catalysis were identified (**Table 1**): Prp5 and Sub2/UAP56 that facilitate E to A (pre-spliceosome) complex transition; p68, and Prp28, that promote transition from A complex to pre-catalytic (B) spliceosome; two alleles of Brr2, and Snu114, required for spliceosome activation (B to B^{act}); Prp2, that catalytically activates the spliceosome (B^{act} to B* complex); Prp16, that proof-reads the second step of splicing from the catalytic complex (C); the post-splicing complex helicase Prp22; and three alleles of the disassembly Prp43 helicase (Marchat et al., 2008; Valdés et al., 2014). The fact that all proofreading RNA helicases are present in *E. histolytica*, contrasts with the multiple splicing products repeatedly detected in deep RNA-seq data (Hon et al., 2013) indicating that additional cues control the splicing and alternative splicing of the majority of *Entamoeba* introns.

The components of the post-catalytic and of the intron lariat splicing complexes (collectively, PILC) have been recently identified (Fourmann et al., 2013). From our published data and the ProteomeXchange repository PXD001080, we identified the corresponding *E. histolytica* PILC factors: SF3a60/Prp9, SF3b1, SF3b3, Snu114, Brr2, 220K/Prp8, Prp19, CDC5, Syfl, RBM22, CWC22, MGC13125, and Prp22 (**Table 1**). Furthermore, the HA-tagged CLIP assays (Valdés et al., 2014) allowed the unprecedented identification of numerous messenger ribonucleoparticles factors, among them additional splicing-related factors, as well as components of the transcription (large subunit of RNA pol II, and various transcription factors), and polyadenylation (EhCstF64) machineries, evidencing the complexity of this co-transcriptional process (**Figure 1**).

Finally, since most *Entamoeba* pre-mRNAs are mono-intronic, and bioinformatic predictions and deep RNA-Seq data indicate that intron retention is the main route for alternative splicing (Davis et al., 2007; McGuire et al., 2008; Hon et al., 2013), splicing events impact both proteome expansion and gene expression regulation in this parasite.

Intron Lariat Debranching Enzyme

Intron lariat debranching enzyme, or Dbr1, is a member of the calcineurin-like metallophosphoesterases (MPEs) superfamily of binuclear metal-ion-center-containing enzymes that hydrolyse phosphomono-, phosphodi-, or phosphotri-esters in a metal-dependent manner. From bacteriophages to humans, the MPE domain is found in Mre11/SbcD DNA-repair enzymes, mammalian phosphoprotein phosphatases, acid sphingomyelinases, purple acid phosphatases, nucleotidases, and bacterial cyclic nucleotide phosphodiesterases. Despite this functional diversity, MPEs show a remarkably similar structural fold and active-site architecture composed of five sequence blocks that allow metal coordination in the conserved motif D[X]H[x]nGD[x]nGNH[D/E] [x]nH[x]nGH[X]H (Matange et al., 2015). Alanine scanning assays identified the yeast Dbr1 RNA debranching active-site *in vivo* and *in vitro*, which in *E. histolytica* correspond to residues Cys14, His16, Asp45, Asn90, His91, His180, His230, and His232; in all debranching enzymes in nature, cysteine substitutes an aspartic acid residue in position 14 (Matange et al., 2015; Schwer et al., 2016).

Compared to different Dbr1 orthologs, *E. histolytica* Dbr1 is the shortest protein due to its truncated C-terminus; i.e., it is ≈50 residues shorter that *S. cerevisiae* Dbr1. Thanks to its small size, *Entamoeba* Dbr1 has been able to co-crystalize with synthetic branched RNAs and analogs, providing insights of enzyme-lariat interactions. Initial structural studies confirmed the MPE β metal binding pocket (Montemayor et al., 2014) however there was no metal in the A pocket. Subsequent structures revealed the 2nd metal ion in the A pocket (Clark et al., 2016; Ransey et al., 2017). Importantly, this approach identified within the MPE the lariat recognition loop (LRL) whose recognition module, unique to Dbr1 enzymes, comprises residues Ile132, Tyr133, Glu138, Pro141, Tyr144, and Pro148. Dbr1-analogs co-crystals showed that Dbr1 prefers 2′ purines in the branch, although the pocket could accommodate pyrimidines. In addition, there are few sequence-specific interactions at the BS, confirming recognition of atypical BS. Finally, the interactions between RNA and the LRL are stabilized by secondary contacts between residues 141–144 of the LRL and residues Phe292, Pro293, and Phe337 of the carboxy-terminal domain (CTD) of Dbr1; and intricate hydrogen bonds centered in Arg158 aid to stabilize further the conformation of the LRL (Montemayor et al., 2014). The structural data was confirmed by Dbr1 activity *in vivo*. Whereas, *E. histolytica* wild type Dbr1 was able to complement *Saccharomyces cerevisiae* Dbr1-deletant strains relieving intron lariat accumulation, none of the constructs carrying Cys14Ala/Ser substitutions or 141-146Ala substitutions, or CTD or LRL deletions relieved intron lariat accumulation (Montemayor et al., 2014). The presence of *E. histolytica* Dbr1 in intron large post-spliceosomal complexes along with U2, U5 and U6 snRNP components, and the proteins Ntr1/TFIP11 and Prp43 (Yoshimoto et al., 2009) or the Drn1/Ygr093w protein that transiently binds Dbr1 to post-spliceosomal complexes is still unproven (Garrey et al., 2014), although our previous findings point to this possibility (Valdés et al., 2014).

UNDERSTANDING POLYADENYLATION IN *E. HISTOLYTICA*

Cis-Elements for Pre-mRNA 3′ End Formation

One of the first reports about mRNA polyadenylation in *E. histolytica* was published in 1993 and describes the existence of a putative polyadenylation motif TAATT and a 12 pyrimidine stretch in the 3′UTR of parasite genes (Bruchhaus et al., 1993). Then, other groups showed that alternative polyadenylation sites and poly(A) tail size represent efficient postranscriptional mechanisms for gene expression regulation (Urban et al., 1996; López-Camarillo et al., 2003). But the publication of the first version of the *E. histolytica* genome sequence in 2005 (assembly of

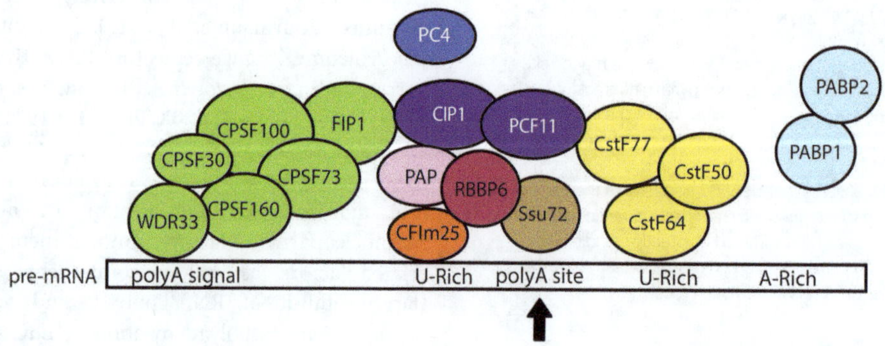

FIGURE 2 | Model of the pre-mRNA 3′ processing complex in *E. histolytica*. The core 3′ processing complex is composed of four main complexes: CPSF (green), CstF (yellow), CFIm (orange), and CFIIm (purple) that bind *cis*-elements within pre-mRNA 3′ UTR. Based on the current knowledge in other eukaryotic cells, we hypothesize that the WDR33 subunit of CPSF complex recognizes the polyadenylation signal (polyA signal) located upstream of the cleavage site (polyA site marked here with a black arrow), while CstF64 recognizes the U-rich downstream element. We also propose that the binding of CFIm25 to the upstream U-rich motif promotes the recruitment of CFIIm subunits (CIP1 and PCF11) and interactions between CPSF and CstF, allowing the RNA cleavage by CPSF73 and the poly(A) tail synthesis by PAP. Additional factors, such as FIP1, PC4, RBBP6, Ssu72, and PABP, would also contribute to the regulation of cleavage/polyadenylation reaction (López-Camarillo et al., 2005). Interactions between EhCFIm25 and EhPAP have been experimentally confirmed *in vitro* (Pezet-Valdez et al., 2013). Interestingly, the interaction of EhCstF77 with U1-A provided the first evidence for a link between mRNA polyadenylation and splicing in *Entamoeba* (Valdés et al., 2014).

~23 Mb that predicted 9938 coding genes comprising 49% region of the genome) (Loftus et al., 2005) represented the critical step to identify motifs in the mRNA 3′UTR and the polyadenylation machinery in this parasite.

A small-scale *in silico* analysis of cDNA and genomic sequences revealed that *E. histolytica* 3′ UTRs contain three conserved motifs: (i) the consensus UA(A/U)UU polyadenylation signal or variants located 10–30 nt upstream the poly(A) site, (ii) the U-rich tract located 1–30 nt upstream the poly(A) site, and (iii) a U-rich element located 3–30 nt downstream the poly(A) site (López-Camarillo et al., 2005). Computational examination of a larger number of cDNA and genomic sequences confirmed this molecular array and suggested the presence of an additional distal A-rich element (**Figure 2**) (Zamorano et al., 2008). Study of the alternative usage of poly(A) sites using RNA-Seq indicated that microheterogeneity in poly(A) sites is likely to be stochastic in *E. histolytica* and only a small fraction of alternative polyadenylation isoforms appeared to be genuine (Hon et al., 2013). Interestingly, genes with alternative poly(A) sites may have a large impact on global gene expression in *E. histolytica* since most of them participate in DNA condensation, DNA binding, translation, splicing, mRNA binding, protein folding and protein transport; other genes are related to signaling, oxidation/reduction, calcium ion binding, cell cycle, and intracellular transport. Indeed, the upstream shift in poly(A) site selection resulting from the silencing of the polyadenylation factor EhCFIm25, was confirmed for thioredoxin and 60S ribosomal protein L7 transcripts and related to specific phenotypical changes and parasite death (Ospina-Villa et al., 2017).

Polyadenylation Factors

Analyses of the 9938 coding genes predicted in the first version of the genome indicated that *E. histolytica* has genes that encode proteins with homology to the majority of polyadenylation factors described in human and yeast (**Table 2**): the cleavage and specificity factor (CPSF160, 100, 73, and 30), the cleavage stimulating factor (CstF77, 64, and 50), the 25 kDa subunit of the cleavage factor Im (CFIm) and both C1P1 and PCF11 subunits of CFIIm, as well as FIP1, poly(A) polymerase (PAP), poly(A) binding protein (PABP), RBBP6 (Mpel in yeast), WDR33 (Psf2 in yeast), PNAS-120 (Ssu72 in yeast), and PC4 (Sub1 in yeast) (**Figure 2**) (López-Camarillo et al., 2005, 2014). In human cells, WDR33 and CPSF30 are the CPSF subunits that binds the polyadenylation signal (Chan et al., 2014; Schonemann et al., 2014). CPSF73 is the endonuclease responsible for RNA cleavage (Mandel et al., 2006). CstF77 interacts with CPSF160, promoting their cooperative RNA binding during the assembly process (Murthy and Manley, 1995). CFIm25 regulates the selection of distal poly(A) sites, contributes to the recruitment of polyadenylation factors and is necessary for poly(A) tail synthesis (Brown and Gilmartin, 2003; Kubo et al., 2006). Although CFIIm subunits are the less characterized polyadenylation factors, evidence suggest that Pcf11 is required for degradation of the 3′ product following cleavage (West and Proudfoot, 2008), while Clp1 interacts with both CPSF and CFIm and likely tethers them to CFIIm (de Vries et al., 2000). PAP is responsible for the addition of the polyadenosine tail (Raabe et al., 1991) and its activity is accelerated by PABP (Wahle, 1991). RBBP6 associates with other core polyadenylation factors through its unusual ubiquitin-like domain and modulates expression of mRNAs with AU-rich 3' UTR (Di Giammartino et al., 2014). PC4 (Sub1 in yeast) associates with the polyadenylation factor CstF64 to modulate transcription termination and polyadenylation initiation (Calvo and Manley, 2001, 2003).

TABLE 2 | Polyadenylation factors in human and *E. histolytica*.

H. sapiens		***E. histolytica***		
Protein	**Access number[a]**	**Locus[b]**	**Protein**	**Access number[a]**
CLEAVAGE AND POLYADENYLATION SPECIFIC FACTORS				
CPSF160	Q10570	EHI_160110	CPSF160	C4M386
CPSF100	Q9P2I0	EHI_033130	CPSF100	C4M6Y0
CPSF73	Q9UKF6	EHI_136700	CPSF73	C4M297
CPSF30	O95639	EHI_067580	CPSF30	C4M9G4
FIP1	Q6UN15	EHI_052180	FIP1	C4M765
WDR33	Q9C0J8	EHI_170080	WDR33	C4M1D0
CLEAVAGE STIMULATING FACTORS				
CstF77	Q12996	EHI_098370	CstF-77	B1N2W3
CstF64	P33240	EHI_151900	CstF-64	C4LSN8
CstF50	Q05048	EHI_152770	CstF-50	C4LSW0
CLEAVAGE FACTORS IM				
CFIm68	Q16630	–	–	–
CFIm59	Q8N684	–	–	–
CFIm25	O43809	EHI_077110	CFIm25	C4M2T1
CLEAVAGE FACTORS IIM				
CIP1	Q92989	EHI_008100	CIP1	C4LYE5
PCF11	O94913	EHI_045130	PCF11	C4LTC6
OTHER POLYADENYLATION FACTORS				
PAP-B	Q9NRJ5	EHI_012040	PAP	Q51D88
Ssu72	Q9BZS6	EHI_027340	Ssu72	C4M1T3
PC4	P53999	EHI_192520	PC4	C4M1H2
PABP1	P11940	EHI_198750	PABP1	C4LWS1
		EHI_033250	PABP2	C4M6Y2
RRBP6	Q7Z6E9	EHI_014000	RRBP6	C4LXP1
Symplekin	Q92797	–	–	–

[a]*UniProtKB;* [b]*AmoebaDB. Data about parasite proteins were obtained from (López-Camarillo et al., 2005, 2014).*

The presence of these proteins in *E. histolytica* suggests that 3′ end processing of parasite mRNA could be performed as it has been described in other eukaryotic cells. Accordingly, EhPAP has the conserved PAP central catalytic domain with the three invariant aspartate residues involved in nucleotide transfer and the F/YGS motif responsible for ATP binding, confirming that it belongs to the polymerases-like superfamily of nucleotidyl transferases (García-Vivas et al., 2005). In the predicted three-dimensional model, both functional domains fold as a U-shaped structure that likely orients the incoming ATP and RNA molecules for poly(A) tail extension. In agreement with its expected role in the poly(A) tail synthesis, EhPAP was able to bind RNA 3′ end although it has a divergent RNA-binding domain (RBD). Moreover, it was located in punctuate nuclear *foci* and in cytoplasmic dots, as it has been described for other polyadenylation factors (García-Vivas et al., 2005; López-Camarillo et al., 2007).

As the human homolog, the EhCFIm25 protein is an unconventional Nudix protein lacking three of the four conserved E residues and the last G residue of the Nudix box, which suggests that it is not able to cleave RNA. Despite the absence of a classical RBD, EhCFIm25 is able to bind the 3′ UTR of *E. histolytica* transcripts and this interaction involves the participation of the conserved Leu135 and Tyr236 residues (Ospina-Villa et al., 2015). EhCFIm25 recognizes the GUUG motif in mRNA 3′end, while the human protein binds the UGUA sequence; consequently, aptamers containing this motif specifically identify the parasite protein, suggesting that they could be used as molecular tools for diagnosis or therapeutic purposes (Ospina-Villa et al., 2018). Interestingly, EhCFIm25 interacts with EhPAP (Pezet-Valdez et al., 2013), which indicates that it may be introduced into the processing complex in the early steps of the cleavage/polyadenylation reaction. EhCFIm25 controls the selection of the distal poly(A) site during mRNA 3′ end formation; consequently, its silencing by dsRNA or its blocking by aptamers alter parasite proliferation and virulence, demonstrating for the first time the relevance of polyadenylation factors as biochemical targets in *E. histolytica* (Ospina-Villa et al., 2017, 2018). Other works have also recently reported that targeting polyadenylation factors represents a valuable strategy for the control of the protozoan parasites *Trypanosoma brucei* (CPSF-30), *Toxoplama gondii,* and *Plasmodium falciparum* (CPSF-73) (Hendriks et al., 2003; Sidik et al., 2016; Palencia et al., 2017; Sonoiki et al., 2017).

EhPC4 is the homolog of the human positive coactivator 4, a multifunctional protein that establishes an important link between transcription and polyadenylation. On one hand, its binding to promoters facilitates the recruitment of transcription factors to stimulate the pre-initiation complex assembly (Conesa and Acker, 2010); on the other hand, its interaction with EhCstF64 avoids premature transcription termination and polyadenylation initiation until the polyadenylation motifs have been transcribed (Calvo and Manley, 2001). Moreover, it mediates chromatin organization and heterochromatin gene silencing by interacting with histones H3 and H2B (Das et al., 2006, 2010). As homologous proteins, the EhPC4 protein contains a single-strand DNA (ssDNA) binding region whose residue K127 is required for DNA interaction, and a dimerization domain in the so-called PC4 domain at the C-terminus (Hernandez de la Cruz et al., 2014). Interestingly EhPC4 and its potential partner, EhCstf-64, were significantly up-regulated in virulent trophozoites (Santi-Rocca et al., 2008). Consistently,

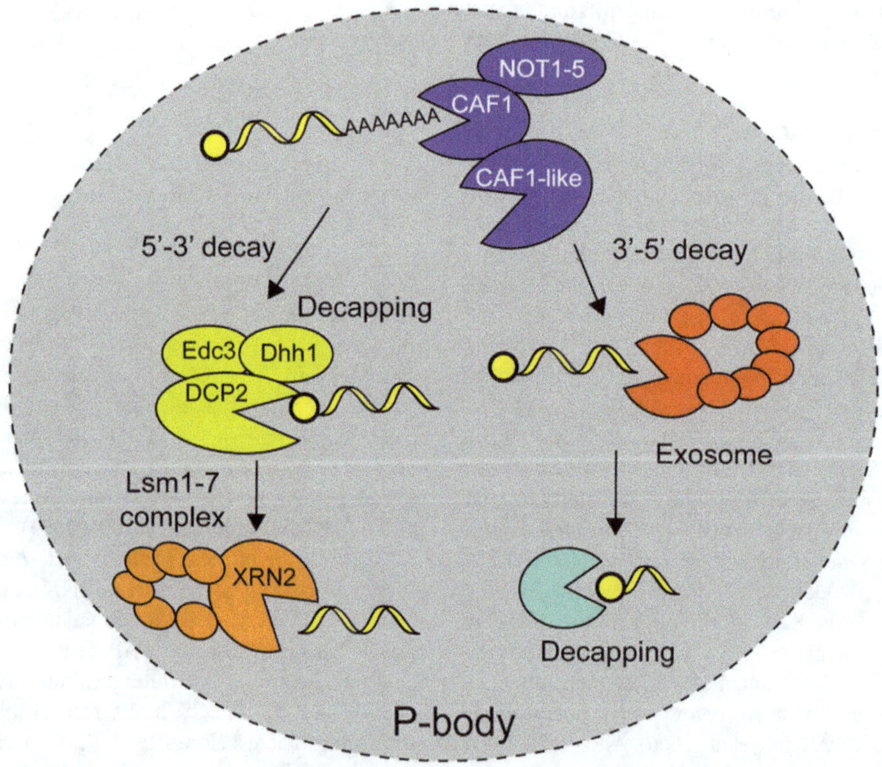

FIGURE 3 | Model for mRNA decay in *E. histolytica.* After mature mRNAs are exported to the cytoplasm where they are eventually translated in a regulated manner, they are later degraded in cytoplasmic P-bodies like structures. The mRNA degradation pathway starts with transcript deadenylation by the CAF1/NOT complex. Then, DCP2 mRNA decapping enzyme removes the cap structure from the 5′ end of the mRNA with the help of accessories proteins Edc3 and Dhh1, which allows 5′-3′ exoribonuclease XRN2 with Lsm protein complex to degrade the rest of mRNA body. Alternatively, the deadenylated transcript is degraded in a 3′-5′ direction by the catalytic subunit Dis3 of the exosome complex and the cap structure is eliminated by DCPs protein (López-Rosas et al., 2012, 2014).

the overexpression of EhPC4 induced the modulation of proteins with key functions in cytoskeleton dynamics, cell migration and invasion in trophozoites. Among them, the up-regulation of a 16-kDa actin-binding protein (EhABP16) which is a putative member of the cofilin/tropomyosin family involved in actin polymerization was associated with an increase in parasite migration of trophozoites and destruction of human SW480 colon cells, confirming that EhPC4 has an impact on parasite virulence (Hernandez de la Cruz et al., 2014). On the other hand, the overexpression of EhPC4 significantly increased cell proliferation, DNA replication and DNA content of trophozoites, promoting the formation of giant multinucleated trophozoites. EhPC4 modulates the expression of genes involved in carbohydrate and nucleic acid metabolism, chromosome segregation and cytokinesis, evidencing the relevance of this factor in polyploidy and genome stability in *E. histolytica* (Hernández de la Cruz et al., 2016). The role of EhPC4 in mRNA 3′end formation and its relevance for the events mentioned above remain to be investigated.

TABLE 3 | Comparison of mRNA decay machineries between human and *E. histolytica*.

H. sapiens		*E. histolytica*			
Protein	**Access number**[a]	**Locus**[b]	**Protein**	**Access number**[a]	**References**
DECAPPING FACTORS					
DCP2	Q8IU60	EHI_058810	EhDCP2	C4M5G6	López-Rosas et al., 2012
Lsm1	O15116	EHI_188020	EhLsm 1	B1N3A8	
Lsm2	Q9Y333	EHI_068580	EhLsm2	C4LU49	
Lsm3	P62310	EHI_151310	EhLsm3	C4LSH4	
Lsm4	Q9Y4Z0	EHI_049370	EhLsm4	C4LUD9	
Lsm5	Q9Y4Y9	EHI_076840	EhLsm5	B1N3I3	
Lsm6	P62312	EHI_188130	EhLsm6	C4M187	
Lsm7	Q9UK45	EHI_025840	EhLsm7	C4M939	
Edc3	Q96F86	EHI_198940	Ehedc3	C4LWU0	
Dhh1	P26196	EHI_093900	Ehdhh1	C4LYI1	
XRN2	Q9H0D6	EHI_133330	EhXRN2	C4MB40	
DEADENYLATION FACTORS					
CAF1	Q9UIV1	EHI_ 048150	EhCAF1	Q56AY2	López-Rosas et al., 2012, 2014
CALIF	Q9UFF9	EHI_039000	EhCAF1-like	C4LZS1	López-Rosas et al., 2012
NOT1	A5YKK6	EHI_200810	EhNOT1	C4M3Y6	
NOT2	Q9NZN8	EHI_044180	EhNOT2	C4M790	
NOT3	O75175	EHI_119550	EhNOT3	C4M7Y3	
NOT4	O95628	EHI_080710	EhNOT4	C4M9N9	
EXOSOME FACTORS					
RRP4	Q13868	EHI_163510	EhRRP4	C4M3T2	López-Camarillo et al., 2014
RRP6	Q01780	EHI_021400	EhRRP6	C4M054	
RRP40	Q9NQT5	EHI_004770	EhRRP40	C4M073	
RRP41	Q9NPD3	EHI_040320	EhRRP41	C4M2G1	
RRP42	Q15024	EHI_000580	EhRRP42	C4LZA9	
RRP43	Q96B26	EHI_188080	EhRRP43	C4M182	
RRP46	Q9NQT4	EHI_086520	EhRRP46	C4M8Y9	
MTR3	Q5RKV6	EHI_126330	EhMTR3	C4LW17	
DIS3	Q9Y2L1	EHI_160720	EhDIS3	C4MAJ9	
NON-SENSE MEDIATED DECAY FACTOR					
UPF1	Q92900	EHI_035550	EhUpf1	C4LXY5	López-Rosas et al., 2012
RNA INTERFERENCE FACTORS					
AGO2	Q9UKV8	EHI_186850	EhAGO2-1	C4LVQ2	Zhang et al., 2008
–	–	EHI_125650	EhAGO2-2	C4LVV2	
–	–	EHI_177170	EhAGO2-3	C4LY31	
–	–	EHI_139420	EhRdRP	C4M6W7	
–	–	EHI_179800	EhRdRP	C4M631	
DICER	Q9UPY3	EHI_068740	EhRNAseIII	C4LU64	Abed and Ankri, 2005; Zhang et al., 2008

[a]*UniProtKB;* [b]*AmoebaDB.*

MOLECULAR EVENTS FOR MRNA DECAY IN *E. HISTOLYTICA*

mRNA Degradation Machineries

E. histolytica has most of the factors that are involved in mRNA degradation in eukaryotic cells, including proteins involved in deadenylation, decapping, and exonuclease activity, but it lacks several components (**Table 3**) (López-Rosas et al., 2012). The reduced mRNA deadenylation machinery includes the CAF1/NOT complex with the five NOT proteins and the poly-A specific ribonucleases CAF1 and CAF1-like, but the carbon catabolite repressor 4 (CCR4) described in yeast and human, as well as PAN2, PAN3, and PARN deadenylases, are missing (**Figure 3**). EhCAF1 is a ribonuclease D family member, having the CAF1 nuclease domain and the conserved DEDD residues ($D_{84}E_{86}D_{206}D_{276}$) that are important for 3′ to 5′ exonuclease activity in homologous proteins (Daugeron et al., 2001). Consequently, EhCAF1 is a functional deadenylase that binds 3′UTR and degrades the poly(A) tail of parasite transcripts in *in vitro* assays (López-Rosas et al., 2014).

Although capping has not been described in *E. histolytica*, bioinformatics analyses revealed the existence of a decapping complex that is formed by the catalytic subunit EhDCP2, and EhXRN2, EhLSM1-6, EhEDC3, and EhDHH1 as decapping associated proteins, whereas it also includes DCP1, SCD6, PAT1, and LSM7 in yeast and animals (**Table 3**; **Figure 3**) (López-Rosas et al., 2012). EhXRN2 and EhDCP2 have the typical architecture of homologous proteins. Notably, EhXRN2 has the XRN_N nuclease domain and the internal tower domain with the active site motif KX_2QQX_2RR, which is critical for ribonuclease function (Xiang et al., 2009). EhDCP2 has the conserved DCP2 box A domain and the conserved nudix Box ($GX_5EX_7REUXEEXGU$) that are both responsible for cap structure removal (She et al., 2008). In eukaryotic cells, the elimination of the 5′ cap compromises mRNA to 5′ to 3′ exonucleolytic decay, apparently in an irreversible way, hence, decapping activity is tightly regulated (Li and Kiledjian, 2010). The heptameric Lsm1-7 complex associates with the 3' end of deadenylated mRNAs and promotes decapping (Tharun et al., 2000; Tharun and Parker, 2001). The activity of the decapping enzyme is stimulated by accessory proteins, such as Edc proteins, the DExD/H-box RNA helicases Dhh1 and Pat1 (Bonnerot et al., 2000; Schwartz et al., 2003).

E. histolytica contains seven exosome encoding genes including Rrp41, Rrp43, Rrp46, Mtr3-Rrp42 and the catalytic subunit Dis3, as well as accessory stabilizing Rrp4, and Rrp40 proteins; but it lacks Rrp45 and Csl4 genes (**Table 3**; **Figure 3**) (López-Rosas et al., 2012). The EhRRP41 protein colocalizes and physically interacts with EhL-PSP, which also interacts and colocalizes with the EhCAF1 deadenylase. But the fact that EhRRP41 did not coimmunoprecipitate with EhCAF1, suggests the existence of two EhL-PSP-containing complexes. The colocalization of exosome factors (EhRrp41) with EhCAF1 and EhL-PSP in trophozoites showed novel interactions between mRNA degradation protein and suggests the existence of cooperative interactions between mRNA decay machineries in *E. histolytica* (López-Rosas et al., 2014). In yeast and human, the nine subunits of the exosome complex form a ring structure in which Dis3 (RRP44) is the key player in mRNA turnover being the catalytic subunit responsible for exonucleolytic and endonucleolytic activities in the 3′-5′ decay of deadenylated transcripts in cytoplasm (Ibrahim et al., 2008). Additionally, the nuclear exosome is involved in 3′-end trimming of rRNA, snRNA, and snoRNA, as well as mRNA surveillance and degradation of cryptic unstable transcripts (Parker and Song, 2004).

E. histolytica genome also contains genes for components of the NMD and RNA interference (RNAi) pathways, namely three Ehupf genes (López-Rosas et al., 2012), as well as two EhRdRP, one EhRNAseIII and three EhAGO2 proteins (Abed and Ankri, 2005; Zhang et al., 2008, 2011), respectively (**Table 3**). The absence of DICER and GW182 homologs suggests that RNA interference may use DICER-independent mechanisms in *E. histolytica* (Zhang et al., 2011). Pompey et al. (2015) recently showed that EhRNAseIII is able to cleave dsRNA to generate shorter fragments in a heterologous system. This suggests that EhRNAseIII in conjunction with other amoebic factors might reconstitute an active DICER-like complex. Congruently, numerous reports involving gene-silencing assays confirmed the functionality of the RNAi pathway in *E. histolytica*.

P-Body-Like Structures

Several experiments suggest that mRNA decay reactions, namely deadenylation, decapping, and 5′-exonucleolytic decay, take place in microscopically detectable cytoplasmic P-bodies like structures in *E. histolytica* (López-Rosas et al., 2012), as it has been described in other eukaryotic cells (Sheth and Parker, 2003). The EhCAF1 deadenylase, EhXRN2 exoribonuclease and EhDCP2 decapping proteins, as well as the EhAGO2-2 protein, were detected in cytoplasmic foci in immunofluorescence and confocal microscopy experiments (López-Rosas et al., 2012). Additionally biochemical analysis revealed that EhCAF1 co-immunoprecipitated with EhXRN2, thus linking deadenylation to 5'-to-3' mRNA degradation. Interestingly, these cytoplasmic structures also contain polyadenylated transcripts and dsRNA, which is congruent with their role in RNA decay. Moreover their formation depends on the presence of active transcription and translation (López-Rosas et al., 2012), as well as cellular stress, such as DNA damage, heat shock, and nitric oxide (López-Rosas et al., 2014), which make them *bona fide* P-body structures (**Figure 3**). Altogether, these data suggest that, as in human cells, the accumulation of transcripts in cytoplasmic P-bodies like structures for silencing or decay, represents a key regulatory process for gene expression regulation in response to specific conditions or signals in *E. histolytica*.

CONCLUSION

Besides the evolutionary distance between *E. histolytica* and its human host, the screening of parasite genome sequences and the functional characterization of specific factors, revealed that molecular mechanisms regulating mRNA processing and degradation seem to be roughly similar in both organisms. Several subtle differences exist, but canonical factors involved in splicing, polyadenylation and decay are generally conserved in this primitive eukaryote, which highlights that these events are key players for gene expression regulation in eukaryotic cells. The study of a larger number of factors involved in splicing, polyadenylation or mRNA degradation remains to be addressed to elucidate all the relationship among these reactions. In addition to contribute to the better understanding of posttranscriptional regulation in *E. histolytica*, the characterization of these factors and events may also lead to the identification of a biochemical target involved in various mRNA processing pathways, whose inhibition would have a massive impact on parasite survival. On the other hand, recent data indicated the potential of factors involved in polyadenylation as biochemical targets for parasite control, which may open the way for the design of new molecules for the control of this parasitic disease. In this context, the results of the proof-of-concept study in *E. histolytica* may promote the use of aptamers to control *E. histolytica* during the development of amoebiasis or to eradicate residual trophozoites during antibiotic treatment. Further experiments are required to confirm their affinity, evaluate their effect *in vivo* and improve their bioavailability.

FUNDING

This study was supported by the Mexico-France program grants ECOS NORD (M14S02) and SEP-CONACYT-ANUIES (249554), and Mexican grants from SIP-IPN (20170969) and CONACyT (178550), Mexico. JO-V was a scholarship recipient of Mexican BEIFI-IPN and CONACyT programs. LM is supported by COFAA-IPN.

AUTHOR CONTRIBUTIONS

JV-F, IL-R, CL-C, ER-M, and JO-V reviewed data about mRNA splicing, polyadenylation and decay, respectively. JO-V designed the figures. CL-C and LM designed the review organization, revised and integrated the different parts of the manuscript.

REFERENCES

Abed, M., and Ankri, S. (2005). Molecular characterization of *Entamoeba histolytica* RNase, III and AGO2, two RNA interference hallmark proteins. *Exp. Parasitol.* 110, 265–269. doi: 10.1016/j.exppara.2005.02.023

Bartschat, S., and Samuelsson, T. (2010). U12 type introns were lost at multiple occasions during evolution. *BMC Genomics* 11:106. doi: 10.1186/1471-2164-11-106

Bonnerot, C., Boeck, R., and Lapeyre, B. (2000). The two proteins Patlp (Mrtlp) and Spb8p interact *in vivo*, are required for mRNA decay, and are functionally linked to Pablp. *Mol. Cell. Biol.* 20, 5939–5946. doi: 10.1128/MCB.20.16.5939-5946.2000

Brown, K. M., and Gilmartin, G. M. (2003). A mechanism for the regulation of pre-mRNA 3' processing by human cleavage factor Im. *Mol. Cell* 12, 1467–1476. doi: 10.1016/S1097-2765(03)00453-2

Bruchhaus, I., Leippe, M., Lioutas, C., and Tannich, E. (1993). Unusual gene organization in the protozoan parasite *Entamoeba histolytica. DNA Cell. Biol.* 12, 925–933.

Calvo, O., and Manley, J. L. (2001). Evolutionarily conserved interaction between CstF-64 and PC4 links transcription, polyadenylation, and termination. *Mol. Cell* 7, 1013–1023. doi: 10.1016/S1097-2765(01)00236-2

Calvo, O., and Manley, J. L. (2003). Strange bedfellows: polyadenylation factors at the promoter. *Genes Dev.* 17, 1321–1327. doi: 10.1101/gad.10 93603

Chan, S. L., Huppertz, I., Yao, C., Weng, L., Moresco, J. J., Yates, J. R. III., et al. (2014). CPSF30 and Wdr33 directly bind to AAUAAA in mammalian mRNA 3' processing. *Genes Dev.* 28, 2370–2380. doi: 10.1101/gad.250993.114

Christie, M., Brosnan, C. A., Rothnagel, J. A., and Carroll, B. J. (2011). RNA decay and RNA silencing in plants: competition or collaboration? *Front. Plant Sci.* 2:99. doi: 10.3389/fpls.2011.00099

Clark, N. E, Katolik, A., Roberts, K. M., Taylor, A. B., Holloway, S. P., Schuermann, J. P., et al. (2016). Metal dependence and branched RNA cocrystal structures of the RNA lariat debranching enzyme Dbr1. *Proc. Natl. Acad. Sci. U.S.A.* 113, 14727–14732. doi: 10.1073/pnas.1612729114

Collins, L., and Penny, D. (2005). Complex spliceosomal organization ancestral to extant eukaryotes. *Mol. Biol. Evol.* 22,1053–1066. doi: 10.1093/molbev/msi091

Conesa, C., and Acker, J. (2010). Subl/PC4 a chromatin associated protein with multiple functions in transcription. *RNA Biol.* 7, 287–290. doi: 10.4161/rna.7.3.11491

Cowling, V. H. (2010). Regulation of mRNA cap methylation. *Biochem. J. 425*, 295–302. doi: 10.1042/BJ20091352

Das, C., Gadad, S. S., and Kundu, T. K. (2010). Human positive coactivator 4 controls heterochromatinization and silencing of neural gene expression by interacting with REST/NRSF and Corest. *J. Mol. Biol.* 397, 1–12. doi: 10.1016/j.jmb.2009.12.058

Das, C., Hizume, K., Batta, K., Kumar, B. R., Gadad, S. S., Ganguly, S., et al. (2006). Transcriptional coactivator pc4, a chromatin-associated protein, induces chromatin condensation. *Mol. Cell. Biol.* 26, 8303–8315. doi: 10.1128/MCB.00887-06

Daugeron, M. C., Mauxion, F., and Séraphin, B. (2001). The yeast POP2 gene encodes a nuclease involved in mRNA deadenylation. *Nucleic Acids Res.* 29, 2448–2455. doi: 10.1093/nar/29.12.2448

David, C.J., Boyne, A. R., Millhouse, S. R., and Manley, J. L. (2011). The RNA polymerase II C-terminal domain promotes splicing activation through recruitment of a U2AF65-Prp19 complex. *Genes Dev.* 25, 972–983. doi: 10.1101/gad.2038011

Dávila López, M., Rosenblad, M. A., and Samuelsson, T. (2008). Computational screen for spliceosomal RNA genes aids in defining the phylogenetic distribution of major and minor spliceosomal components. *Nucleic Acids Res.* 36, 3001–3010. doi: 10.1093/nar/gkn142

Davis, C. A., Brown, M. P., and Singh, U. (2007). Functional characterization of spliceosomal introns and identification of U2, U4, and U5 snRNAs in the deep-branching eukaryote *Entamoeba histolytica*. *Eukaryotic Cell* 6, 940–948. doi: 10.1128/EC.00059-07

de Vries, H., Rüegsegger, U., Hübner, W., Friedlein, A., Langen, H., and Keller, W. (2000). Human pre-mRNA cleavage factor II(m) contains homologs of yeast proteins and bridges two other cleavage factors. *EMBO J.* 19, 5895–5904. doi: 10.1093/emboj/19.21.5895

Di Giammartino, D. C., Li, W., Ogami, K., Yashinskie, J. J., Hoque, M., Tian, B., et al. (2014). RBBP6 isoforms regulate the human polyadenylation machinery and modulate expression of mRNAs with AU-rich 3' UTRs. *Genes Dev.* 28, 2248–2260. doi: 10.1101/gad.245787.114

Eulalio, A., Behm-Ansmant, I., and Izaurralde, E. (2007). P-bodies: at the crossroads of post-transcriptional pathways. *Nat. Rev. Mol. Cell Biol.* 8, 9–22. doi: 10.1038/nrm2080

Förch, P., Puig, O., Martínez, C., Séraphin, B., and Valcárcel, J. (2002). The splicing regulator TIA-1 interacts with U1-C to promote U1 snRNP recruitment to 5' splice sites. *EMBO J.* 21, 6882–6892. doi: 10.1093/emboj/cdf668

Fourmann, J. B., Schmitzová, J., Christian, H., Urlaub, H., Ficner, R., Boon, K. L., et al. (2013). Dissection of the factor requirements for spliceosome disassembly and the elucidation of its dissociation products using a purified splicing system. *Genes Dev.* 27, 413–428. doi: 10.1101/gad.207779.112

Furth, P. A., Choe, W. T., Rex, J. H., Byrne, J. C., and Baker, C. C. (1994). Sequences homologous to 5' splice sites are required for the inhibitory activity of papillomavirus late 3' untranslated regions. *Mol. Cell. Biol.* 14, 5278–5289.

García-Vivas, J., López-Camarillo, C., Azuara-Liceaga, E., Orozco, E., and Marchat, L. A. (2005). *Entamoeba histolytica*: cloning and expression of the poly(A) polymerase EhPAP. *Exp. Parasitol.* 110, 226–232. doi: 10.1016/j.exppara.2005.02.017

Garrey, S. M., Katolik, A., Prekeris, M., Li, X., York, K., Bernards, S., et al. (2014). A homolog of lariat-debranching enzyme modulates turnover of branched RNA. *RNA* 20, 1337–1348. doi: 10.1261/rna.044602.114

Gu, B., Eick, D., and Bensaude, O. (2013). CTD serine-2 plays a critical role in splicing and termination factor recruitment to RNA polymerase II *in vivo*. *Nucleic Acids Res.* 41, 1591–1603. doi: 10.1093/nar/gks1327

Gunderson, S.I., Beyer, K., Martin, G., Keller, W., Boelens,W. C., and Mattaj, L. W. (1994). The human U1A snRNP protein regulates polyadenylation via a direct interaction with poly(A) polymerase. *Cell* 76, 531–541. doi: 10.1016/0092-8674(94)90116-3

Gunderson, S. I., Vagner, S., Polycarpou-Schwarz, M., and Mattaj, I. W. (1997). Involvement of the carboxyl terminus of vertebrate poly(A) polymerase in U1A autoregulation and in the coupling of splicing and polyadenylation. *Genes Dev.* 11, 761–773. doi: 10.1101/gad.11.6.761

Hahn, D., Kudla, G., Tollervey, D., and Beggs, J. D. (2012). Brr2p-mediated conformational rearrangements in the spliceosome during activation and substrate repositioning. *Genes Dev.* 26, 2408–2421. doi: 10.1101/gad.199307.112

Hendriks, E. F., Abdul-Razak, A., and Matthews, K. R. (2003). tbCPSF30 depletion by RNA interference disrupts polycistronic RNA processing in *Trypanosoma* brucei. *J. Biol. Chem.* 278, 26870–26878. doi: 10.1074/jbc.M302405200

Hernández de la Cruz, O., Marchat, L. A., Guillén, N., Weber, C., López Rosas, I., Díaz-Chávez, J., et al. (2016). Multinucleation and polykaryon formation is promoted by the EhPC4 transcription factor in *Entamoeba histolytica. Sci. Rep.* 6:19611. doi: 10.1038/srep19611

Hernandez de la Cruz, O. N., Muñiz-Lino, M., Guillén, N., Weber, C., Marchat, L. A., López-Rosas, I., et al. (2014). Proteomic profiling reveals that EhPC4 transcription factor induces cell migration through upregulation of the 16-kDa actin-binding protein EhABP16 in *Entamoeba histolytica*. *J. Proteomics* 111, 46–58. doi: 10.1016/j.jprot.2014.03.041

Hernández-Rivas, R., Ramírez, C., Guillén, N., and Vargas, M. (2000). DNA cloning of the *Entamoeba histolytica* PRP6 gene: a putative U4/U6 small nuclear ribonucleoprotein particle (snRNP). *Arch. Med. Res.* 31, S294–295. doi: 10.1016/S0188-4409(00)00119-3

Hon, C. C., Weber, C., Sismeiro, O., Proux, C., Koutero, M., Deloger, M., et al. (2013). Quantification of stochastic noise of splicing and polyadenylation in *Entamoeba histolytica*. *Nucleic Acids Res.* 41, 1936–1952. doi: 10.1093/nar/gks1271

Huang, S. C., Ou, A. C., Park, J., Yu, F., Yu, B., Lee, A., et al. (2012). RBFOX2 promotes protein 4.1R exon 16 selection via U1 snRNP recruitment. *Mol. Cell. Biol.* 32, 513–526. doi: 10.1128/MCB.06423-11

Ibrahim, H., Wilusz, J., and Wilusz, C. J. (2008). RNA recognition by 3'-to-5' exonucleases: the substrate perspective. *Biochim. Biophys. Acta* 1779, 256–265. doi: 10.1016/j.bbagrm.2007.11.004

Isken, O., and Maquat, L. E. (2008). The multiple lives of NMD factors: balancing roles in gene and genome regulation. *Nat. Rev. Genet.* 9, 699–712. doi: 10.1038/nrg2402

Kandels-Lewis, S., and Séraphin, B. (1993). Involvement of U6 snRNA in 5' splice site selection. *Science* 262, 2035–2039. doi: 10.1126/science.8266100

Kubo, T., Wada, T., Yamaguchi, Y., Shimizu, A., and Handa, H. (2006). Knock-down of 25 kDa subunit of cleavage factor Im in Hela cells alters alternative polyadenylation within 30-UTRs. *Nucleic Acids Res.* 34, 6264–6271. doi: 10.1093/nar/gkl794

Kyburz, A., Friedlein, A., Langen, H., and Keller, W. (2006). Direct interactions between subunits of CPSF and the U2 snRNP contribute to the coupling of pre-mRNA 3' end processing and splicing. *Mol. Cell* 23, 195–205. doi: 10.1016/j.molcel.2006.05.037

Łabno, A., Tomecki, R., and Dziembowski, A. (2016). Cytoplasmic RNA decay pathways - Enzymes and mechanisms. *Biochim. Biophys. Acta* 1863, 3125–3147. doi: 10.1016/j.bbamcr.2016.09.023

Larson, J. D., and Hoskins, A. A. (2017). Dynamics and consequences of spliceosome E complex formation. *Elife* 6:e27592. doi: 10.7554/eLife.27592

Li, Y., and Kiledjian, M. (2010). Regulation of mRNA decapping. *Wiley Interdiscip. Rev. RNA* 1, 253–265. doi: 10.1002/wrna.15

Liu, Z. R. (2002). p68 RNA helicase is an essential human splicing factor that acts at the U1 snRNA-5' splice site duplex. *Mol. Cell. Biol.* 22, 5443–5450. doi: 10.1128/MCB.22.15.5443-5450.2002

Loftus, B., Anderson, I., Davies, R., Alsmark, U. C., Samuelson, J., Amedeo, P., et al. (2005). The genome of the protist parasite *Entamoeba histolytica*. *Nature* 433, 865–868. doi: 10.1038/nature03291

López-Camarillo, C., López-Rosas, I., Ospina-Villa, J. D., and Marchat, L. A. (2014). Deciphering molecular mechanisms of mRNA metabolism in the deep-branching eukaryote *Entamoeba histolytica*. *Wiley Interdiscip. Rev. RNA* 5, 247–262. doi: 10.1002/wrna.1205

López-Camarillo, C., Luna-Arias, J. P., Marchat, L. A., and Orozco,. E. (2003). EhPgp5 mRNA stability is a regulatory event in the *Entamoeba histolytica* multidrug resistance phenotype. *J. Biol. Chem.* 278, 11273–11280. doi: 10.1074/jbc.M211757200

López-Camarillo, C., Marchat, L. A., Orozco, E., Azuara-Liceaga, E., and García-Vivas, J. (2007). "Canonical and non canonical poly(A) polymerases: from human to the protozoan parasite *Entamoeba histolytica*," in *Messenger RNA Research Perspectives*, ed T. Takeyama (Hauppauge, NY: Nova Publishers), 125–144.

López-Camarillo, C., Orozco, E., and Marchat, L. A. (2005). *Entamoeba histolytica*: comparative genomics of the pre-mRNA 3' end processing machinery. *Exp. Parasitol.* 110, 184–190. doi: 10.1016/j.exppara.2005.02.024

López-Rosas, I., Marchat, L. A., Olvera, B. G., Guillen, N., Weber, C., Hernández de la Cruz, O., et al. (2014). Proteomic analysis identifies endoribouclease EhL-PSP and EhRRP41 exosome protein as novel interactors of EhCAF1 deadenylase. *J. Proteomics* 111, 59–73. doi: 10.1016/j.jprot.2014.06.019

López-Rosas, I., Orozco, E., Marchat, L. A., García-Rivera, G., Guillen, N., Weber, C., et al. (2012). mRNA decay proteins are targeted to poly(A)+RNA and dsRNA-containing cytoplasmic foci that resemble P-bodies in Entamoeba histolytica. *PLoS ONE* 7:e45966. doi: 10.1371/journal.pone.0045966

Lutz, C. S., Murthy, K. G., Schek, N., O'Connor, J. P., Manley, J. L., and Alwine, J. C. (1996). Interaction between the U1 snRNP-A protein and the 160-kD subunit of cleavage-polyadenylation specificity factor increases polyadenylation efficiency *in vitro*. *Genes Dev.* 10, 325–337.

Mandel, C. R., Kaneko, S., Zhang, H., Gebauer, D., Vethantham, V., Manley, J. L., et al. (2006). Polyadenylation factor CPSF-73 is the pre-mRNA 3'-end-processing endonuclease. *Nature* 444, 53–56. doi: 10.1038/nature05363

Marchat, L. A., Orozco, E., Guillen, N., Weber, C., and López-Camarillo, C. (2008). Putative DEAD and DExH-box RNA helicases families in Entamoeba histolytica. *Gene* 424, 1–10. doi: 10.1016/j.gene.2008.07.042

Matange, N., Podobnik, M., and Visweswariah, S. S. (2015). Metallophosphoesterases: structural fidelity with functional promiscuity. *Biochem. J.* 467, 201–216. doi: 10.1042/BJ20150028

McGuire, A. M., Pearson, M. D., Neafsey, D. E., and Galagan, J. E. (2008). Cross-kingdom patterns of alternative splicing and splice recognition. *Genome Biol.* 9:R50. doi: 10.1186/gb-2008-9-3-r50

Millevoi, S., Loulergue, C., Dettwiler, S., Karaa, S. Z., Keller, W., Antoniou, M., et al. (2006). An interaction between U2AF 65 and CF I(m) links the splicing and 3' end processing machineries. *EMBO J.* 25, 4854–4864. doi: 10.1038/sj.emboj.7601331

Miranda, R., Salgado, L. M., Sánchez-López, R., Alagón, A., and Lizardi, P. M. (1996). Identification and analysis of the u6 small nuclear RNA gene from *Entamoeba histolytica*. *Gene* 180, 37–42. doi: 10.1016/S0378-1119(96)003 97-6

Montemayor, E. J., Katolik, A., Clark, N. E., Taylor, A. B., Schuermann, J.P., Combs, D. J., et al. (2014). Structural basis of lariat RNA recognition by the intron debranching enzyme Dbr1. *Nucleic Acids Res.* 42, 10845–10855. doi: 10.1093/nar/gku725

Murthy, K. G., and Manley, J. L. (1995). The 160-kD subunit of human cleavage-polyadenylation specificity factor coordinates pre-mRNA 3'-end formation. *Genes Dev.* 9, 2672–2683. doi: 10.1101/gad.9.21.2672

Ospina-Villa, J. D., Dufour, A., Weber, C., Ramirez-Moreno, E., Zamorano-Carrillo, E., Guillen, N., et al. (2018). Targeting the polyadenylation factor EhCFIm25 with RNA aptamers controls survival in *Entamoeba histolytica*. *Sci. Rep.* 8:5720. doi: 10.1038/s41598-018-23997-w

Ospina-Villa, J. D., Guillén, N., Lopez-Camarillo, C., Soto-Sanchez, J., Ramirez-Moreno, E., Garcia-Vazquez, R., et al. (2017). Silencing the cleavage factor CFIm25 as a new strategy to control *Entamoeba histolytica* parasite. *J. Microbiol.* 55, 783–791. doi: 10.1007/s12275-017-72 59-9

Ospina-Villa, J. D., Zamorano-Carrillo, A., Lopez-Camarillo, C., Castañon-Sanchez, C. A., Soto-Sanchez, J., Ramirez-Moreno, E., et al. (2015). Amino acid residues Leu135 and Tyr236 are required for RNA binding activity of CFIm25 in Entamoeba histolytica. *Biochimie* 115, 44–51. doi: 10.1016/j.biochi.2015.04.017

Palencia, A., Bougdour, A., Brenier-Pinchart, M. P., Touquet, B., Bertini, R. L., Sensi, C., et al. (2017). Targeting *Toxoplasma gondii* CPSF3 as a new approach to control toxoplasmosis. *EMBO Mol. Med.* 9, 385–394. doi: 10.15252/emmm.201607370

Parker, R., and Song, H. (2004). The enzymes and control of eukaryotic mRNA turnover. *Nat. Struct. Mol. Biol.* 11, 121–127. doi: 10.1038/nsmb724

Pezet-Valdez, M., Fernández-Retana, J., Ospina-Villa, J. D., Ramírez-Moreno, M. E., Orozco, E., Charcas-López, S., et al. (2013). The 25 kDa subunit of cleavage factor Im Is a RNA-binding protein that interacts with the poly(A) polymerase in *Entamoeba histolytica*. *PLoS ONE* 8:e67977. doi: 10.1371/journal.pone.0067977

Pompey, J. M., Foda, B., and Singh, U. (2015). A Single RNaseIII Domain Protein from *Entamoeba histolytica* Has dsRNA cleavage activity and can help mediate RNAi gene silencing in a heterologous system. *PLoS ONE* 10:e0133740. doi: 10.1371/journal.pone.0133740

Raabe, T., Bollum, F. J., and Manley, J. L. (1991). Primary structure and expression of bovine poly(A) polymerase. *Nature* 353, 229–234.

Ramanathan, A., Robb, G. B., and Chan, S. H. (2016). mRNA capping: biological functions and applications. *Nucleic Acids Res.* 44, 7511–7526. doi: 10.1093/nar/gkw551

Ransey, E., Paredes, E., Dey, S. K., Das, S. R., Heroux, A., and Macbeth, M. R. (2017). Crystal structure of the *Entamoeba histolytica* RNA lariat debranching enzyme EhDbr1 reveals a catalytic Zn(2+) /Mn(2+) heterobinucleation. *FEBS Lett.* 591, 2003–2010. doi: 10.1002/1873-3468.12677

Rebbapragada, I., and Lykke-Andersen, J. (2009). Execution of nonsense-mediated mRNA decay: what defines a substrate? *Curr. Opin. Cell Biol.* 21, 394–402. doi: 10.1016/j.ceb.2009.02.007

Rhode, B.M., Hartmuth, K., Westhof, E., and Lührmann R. (2006). Proximity of conserved U6 and U2 snRNA elements to the 5' splice site region in activated spliceosomes. *EMBO J.* 25, 2475–2486. doi: 10.1038/sj.emboj.76 01134

Santi-Rocca, J., Weber, C., Guigon, G., Sismeiro, O., Coppée, J. Y., and Guillén, N. (2008). The lysine- and glutamic acid-rich protein KERP1 plays a role in *Entamoeba histolytica* liver abscess pathogenesis. *Cell. Microbiol.* 10,202–217. doi: 10.1111/j.1462-5822.2007.01030.x

Schonemann, L., Kuhn, U., Martin, G., Schafer, P., Gruber, A. R., Keller, W., et al. (2014). Reconstitution of CPSF active in polyadenylation: recognition of the polyadenylation signal by WDR33. *Genes Dev.* 28, 2381–2293. doi: 10.1101/gad.250985.114

Schwartz, D., Decker, C. J., and Parker, R. (2003). The enhancer of decapping proteins, Edc1p and Edc2p, bind RNA and stimulate the activity of the decapping enzyme. *RNA* 9, 239–251. doi: 10.1261/rna.2171203

Schwer, B., Khalid, F., and Shuman, S. (2016). Mechanistic insights into the manganese-dependent phosphodiesterase activity of yeast Dbr1 with bis-p-nitrophenylphosphate and branched RNA substrates. *RNA* 22, 1819–1827. doi: 10.1261/rna.05855 2.116

She, M., Decker, C. J., Svergun, D. I., Round, A., Chen, N., Muhlrad D., et al. (2008). Structural basis of dcp2 recognition and activation by dcp1. *Mol. Cell.* 29, 337–349. doi: 10.1016/j.molcel.2008.01.002

Sheth, U., and Parker, R. (2003). Deccaping and decay of RNAs occur in cytoplasmic processing bodies. *Science* 300, 805–808. doi: 10.1126/science.1082320

Shi, Y. (2017). Mechanistic insights into precursor messenger RNA splicing by the spliceosome. *Nat. Rev. Mol. Cell Biol.* 18, 655–670. doi: 10.1038/nrm.20 17.86

Sidik, S. M., Huet, D., Ganesan, S. M., Huynh, M. H., Wang, T., Nasamu, A. S., et al. (2016). A Genome-wide CRISPR Screen in Toxoplasma identifies essential apicomplexan genes. *Cell* 166, 1423–1435. doi: 10.1016/j.cell.2016.0 8.019

Sonoiki, E., Ng, C. L., Lee, M. C., Guo, D., Zhang, Y. K., Zhou, Y., et al. (2017). A potent antimalarial benzoxaborole targets a *Plasmodium falciparum* cleavage and polyadenylation specificity factor homologue. *Nat. Commun.* 8:14574. doi: 10.1038/ncomms14574

Tharun, S., He, W., Mayes, A. E., Lennertz, P., Beggs, J. D., and Parker, R. (2000). Yeast Sm-like proteins function in mRNA decapping and decay. *Nature* 404, 515–518. doi: 10.1038/35006676

Tharun, S., and Parker, R. (2001). Targeting an mRNA for decapping: displacement of translation factors and association of the Lsm1p−7p complex on deadenylated yeast mRNAs. *Mol. Cell* 8, 1075–1083. doi: 10.1016/S1097-2765(01)00395-1

Urban, B., Blasig, C., Förster, B., Hamelmann, C., and Horstmann, R.D. (1996). Putative serine/threonine protein kinase expressed in complement-resistant forms of *Entamoeba histolytica*. *Mol. Biochem. Parasitol.* 80, 171–178. doi: 10.1016/0166-6851(96)02684-9

Vagner, S., Vagner, C., and Mattaj, I. W. (2000). The carboxyl terminus of vertebrate poly(A) polymerase interacts with U2AF 65 to couple 3'-end processing and splicing. *Genes Dev.* 14, 403–413.

Valdés, J., Nozaki, T., Sato, E., Chiba, Y., Nakada-Tsukui, K., Villegas-Sepúlveda, N., et al. (2014). Proteomic analysis of *Entamoeba histolytica in vivo* assembled pre-mRNA splicing complexes. *J. Proteomics* 111, 30–45. doi: 10.1016/j.jprot.2014.07.027

Wahl, M. C., and Luhrmann, R. (2015). SnapShot: spliceosome dynamics, I. *Cell* 162:690.e1. doi: 10.1016/j.cell.2015.07.033

Wahle, E. (1991). A novel poly(A)-binding protein acts as a specificity factor in the second phase of messenger RNA polyadenylation. *Cell* 66, 759–768. doi: 10.1016/0092-8674(91)90119-J

Weedall, G. D., and Hall, N. (2011). Evolutionary genomics of *Entamoeba*. *Res. Microbiol.* 162, 637–645. doi: 10.1016/j.resmic.2011.01.007

West, S., and Proudfoot, N. J. (2008). Human Pcf11 enhances degradation of RNA polymerase II-associated nascent RNA and transcriptional termination. *Nucleic Acids Res.* 36, 905–914. doi: 10.1093/nar/gkm1112

Wilihoeft, U., Campos-Góngora, E., Touzni, S., Bruchhaus, I., and Tannich, E. (2001). Introns of *Entamoeba histolytica* and *Entamoeba dispar*. *Protist* 152, 149–156. doi: 10.1078/1434-4610-00053

Xiang, K., Tong, L., and Manley, J. L. (2014). Delineating the structural blueprint of the pre-mRNA 3'-end processing machinery. *Mol. Cell. Biol. J.* 34, 1894–1910. doi: 10.1128/MCB.00084-14

Xiang, S., Cooper-Morgan, A., Jiao, X., Kiledjian, M., Manley, J. L., Tong L et al. (2009). Structure and function of the 5'→ 3' exoribonuclease Rat1 and its activating partner Rai1. *Nature* 458, 784–788. doi: 10.1038/nature07731

Yang, Q., Gilmartin, G. M., and Doublié. S. (2011). The structure of human cleavage factor I(m) hints at functions beyond UGUA-specific RNA binding: a role in alternative polyadenylation and a potential link to 5' capping and splicing. *RNA Biol.* 8, 748–753. doi: 10.4161/rna.8.5.16040

Yoshimoto, R., Kataoka, N., Okawa, K., and Ohno, M. (2009). Isolation and characterization of post-splicing lariat-intron complexes. *Nucleic Acids Res.* 37, 891–902. doi: 10.1093/nar/gkn1002

Zamorano, A., López-Camarillo, C., Orozco, E., Weber, C., Guillen, N., and Marchat, L A. (2008). *In silico* analysis of EST and genomic sequences allowed the prediction of cis-regulatory elements for *Entamoeba histolytica* mRNA polyadenylation. *Comput. Biol. Chem.* 32, 256–263. doi: 10.1016/j.compbiolchem.2008.03.019

Zhang, H., Ehrenkaufer, G. M., Pompey, J. M., Hackney, J. A., and Singh, U (2008). Small RNAs with 5′ -polyphosphate termini associate with a piwi-related protein and regulate gene expression in the single-celled eukaryote *Entamoeba histolytica*. *PLoS Pathog.* 4:e1000219. doi: 10.1371/journal.ppat.1000219

Zhang, H., Pompey, J. M., and Singh, U (2011). RNA interference in *Entamoeba histolytica*: implications for parasite biology and gene silencing. *Future Microbiol.* 61, 103–117. doi: 10.2217/fmb.10.154

12

Epithelial Cells Expressing EhADH, An *Entamoeba histolytica* Adhesin, Exhibit Increased Tight Junction Proteins

Abigail Betanzos[1,2*]*, Dxinegueela Zanatta*[2]*, Cecilia Bañuelos*[3]*,*
Elizabeth Hernández-Nava[4]*, Patricia Cuellar*[5] *and Esther Orozco*[2*]

[1] *Consejo Nacional de Ciencia y Tecnología, Mexico City, Mexico,* [2] *Departamento de Infectómica y Patogénesis Molecular, Centro de Investigación y de Estudios Avanzados del Instituto Politécnico Nacional, Mexico City, Mexico,* [3] *Coordinación General de Programas de Posgrado Multidisciplinarios, Programa de Doctorado Transdisciplinario en Desarrollo Científico y Tecnológico para la Sociedad, Centro de Investigación y de Estudios Avanzados del Instituto Politécnico Nacional, Mexico City, Mexico,* [4] *Programa de Cáncer de Ovario, Instituto Nacional de Cancerología, Mexico City, Mexico,* [5] *Centro Regional de Educación Superior, Universidad Autónoma de Guerrero, Chilpancingo, Mexico*

***Correspondence:**
Abigail Betanzos
abetanzosfe@conacyt.mx
Esther Orozco
esther@cinvestav.mx

In *Entamoeba histolytica*, the EhADH adhesin together with the EhCP112 cysteine protease, form a 124 kDa complex named EhCPADH. This complex participates in trophozoite adherence, phagocytosis and cytolysis of target cells. EhCPADH and EhCP112 are both involved on epithelium damage, by opening tight junctions (TJ) and reaching other intercellular junctions. EhADH is a scaffold protein belonging to the ALIX family that contains a Bro1 domain, expresses at plasma membrane, endosomes and cytoplasm of trophozoites, and is also secreted to the medium. Contribution of EhADH to TJ opening still remains unknown. In this paper, to elucidate the role of EhADH on epithelium injury, we followed two strategies: producing a recombinant protein (rEhADH) and transfecting the *ehadh* gene in MDCK cells. Results from the first strategy revealed that rEhADH reached the intercellular space of epithelial cells and co-localized with claudin-1 and occludin at TJ region; later, rEhADH was mainly internalized by clathrin-coated vesicles. In the second strategy, MDCK cells expressing EhADH (MDCK-EhADH) showed the adhesin at plasma membrane. In addition, MDCK-EHADH cells exhibited adhesive features, producing epithelial aggregation and adherence to erythrocytes, as described in trophozoites. Surprisingly, the adhesin expression produced an increase of claudin-1, occludin, ZO-1 and ZO-2 at TJ, and also the transepithelial electric resistance (TEER), which is a measure of TJ gate function. Moreover, MDCK-EhADH cells resulted more susceptible to trophozoites attack, as showed by TEER and cytopathic experiments. Overall, our results indicated that EhADH disturbed TJ from the extracellular space and also intracellularly, suggesting that EhADH affects by itself TJ proteins, and possibly synergizes the action of other parasite molecules during epithelial invasion.

Keywords: MDCK cells, EhCPADH, amoebiasis, trophozoites, epithelial barrier, transepithelial electrical resistance, intercellular junctions

INTRODUCTION

Entamoeba histolytica is the protozoan responsible for human amoebiasis that infects 50 million people and kills between 30 and 100 thousand individuals around the world (Singh et al., 2016). Amoebiasis is characterized by acute diarrhea due to the substantial damage of the colonic epithelium produced by *E. histolytica* trophozoites (Cornick and Chadee, 2017). Trophozoites attach to and displace over the epithelium, contacting the epithelial cell surface. Then, they open the intercellular spaces by gradual separation of adjacent cells. Subsequently, epithelial cells are detached from the substrate and phagocytosed by the parasite (Martínez-Palomo et al., 1985). Several molecules are involved in this process, such as Gal/GalNAc lectin, amoebapores, cysteine and serine proteases, prostaglandin E2 (PGE2), the EhCPADH complex, among others (Chadee et al., 1987; Leippe, 1997; García-Rivera et al., 1999; Meléndez-López et al., 2007; Lejeune et al., 2011; Cornick et al., 2016).

Tight junctions (TJ) regulate ion and macromolecules flux across the epithelium, and also constitute the first barrier that pathogens face during host invasion. TJ are composed by integral proteins (e.g., claudins, occludin and junctional adhesion molecules) bound to the actin-cytoskeleton by cortical proteins, such as ZO-1,−2, and−3 (Capaldo et al., 2014).

The initial epithelial damage produced by *E. histolytica* is characterized by TJ opening, reflected as a dramatic drop of transepithelial electrical resistance (TEER) (Martínez-Palomo et al., 1985; Leroy et al., 2000; Betanzos et al., 2013), with the participation of PGE2 (Lejeune et al., 2011) and EhCPADH (Betanzos et al., 2013). PGE2 increases ion permeability by altering claudin-4 (Lejeune et al., 2011), while the EhCPADH complex affects claudin-1 and occludin (Betanzos et al., 2013). EhCPADH also damages adherens junctions (AJ) and desmosomes (DSM) (Hernández-Nava et al., 2017), structures that reinforce adhesion among epithelial cells, participate in cell polarity establishment and constitute centers of intracellular signaling (Capaldo et al., 2014).

The EhCPADH complex (Arroyo and Orozco, 1987), formed by an adhesin (EhADH) and a cysteine protease (EhCP112), participates in adhesion, cytolysis and phagocytosis of target cells (García-Rivera et al., 1999). EhCPADH, EhADH, and EhCP112 are secreted during trophozoite attack (Ocádiz et al., 2005; Bolaños et al., 2016). Moreover, an EhCP112 recombinant protein drops TEER of epithelial cells, and dislocates and degrades junctional molecules, including claudin-1, claudin-2, β-catenin, E-cadherin, desmoplakin-I/II and desmoglein-2 (Cuellar et al., 2017; Hernández-Nava et al., 2017).

EhADH contains a Bro1 domain (residues 9–349), characteristic of ALIX family members which are scaffold and multifunctional proteins (Odorizzi, 2006; Morita et al., 2007; Bissig and Gruenberg, 2014). Besides to its adhesive properties, EhADH is also an accessory protein of the endosomal sorting complex required for transport (ESCRT) machinery, whose components are pivotal players during phagocytosis in trophozoites (Avalos-Padilla et al., 2015, 2018). EhADH is localized at plasma membrane and endosomal compartments, and together with ESCRT members, contributes to multivesicular bodies formation (Bañuelos et al., 2012; Avalos-Padilla et al., 2015). Moreover, EhADH associates to cholesterol-trafficking proteins EhNPC1 and EhNPC2, suggesting an extra role in the uptake and transport of this essential lipid toward cellular membranes (Bolaños et al., 2016). Monoclonal antibodies (mAbAdh) against the C-terminal adherence domain (residues 480–600) of this protein (Montaño et al., 2017), inhibit trophozoite adhesion to and phagocytosis of erythrocytes, as well as destruction of MDCK cell monolayers (García-Rivera et al., 1999). However, the specific role of EhADH on epithelium damage has not been fully studied. What does the parasite protein do when it reaches the epithelium? Does it penetrate the target cell? If so, what does the adhesin carry out inside the cell? To approach these questions, we followed two different strategies: (i) we produced a recombinant protein (rEhADH) to scrutinize the effects of EhADH alone on epithelial cell monolayers, and (ii) we generated epithelial cells stably transfected with the *ehadh* gene (MDCK-EhADH) to evaluate EhADH effects within the cells.

Our findings showed rEhADH reaching the intercellular space of epithelial cells, co-localizing at TJ with claudin-1 and occludin. This protein was mainly internalized by clathrin-coated vesicles to MDCK cells. Meanwhile, MDCK cells expressing EhADH, exhibited epithelial aggregation and an increased adhesion to erythrocytes. Furthermore, EhADH mainly altered the amount of claudin-1 and occludin, reflected as an increase of TEER. Interestingly, we found that MDCK-EhADH cells resulted more susceptible to live trophozoites during TEER and cytopathic assays, than control cells. Thus, we suspect that EhADH, which preserved its adhesive properties within MDCK-EhADH cells, could be in some way preparing to epithelial cells for the trophozoites attack mediated by other virulence factors, whose identity and role on the concerted mechanism of epithelium damage should be further addressed.

MATERIALS AND METHODS

Antibodies

For EhADH immunodetection, we obtained rabbit polyclonal antibodies (α-EhADH) against a specific EhADH peptide (N-566 QCVINLLKEFDNTKNI 582-C) localized within the adherence domain. New Zealand male rabbits were immunized three times (each 2 weeks) with 300 μg of this peptide diluted in TiterMax® Gold Adjuvant liquid (Sigma). Other primary antibodies used were: mouse against EhADH (mAbAdh) (Arroyo and Orozco, 1987), α-actin (kindly donated by Dr. José Manuel Hernández from Department of Cellular Biology, CINVESTAV, Mexico), α-claudin-1 (Invitrogen), α-occludin (Invitrogen) and α-caveolin-1 (Santa Cruz Biotechnology); rabbit α-ZO-2 (Invitrogen), α-ZO-1 (Invitrogen), α-occludin (Invitrogen), α-α/β tubulin (Cell Signaling), and α-PCNA (Azuara-Liceaga et al., 2018); and goat α-clathrin (Santa Cruz Biotechnology) and α-GAPDH (Santa Cruz Biotechnology). For some experiments, mouse IgM isotype control (Thermo Fisher) was used. Secondary antibodies included: α-rabbit, α-mouse and α-goat HRP-labeled IgG (1:10,000) (Life technologies); and α-rabbit, α-mouse and α-goat FITC-, TRITC- and Cy5-labeled IgM, and IgG (1:100) (Zymed) antibodies.

Cell Cultures

Trophozoites of *E. histolytica* strain HM1:IMSS clone A (Orozco et al., 1983) were axenically cultured at 37°C in TYI-S-33 medium and harvested during the logarithmic growth phase by chilling the culture tubes for 10 min in an ice-water bath. Then, trophozoites were collected by centrifugation at 360 × g for 5 min (Diamond et al., 1978).

Madin Darby canine kidney (MDCK) epithelial cells type I (Cereijido et al., 1978) and human colorectal adenocarcinoma (Caco-2) from the C2BBe1 lineage (Sambuy et al., 2005) were grown in DMEM medium (Gibco) supplemented with 100 IU/ml penicillin (*in vitro*), 100 mg/ml streptomycin (*in vitro*), 10% fetal bovine serum (Gibco), and 0.08 U/ml rapid-acting insulin (Eli Lilly), at 37°C in a 95% air and 5% CO_2 atmosphere (Betanzos et al., 2013). Transfected MDCK cells were cultured in DMEM medium supplemented with 0.5 mg/ml G-418 (Gibco), a neomycin derivative.

Construction of Plasmids and Production of rEhADH

A DNA fragment of 2061 bp encoding the full-length of *E. histolytica ehadh* gene, was PCR amplified from the *pExEhNeo-Ehadh112* plasmid (Bañuelos et al., 2005) using the oligonucleotides described in **Table 1**. The *ehadh* gene was cloned into the *pGEX6P1* and *pcDNA3* plasmids (Invitrogen) between *BamHI* and *Xho1*, or *KpnI* and *BamH1* digestion sites, respectively. *Escherichia coli* C43 (DE3) and -DH5α bacteria (Invitrogen) were transformed with *pGEX6P1-ehadh* and *pcDNA3-ehadh*, respectively. Plasmids were purified by an affinity column (Qiagen) and automatically sequenced to corroborate the *ehadh* gene sequence.

To produce an EhADH recombinant protein (rEhADH), *E. coli* C43 (DE3) bacteria were transformed with the *pGEX6P1-ehadh* plasmid. The recombinant protein was induced with 1 mM IPTG and purified as described (Bañuelos et al., 2012).

Transfection Assays

Transfection of *pcDNA3-ehadh* or *pcDNA3* plasmids into MDCK cells was performed with the Lipofectamine® 2,000 transfection reagent (Invitrogen), following the manufacturer's instructions. Positive clones were selected after 48 h transfection using 1 mg/ml of G-418 in the culture medium. After 3 weeks, the antibiotic was diminished to 0.5 mg/ml.

RT-PCR Experiments

Total RNA from non-transfected and transfected MDCK cells was isolated by TRIzol® Reagent (Invitrogen). cDNAs were reverse-transcribed from 1 μg of total RNAs using M-MLV Reverse Transcriptase (Promega) and following the manufacturer's instructions. Then, PCR for *ehadh, neo,* and *gapdh* (as internal control) genes were performed with the oligonucleotides described in **Table 1**. PCR amplifications were done following standard procedures for cycling conditions that included an initial denaturing step at 94°C for 1 min, followed by 30 cycles of 94°C for 1 min, 50, 60, or 65°C (according to respective Tm) for 1 min, and 72°C for 1 min, with a final extension step at 72°C for 7 min. Products were separated by electrophoresis in 1% agarose gels and revealed by ethidium bromide staining (Bolaños et al., 2016).

Cellular Extracts

Bacteria were lysed with 2% sarcosyl and 0.5% Triton X-100 in PBS by sonication at 4°C.

Trophozoites were washed twice with ice-cold PBS (140 mM NaCl, 2.7 mM KCl, 10 mM Na_2HPO_4, 1.8 mM KH_2PO_4, pH 7.4) and lysed by freeze-thawing in the presence of 100 mM p-hydroxymercuribenzoate (PHMB) and 40 μg/ml of E-64 (García-Rivera et al., 1999).

MDCK cells were collected with a rubber policeman, washed three times with ice-cold PBS and lysed for 30 min in RIPA buffer (40 mM Tris-HCl pH 7.6, 150 mM NaCl, 2 mM EDTA, 10% glycerol, 1% Triton X-100, 0.5% sodium deoxycholate, 0.2% SDS, 1 mM PMSF and the Complete™ [Roche] protease inhibitor cocktail) under continuous and vigorous shaking. Extracts were

TABLE 1 | Oligonucleotide sequences.

Complete gene		Sequence primer	TM (°C)	Restriction enzyme	Plasmid
ehadh	F	GG<u>GGTACC</u>TATGAATAGACAATTCATTCCTGAA	69	*KpnI*	*pGEX6P1*
	R	CG<u>GGATCC</u>TTAAAGAGATGGAAACATAGGATTG		*BamH1*	
ehadh	F	CG<u>GGATCC</u>ATGAATAGACAATTCATTCCT	72	*BamH1*	*pcDNA3*
	R	AG<u>CTCGAG</u>TTAAAGAGATGGA		*Xho1*	

RT-PCR		Sequence primer	TM (°C)	Amplicon size (bp)
ehadh	F	CATACCAATGAGAAAGTCAGATCC	65	796
	R	C GAGCACATCCTAACGCTAAGG		
neo	F	ATGATTGAACAAGATGG	50	650
	R	TTAGAAGAACTCGTC		
gapdh	F	TCCTGCACCACCAACTGCTT	60	100
	R	GGCATGGACGGTGGTCATGA		

Restriction enzyme sites are underlined. F, forward; R, reverse.

sonicated three times for 30 s and centrifuged for 15 min at 25,000 × g to eliminate undissolved cellular debris (Betanzos et al., 2013).

Western Blot Assays

Protein samples were separated by 6, 8, 10, or 15% sodium dodecyl sulfate polyacrylamide gel electrophoresis (SDS-PAGE), subsequently transferred onto nitrocellulose membranes and incubated 1 h with 5% non-fat milk. Blotting were performed overnight (ON) with mouse mAbAdh (1:50), α-claudin-1 (1:1,000) or α-actin (1:1,500); rabbit α-EhADH (1:3,000), α-occludin (1:1,000), α-ZO-1 (1:500), α-ZO-2 (1:800) or α-tubulin (1:3,000); or goat α-GAPDH (1:10,000) antibodies. Then, we used HRP-conjugated secondary antibodies against mouse IgM and IgG, rabbit IgG or goat IgG, followed by a chemiluminiscence detection system (ECL-Plus kit; Amersham Pharmacia Biotech). Protein bands were visualized on a MicroChemi System (DNR Bio-Imaging), and densitometry analysis were performed using the ImageJ software.

Interaction of Epithelial Cells With Recombinant Proteins

Confluent and sparse MDCK and Caco-2 cell monolayers were apically incubated with 10 $\mu g/cm^2$ of rEhADH or rEhPCNA (Cardona-Felix et al., 2011) for different times at 37°C. After interaction, epithelial cells were washed five times with PBS (140 mM NaCl, 2.7 mM KCl, 10 mM Na_2HPO_4, 1.8 mM KH_2PO_4, pH 6.8) to eliminate unbound molecules, and treated for immunofluorescence assays as described below.

In the case of rEhADH, it was Alexa Fluor 647-labeled using the Antibodies Labeling Kit (Molecular Probes), following the manufacturer's instructions. Briefly, 100 μg of rEhADH were equilibrated with 0.1 M sodium bicarbonate to allow the adequate succinimidyl ester reaction with primary amines of the protein, to form stable dye-protein conjugates (Cuellar et al., 2017).

Immunofluorescence Assays

MDCK and Caco-2 cell monolayers grown on glass coverslips were fixed and permeabilized with absolute ethanol for 30 min at −20°C. Cells were blocked for 30 min with 0.5% BSA and 0.05% saponin, and then incubated ON at 4°C with mouse α-claudin-1 (1:25), mouse α-occludin (1:1,000), rabbit α-EhADH (1:100), rabbit α-ZO-1 (1:100) or rabbit α-ZO-2 (1:100) antibodies. For co-localization experiments, monolayers were incubated with mouse mAbAdh (1:10), rabbit α-EhADH (1:100) or rabbit α-PCNA (1:100), and mouse α-caveolin-1 (1:100), goat α-clathrin (1:100), mouse α-claudin-1 (1:25), mouse α-occludin (1:1,000), rabbit α-ZO-1 (1:100) or rabbit α-ZO-2 (1:100) antibodies. After three-times washing with PBS, preparations were accordingly incubated for 1 h at room temperature (RT) with FITC-, TRITC- and Cy5-conjugated secondary antibodies. For cells in suspension, the procedure was performed in Eppendorf tubes and finally placed on coverslips. In some cases, nuclei were counterstained with 2.5 μg/ml of 4′,6-diamidino-2-phenylindole (DAPI) (Zymed) during 5 min. Preparations were mounted with the antifade reagent Vectashield (Vector laboratories) and examined through a confocal microscope (Leica TCS_SP5_MO) in *Z*-stack optical sections of 0.5 μm and *xz*- and *zy*-planes. In all cases, 10 fields per condition were analyzed and representative images were selected for each time.

For inhibition of clathrin-coated vesicles transport, MDCK cells were pre-incubated with 300 mM sucrose diluted in DMEM medium at 37°C for 1 h or DMEM medium as a control (Mosso et al., 2008). Then, cells were processed for immunofluorescence as above.

Aggregation and Adhesion Assays

Transfected MDCK cells were trypsinysed, washed twice in PBS, diluted in DMEM and suspended as hanging drops from the lid of a 24 well culture dish. Wells were filled with sterile water to prevent drops drying (Thoreson et al., 2000). Culture dishes were kept in a humid 5% CO_2 incubator at 37°C and cell aggregation was determined 4 h after plating. Cells in each drop were passed 10 times through a standard 200 μl Gilson pipet tip and photographed through a Nikon E600 microscope, using a 20X phase contrast objective. The number of isolated cells and cells forming aggregates were counted in five random fields from three independent experiments.

Adhesion assays were lightly modified from previously described (Orozco et al., 1983). Briefly, MDCK cells in suspension were mixed with washed erythrocytes (1:100 ratio). Cell mixture was incubated for 0.5, 1 and 2 h at 37°C, fixed with 2.5% glutaraldehyde for 30 min at 37°C and washed three-times with PBS. Erythrocytes were counterstained with 4.5 mM diaminobenzidine for 30 min at 37°C. Finally, adhered erythrocytes to each MDCK cell in ten random fields from three independent experiments were counted through a Nikon E600 microscope.

For inhibiting cell aggregation and erythrocytes adhesion, before experiments, 2×10^5 MDCK cells were incubated with 10 μg mAbAdh antibody or IgM isotype for 30 min at 37°C.

Measurement of Transepithelial Electrical Resistance (TEER)

Transfected MDCK cells were seeded on Transwell filter supports (6.5 mm diameter and 0.4 μm pore; Corning). Three days after plating, and after confirming through an inverted microscope that monolayers reached confluency, the TEER was measured using an EVOM epithelial voltmeter (World Precision Instruments) (Betanzos et al., 2013). TEER values were obtained by subtracting cell-free filter readings.

For some experiments, transfected MDCK cells were apically incubated with live trophozoites ($10^5/cm^2$) and TEER was monitored during 90 min.

Paracellular Flux Assays

TRITC-dextran (3 mg/ml) of 4 kDa (Sigma Aldrich) was added to the apical side of transfected epithelial cells in confluency, seeded in Transwell filters. After 90 min incubation at 37°C with gentle shaking and darkness, samples from the basal chamber were collected and the diffused fluorescent tracer was measured in a fluorimeter (excitation λ = 547 nm; emission λ = 572 nm). Emission values were converted to TRITC-dextran concentration, using a standard curve (Cuellar et al., 2017). As a positive control, before tracer addition, cells were incubated for 30 min with 5 mM EDTA.

Cytopathic Assays

Transfected MDCK cells in confluency, seeded in 24-well plates, were twice-washed with PBS to remove traces of serum and then incubated with live trophozoites (50, 100, and 250 × 10^3) suspended in TYI-S-33 medium without serum. Incubation was carried out for 2 h at 37°C in a CO_2 containing incubator. The reaction was stopped by cooling cell culture plates in an ice-water bath, to release adhered trophozoites. Epithelial cells were carefully washed with cold PBS and monolayer destruction was measured as described (Bracha and Mirelman, 1984).

Statistical Analysis

All data shown in this work, were representative from three independent experiments performed at least by triplicate. Results were displayed as mean and standard error. For statistical analysis, we followed the two-tailed Student *t*-test and two-ways ANOVA using the GraphPad Prism 5 software. Statistical significance was assumed when $^*p < 0.05$, $^{**}p < 0.01$, or $^{***}p < 0.001$.

Ethics Statement

The Centre for Research and Advanced Studies (CINVESTAV) fulfilled the standard of the Mexican Official Norm (NOM-062-ZOO-1999) and Technical Specifications for the Care and Use of Laboratory Animals based on the Guide for the Care and Use of Laboratory Animals The Guide, 2011, NRC, USA with the Federal Register Number BOO.02.03.02.01.908. This is awarded by the National Health Service, Food Safety and Quality (SENASICA) belonging to the Animal Health Office of the Secretary of Agriculture, Livestock, Rural Development, Fisheries and Food (SAGARPA), an organization that verifies the state compliance of such Mexican Official Norm (NOM) in Mexico. The Institutional Animal Care and Use Committee (IACUC/ethics committee) of CINVESTAV, as the regulatory office for the approval of research protocols involving the use of laboratory animals and, in fulfillment of the NOM, has reviewed and approved all animal experiments (Protocol Number 0505-12, CICUAL 001).

RESULTS

Recombinant EhADH (rEhADH) Penetrates Epithelial Cells Through the Paracellular Route

The EhCPADH complex is a virulence factor involved in adhesion, phagocytosis and cytolysis of target cells by *E. histolytica* trophozoites. This protein, as well as EhCP112 and EhADH, are secreted during host invasion, and from the medium they reach the target cell surface (García-Rivera et al., 1999; Ocádiz et al., 2005). To investigate the role of EhADH on epithelium damage without the interference of other trophozoite proteins, we produced an EhADH recombinant protein (rEhADH). The *ehadh* gene was cloned into the *pGEX6P1* plasmid, and *pGEX6P1-ehadh* transformed bacteria were induced for EhADH expression as a recombinant protein tagged to GST (**Figure 1A**). After purification by a glutathione-sepharose resin, the purity of rEhADH was visualized in silver-stained gels. A single 101 kDa band corresponding to the expected molecular weight for EhADH (75 kDa) (García-Rivera et al., 1999) plus GST (26 kDa) was evidenced (**Figure 1B**). The identity of the recombinant protein was probed by western blot assays using α-GST and mAbAdh antibodies. Both antibodies recognized the same 101 kDa band (**Figure 1B**); whereas in trophozoites lysates, the polyclonal α-EhADH antibody directed against a EhADH polypeptide (residues 566–582) located within the adherence domain, recognized the 75 kDa band (**Figure 1C**). Purified rEhADH coupled to the Alexa 647 fluorescent dye, was added to the apical side of confluent MDCK cells. Confocal microscopy images showed that immediately after rEhADH addition, the protein located at cellular borders, then, it appeared co-localizing with occludin and claudin-1 at the TJ region (**Figures 2, 3**). *xz*-planes images revealed that rEhADH was posed firstly on the apical surface of cells. Next, it penetrated through the intercellular space to be later found inside the cells. During these experiments, monolayers seemed intact under phase contrast images, even at 60 min rEhADH incubation. However, confocal images revealed that after cells contact with rEhADH (1 and 5 min), occludin and claudin-1 were delocalized from the cellular borders and eventually, both proteins were internalized to the cytoplasm (15 min). Afterwards, at 30 and 60 min these proteins partially recovered their TJ localization. Another *E. histolytica* recombinant protein, rEhPCNA (Cardona-Felix et al., 2011), did not bind to epithelial cells and neither produced modifications on TJ proteins (**Figure 2B**), indicating that the rEhADH effects were specific. We also investigated the effect of rEhADH on sparse MDCK cultures, where TJ structure and functions are not yet well stablished. Results evidenced claudin-1 at cellular borders in a discontinuous pattern, and this protein was not diminished neither internalized during all rEhADH incubation times (**Figure S1**). Whilst, at the beginning of incubation, rEhADH was mainly localized at the borders of cellular groups in growth. Nevertheless, at 30 min incubation, rEhADH was found at plasma membrane and cytoplasm (**Figure S1**), in accordance to the effect of this protein on confluent cells at 15 min (**Figure 3**). To analyse the effect produced by rEhADH on the natural colonization site in the host, we assessed its localization on human intestinal Caco-2 cells. Confocal images showed similar results in Caco-2 (**Figure 4**) and MDCK cells, confirming that rEhADH contacts epithelial cells, then displaces along the intercellular space, penetrates the cells and delocalizes occludin and claudin-1.

rEhADH Is Internalized by Clathrin-Coated Vesicles

Some pathogens and their secreted molecules enter the host cell by lipid microdomains known as caveolae and clathrin-coated vesicles (Rosenberger et al., 2000; Moreno-Ruiz et al., 2009; Machado et al., 2012). In fact, we have reported that EhCP112, the other part of the EhCPADH complex, is introduced to epithelial

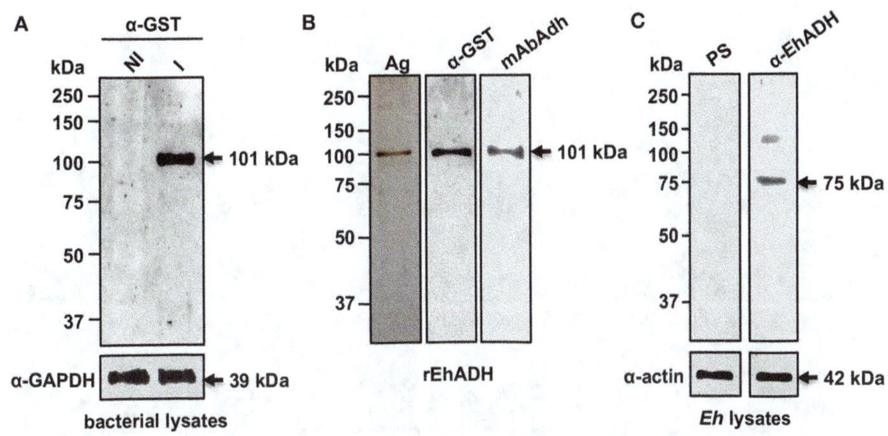

FIGURE 1 | Production of rEhADH. **(A)** Lysates of *E. coli* C43 (DE3) bacteria transformed with the *pGEX6P1-ehadh* plasmid. The recombinant GST-EhADH (rEhADH) expression was induced in bacteria by 1 mM IPTG and analyzed by western blot assays using the α-GST or α-GAPDH (loading control) antibodies. NI: non-induced. I: induced. **(B)** rEhADH purity was analyzed by silver gel staining (Ag) and western blot assays using α-GST and mAbAdh antibodies. **(C)** Trophozoites (*Eh*) lysates were analyzed by western blot using pre-immune serum (PS), α-EhADH or α-actin (loading control) antibodies. Numbers at left: molecular weight standards. Arrows: expected molecular weight of proteins.

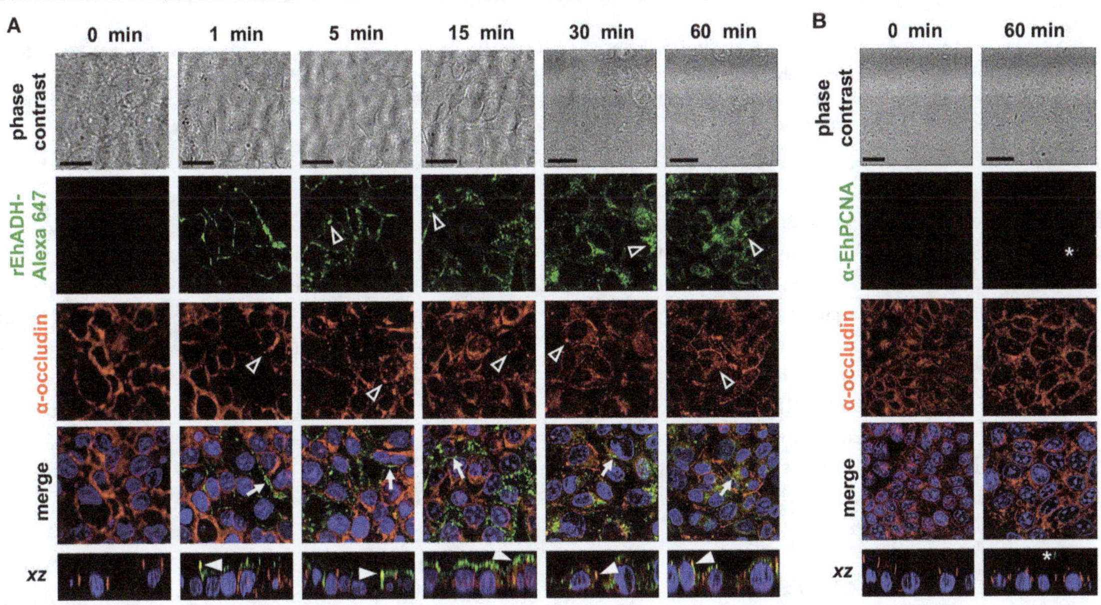

FIGURE 2 | Co-localization of rEhADH with occludin on MDCK cells. **(A)** rEhADH coupled to Alexa 647 (green) or **(B)** rEhPCNA were apically added to confluent MDCK cells and incubated for different times, then, cells were fixed and processed for immunofluorescence assays using the α-occludin antibody (red). rEhPCNA was detected by α-EhPCNA antibody (green). Nuclei were counterstained with DAPI (blue) and preparations were analyzed through a confocal microscope at *xy*- and *zy*-planes. Arrows: co-localization at cellular borders. Full arrowheads: co-localization at lateral membrane. Empty arrowheads: localization of EhADH (green) and occludin (red) at cytoplasm. Asterisks: EhPCNA localization. Bar = 20 μm.

cells by these kind of vesicles (Hernández-Nava et al., 2017). To explore whether rEhADH was internalized into MDCK cells through any of these mechanisms, we used antibodies against human clathrin−1 and caveolin. MDCK cells were incubated with fluorescence-labeled rEhADH and followed by confocal microscopy. Images evidenced that rEhADH strongly localized at clathrin-coated vesicles, whereas its localization at caveolae was poor (**Figure 5A**). Next, to confirm rEhADH endocytosis mediated by clathrin-coated vesicles, we used sucrose to inhibit this type of transport (Mosso et al., 2008). MDCK cells treated for 1 h with sucrose diminished clathrin-coated vesicles (**Figure 5B**). These cells now incubated for 1 (**Figure S2**) and 5 min (**Figure 5B**) with rEhADH, poorly bound it and were not able to internalize this protein, while sucrose-untreated cells presented

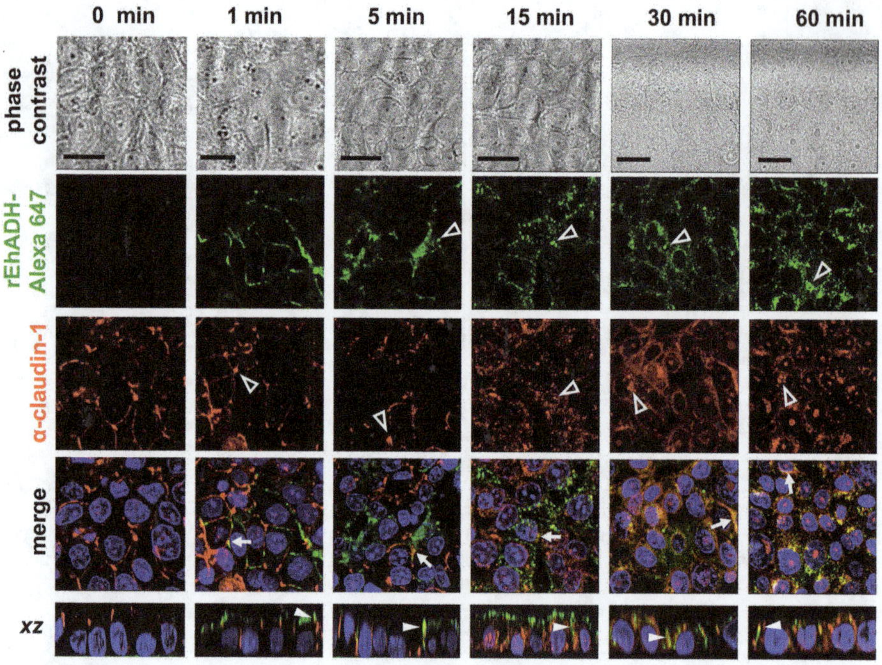

FIGURE 3 | Co-localization of rEhADH with claudin-1 on MDCK cells. rEhADH coupled to Alexa 647 (green) was apically added to confluent MDCK cells and incubated for different times, then, cells were fixed and processed for immunofluorescence assays using the α-claudin-1 antibody (red). Nuclei were counterstained with DAPI (blue) and preparations were analyzed through a confocal microscope at *xy*- and *zy*-planes. Arrows: co-localization at cellular borders. Full arrowheads: co-localization at lateral membrane. Empty arrowheads: localization of EhADH (green) and claudin-1 (red) at cytoplasm. Bar = 20 μm.

rEhADH at cellular borders and inside the cells, co-localizing with clathrin (**Figure 5B**). In rEhADH-untreated MDCK cells, the sucrose treatment also affected the occludin pattern at TJ region, lightly reducing its localization at cellular borders. As mentioned above, in sucrose-untreated MDCK cells and incubated with rEhADH, occludin was delocalized (**Figure 2A**), however after 5 min rEhADH incubation, when clathrin-transport is inhibited, occludin remained in its characteristic localization (**Figure 5B**). These findings robustly suggested that rEhADH is internalized to target cells by clathrin-coated vesicles.

E. histolytica EhADH Is Expressed by *pcDNA3-ehadh* Transfected MDCK Cells

To study the effect produced by EhADH inside epithelial cells, we expressed this protein in MDCK cells that were transfected with the *pcDNA3-ehadh* plasmid, which contains a promoter for expressing exogenous genes in mammalian cells. Stably transfected cells were selected with G-418. To evidence the presence of the *ehadh* transcript, we performed RT-PCR assays. Results revealed that only MDCK cells transfected with *pcDNA3-ehadh* (MDCK-EhADH), expressed the *ehadh* transcript, in contrast to *pcDNA3* transfected (MDCK-3) or non-transfected (MDCK) cells (**Figure 6A**). The stable gene transfection in these cells was also demonstrated by RNA expression of the *neomycin* resistance gene, which was also expressed by MDCK-3 cells. The expression of the EhADH protein was verified by western blot assays, using total extracts of MDCK-EhADH cells and a specific polyclonal antibody against the adhesin (α-EhADH). The α-EhADH antibody recognized a single 75 kDa band (**Figure 6B**), as reported (García-Rivera et al., 1999), and did not detect any protein in MDCK-3 and non-transfected cells (**Figure 6B**). In general, growth rates for all cell types were similar (**Figure 6C**). Thus, MDCK cells constitutively expressed *E. histolytica* EhADH and apparently, by itself the adhesin did not affect the viability and growth of epithelial cells.

EhADH Is Localized at the MDCK Cellular Membrane

Protein function is closely related to its location in cellular structures. In trophozoites, EhADH is localized at plasma membrane, endosomes and cytoplasm (Avalos-Padilla et al., 2015; Montaño et al., 2017). The location of the EhADH protein in MDCK-EhADH cells was studied at different stages of the cell monolayer formation through immunofluorescence assays using the mAbAdh antibody. In MDCK-EhADH cells in suspension, EhADH mainly appeared at the plasma membrane (**Figure 6D**). In sparse cultures, when cell polarization begins, EhADH was predominantly concentrated at borders of the growing cellular groups, where the cell monolayer was extending (**Figure 6D**). This pattern correlated with that observed in sparse non-transfected cultures incubated with rEhADH (**Figure S1**). Interestingly, MDCK-EhADH confluent monolayers presented EhADH at cellular borders (**Figure 6D**), which is in concordance with the localization of its rat homolog (Alix), present at cellular borders of immortalized epithelial cells from rat choroid plexus

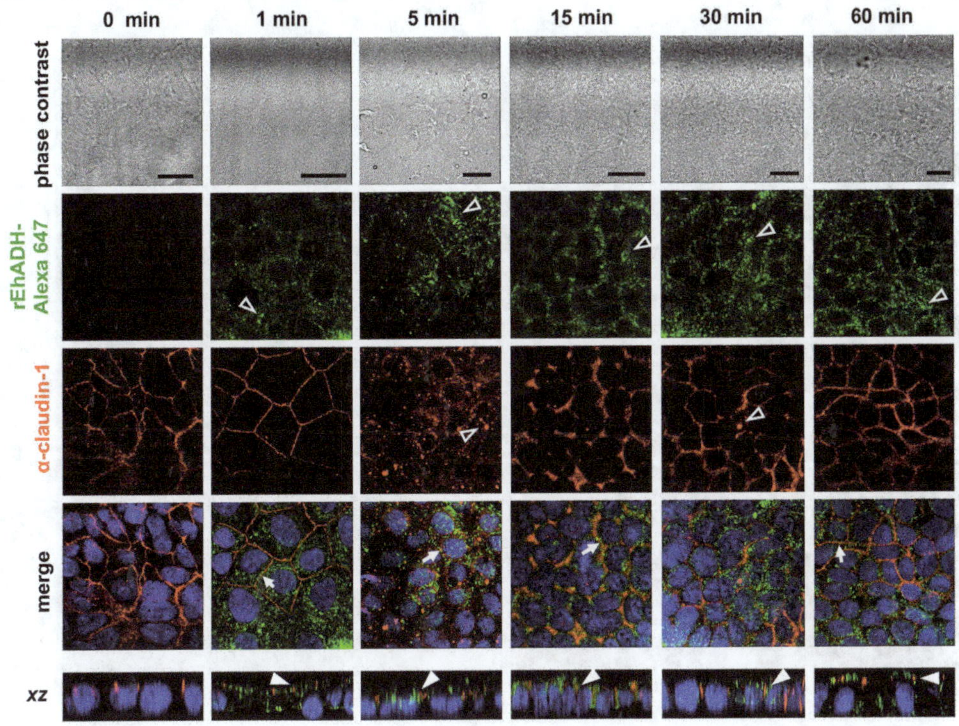

FIGURE 4 | Co-localization of rEhADH with claudin-1 on Caco-2 cells. rEhADH coupled to Alexa 647 (green) was apically added to confluent Caco-2 cells and incubated for different times, then, cells were fixed and processed for immunofluorescence assays using the α-claudin-1 antibody (red). Nuclei were counterstained with DAPI (blue) and preparations were analyzed through a confocal microscope at *xy*- and *xz*-planes. Arrows: co-localization at cellular borders. Full arrowheads: co-localization at lateral membrane. Empty arrowheads: localization of EhADH (green) and claudin-1 (red) at cytoplasm. Bar = 20 μm.

(Campos et al., 2016). EhADH was also abundantly detected around nuclei, probably in the endoplasmic reticulum, where adhesin is being synthesized (**Figure 6D**). As expected, EhADH was not present in MDCK-3 cells. These results indicated that as in trophozoites, EhADH localized at the plasma membrane and cytoplasm of transfected epithelial cells. Additionally, these experiments corroborated that EhADH stable expression did not modify the morphology of MDCK cells.

EhADH Induces Aggregation of Target Cells

In *E. histolytica* trophozoites, EhADH is involved in target cell adherence (García-Rivera et al., 1999; Madriz et al., 2004; Martinez-Lopez et al., 2004). Therefore, we analyzed whether EhADH expressed by MDCK cells, evoked its adhesin function to target cells. For these experiments, transfected epithelial cells were trypsinysed and incubated in PBS at 37°C for 4 h, then, we counted the number of clumps formed and the number of cells contained in each one. Optical microscopy images clearly evidenced that MDCK-EhADH cells formed more clumps with a higher number of cells than MDCK-3 cells that did not express the adhesin (**Figure 7A**). For quantification, clumps were grouped according to the number of contained cells (1–5, 6–10, 11–20, 21–40, and more than 40 cells) and their frequencies were determined. Whilst MDCK-3 cells formed 82% of clumps containing 1–5 cells, only 43% of clumps were constituted by MDCK-EhADH cells (**Figure 7B**). In contrast, MDCK-EhADH and MDCK-3 cells formed 30% and 6% of clumps containing more than 40 cells, respectively. To confirm the adhesive role of EhADH in MDCK cells, before aggregation assays, transfected cells were pre-incubated with the mAbAdh antibody to inhibit clumps formation. Results showed that the antibody treatment, reduced the frequency of clumps with a higher number of cells in MDCK-EhADH, but not in MDCK-3 cells (**Figure 7B**). In contrast, an IgM isotype used as control, did not modify clumps frequency. These results suggested that MDCK-EhADH cells displayed stronger associations among them than MDCK-3 cells.

In trophozoites, EhADH also participates in erythrocytes adhesion (Avalos-Padilla et al., 2015; Bolaños et al., 2016). Thus, we studied whether MDCK-EhADH cells were able to bind erythrocytes. Transfected MDCK cells were incubated for different times with red blood cells and adhered erythrocytes were counted. Surprisingly, both types of transfected MDCK cells were able to attach erythrocytes (**Figure 7C**). However, after 1 and 2 h incubation, MDCK-EhADH cells adhered twice more erythrocytes than MDCK-3 cells (**Figure 7D**). To inhibit erythrocytes adhesion, again, before assays, transfected cells were pre-incubated with the mAbAdh antibody, resulting in a decreased number of red blood cells adhered to MDCK-EhADH, but not to MDCK-3 cells (**Figure 7D**). The IgM isotype presented a similar effect than in control transfected MDCK cells. These experiments showed that

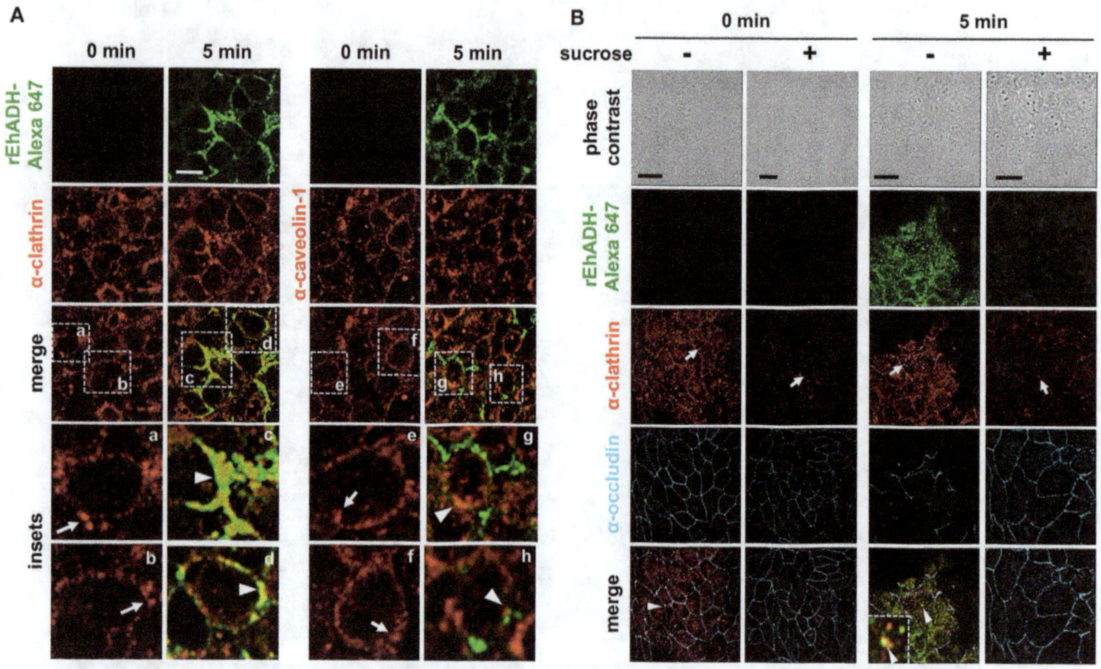

FIGURE 5 | Co-localization of rEhADH with clathrin and caveolin-1 on MDCK cells. **(A)** rEhADH coupled to Alexa 647 (green) was apically added to confluent MDCK cells and incubated for 5 min, then, cells were fixed and processed for immunofluorescence assays using α-clathrin or α-caveolin-1 antibodies (red). Preparations were analyzed through a confocal microscope at the *xy*-plane. Insets: magnification of squares (a–h) from merge images. **(B)** MDCK cells were incubated for 1 h with DMEM medium (–) or 300 mM sucrose (+) at 37°C and then processed as in **(A)**, but also using the α-occludin antibody (cyan). Inset: magnification of rEhADH and clathrin co-localization. Arrows: vesicles close to cellular borders. Arrowheads: co-localization. Bar = 20 μm.

EhADH preserved its adhesive properties within MDCK-EhADH cells.

MDCK-EhADH Cells Present an Increased TEER

Previously, we reported that EhCPADH and EhCP112 affect the gate function of TJ in epithelial cells (Cuellar et al., 2017; Hernández-Nava et al., 2017). Therefore, we wondered if EhADH expression on MDCK cells may alter this function, characterized by the regulation of ion and macromolecules flux. To evaluate this, we used transfected epithelial cells cultured in Transwell filters. MDCK-EHADH cells exhibited approximately twice higher TEER values compared to MDCK-3 cells (**Figure 8A**). To measure the macromolecules flux, the non-ionic dextran marker coupled to the TRITC-fluorescent dye was added to the apical side of epithelial monolayers and then, we quantified the tracer diffusion across the paracellular pathway from the apical to the basolateral side. MDCK-EhADH and MDCK-3 cells presented a low dextran permeability, similar to non-transfected MDCK cells (**Figure 8B**). As a positive control, cells were incubated with EDTA that disassembles epithelial junctions (Deli, 2009). MDCK cells treated with EDTA allowed the free passage of dextran between intercellular spaces. Our data showed that EhADH enhanced the electrical tightness of MDCK monolayers, but it had not impact on macromolecules permeability.

EhADH Co-localizes and Increases the Amount of TJ Proteins in MDCK-EhADH Cells

The above results evidenced that MDCK-EhADH monolayers have a higher TEER than MDCK-3 cells. TJ functions depend on the localization and amount of proteins in the intercellular space. Thus, to analyse the effect of EhADH expression in the localization of junctional proteins, we performed immunofluorescence assays using α-claudin-1, α-occludin, α-ZO-1, α- ZO-2, and α-EhADH antibodies. In contrast to the results obtained using the rEhADH added to the apical side of cell monolayers (**Figures 2**, **3**), confocal images showed that EhADH expression in MDCK cells did not affect the localization of proteins at TJ region, as it was clearly evidenced at *xz*-planes (**Figure 9A**). However, MDCK-EhADH cells presented an increase of the fluorescence corresponding to claudin-1, occludin, ZO-1 and ZO-2 (**Figure 9A**). As expected, all TJ proteins studied here co-localized with EhADH at the TJ region (**Figure 9B**). These results suggested that the stable presence of EhADH in transfected cells provoked an increase of claudin-1, occludin, ZO-1, and ZO-2 at TJ.

To further confirm the increased amount of TJ proteins in transfected cells, we analyzed their expression by western blot assays using the corresponding antibodies. Quantification of western blot results revealed that the amount of claudin-1 and occludin increased around 2.5 times in MDCK-EhADH cells, in comparison to MDCK-3 cells (**Figure 10**). Meanwhile, ZO-1

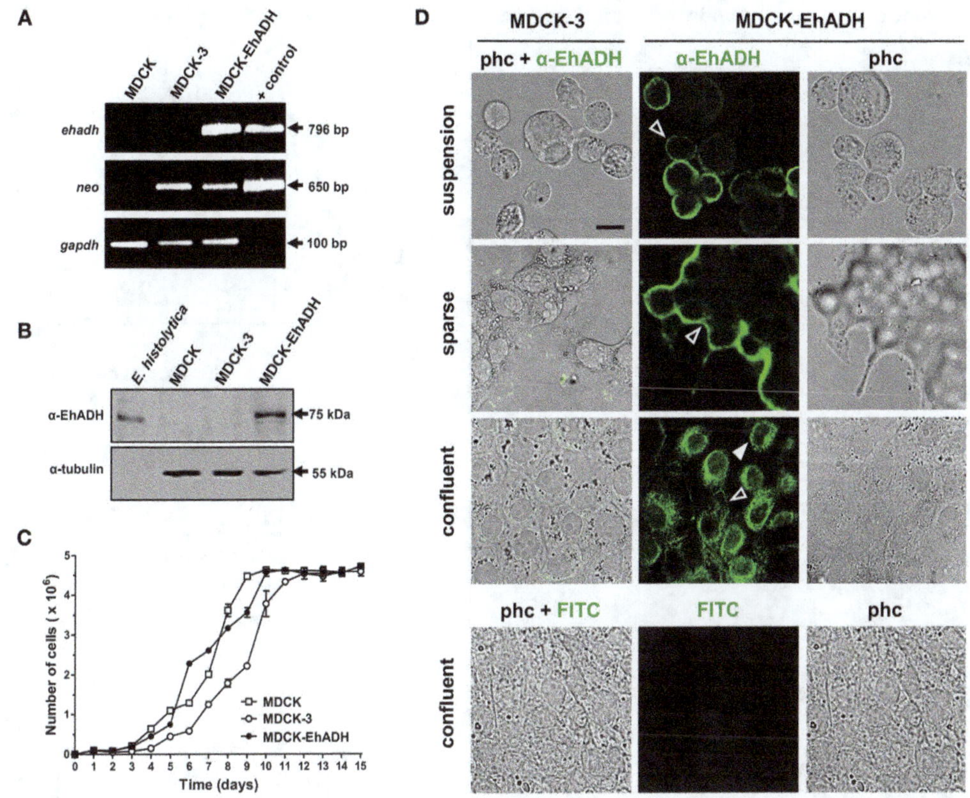

FIGURE 6 | Expression of the *E. histolytica* EhADH protein in MDCK epithelial cells. MDCK cells were transfected with the *pcDNA3* (MDCK-3) or *pcDNA3-ehadh* (MDCK-EhADH) plasmids and EhADH expression and localization were analyzed. **(A)** RT-PCR assays of non-transfected (MDCK) or transfected MDCK cells, using specific primers for *ehadh*, *neo* and *gapdh* (as internal control) genes. As positive control, the *pcDNA3-ehadh* plasmid was used as template in PCR experiments. Numbers at right: amplicon size. **(B)** Western blot experiments of epithelial lysates, employing α-EhADH and α-tubulin (as loading control) antibodies. Trophozoites lysates were used as positive control. Numbers at right: expected molecular weight of proteins. **(C)** Growth curves of MDCK cells. After 48 h of plasmid transfection into cells, growth medium was supplemented with 1 mg/ml G-418, whereas non-transfected cells were grown in normal medium. The number of cells were counted in a Neubauer haemocytometer. Each point represents the mean and standard error of three independent experiments. **(D)** Suspension, sparse and confluent transfected MDCK cells were fixed, permeabilized and processed for immunofluorescence assays using the mAbAdh antibody. Bottom panel: MDCK-EhADH cells treated only with the secondary antibody (FITC). All images represent *xy*-optical sections. Empty arrowheads: plasma membrane. Full arrowhead: perinuclear localization. phc: phase contrast. Bar = 20 μm.

and ZO-2 showed a slight increase in MDCK-EhADH cells without significant differences when compared to MDCK-3 cells. Actin was used as loading control and all densitometric analysis were normalized regarding this protein. These results correlated with the immunofluorescence findings, confirming that EhADH expression provoked a significant increase of claudin-1 and occludin, which are mainly responsible for the TJ gate function.

EhADH Expression in MDCK Cells Facilitates Epithelial Destruction by Trophozoites

One of the first signs of damage to MDCK cell monolayers during *E. histolytica* invasion is TEER dropping. After this, cells are detached from the substrate and destroyed by the parasite (Martínez-Palomo et al., 1985). To evaluate the effect of *E. histolytica* trophozoites over transfected MDCK cells, epithelial cells were grown in Transwell filters until confluence, and live trophozoites were added in the apical side of monolayers, then, TEER was monitored during 90 min. To compare the TEER behavior of transfected cells, we normalized each TEER value regarding the one registered at 0 min. Results showed a stable TEER performance by MDCK-EhADH and MDCK-3 cells non-incubated with parasites (**Figure 11A**). Meanwhile, a TEER drop was evident when transfected cells were incubated with trophozoites. However, TEER values were lower in MDCK-EhADH than in MDCK-3 cells, from 5 to 30 min incubation. After this time, the effect of trophozoites on TEER seemed indistinct between MDCK-3 and MDCK-EhADH cells, reaching a stable behavior from 45 to 90 min.

To visualize and determine epithelial destruction by live trophozoites on transfected MDCK cells, confluent monolayers were apically incubated with different number of parasites. Live trophozoites destroyed 33, 65, and 100% (using 50, 100, and 250 × 10^3 amoebas, respectively) more MDCK-EhADH than MDCK-3 cells monolayers (**Figure 11B**). Representatives images of methylene blue-stained monolayers evidenced the damage produced by parasites. Surprisingly, trophozoites displayed more

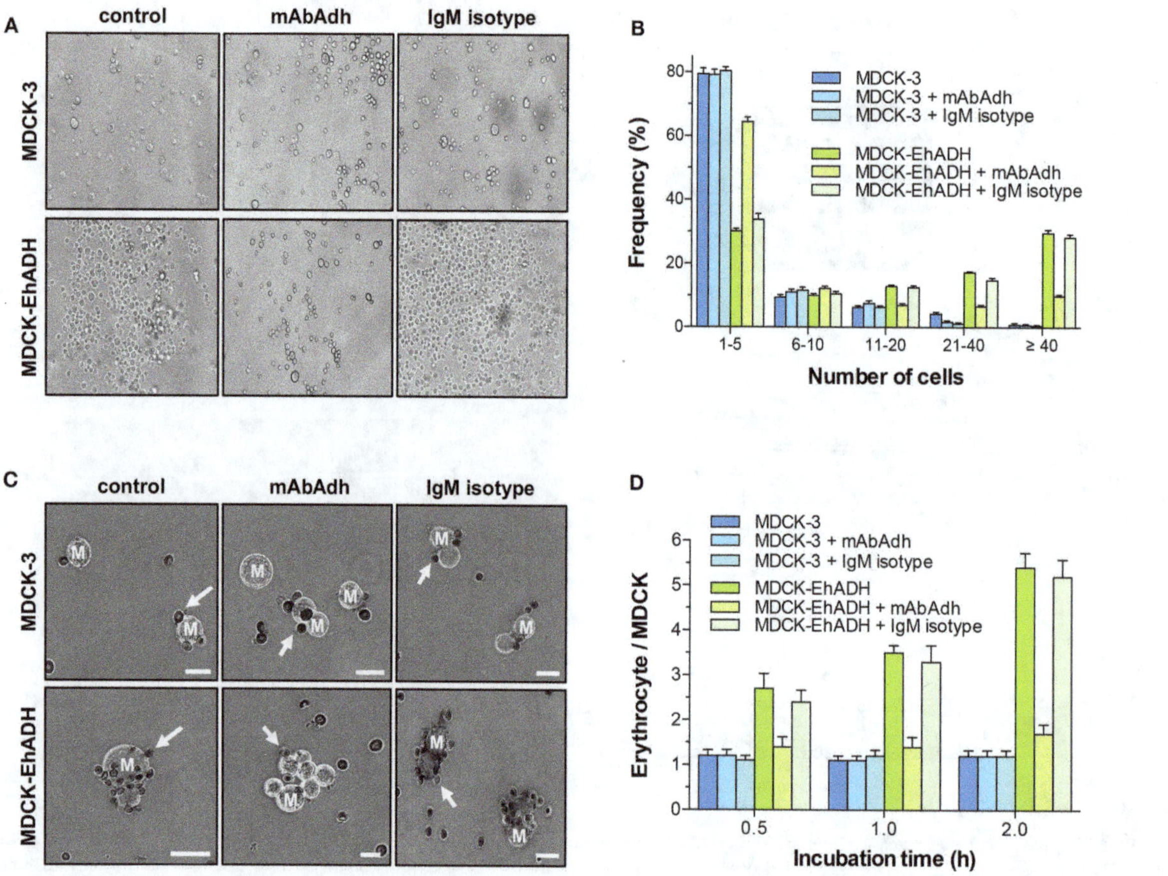

FIGURE 7 | Adherence properties of MDCK-EhADH cells. **(A)** Transfected MDCK cells were trypsinysed, incubated with PBS (control), mAbAdh antibody or IgM isotype for 30 min at 37°C and suspended as hanging drops from the lid of a 24 well culture dish. Four hours after plating, cells in drops were resuspended and photographed in an optical microscope with 20X phase contrast objective (representative images). **(B)** Single cells and cellular clusters showed in **(A)** were counted, and frequency for each group with similar cell numbers were graphed. Data represent the mean and standard error of five fields quantified from three independent experiments. **(C)** Transfected MDCK cells were trypsinysed, incubated with PBS (control), mAbAdh antibody or IgM isotype for 30 min at 37°C, and mixed with erythrocytes. After 0.5, 1 and 2 h of incubation, erythrocytes were stained with diaminobenzidine and adhered erythrocytes (arrows) to MDCK cells (M) were photographed. Representative images from 2 h incubation are shown. Bar = 10 μm. **(D)** Adhered erythrocytes to each MDCK cell were counted. Values represent the mean and standard error from three independent experiments by triplicate. Differences found between groups were statistically significant (***$p < 0.001$), according to two-ways ANOVA test.

damage on MDCK cells expressing EhADH than MDCK-3 cells, suggesting that this protein facilitated the epithelial injury.

In summary, all results of this work suggested that EhADH altered TJ of the host epithelium, reaching the paracellular space, being internalized mainly by clathrin-coated vesicles, delocalizing and increasing TJ proteins, for eventually making epithelial cells more susceptible to other trophozoite effector proteins. Nevertheless, this hypothesis should be further addressed to get in depth on EhADH action mechanisms in this event.

DISCUSSION

E. histolytica trophozoites use several molecules to invade the host epithelium. Among them, our group has been investigating the participation of the EhCPADH complex in the breaking of intercellular junctions. We have found that EhCPADH and also EhCP112 reach the paracellular pathway by opening intercellular junctions and eventually, both proteins penetrate epithelial cells. The damage begins by affecting proteins and functions of TJ, and then, it continues degrading AJ and DSM proteins (Betanzos et al., 2013; Cuellar et al., 2017; Hernández-Nava et al., 2017). Nevertheless, the EhADH contribution to epithelium impairment during trophozoite invasion, had not been yet elucidated. In this work, by using a recombinant protein we revealed that EhADH gets first into the intercellular space, and next, it enters into the epithelial cells mainly by clathrin-coated vesicles. To analyse the effect of EhADH inside host cells, we generated MDCK cells stably expressing this adhesin. The EhADH expression produced more adhesiveness to target cells and an enhanced TEER due to a higher amount of claudin-1 and occludin. Interestingly, the EhADH expression in MDCK cells facilitated the epithelial damage produced by

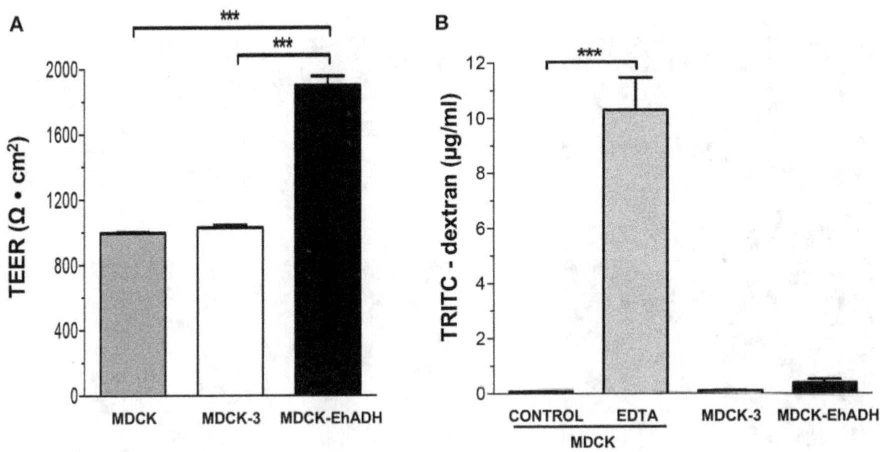

FIGURE 8 | Permeability of MDCK-EhADH cells. **(A)** Non-transfected and transfected MDCK cells were seeded in Transwell filters and when they reached confluence, TEER was monitored. Background resistance from empty filters was deducted for each value. **(B)** Non-transfected and transfected MDCK cells were seeded in Transwell filters and when they reached confluence, the paracellular flux of 4 kDa TRITC-dextran was measured from the apical to the basolateral direction. MDCK cells treated with 5 mM EDTA were used as positive control. Data represent the mean and standard error from three independent experiments by triplicate. ***$p < 0.001$, according to two-tailed Student *t*-test.

live trophozoites, suggesting a putative role for EhADH in synergizing the effect of other *E. histolytica* molecules during host invasion.

EhCPADH and its components are secreted to the medium (García-Rivera et al., 1999; Ocádiz et al., 2005; Bolaños et al., 2016), and together with other parasite molecules (Lejeune et al., 2011; Cornick et al., 2016) constitute an efficient mechanism to reach and effectively damage the host epithelium. We previously demonstrated that the EhCPADH complex drops TEER and interacts with claudin-1 and occludin, to eventually degrade them along with ZO-1 and ZO-2 (Betanzos et al., 2013). Besides, we evaluated the participation of EhCP112, the proteolytic part of this complex, by producing a recombinant enzyme (rEhCP112) which reaches the apical side of epithelium and then invade it through intercellular junctions (Cuellar et al., 2017; Hernández-Nava et al., 2017). Here, we investigated if the other part of the EhCPADH complex, the EhADH adhesin, also extended into the paracellular pathway, by using a recombinant protein (rEhADH, **Figure 1**) and characterizing its effect on epithelial cells. When rEhADH was added to the apical side of MDCK cells, it was at cellular borders co-localizing with occludin and claudin-1 at TJ, and eventually penetrated the cell (**Figures 2, 3**). These findings were consistent to that observed in Caco-2 cells (**Figure 4**), which have been used in other works for resembling the *E. histolytica* natural colonization site in host (Li et al., 1994; Ralston et al., 2014). Here, we preferred the MDCK cells model because this cell line is a friendly and easy system to study molecules and functions of TJ, and also to stably and efficiently transfect heterologous genes (Cereijido et al., 1978; Furuse et al., 2001; Dukes et al., 2011). In addition, they have been widely used as a model to characterize trophozoites damage and TEER dropping during epithelial invasion (Martínez-Palomo et al., 1985; Dolabella et al., 2012; Betanzos et al., 2013; Hernández-Nava et al., 2017).

To investigate the EhADH internalization mechanism, we followed this adhesin together with clathrin and caveolin-1, resulting in a higher co-localization with clathrin than with caveolin-1 (**Figure 5A**). The rEhADH endocytosis mediated by clathrin-coated vesicles was confirmed by using sucrose as an inhibitor (Mosso et al., 2008), which diminished these vesicles and rEhADH internalization, thus preventing occludin delocalization from the membrane (**Figure 5B**). The endocytosis mechanism mediated by clathrin-coated vesicles has been observed for other pathogens adhesins, such as AfaD of diarrhea-associated *E. coli* strains or HadA of *Haemophilus influenzae* (Jouve et al., 1997; Serruto et al., 2009). Moreover, similarly to EhADH, EhCP112 is transported by clathrin-coated vesicles, although this enzyme is also internalized by caveolae (Hernández-Nava et al., 2017).

In order to analyse the role of EhADH inside epithelial cells and also to eliminate the noise coming from other amoebic proteins that produce host cell damage, we performed the heterologous expression of this adhesin by transfecting MDCK cells with the *pcDNA3-ehadh* construct. MDCK-EhADH cells efficiently expressed the *ehadh* transcript and the corresponding protein with the expected 75 kDa molecular weight, maintaining a similar growing rate than control cells (**Figures 6A–C**). As well as in trophozoites (García-Rivera et al., 1999; Avalos-Padilla et al., 2015), EhADH was localized in cytoplasmic vesicles and at the plasma membrane of epithelial cells (**Figure 6D**).

EhADH possesses adhesive properties, facilitating trophozoites adhesion to target cells (García-Rivera et al., 1999; Bañuelos et al., 2012). Here, we demonstrated that MDCK-EhADH cells aggregated more among them, and adhered more erythrocytes than control cells (**Figure 7**). The observed adhesive features were specific, since the mAbAdh antibody directed against EhADH inhibited them (**Figure 7**). Our findings suggested that MDCK-EhADH cells acquired the adhesive

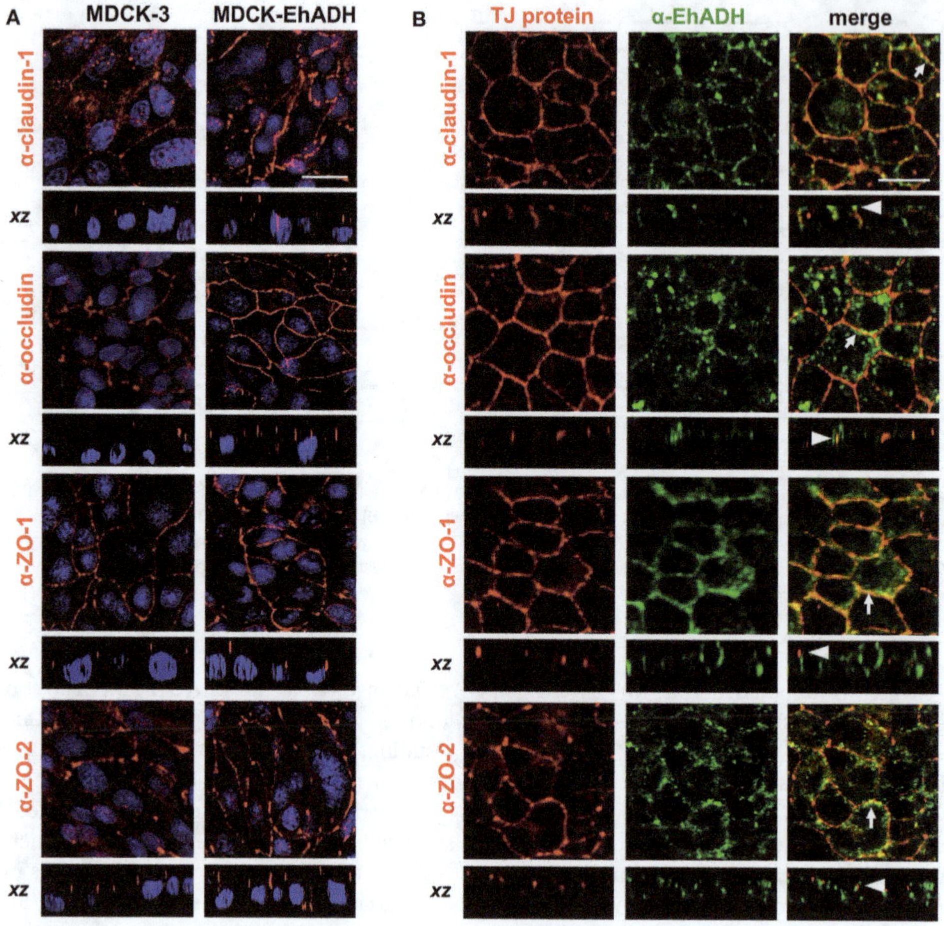

FIGURE 9 | Effect of EhADH expression on TJ proteins localization. **(A)** Confluent transfected MDCK cells were fixed, permeabilized and stained with α-claudin-1, α-occludin, α-ZO-1 or α-ZO-2 antibodies, followed by the corresponding TRITC-secondary antibodies. Nuclei were counterstained with DAPI (blue). **(B)** MDCK-EhADH cells were stained with α-claudin-1, α-occludin, α-ZO-1 or α-ZO-2 (red) and α-EhADH (green) antibodies, followed by the corresponding TRITC- and FITC-secondary antibodies, respectively. Arrows: co-localization at the plasma membrane. Arrowheads: co-localization at the TJ region. Representative images of *xy*- and *xz*-optical planes observed by confocal microscopy. Bar = 20 μm.

properties displayed by this trophozoite protein. A similar effect was also reported for the *H. influenzae* HadA adhesin during its heterologous expression in a non-invasive *E. coli* strain, which gained properties for aggregation and adherence to human epithelial cells and to extracellular matrix proteins (collagens I and III, fibronectin and laminin) (Serruto et al., 2009). On the other hand, it was not surprising that MDCK cells adhered erythrocytes, since epithelial cells are similar to erythroid cells and both contain similar membrane-cytoskeletal components (Bennett and Lorenzo, 2013). In addition, both cell types contain ankyrin and fodrin, involved in lateral membrane association upon cell-cell contact induction (Glenney and Glenney, 1983; Bennett and Lorenzo, 2013).

The increased adhesiveness among MDCK-EhADH cells and the presence of EhADH at cellular borders, affected the TJ gate function evidenced as an augment of TEER (**Figure 8**). In agreement, macromolecules flux by the paracellular pathway remained low. Other amoeba as *Acanthamoeba* also produced a high TEER in MDCK cells, probably because claudin-4 was increased and re-targeted to TJ, while claudin-2 diminished and was removed from the cellular borders (Flores-Maldonado et al., 2017). TEER is a measurement of ions flux through the paracellular pathway, and this flux is mainly regulated by claudins in different fashions; for example, claudin-4 promotes a barrier function by forming an ion channel, whereas claudin-2, constitutively expressed in the most leaky-epithelia, makes paracellular cation and water channels (Barmeyer et al., 2017). Therefore, we evaluated the localization and expression of TJ integral (claudin-1 and occludin) and scaffold (ZO-1 and ZO-2) proteins. According to TEER results, by immunofluorescence and western blot assays in MDCK-EhADH cells we observed an increase of the analyszd proteins at cellular borders, co-localizing with EhADH at the TJ region (**Figure 9**), although the augment was only significant for claudin-1 and occludin (**Figure 10**), molecules responsible for the gate function (Liang and Weber, 2014). Thereby, the delicate nature of the molecular composition of junctions and their balance, could be influencing the

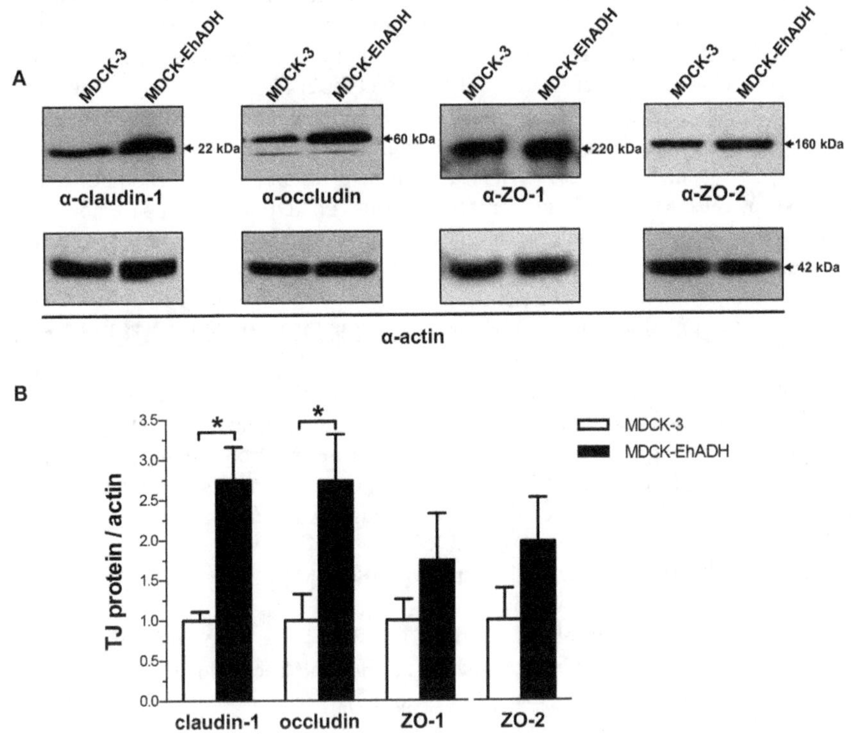

FIGURE 10 | Effect of EhADH expression on the amount of TJ proteins. **(A)** Total extracts of confluent transfected MDCK cells were separated on SDS-PAGE, transferred to nitrocellulose membranes and blotted with α-claudin-1, α-occludin, α-ZO-1 or α-ZO-2 antibodies (upper panels). Lower panels: as loading controls, same membranes were stripped and blotted with the α-actin antibody (representative images). **(B)** The specific amount of TJ proteins was obtained as the ratio of TJ proteins between actin densitometric evaluations from **(A)**. Data represent the mean values and standard error from three independent experiments. $^*p < 0.05$, according to two-tailed Student *t*-test.

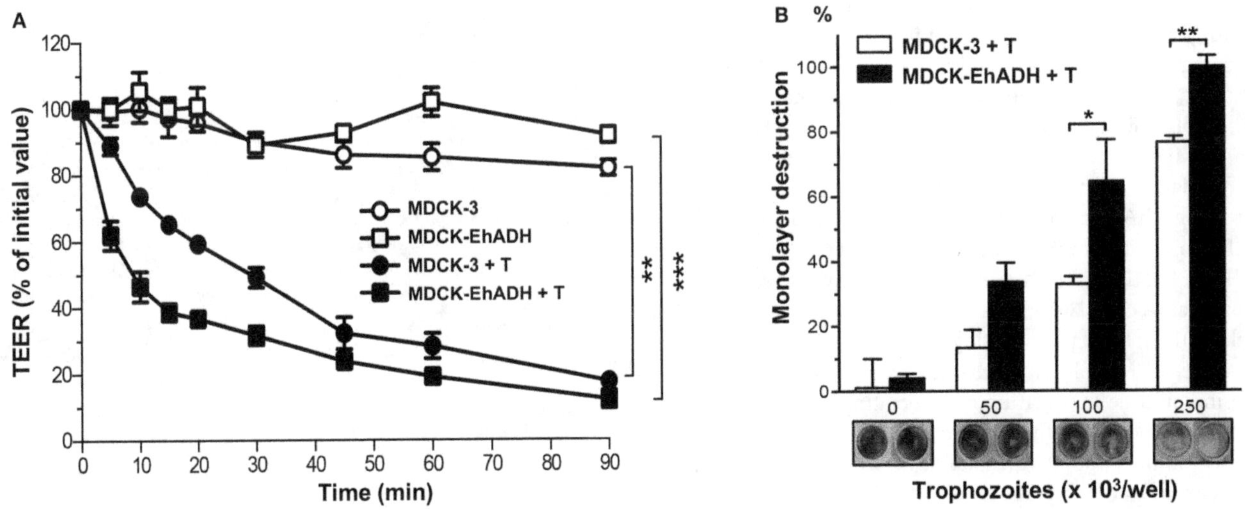

FIGURE 11 | Effect of trophozoites on MDCK cells expressing EhADH. **(A)** Transfected MDCK cells were seeded in Transwell filters and when they reached confluence, trophozoites ($10^5/cm^2$) were apically added. TEER was monitored for 2 h and data were normalized according to the initial value given by each Transwell. Means and standard errors represent each time point from three independent assays performed by triplicate. $^{**}p < 0.01$ and $^{***}p < 0.001$, according to two-tailed Student *t*-test. **(B)** Transfected confluent MDCK cells were incubated with 0, 50, 100, and 250 × 10^3 live trophozoites. Monolayers cell destruction was determined after 2 h incubation by methylene blue staining. Then, dye was eluted and quantified by spectrophotometry. Data represent the mean and standard error of three independent experiments by triplicate statistically analyzed by two-tailed Student *t*-test. $^*p < 0.05$, $^{**}p < 0.01$. Representative images of monolayers destruction are showed below the graph.

epithelium susceptibility for alterations due to pathogens and their molecules.

The effect produced by EhADH inside epithelial cells could be explained by its scaffold properties, characteristic of ALIX family protein members (Bissig and Gruenberg, 2014). TJ peripheral scaffold proteins link transmembrane and functional barrier proteins to the actomyosin-ring (Liang and Weber, 2014). In fact, in immortalized rat choroid plexus cells, Alix protein guarantees the proper assembly and actomyosin-ring positioning at the TJ region by interacting with F-actin, Par-3 and ZO-1, thus contributing to the maintenance of epithelial cell polarity and barrier function (Campos et al., 2016). Otherwise, from previous experiments, we demonstrated that an EhADH recombinant protein including the adherence epitope, interacts with a 97 kDa membrane protein of MDCK cells (Martinez-Lopez et al., 2004). We hypothesized this protein could correspond to a claudin-1 tetramer, since claudins are capable to form oligomers, which are responsible for junction selectivity (Coyne et al., 2003). Furthermore, EhCPADH binds to claudin-1, occludin, ZO-1 and ZO-2 in MDCK cells (Betanzos et al., 2013). Thus, our findings in this work suggested that EhADH could be acting as a peripheral scaffolding protein to reinforce the attachment of claudin-1 and occludin to the TJ region, probably tightening cell-cell contacts. This assumption can be reinforced by the fact that other amoeba proteins also act as intercellular junction molecules. *Dictyostelium discoideum* amoeba contains an adhesion molecule named Aardvark, which is similar to the AJ scaffold protein β-catenin, suggesting the presence of a rudimentary cell-cell adhesion during the formation of the fruiting body that develops in colonies deprived of nutrients (Grimson et al., 2000). Even more, *E. histolytica* expresses an occludin-like protein that can alter the colonic epithelial barrier (Goplen et al., 2013).

Interestingly, MDCK-EhADH cells incubated with live trophozoites were more susceptible to parasites damage, according to TEER and cytopathic experiments (**Figure 11**). Although, these cells developed higher TEER values than control cells, trophozoites dropped TEER in MDCK-EhADH cells more than in MDCK-3 cells (from 5 to 30 min amoeba incubation); in accordance, parasites caused more damage on monolayers expressing EhADH. In trophozoites, it has been reported that EhADH binds to diverse molecules such as EhCP112, EhVps32, EhNPC1, EhNPC2, LBPA and cholesterol (Avalos-Padilla et al., 2015; Bolaños et al., 2016; Castellanos-Castro et al., 2016; Cuellar et al., 2017), thus participating in distinct virulence events. Therefore, in MDCK-EhADH cells, we hypothesized that this adhesin could be modulating or associating to these molecules or others, to facilitate their participation on epithelial damage. Identity of these putative molecules and related mechanisms should be further investigated.

Summarizing our findings from previous reports and those obtained in this paper, we demonstrated that EhCPADH and its components by separate, could reach the intercellular space and affect the epithelial barrier function. In the case of EhADH, when it is secreted by trophozoites to the medium, extends toward the paracellular pathway and later, after its internalization, modulates the expression and localization of claudin-1 and occludin. Once inside, EhADH could prepare host cells for the action of other virulence factors, making the epithelium more susceptible to the trophozoite attack.

AUTHOR CONTRIBUTIONS

AB and EO: Designed, performed and analyzed experiments, and wrote the manuscript. DZ: Carried out immunofluorescence assays. EH-N: Produced the recombinant protein. PC: Performed RT-PCR experiments. CB: Contributed to experiments analysis, discussion and manuscript writing.

FUNDING

This work was financed by the Mexican National Council for Science and Technology (CONACYT, 284477 to AB and 220049 to EO).

ACKNOWLEDGMENTS

We are grateful to Dr. Guillermina García-Rivera, Dr. Miriam Huerta-Pérez and Ricardo Ceja for their assistance with *E. histolytica* assays and Alejandrina Reyes for her technical support.

SUPPLEMENTARY MATERIAL

Figure S1 | Co-localization of rEhADH with claudin-1 on sparse MDCK cells. rEhADH coupled to Alexa 647 (green) was apically added to sparse MDCK cells and incubated for different times, then, cells were fixed and processed for immunofluorescence assays using the α-claudin-1 antibody (red). Nuclei were counterstained with DAPI (blue) and preparations were analyzed through a confocal microscope at *xy*- and *zy*-planes. Arrows: co-localization at cellular borders. Full arrowheads: co-localization at lateral membrane. Empty arrowheads: localization of EhADH (green) and claudin-1 (red) at cytoplasm. Bar = 20 μm.

Figure S2 | rEhADH localization in MDCK cells where clathrin-transport was inhibited. MDCK cells were incubated for 1 h with DMEM medium (–) or 300 mM sucrose (+) at 37°C and then rEhADH coupled to Alexa 647 (green) was apically added for 1 min. Preparations were analyzed through a confocal microscope at *xy*- and *xz*-planes. Arrows: rEhADH localization. Bar = 20 μm.

REFERENCES

Arroyo, R., and Orozco, E. (1987). Localization and identification of an *Entamoeba histolytica* adhesin. *Mol. Biochem. Parasitol.* 23, 151–158. doi: 10.1016/0166-6851(87)90150-2

Avalos-Padilla, Y., Betanzos, A., Javier-Reyna, R., Garcia-Rivera, G., Chávez-Munguía, B., Lagunes-Guillen, A., et al. (2015). EhVps32 is a vacuole-associated protein involved in pinocytosis and phagocytosis of *Entamoeaba histolytica*. *PLoS Pathog.* 11:e1005079. doi: 10.1371/journal.ppat.1005079

Avalos-Padilla, Y., Knorr, R. L., Javier-Reyna, R., García-Rivera, G., Lipowsky, R., Dimova, R., et al. (2018). The Conserved ESCRT-III machinery participates in the phagocytosis of *Entamoeba histolytica*. *Front. Cell. Infect. Microbiol.* 8:53. doi: 10.3389/fcimb.2018.00053

Azuara-Liceaga, E., Betanzos, A., Cardona-Felix, C. S., Castañeda-Ortiz, E. J., Cárdenas, H., Cárdenas-Guerra, R. E., et al. (2018). The Sole DNA ligase in *Entamoeba histolytica* is a high-fidelity DNA ligase involved in DNA damage repair. *Front. Cell. Infect. Microbiol.* 8:214. doi: 10.3389/fcimb.2018.00214

Bañuelos, C., García-Rivera, G., López-Reyes, I., Mendoza, L., González-Robles, A., Herranz, S., et al. (2012). EhADH112 Is a Bro1 domain-containing protein involved in the *Entamoeba histolytica* multivesicular bodies pathway. *J. Biomed. Biotechnol.* 2012:657942. doi: 10.1155/2012/657942

Bañuelos, C., García-Rivera, G., López-Reyes, I., and Orozco, E. (2005). Functional characterization of EhADH112: an *Entamoeba histolytica* Bro1 domain-containing protein. *Exp Parasitol.* 110, 292–297. doi: 10.1016/j.exppara.2005.03.005

Barmeyer, C., Fromm, M., and Schulzke, J. D. (2017). Active and passive involvement of claudins in the pathophysiology of intestinal inflammatory diseases. *Pflugers Arch. Eur. J. Physiol.* 469, 15–26. doi: 10.1007/s00424-016-1914-6

Bennett, V., and Lorenzo, D. N. (2013). Spectrin- and ankyrin-based membrane domains and the evolution of vertebrates. *Curr. Top. Membr.* 72, 1–37. doi: 10.1016/B978-0-12-417027-8.00001-5

Betanzos, A., Javier-Reyna, R., García-Rivera, G., Bañuelos, C., González-Mariscal, L., Schnoor, M., et al. (2013). The EhCPADH112 Complex of *Entamoeba histolytica* interacts with tight Junction proteins occludin and claudin-1 to produce epithelial damage. *PLoS ONE* 8:e065100. doi: 10.1371/journal.pone.0065100

Bissig, C., and Gruenberg, J. (2014). ALIX and the multivesicular endosome: ALIX in Wonderland. *Trends Cell Biol.* 24, 19–25. doi: 10.1016/j.tcb.2013.10.009

Bolaños, J., Betanzos, A., Javier-Reyna, R., García- Rivera, G., Huerta, M., Pais-Morales, J., et al. (2016). EhNPC1 and EhNPC2 proteins participate in trafficking of exogenous cholesterol in *Entamoeba histolytica* trophozoites: relevance for phagocytosis. *PLoS Pathog.* 12:e1006089. doi: 10.1371/journal.ppat.1006089

Bracha, R., and Mirelman, D. (1984). Virulence of *Entamoeba histolytica* trophozoites. Effects of bacteria, microaerobic conditions, and metronidazole. *J. Exp. Med.* 160, 353–368. doi: 10.1084/jem.160.2.353

Campos, Y., Qiu, X., Gomero, E., Wakefield, R., Horner, L., Brutkowski, W., et al. (2016). Alix-mediated assembly of the actomyosin-tight junction polarity complex preserves epithelial polarity and epithelial barrier. *Nat. Commun.* 7:11876. doi: 10.1038/ncomms11876

Capaldo, C. T., Farkas, A. E., and Nusrat, A. (2014). Epithelial adhesive junctions. *F1000Prime Rep.* 6:1. doi: 10.12703/P6-1

Cardona-Felix, C. S., Lara-Gonzalez, S., and Brieba, L. G. (2011). Structure and biochemical characterization of proliferating cellular nuclear antigen from a parasitic protozoon. *Acta Crystallogr. D Biol. Crystallogr.* 67, 497–505. doi: 10.1107/S0907444911010547

Castellanos-Castro, S., Cerda-García-Rojas, C. M., Javier-Reyna, R., Pais-Morales, J., Chávez-Munguía, B., and Orozco, E. (2016). Identification of the phospholipid lysobisphosphatidic acid in the protozoan *Entamoeba histolytica*: an active molecule in endocytosis. *Biochem. Biophys. Rep.* 5, 224–236. doi: 10.1016/j.bbrep.2015.12.010

Cereijido, M., Robbins, E. S., Dolan, W. J., Rotunno, C. A., and Sabatini, D. D. (1978). Polarized monolayers formed by epithelial cells on a permeable and translucent support. *J. Cell Biol.* 77, 853–880. doi: 10.1083/jcb.77.3.853

Chadee, K., Petri, Jr., W. A., Innes, D. J., and Ravdin, J. I. (1987). Rat and human colonic mucins bind to and inhibit adherence lectin of *Entamoeba histolytica*. *J. Clin. Invest.* 80, 1245–1254. doi: 10.1172/JCI113199

Cornick, S., and Chadee, K. (2017). *Entamoeba histolytica*: Host parasite interactions at the colonic epithelium. *Tissue Barriers* 5:e1283386. doi: 10.1080/21688370.2017.1283386

Cornick, S., Moreau, F., and Chadee, K. (2016). *Entamoeba histolytica* cysteine proteinase 5 evokes mucin exocytosis from colonic goblet cells via αvβ3 integrin. *PLoS Pathog.* 12:e1005579. doi: 10.1371/journal.ppat.1005579

Coyne, C. B., Gambling, T. M., Boucher, R. C., Carson, J. L., and Johnson, L. G. (2003). Role of claudin interactions in airway tight junctional permeability. *Am. J. Physiol. Lung Cell. Mol. Physiol.* 285, L1166–L1178. doi: 10.1152/ajplung.00182.2003

Cuellar, P., Hernández-Nava, E., García-Rivera, G., Chávez-Munguía, B., Schnoor, M., Betanzos, A., et al. (2017). *Entamoeba histolytica* EhCP112 dislocates and degrades claudin-1 and claudin-2 at tight junctions of the intestinal epithelium. *Front. Cell. Infect. Microbiol.* 7:372. doi: 10.3389/fcimb.2017.00372

Deli, M. A. (2009). Potential use of tight junction modulators to reversibly open membranous barriers and improve drug delivery. *Biochim. Biophys. Acta - Biomembr.* 1788, 892–910. doi: 10.1016/j.bbamem.2008.09.016

Diamond, L. S., Harlow, D. R., and Cunnick, C. C. (1978). A new medium for the axenic cultivation of *Entamoeba histolytica* and other Entamoeba. *Trans. R Soc. Trop. Med. Hyg.* 72, 431–432. doi: 10.1016/0035-9203(78)90144-X

Dolabella, S. S., Serrano-Luna, J., Navarro-García, F., Cerritos, R., Ximénez, C., Galván-Moroyoqui, J. M., et al. (2012). Amoebic liver abscess production by entamoeba dispar. *Ann. Hepatol.* 11, 107–117.

Dukes, J. D., Whitley, P., and Chalmers, A. D. (2011). The MDCK variety pack: Choosing the right strain. *BMC Cell Biol.* 12:43. doi: 10.1186/1471-2121-12-43

Flores-Maldonado, C., González-Robles, A., Salazar-Villatoro, L., Omaña-Molina, M., Gallardo, J. M., González-Lázaro, M., et al. (2017). Acanthamoeba (T4) trophozoites cross the MDCK epithelium without cell damage but increase paracellular permeability and transepithelial resistance by modifying tight junction composition. *Exp. Parasitol.* 183, 69–75. doi: 10.1016/j.exppara.2017.10.013

Furuse, M., Furuse, K., Sasaki, H., and Tsukita, S. (2001). Conversion of zonulae occludentes from tight to leaky strand type by introducing claudin-2 into madin-darby canine kidney I cells. *J. Cell Biol.* 153, 263–272. doi: 10.1083/jcb.153.2.263

García-Rivera, G., Rodríguez, M. A., Ocadiz, R., Martinez-Lopez, M. C., Arroyo, R., Gonzalez-Robles, A., et al. (1999). *Entamoeba histolytica* : a novel cysteine protease and an adhesin form the 112 kDa surface protein. *Mol. Microbiol.* 33, 556–568. doi: 10.1046/j.1365-2958.1999.01500.x

Glenney, J. R., and Glenney, P. (1983). Fodrin is the general spectrin-like protein found in most cells whereas spectrin and the TW protein have a restricted distribution. *Cell* 34, 503–512. doi: 10.1016/0092-8674(83)90383-5

Goplen, M., Lejeune, M., Cornick, S., Moreau, F., and Chadee, K. (2013). *Entamoeba histolytica* contains an occludin-like protein that can alter colonic epithelial barrier function. *PLoS ONE* 8:e73339. doi: 10.1371/journal.pone.0073339

Grimson, M. J., Coates, J. C., Reynolds, J. P., Shipman, M., Blanton, R. L., and Harwood, A. J. (2000). Adherens junctions and beta-catenin-mediated cell signalling in a non-metazoan organism. *Nature* 408, 727–731. doi: 10.1038/35047099

Hernández-Nava, E., Cuellar, P., Nava, P., Chávez-Munguía, B., Schnoor, M., Orozco, E., et al. (2017). Adherens junctions and desmosomes are damaged by *Entamoeba histolytica*: participation of EhCPADH complex and EhCP112 protease. *Cell Microbiol.* 19:e12761. doi: 10.1111/cmi.12761

Jouve, M., Garcia, M. I., Courcoux, P., Labigne, A., Gounon, P., and Le Bouguénec, C. (1997). Adhesion to and invasion of HeLa cells by pathogenic Escherichia coli carrying the afa-3 gene cluster are mediated by the AfaE and AfaD proteins, respectively. *Infect. Immun.* 65, 4082–4089.

Leippe, M. (1997). Amoebapores. *Parasitol. Today* 13, 178–183. doi: 10.1016/S0169-4758(97)01038-7

Lejeune, M., Moreau, F., and Chadee, K. (2011). Prostaglandin E2 produced by *Entamoeba histolytica* signals via EP4 receptor and alters claudin-4 to increase ion permeability of tight junctions. *Am. J. Pathol.* 179, 807–818. doi: 10.1016/j.ajpath.2011.05.001

Leroy, A., Lauwaet, T., De Bruyne, G., Cornelissen, M., and Mareel, M. (2000). *Entamoeba histolytica* disturbs the tight junction complex in human enteric T84 cell layers. *FASEB J.* 14, 1139–1146. doi: 10.1096/fasebj.14.9.1139

Li, E., Stenson, W. F., Kunz-Jenkins, C., Swanson, P. E., Duncan, R., and Stanley, S. L. Jr. (1994). *Entamoeba histolytica* interactions with polarized human intestinal Caco-2 epithelial cells. *Infect. Immun.* 62, 5112–5119.

Liang, G. H., and Weber, C. R. (2014). Molecular aspects of tight junction barrier function. *Curr. Opin. Pharmacol.* 19, 84–89. doi: 10.1016/j.coph.2014.07.017

Machado, F. S., Rodriguez, N. E., Adesse, D., Garzoni, L. R., Esper, L., Lisanti, M. P., et al. (2012). Recent developments in the interactions between caveolin and pathogens. *Adv. Exp. Med. Biol.* 729, 65–82. doi: 10.1007/978-1-4614-1222-9_5

Madriz, X., Martínez, M. B., Rodríguez, M. A., Sierra, G., Martínez-López, C., Riverón, A. M., et al. (2004). Expression in fibroblasts and in live animals of *Entamoeba histolytica* polypeptides EhCP112 and EhADH112. *Microbiology* 150, 1251–1260. doi: 10.1099/mic.0.26938-0

Martinez-Lopez, C., Orozco, E., Sanchez, T., Garcia-Perez, R. M., Hernandez-Hernandez, F., and Rodriguez, M. A. (2004). The EhADH112 recombinant polypeptide inhibits cell destruction and liver abscess formation by *Entamoeba histolytica* trophozoites. *Cell Microbiol.* 6, 367–376. doi: 10.1111/j.1462-5822.2004.00363.x

Martínez-Palomo, A., Gonzalez-Robles, A., Chávez, B., Orozco, E., Fernandez-Castelo, S., and Cervantes, A. (1985). Structural bases of the cytolytic mechanisms of *Entamoeba histolytica*. *J. Protozool.* 32, 166–175. doi: 10.1111/j.1550-7408.1985.tb03033.x

Meléndez-López, S. G., Herdman, S., Hirata, K., Choi, M. H., Choe, Y., Craik, C., et al. (2007). Use of recombinant *Entamoeba histolytica* cysteine proteinase 1 to identify a potent inhibitor of amebic invasion in a human colonic model. *Eukaryot. Cell* 6, 1130–1136. doi: 10.1128/EC.00094-07

Montaño, S., Orozco, E., Correa-Basurto, J., Bello, M., Chávez-Munguía, B., and Betanzos, A. (2017). Heterodimerization of the *Entamoeba histolytica* EhCPADH virulence complex through molecular dynamics and protein–protein docking. *J. Biomol. Struct. Dyn.* 35, 486–503. doi: 10.1080/07391102.2016.1151831

Moreno-Ruiz, E., Galán-Díez, M., Zhu, W., Fernández-Ruiz, E., D'Enfert, C., Filler, S. G., et al. (2009). Candida albicans internalization by host cells is mediated by a clathrin-dependent mechanism. *Cell Microbiol.* 11, 1179–1189. doi: 10.1111/j.1462-5822.2009.01319.x

Morita, E., Sandrin, V., Chung, H. Y., Morham, S. G., Gygi, S. P., Rodesch, C. K., et al. (2007). Human ESCRT and ALIX proteins interact with proteins of the midbody and function in cytokinesis. *EMBO J.* 26, 4215–4227. doi: 10.1038/sj.emboj.7601850

Mosso, C., Galván-Mendoza, I. J., Ludert, J. E., and del Angel, R. M. (2008). Endocytic pathway followed by dengue virus to infect the mosquito cell line C6/36 HT. *Virology* 378, 193–199. doi: 10.1016/j.virol.2008.05.012

Ocádiz, R., Orozco, E., Carrillo, E., Quintas, L. I., Ortega-Lopez, J., Garcia-Perez, R. M., et al. (2005). EhCP112 is an *Entamoeba histolytica* secreted cysteine protease that may be involved in the parasite-virulence. *Cell Microbiol.* 7, 221–232. doi: 10.1111/j.1462-5822.2004.00453.x

Odorizzi, G. (2006). The multiple personalities of Alix. *J. Cell Sci.* 119, 3025–3032. doi: 10.1242/jcs.03072

Orozco, E., Guarneros, G., Martinez-Palomo, A., and Sanchez, T. (1983). *Entamoeba histolytica*. Phagocytosis as a virulence factor. *J. Exp. Med.* 158, 1511–1521. doi: 10.1084/jem.158.5.1511

Ralston, K. S., Solga, M. D., Mackey-Lawrence, N. M., Somlata, Bhattacharya, A., and Petri, W. A. (2014). Trogocytosis by *Entamoeba histolytica* contributes to cell killing and tissue invasion. *Nature* 508, 526–530. doi: 10.1038/nature13242

Rosenberger, C. M., Brumell, J. H., and Finlay, B. B. (2000). Microbial pathogenesis: lipid rafts Rosenberger et al., 2000 as pathogen portals. *Curr. Biol.* 10, R823–R825. doi: 10.1016/S0960-9822(00)00788-0

Sambuy, Y., De Angelis, I., and Ranaldi, G. (2005). The Caco-2 cell line as a model of the intestinal barrier: influence of cell and culture-related factors on Caco-2 cell functional characteristics. *Cell Biol.* 21, 1–26. doi: 10.1007/s10565-005-0085-6

Serruto, D., Spadafina, T., Scarselli, M., Bambini, S., Comanducci, M., Höhle, S., et al. (2009). HadA is an atypical new multifunctional trimeric coiled-coil adhesin of Haemophilus influenzae biogroup aegyptius, which promotes entry into host cells. *Cell Microbiol.* 11, 1044–1063. doi: 10.1111/j.1462-5822.2009.01306.x

Singh, R. S., Walia, A. K., Kanwar, J. R., and Kennedy, J. F. (2016). Amoebiasis vaccine development: a snapshot on *E. histolytica* with emphasis on perspectives of Gal/GalNAc lectin. *Int. J. Biol. Macromol.* 91, 258–268. doi: 10.1016/j.ijbiomac.2016.05.043

Thoreson, M. A., Anastasiadis, P. Z., Daniel, J. M., Ireton, R. C., Wheelock, M. J., Johnson, K. R., et al. (2000). Selective uncoupling of p120(ctn) from E-cadherin disrupts strong adhesion. *J. Cell Biol.* 148, 189–201. doi: 10.1083/jcb.148.1.189

13

Unexplored Molecular Features of the *Entamoeba histolytica* RNA Lariat Debranching Enzyme Dbr1 Expression Profile

Jesús Valdés[1], *Carlos Ortuño-Pineda*[2], *Odila Saucedo-Cárdenas*[3,4] *and María S. Mendoza-Figueroa*[1,5*]

[1] Departamento de Bioquímica, Centro de Investigación y de Estudios Avanzados del Instituto Politécnico Nacional, Mexico City, Mexico, [2] Unidad Académica de Ciencias Químico Biológicas, Universidad Autónoma de Guerrero, Chilpancingo, Mexico, [3] Histología, Facultad de Medicina, Universidad Autónoma de Nuevo León, San Nicolás de los Garza, Mexico, [4] División de Genética, Centro de Investigación Biomédica del Noreste, Instituto Mexicano del Seguro Social, Monterrey, Mexico, [5] Departamento de Atención a la Salud, Universidad Autónoma Metropolitana-Xochimilco, Mexico City, Mexico

***Correspondence:**
María S. Mendoza-Figueroa
msmendozafigueroa@gmail.com

The RNA lariat debranching enzyme (Dbr1) has different functions in RNA metabolism, such as hydrolyzing the 2′-5′ linkage in intron lariats, positively influencing Ty1 and HIV-1 retrotransposition, and modulating snRNP recycling during splicing reactions. It seems that Dbr1 is one of the major players in RNA turnover. It is remarkable that of all the studies carried out to date with Dbr1, to our knowledge, none of them have evaluated the expression profile of the endogenous *Dbr1* gene. In this work, we describe, for the first time, that *Entamoeba histolytica EhDbr1* mRNA has a very short half-life (less than 30 min) and encodes a very stable protein that is present until trophozoite cultures die. We also show that the EhDbr1 protein is present in the nuclear periphery on the cytoplasmic basal side, contrary to the localization of human Dbr1. Comparing these results with previous hypotheses and with results from different organisms suggests that *Dbr1* gene expression is finely tuned and conserved across eukaryotes. Experiments describing the aspects of *Dbr1* gene expression and *Dbr1* mRNA turnover as well as other functions of the protein need to be performed. Particularly, a special emphasis is needed on the protozoan parasite *E. histolytica,* the causative agent of amoebiasis, since even though it is a unicellular organism, it is an intron-rich eukaryote whose intron lariats seem to be open to avoid intron lariat accumulation and to process them in non-coding RNAs that might be involved in its virulence.

Keywords: *Entamoeba histolytica*, lariat, Dbr1, mRNA, splicing

INTRODUCTION

The spliceosome mediates intron removal and exon ligation of pre-mRNA through two consecutive trans-esterification reactions, resulting in a 2′-5′ linked lariat and in mRNA molecules (Padgett et al., 1984; Ruskin et al., 1984; Ruskin and Green, 1985; Konarska et al., 2006; Smith et al., 2009). Intron turnover is carried out by the RNA lariat debranching enzyme (Dbr1) that hydrolyzes the 2′-5′ linkage, opening the lariats (Ruskin and Green, 1985) either to be degraded or processed in non-coding RNAs (Ooi et al., 1998). After splicing, lariat RNA is present in two different post-splicing complexes, Intron Large (IL) and Intron Small (IS), but Dbr1 is not associated with either of them, indicating that Dbr1 association with lariat molecules is transitory (Yoshimoto et al., 2009; Garrey et al., 2014). Consistent with its function, the *Homo sapiens* Dbr1 (HsDbr1) in HeLa cells is localized in the nucleoplasm (Kataoka et al., 2013).

Dbr1 protein sequences from different organisms show high homology (Nam et al., 1997; Kim et al., 2000; Kataoka et al., 2013), suggesting that Dbr1 both in structure and in function is phylogenetically conserved. Dbr1 enzymes belong to the metallophosphoesterase (MPE) family (Koonin, 1994), showing a conserved N-terminal domain, a C-terminal domain (CTD) that does not show sequence similarity to any other class of proteins; a third domain between them, the lariat recognition loop (LRL) adjacent to the active site, is not present in other MPEs (Kim et al., 2000). As MPEs, Dbr1 enzymes use divalent metals for their activity (Arenas and Hurwitz, 1987), such as manganese in the case of the *Saccharomyces cerevisiae* Dbr1 (ScDbr1) (Khalid et al., 2005) or Fe^{2+}, Zn^{2+}, or Mn^{2+} in the case of *Entamoeba histolytica* Dbr1 (EhDbr1) (Clark et al., 2016; Ransey et al., 2017), suggesting a different requirement of metal cofactors.

To date, only the protozoan EhDbr1 has been crystallized (Montemayor et al., 2014; Clark et al., 2016; Ransey et al., 2017) from these structures, with the observation that a trinucleotide formed by the adenosine branch point flanked by 2′-5′ and 5′-3′ bonds is the minimal substrate for the debranching enzyme (Arenas and Hurwitz, 1987), Montemayor and coworkers proposed that the lariat molecule seems to be the determinant instead of a specific sequence for substrate recognition by Dbr1, allowing for the debranching of a diverse set of lariat RNA molecules (Montemayor et al., 2014). It is proposed that the hydrolysis of the debranching reaction is a SN2 mechanism via a trigonal bipyramidal pentacoordinate intermediate that results in an investment of the configuration, after which the 2′-O leaving group is protonated (Clark et al., 2016).

It has been observed that in *S. cerevisiae Dbr1* mutants that exhibit intron accumulation (Chapman and Boeke, 1991) and complementation with HsDbr1 (Kim et al., 2000), with the *Caenorhabditis elegans* Dbr1 (CeDbr1) (Nam et al., 1997), or with EhDbr1 (Montemayor et al., 2014), such a phenotype is rescued.

In the present work, we describe unstudied traits of the *E. histolytica* Dbr1 protein, whose structure has been determined recently (Montemayor et al., 2014). We found that the *EhDbr1* mRNA half-life is less than 30 min, but in contrast, it encodes a very stable protein that seems to be present until trophozoite cell cultures die. Additionally, we show that contrary to HsDbr1, EhDbr1 protein is present in the nuclear periphery on the cytoplasmic basal side, indicating that lariat opening in *E. histolytica* is carried out in a different cell compartment and suggesting that intron turnover in this organism might be regulated in a different way than humans. These data and data from other organisms suggest that *Dbr1* gene expression is finely tuned and conserved across eukaryotes. Thus, studies with an emphasis on *Dbr1* gene expression need to be performed. Particularly, in the protozoan parasite *E. histolytica*, EhDbr1 is possibly needed to open intron lariats that seem to be precursors of non-coding RNAs with unknown functions and is expressed from virulence genes (Mendoza-Figueroa et al. this issue).

MATERIALS AND METHODS

Entamoeba histolytica Cell Cultures

E. histolytica trophozoites from HMI: IMSS strain were axenically grown at 37°C in TYI-S-33 medium (Diamond et al., 1978) until they reached the exponential growth phase. Cells were harvested first by incubating them in an ice-water bath and then collected by centrifugation. Trophozoites were used immediately to extract total RNA or proteins by the TRIzol method (Invitrogen) according to the manufacturer's instructions.

HeLa and MRC-5 Cell Cultures

Human cervical carcinoma (HeLa) cells were grown on coverslips inside Petri dishes and cultured in DMEM (Life Technologies). MRC-5 cells were grown in RPMI (Life Technologies). Both cultures were supplemented with 10% fetal bovine serum and were incubated at 37°C in a humid atmosphere of 5% CO_2.

RT-PCRs

Retrotranscription (RT) reactions were carried out with the M-MLV retrotranscriptase (Invitrogen) according to manufacturer's instruction. As template 10, 0.5, and 0.5 μg of total RNA were used in order to produce the *EhDbr1*, *18S rRNA*, and *EhActin* cDNAs, respectively. Polymerase Chain Reactions (PCR) were carried out with 10% cDNA and the Taq DNA Polymerase (Invitrogen) according to manufacturer's instruction. Primers and PCR conditions are indicated in Table S1. As control in each experiment, PCR reactions with total RNA as template were carried out. Amplicons were analyzed in agarose gels and stained with ethidium bromide.

EhDbr1 mRNA Half-life

Eighty percent confluent cell cultures of *E. histolytica* trophozoites were incubated in the presence of Actinomycin D to a final concentration of 1.3 nM (Ayala et al., 1990; Lopez-Camarillo et al., 2003) during the periods indicated in **Figure 1A**. Then, total RNA was extracted and *EhDbr1* gene expression was analyzed by RT-PCR. As control *EhActin* and *18S rRNA* gene expression were analyzed. The treatment was made by triplicate.

EhDbr1 Protein Half-life

Eighty percent confluent cell cultures of *E. histolytica* trophozoites were incubated with the protein synthesis inhibitor emetine (Sigma-Aldrich) to a final concentration of 25 μM (Grollman, 1966) during the periods indicated in **Figures 1C,D**. After that, cells were counted (**Figure 1C**) and total proteins extracted by incubating cells in extraction buffer [10 mM HEPES-KOH, pH 7.2, 24 mM KCl, 10 mM $MgCl_2$, 1 mM PMSF, 2 mM DTT, 1% NP-40, in the presence of the protease inhibitor cocktail "Complete" (Roche)] during 30 min with gentle agitation on ice. Samples were centrifuged at 6,000 × g 10 min at 4°C and proteins in the supernatant were quantitated with the DC Protein Assay Kit (Bio-Rad). Western blot assays were carried out in order to detect EhDbr1 and EhGAPDH proteins. The

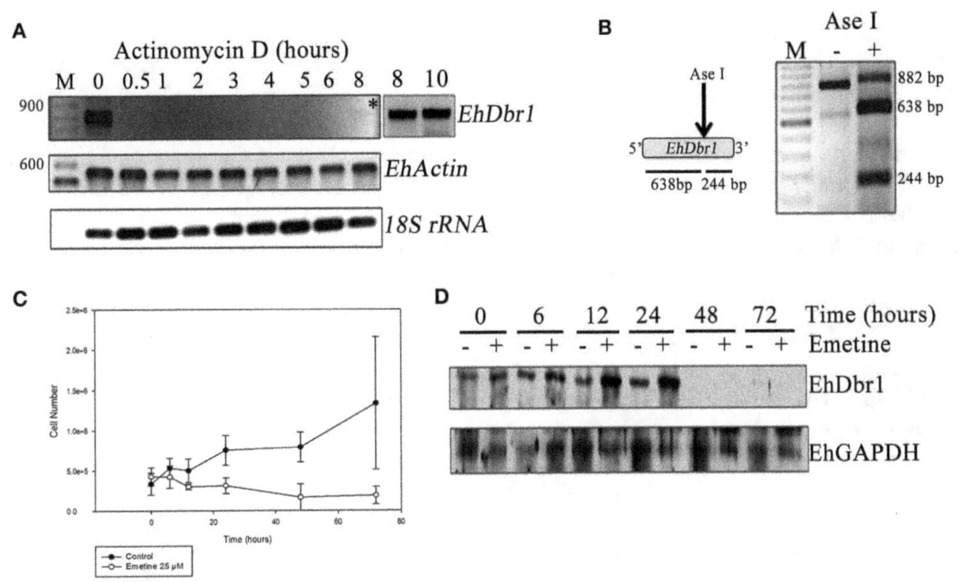

FIGURE 1 | *EhDBR1* mRNA has low abundance, but the EhDbr1 protein has high stability. **(A)** Inhibition of RNA polymerase II transcription in *E. histolytica* trophozoites with Actinomycin D. *EhDbr1*, *EhActin*, and *18S rRNA* gene expression was evaluated to assess the *EhDbr1* mRNA half-life. Recuperation of *EhDbr1* expression is indicated with an asterisk; last two lanes in the left upper panel show PCR reactions of the 8 h sample, with additional (45 and 50) PCR amplification cycles. **(B)** Digestion of the EhDbr1 amplicon obtained in **(A),** with the enzyme AseI as predicted from the restriction map. **(C)** *E. histolytica* trophozoite growth curve without or after 25μM emetine treatment. **(D)** EhDbr1 protein half-life measured by western blots from the previous trophozoite cultures.

antibody Dbrl (ThermoFisher Scientific) was used in a dilution 1:1,500 and the anti GAPDH (Santa Cruz Biotechnology) in a dilution 1: 10,000. The treatment was made by triplicate.

Nuclear and Cytoplasmic Extracts

Nuclear and cytoplasmic extracts were obtained following the Dignam (Dignam et al., 1983) and Rio protocols (Rio et al., 2011). Both extracts were quantitated by the Bradford method and used for western blot assays in order to detect the EhDbrl protein. Also western blots using the antibody EhCPADH (Garcia-Rivera et al., 1999), a gift from Dra. Esther Orozco, in a dilution 1: 40,000 and the antibody Tri-methyl-histone H3 (Lys4) (Cell Signaling) in a dilution 1: 1,000 were carried out as cytoplasmic and nuclear controls, respectively.

EhDbr1 Localization by Confocal Microscopy

E. histolytica trophozoites grown on coverslips were fixed and permeabilized with cold 100% methanol for 5 min and then blocked with 10% adult bovine serum for 1 h at room temperature. Cells were incubated overnight at 4°C with the first antibody Dbrl (1:150) or with PBS (Phosphate Buffered Saline) as negative control. After several washes, samples were incubated with the Goat anti-Rabbit IgG rhodamine conjugated (1:100) (ThermoFischer Scientific). Nuclei were stained with 4′,6-Diamidino-2-Phenylindole (DAPI) and samples were observed through a confocal microscope (Carl Zeiss LSM 700) using the ZEN 2009 software. Observations were performed in approximately 20 optical sections from the top to the bottom of each sample.

RESULTS

EhDbr1 mRNA Abundance Is Low, But the Enzyme Has High Stability

Dbrl cDNA has been isolated and has been used in complementation assays in different organisms (Nam et al., 1997; Kim et al., 2000). However, until now, knowledge about the *Dbrl* mRNA half-life has been missing. To determine the half-life of the *EhDbrl* mRNA, RNA polymerase II transcription was inhibited in *E. histolityca* trophozoites using Actinomycin D (Ayala et al., 1990; Lopez-Camarillo et al., 2003); after different incubation times with the drug, the total RNA was isolated, and the expression of *EhDbrl* was analyzed by RT-PCR. As **Figure 1A** shows, *EhDbrl* mRNA disappeared almost immediately after addition of the drug to the cultures. *EhDbrl* mRNA recuperated after 8 h.

Importantly, to amplify the *EhDbrl* transcript, 10 μg of total RNA was needed in the RT reaction, and extra PCR cycles were employed to better visualize the product at 8 h of Actynomycin D treatment (**Figure 1A**, lanes 8 and 10 to the right of the main panel), suggesting a low level of EhDbrl transcripts. This result is consistent with data from *Arabidopsis thaliana,* where amplification of the *AtDbrl* transcript needed 40 PCR cycles compared to 24 for *AhTUB2,* indicating a low *AtDbrl* mRNA abundance (Wang et al., 2004).

The identity of the PCR product was corroborated by restriction analysis of the amplicon (**Figure 1B**). *EhActin* gene expression was analyzed to control RNA polymerase II inhibition and, the results were consistent with previous work (Lopez-Camarillo et al., 2003); its transcription was not inhibited (half-life >12 h). The expression of the *18S rRNA* was analyzed as a loading control and to control the resistance of RNA polymerase I to Actinomycin D (Oakes et al., 1993).

The EhDbr1 protein half-life was evaluated by inhibition of protein synthesis of *E. histolytica* trophozoites with emetine (Grollman, 1966). After incubation with the drug, the total protein was extracted and analyzed by western blots to detect the enzyme as well as to detect EhGAPDH as a loading control. In **Figure 1C**, the growth curve of *E. histolytica* trophozoites after emetine treatment is shown. Consistent with previous findings (Grollman, 1966), trophozoite growth was inhibited by the drug. Notably, EhDbr1 synthesis was inhibited only after 24 h of treatment (**Figure 1D**); however, protein disappearance coincided with the near absence of cells, suggesting that EhDbr1 disappearance is due to cell death instead of synthesis inhibition. This result indicates that EhDbr1 is present in the cells until trophozoites cultures die. It is interesting to note that the EhDbr1 signal disappears after 48 h, even in the absence of emetine. This result most likely occurs because starting at this time point, cell cultures are over 70% lysed and because at this time point EhDbr1 could be degraded faster than EhGAPDH.

EhDbr1 Localization

Consistent with its function, the HsDbr1 protein is mainly localized in the nucleus (**Figure 2**), but in certain circumstances, it has been observed in the cytoplasm (Kataoka et al., 2013). We set to determine EhDbr1 localization in *E. histolytica* trophozoites. First, nuclear- and cytoplasmic-enriched fractions were obtained, and EhDbr1 was detected by western blot. Unexpectedly, as seen in **Figure 2A**, the EhDbr1 enzyme was localized mainly in the cytoplasm and was nearly absent in the nucleus. As controls of nuclear and cytoplasmic fractionation, histones and the EhCPADH complex (Garcia-Rivera et al., 1999), respectively, were evaluated by western blot, confirming appropriate fractionation.

The Z planes of confocal images suggest that EhDbr1 is in the nuclear periphery on the cytoplasmic side (**Figure 2Ba**), toward the basal-substrate region. Taken together, these results suggest that EhDbr1 might be associated with the nuclear envelope on the cytoplasmic basal side of the *E. histolytica* trophozoites.

DISCUSSION

One of the natural products of pre-mRNA splicing are intron lariat molecules, whose functions are less characterized compared to mRNA. It seems that independent of its function, the 2′-5′ phosphodiester linkage in the intron lariats needs to be opened by the Dbr1 enzyme to process the lariats. It is remarkable that of all the studies carried out to date with Dbr1, to our knowledge, none of them have evaluated the expression profile of the endogenous *Dbr1* gene.

EhDbr1 mRNA appears to have a half-life of less than 30 min, indicating a low abundance of the transcript in the cell under steady state conditions, possibly due to low *EhDbr1* gene transcription, which is consistent with the recuperation of transcription after 8 h of Actinomycin D treatment. Then, once translated, its degradation rate might be increased, resulting in a low accumulation of the *EhDbr1* transcript. In this scenario, the resultant protein should have high stability, such that high quantities of mRNA are not required. In *A. thaliana*, Wang and coworkers observed that the accumulation level of the *AtDbr1* transcript was low (Wang et al., 2004). As in this work, the authors needed a high number of PCR cycles to amplify the *AtDbr1* mRNA. Furthermore, because *S. cerevisiae, C. elegans* and *A. thaliana* contain a single copy of the *Dbr1* gene and because *H. sapiens* contain, at most, two copies (Kim et al., 2000; Wang et al., 2004), it has been proposed that *HsDbr1* mRNA abundance should be extremely low and that the encoded protein should have a high specific activity, perhaps being very stable (Kim et al., 2000). In *E. histolytica*, the *EhDbr1* gene copy number has not yet been determined, but we observed that the EhDbr1 protein is very stable.

First, low *Dbr1* mRNA levels in *E. histolytica*, as in *A. thaliana*, suggest that their RNA turnover is fast. Particularly, in amoeba, the mRNA half-life is influenced by the length of the 3′ end poly(A) tail, modified by stress conditions (Lopez-Camarillo et al., 2003, 2014). The poly(A) tail length of *EhDbr1* mRNA is unknown, but it will be important to determine this signature in the transcript to know if it is a determinant for the low accumulation observed. We do not know if other *E. histolytica* genes carry out a similar rate of RNA turnover.

Second, compared with the forward K_M values of constitutive glycolytic amoebic enzymes such as hexokinase (~33 μM for glucose), GAPDH (~33 μM for glyceraldehyde-3-phosphate) or the fructose bisphosphate aldolases that shows the highest affinities for their substrate Fru(1,6)P_2 (~4 μM) (Saavedra et al., 2005), the K_M value for Dbr1 is 0.2–0.5 μM for short-branched RNAs (Garrey et al., 2014; Clark et al., 2016). These K_M values suggest that debranching enzymes have a high specific activity, as previously proposed (Kim et al., 2000), with turnover rates of ~3 s^{-1} (Clark et al., 2016). This activity is enhanced by Dnr1, a Dbr1 homolog protein, that directly interacts with the lariat (Garrey et al., 2014).

Thus, all of these data support the idea that *EhDbr1* gene expression regulation seems to be finely tuned and conserved across eukaryotes, such that cells synthesize few mRNA molecules that are translated into robust Dbr1 enzymes, constituting one of the key (and probably the most critical) factors that regulate intron lariat turnover.

Surprisingly, the EhDbr1 enzyme is present until trophozoite cultures die, suggesting that the half-life of the EhDbr1 enzyme may be longer than the trophozoite cell doubling time. We suspect that the longer half-life of this enzyme could be due to the absence of additional ubiquitination sites present in HsDbr1 (Figure S1), although this possibility remains to be tested. However, we can envisage the need of a robust EhDbr1 since, even though *E. histolytica* is a unicellular organism, it is an intron-rich eukaryote (Hon et al., 2013); thus, amoebic intron lariats need to be immediately open to degrade them, avoiding lariat accumulation, or to process them in ncRNAs, such as circular RNA molecules (Mendoza-Figueroa et al. this issue).

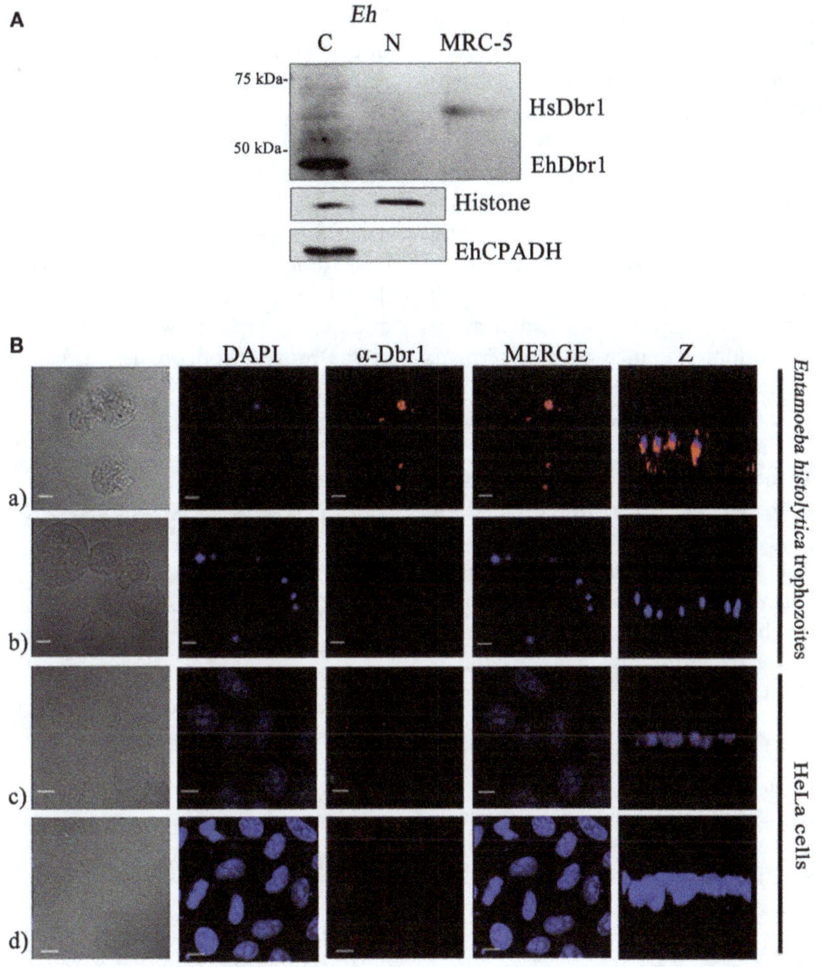

FIGURE 2 | EhDbr1 cellular localization. **(A)** EhDbr1 protein localization was evaluated by cytoplasmic and nuclear fractionation of *E. histolytica* trophozoites. A sample of human (MRC-5 cells) proteins was included in the western blot. EhDbr1 is 42 kDa, and HsDbr1 is 61 kDa. Histone and EhCPADH were analyzed as cytoplasmic and nuclear indicators, respectively. **(B)** Apparently, EhDbr1 localizes in the cytoplasmic-basal nuclear periphery. (a,c) confocal immunofluorescence of *E. histolytica* and HeLa cells, respectively, using the anti-Dbr1 as the primary antibody and goat anti-rabbit IgG rhodamine conjugated secondary antibody (red). (b,d) same as above, without the primary antibody. Nuclei were stained with DAPI (blue). Z plane: lateral image of cells. Bar scale = 10 μm.

Because of the difference in the localization pattern between HsDbr1 and EhDbr1 shown by western blot analysis, we hypothesized that EhDbr1 has a weak nuclear localization signal (NLS), allowing its passage to the nucleus in minute quantities. The EhDbr1 protein sequence alignments with the bipartite NLS (VPLKRLSDEHEPEQRKKIKRRNQAIYAAVDDDDDDAA) of the HsDbr1 C-terminal domain (HsNLS), constituted by 37 amino acid residues (Kataoka et al., 2013) and the three portions (EhNLS1, 2, and 3) of the *E. histolytica* EhNCABP166 tripartite NLS (Uribe et al., 2012), showed that the single EhDbr1 NLS does not match perfectly to any of the NLS tested (Figure S2), supporting the notion of a weak NLS in EhDbr1 compared with the bipartite HsNLS and the tripartite EhNLS. This situation prevented the EhDbr1 from entering the nucleus as efficiently as HsDbr1 does. We do not discard the possibility that in other growth phases, EhDbr1 could be present abundantly inside the nucleus. These possibilities need further evaluation. EhDbr1 localization was analyzed by confocal microscopy. For comparison, nuclear speckles localization of the HsDbr1 in HeLa cells was included (Kataoka et al., 2013). Our results suggest that the EhDbr1 is localized on the cytoplasmic side of the nuclear periphery, appearing concentrated on the basal (toward the substrate) region. Taken together, these results suggest that the EhDbr1 might be associated with the nuclear envelope on the cytoplasmic side of the *E. histolytica* trophozoites, arguing for an inefficient NLS C-terminal EhDbr1 and allowing for minute amounts of nuclear EhDbr1 to be transported. It is also possible that in the growth phase analyzed, EhDbr1 mainly rests on the cytoplasmic side, while in other growth phases, it could be mainly nuclear. These hypotheses need to be evaluated.

The main function attributed to Dbr1 is to hydrolyze the 2′-5′ linkage in RNA lariats (Ruskin and Green, 1985); however, other functions have been associated with Dbr1. For example, the retrotransposon Tyl replicates by retrotranscription, and the resultant cDNA then is then integrated into the host genome. In Δ*dbrl S. cerevisiae* cells, Tyl cDNA accumulates (Chapman and Boeke, 1991; Salem et al., 2003), suggesting that ScDbrl is involved in retrotranscription or cDNA stability (Salem et al., 2003). Experiments carried out by Salem and coworkers ruled out the possibility that the Tyl cDNA had 2′-5′ linkages at the 5′ or 3′ ends since it integrates into the genome in the Δ*dbrl* cells. Additionally, Pratico and Silverman demonstrated that a 2′-5′-branched RNA is not a retrotransposition intermediate, suggesting that Dbrl binds RNA only to stabilize it or that it carries other functions different from the 2′-5′ bond cleavage during the Tyl retrotransposition (Pratico and Silverman, 2007). To gain more insights into the role of Dbrl in Tyl retrotransposition, it will be important to determine if Dbrl associates with Tyl RNA directly in the nucleus or in the retrosomes, the cytoplasmic foci where the virus-like particles are assembled (Pachulska-Wieczorek et al., 2016). Moreover, HIV-1 is a retrovirus resembling retrotransposons. It seems that HIV-1 initiates its cDNA synthesis at the cytoplasm and then completes it in the nucleus or in the perinuclear region. The initial synthesis does not depend on HsDbrl, but its completion does. Currently, it is unknown if a lariat-like structure with a 2′-5′ bond is formed in the HIV-1 RNA such that HsDbrl needs to open it (Galvis et al., 2014).

Recently, Han and coworkers showed that HsDbrl modulates snRNP recycling, allowing the enzymes to dissociate from post-catalytic complexes and to be available to form new spliceosomes complexes. If snRNP availability is compromised, the resulting effect is a change in the alternative splicing pattern that leads to tumorigenesis (Han et al., 2017).

To date, the role of Dbrl in the cytoplasm is not clear; however, from Tyl and HIV-1 data, it seems that Dbrl might have a function different from that of 2′-5′ bond cleavage. EhDbrl, as well as other Dbrl enzymes, may have a conserved cytoplasmic function not described thus far.

CONCLUSION AND FUTURE DIRECTIONS

In this work, we describe that *EhDbrl* mRNA has a very short half-life (less than 30 min) and encodes a very stable protein that is present until trophozoites cultures die. Moreover, in a steady state, *E. histolytica* trophozoite EhDbrl seems to be localized in the nuclear periphery, probably because of the lack of a well-defined nuclear localization signal. These data and data from other organisms suggest that Dbrl gene expression is finely tuned and conserved across eukaryotes. Experiments that describe the aspects of *EhDbrl* gene transcription and *EhDbrl* mRNA turnover, as well as those describing other functions of the protein both in the nucleus and cytosol, need to be performed.

AUTHOR CONTRIBUTIONS

MM-F conceived, designed, acquired data, carried out the experiments, analyzed data and drafted the manuscript; CO-P participated in the design of the study and drafted the manuscript; OS-C drafted the manuscript; JV conceived and designed the study, analyzed data and drafted the manuscript. All authors read and approved the final manuscript.

ACKNOWLEDGMENTS

The authors thank Dr. Esther Orozco from Departamento de Infectómica y Patogénesis Molecular-CINVESTAV for the antibody anti-EhCPADH.

This work was supported by Consejo Nacional de Ciencia y Tecnología (CONACyT, México) grants 127557-M and 236104. MM-F received the CONACyT fellowship 46417.

REFERENCES

Arenas, J., and Hurwitz, J. (1987). Purification of a RNA debranching activity from HeLa cells. *J. Biol. Chem.* 262, 4274–4279.

Ayala, P., Samuelson, J., Wirth, D., and Orozco, E. (1990). *Entamoeba histolytica*: physiology of multidrug resistance. *Exp. Parasitol.* 71, 169–175. doi: 10.1016/0014-4894(90)90019-9

Chapman, K. B., and Boeke, J. D. (1991). Isolation and characterization of the gene encoding yeast debranching enzyme. *Cell* 65, 483–492. doi: 10.1016/0092-8674(91)90466-C

Clark, N. E., Katolik, A., Roberts, K. M., Taylor, A. B., Holloway, S. P., Schuermann, J. P., et al. (2016). Metal dependence and branched RNA cocrystal structures of the RNA lariat debranching enzyme Dbrl. *Proc. Natl. Acad. Sci. U.S.A.* 113, 14727–14732. doi: 10.1073/pnas.1612729114

Diamond, L. S., Harlow, D. R., and Cunnick, C. C. (1978). A new medium for the axenic cultivation of *Entamoeba histolytica* and other Entamoeba. *Trans. R. Soc. Trop. Med. Hyg.* 72, 431–432. doi: 10.1016/0035-9203(78)90144-X

Dignam, J. D., Lebovitz, R. M., and Roeder, R. G. (1983). Accurate transcription initiation by RNA polymerase II in a soluble extract from isolated mammalian nuclei. *Nucleic Acids Res.* 11, 1475–1489. doi: 10.1093/nar/11.5.1475

Galvis, A. E., Fisher, H. E., Nitta, T., Fan, H., and Camerini, D. (2014). Impairment of HIV-1 cDNA synthesis by DBR1 knockdown. *J. Virol.* 88, 7054–7069. doi: 10.1128/JVI.00704-14

García-Rivera, G., Rodríguez, M. A., Ocádiz, R., Martínez-López, M. C., Arroyo, R., González-Robles, A., et al. (1999). *Entamoeba histolytica* : a novel cysteine protease and an adhesin form the 112 kDa surface protein. *Mol. Microbiol.* 33, 556–568. doi: 10.1046/j.1365-2958.1999.01500.x

Garrey, S. M., Katolik, A., Prekeris, M., Li, X., York, K., Bernards, S., et al. (2014). A homolog of lariat-debranching enzyme modulates turnover of branched RNA. *RNA* 20, 1337–1348. doi: 10.1261/rna.044602.114

Grollman, A. P. (1966). Structural basis for inhibition of protein synthesis by emetine and cycloheximide based on an analogy between ipecac alkaloids and glutarimide antibiotics. *Proc. Natl. Acad. Sci. U.S.A.* 56, 1867–1874. doi: 10.1073/pnas.56.6.1867

Han, B., Park, H. K., Ching, T., Panneerselvam, J., Wang, H., Shen, Y., et al. (2017). Human DBR1 modulates the recycling of snRNPs to affect alternative RNA splicing and contributes to the suppression of cancer development. *Oncogene* 36, 5382–5391. doi: 10.1038/onc.2017.150

Hon, C. C., Weber, C., Sismeiro, O., Proux, C., Koutero, M., Deloger, M., et al. (2013). Quantification of stochastic noise of splicing and polyadenylation in *Entamoeba histolytica*. *Nucleic Acids Res.* 41, 1936–1952. doi: 10.1093/nar/gks1271

Kataoka, N., Dobashi, I., Hagiwara, M., and Ohno, M. (2013). hDbr1 is a nucleocytoplasmic shuttling protein with a protein phosphatase-like motif essential for debranching activity. *Sci. Rep.* 3:1090. doi: 10.1038/srep01090

Khalid, M. F., Damha, M. J., Shuman, S., and Schwer, B. (2005). Structure-function analysis of yeast RNA debranching enzyme (Dbr1), a manganese-dependent phosphodiesterase. *Nucleic Acids Res.* 33, 6349–6360. doi: 10.1093/nar/gki934

Kim, J. W., Kim, H. C., Kim, G. M., Yang, J. M., Boeke, J. D., and Nam, K. (2000). Human RNA lariat debranching enzyme cDNA complements the phenotypes of *Saccharomyces cerevisiae* dbr1 and *Schizosaccharomyces pombe* dbr1 mutants. *Nucleic Acids Res.* 28, 3666–3673. doi: 10.1093/nar/28.18.3666

Konarska, M. M., Vilardell, J., and Query, C. C. (2006). Repositioning of the reaction intermediate within the catalytic center of the spliceosome. *Mol. Cell* 21, 543–553. doi: 10.1016/j.molcel.2006.01.017

Koonin, E. V. (1994). Conserved sequence pattern in a wide variety of phosphoesterases. *Protein Sci.* 3, 356–358. doi: 10.1002/pro.5560030218

López-Camarillo, C., López-Rosas, I., Ospina-Villa, J. D., and Marchat, L. A. (2014). Deciphering molecular mechanisms of mRNA metabolism in the deep-branching eukaryote *Entamoeba histolytica*. *Wiley Interdiscip. Rev. RNA* 5, 247–262. doi: 10.1002/wrna.1205

López-Camarillo, C., Luna-Arias, J. P., Marchat, L. A., and Orozco, E. (2003). EhPgp5 mRNA stability is a regulatory event in the *Entamoeba histolytica* multidrug resistance phenotype. *J. Biol. Chem.* 278, 11273–11280. doi: 10.1074/jbc.M211757200

Montemayor, E. J., Katolik, A., Clark, N. E., Taylor, A. B., Schuermann, J. P., Combs, D. J., et al. (2014). Structural basis of lariat RNA recognition by the intron debranching enzyme Dbr1. *Nucleic Acids Res.* 42, 10845–10855. doi: 10.1093/nar/gku725

Nam, K., Lee, G., Trambley, J., Devine, S. E., and Boeke, J. D. (1997). Severe growth defect in a *Schizosaccharomyces pombe* mutant defective in intron lariat degradation. *Mol. Cell. Biol.* 17, 809–818. doi: 10.1128/MCB.17.2.809

Oakes, M., Nogi, Y., Clark, M. W., and Nomura, M. (1993). Structural alterations of the nucleolus in mutants of *Saccharomyces cerevisiae* defective in RNA polymerase I. *Mol. Cell. Biol.* 13, 2441–2455. doi: 10.1128/MCB.13.4.2441

Ooi, S. L., Samarsky, D. A., Fournier, M. J., and Boeke, J. D. (1998). Intronic snoRNA biosynthesis in *Saccharomyces cerevisiae* depends on the lariat-debranching enzyme: intron length effects and activity of a precursor snoRNA. *RNA* 4, 1096–1110. doi: 10.1017/S1355838298980785

Pachulska-Wieczorek, K., Le Grice, S. F., and Purzycka, K. J. (2016). Determinants of genomic RNA encapsidation in the *Saccharomyces cerevisiae* long terminal repeat retrotransposons Ty1 and Ty3. *Viruses* 8:193. doi: 10.3390/v8070193

Padgett, R. A., Konarska, M. M., Grabowski, P. J., Hardy, S. F., and Sharp, P. A. (1984). Lariat RNA's as intermediates and products in the splicing of messenger RNA precursors. *Science* 225, 898–903. doi: 10.1126/science.6206566

Pratico, E. D., and Silverman, S. K. (2007). Ty1 reverse transcriptase does not read through the proposed 2′,5′-branched retrotransposition intermediate *in vitro*. *RNA* 13, 1528–1536. doi: 10.1261/rna.629607

Ransey, E., Paredes, E., Dey, S. K., Das, S. R., Heroux, A., and Macbeth, M. R. (2017). Crystal structure of the *Entamoeba histolytica* RNA lariat debranching enzyme EhDbr1 reveals a catalytic Zn(2+) /Mn(2+) heterobinucleation. *FEBS lett.* 591, 2003–2010. doi: 10.1002/1873-3468.12677

Rio D. C., Ares M. Jr., Hannon G. J., and Nilsen T. W. (2011). *RNA: A laboratory manual.* New York, NY: Cold Spring Harbor Laboratory Press.

Ruskin, B., and Green, M. R. (1985). An RNA processing activity that debranches RNA lariats. *Science* 229, 135–140. doi: 10.1126/science.2990042

Ruskin, B., Krainer, A. R., Maniatis, T., and Green, M. R. (1984). Excision of an intact intron as a novel lariat structure during pre-mRNA splicing *in vitro*. *Cell* 38, 317–331. doi: 10.1016/0092-8674(84)90553-1

Saavedra, E., Encalada, R., Pineda, E., Jasso-Chavez, R., and Moreno-Sanchez, R. (2005). Glycolysis in *Entamoeba histolytica*. Biochemical characterization of recombinant glycolytic enzymes and flux control analysis. *FEBS J.* 272, 1767–1783. doi: 10.1111/j.1742-4658.2005.04610.x

Salem, L. A., Boucher, C. L., and Menees, T. M. (2003). Relationship between RNA lariat debranching and Ty1 element retrotransposition. *J. Virol.* 77, 12795–12806. doi: 10.1128/JVI.77.23.12795-12806.2003

Smith, D. J., Konarska, M. M., and Query, C. C. (2009). Insights into branch nucleophile positioning and activation from an orthogonal pre-mRNA splicing system in yeast. *Mol. Cell* 34, 333–343. doi: 10.1016/j.molcel.2009.03.012

Uribe, R., Almaraz Barrera Mde, J., Robles-Flores, M., Mendoza Hernández, G., González-Robles, A., Hernández-Rivas, R., et al. (2012). A functional study of nucleocytoplasmic transport signals of the EhNCABP166 protein from *Entamoeba histolytica*. *Parasitology* 139, 1697–1710. doi: 10.1017/S0031182012001199

Wang, H., Hill, K., and Perry, S. E. (2004). An Arabidopsis RNA lariat debranching enzyme is essential for embryogenesis. *J. Biol. Chem.* 279, 1468–1473. doi: 10.1074/jbc.M309106200

Yoshimoto, R., Kataoka, N., Okawa, K., and Ohno, M. (2009). Isolation and characterization of post-splicing lariat-intron complexes. *Nucleic Acids Res.* 37, 891–902. doi: 10.1093/nar/gkn1002

14

Entamoeba histolytica Induce Signaling via Raf/MEK/ERK for Neutrophil Extracellular Trap (NET) Formation

Zayda Fonseca[1], *César Díaz-Godínez*[1], *Nancy Mora*[1], *Omar R. Alemán*[1], *Eileen Uribe-Querol*[2], *Julio C. Carrero*[1*] *and Carlos Rosales*[1*]

[1] *Departamento de Inmunología, Instituto de Investigaciones Biomédicas, Universidad Nacional Autónoma de México, Mexico City, Mexico,* [2] *División de Estudios de Posgrado e Investigación, Facultad de Odontología, Universidad Nacional Autónoma de México, Mexico City, Mexico*

***Correspondence:**
Julio C. Carrero
carrero@unam.mx
Carlos Rosales
carosal@unam.mx

Amoebiasis, the disease caused by *Entamoeba histolytica* is the third leading cause of human deaths among parasite infections. *E. histolytica* was reported associated with around 100 million cases of amoebic dysentery, colitis and amoebic liver abscess that lead to almost 50,000 fatalities worldwide in 2010. *E. histolytica* infection is associated with the induction of inflammation characterized by a large number of infiltrating neutrophils. These neutrophils have been implicated in defense against this parasite, by mechanisms not completely described. The neutrophil antimicrobial mechanisms include phagocytosis, degranulation, and formation of neutrophil extracellular traps (NETs). Recently, our group reported that NETs are also produced in response to *E. histolytica* trophozoites. But, the mechanism for NETs induction remains unknown. In this report we explored the possibility that *E. histolytica* leads to NETs formation via a signaling pathway similar to the pathways activated by PMA or the Fc receptor FcγRIIIb. Neutrophils were stimulated by *E. histolytica* trophozoites and the effect of various pharmacological inhibitors on amoeba-induced NETs formation was assessed. Selective inhibitors of Raf, MEK, and NF-κB prevented *E. histolytica*-induced NET formation. In contrast, inhibitors of PKC, TAK1, and NADPH-oxidase did not block *E. histolytica*-induced NETs formation. *E. histolytica* induced phosphorylation of ERK in a Raf and MEK dependent manner. These data show that *E. histolytica* activates a signaling pathway to induce NETs formation, that involves Raf/MEK/ERK, but it is independent of PKC, TAK1, and reactive oxygen species (ROS). Thus, amoebas activate neutrophils via a different pathway from the pathways activated by PMA or the IgG receptor FcγRIIIb.

Keywords: *Entamoeba histolytica*, neutrophil, NETosis, NETs, ROS, ERK, NF-κB

INTRODUCTION

Entamoeba histolytica is a protozoan parasite with high prevalence in developing countries (Verkerke and Petri, 2012; Tellevik et al., 2015; Ghenghesh et al., 2016). Amoebiasis, the disease caused by *E. histolytica* affects the intestine and the liver, and is the third leading cause of human deaths among parasite infections (Walsh, 1986; Lozano et al., 2012). In this context, *E. histolytica* was found responsible for about 100 million cases of amoebiasis that led to some 50,000 global deaths in 2010 (Mortimer and Chadee, 2010). Although there is growing understanding of the immune response against amoebas, a full solution to amoebiasis is still needed (Moonah et al., 2013; Nakada-Tsukui and Nozaki, 2016; Cornick and Chadee, 2017). *E. histolytica* infection of the intestine or liver is associated with a strong inflammation characterized by a large number of infiltrating neutrophils (Prathap and Gilman, 1970; Tsutsumi et al., 1984; Tsutsumi and Martinez-Palomo, 1988; Espinosa-Cantellano and Martínez-Palomo, 2000). Usually, large numbers of neutrophil are seen surrounding trophozoites. Yet, amoebas do not seem to be damaged by this interaction. Neutrophils have been implicated in defense against this parasite playing a crucial protective role (Seydel et al., 1997; Velazquez et al., 1998; Jarillo-Luna et al., 2002; Asgharpour et al., 2005; Estrada-Figueroa et al., 2011). However, neutrophils and other leukocytes have also been reported as major inducers of tissue damage during intestinal and liver amoebiasis (Salata and Ravdin, 1986; Pérez-Tamayo et al., 1991, 2006; Seydel et al., 1998; Olivos-García et al., 2007; Dickson-Gonzalez et al., 2009). Therefore, the role of neutrophils in this parasitic infection remains controversial.

Neutrophils, the most abundant leucocytes in peripheral blood, migrate from the circulation to sites of inflammation. Typically, neutrophils are considered the first line of defense because they are the first cells to arrive at the infected site, and they present several antimicrobial functions (Deniset and Kubes, 2014; Mayadas et al., 2014). Among these functions, phagocytosis, degranulation, and formation of neutrophil extracellular traps (NETs) are the most important (Brinkmann et al., 2004; Yipp et al., 2012). NETs are formed by a process known as "NETosis" that involves activation in most cases of nicotinamide adenine dinucleotide phosphate (NADPH)-oxidase, which produces reactive oxygen species (ROS) (Fuchs et al., 2007; Bianchi et al., 2009; Remijsen et al., 2011). NETs are fibers of DNA decorated with histones (Neeli and Radic, 2012) and antimicrobial proteins, such as elastase, myeloperoxidase, lactoferrin, and metalloprotease 9 (Brinkmann et al., 2004; Fuchs et al., 2007). NETs can block the dissemination of microorganisms because they function as a physical barrier where pathogens get caught, and get also exposed to antimicrobial proteins. Consequently, NETs can eliminate pathogens extracellularly and independently of phagocytosis (Papayannopoulos and Zychlinsky, 2009). Several human protozoan parasites have been reported to induce the formation of NETs, including *Leishmania amazonensis*, *L. major*, *L. chagasi*, *Leishmania donovani* (Guimarães-Costa et al., 2009; Gabriel et al., 2010; Hurrell et al., 2015), *Toxoplasma gondii* (Abi Abdallah et al., 2012), and *Trypanosoma cruzi* (Sousa-Rocha et al., 2015). Recently, *E. histolytica* trophozoites were also demonstrated to induce NETs formation (Ávila et al., 2016; Ventura-Juarez et al., 2016). Yet, the mechanism of NETs induction by any of these parasites remains unknown. Although, many microorganisms can induce NETs, no single receptor for pathogen-associated molecular patterns (PAMPs) has been identified as responsible for inducing this neutrophil response. However, Toll-like receptors (TLRs) have been suggested to participate (Yipp et al., 2012). Only two receptors for antibody molecules are reported to be bona fide activators of NETs release from human neutrophils, the IgA receptor FcαR (Aleyd et al., 2014), and the IgG receptor FcγRIIIb (Behnen et al., 2014; Alemán et al., 2016a).

It was firstly published that signaling activated by phorbol 12-myristate 13-acetate (PMA) in neutrophils for NETs formation involves the Raf/ERK pathway (Hakkim et al., 2011) and requires ROS produced by the NADPH-oxidase (Almyroudis et al., 2013). In contrast, we previously found that signaling activated by the FcγRIIIb for NETs formation is different from the pathway activated by PMA (Alemán et al., 2016a,b). For this receptor, NETs formation is dependent on NADPH-oxidase, and extracellular signal-regulated kinase (ERK) activation (Alemán et al., 2016a), and requires signaling through the kinases spleen tyrosine kinase (Syk) and transforming growth factor-β-activated kinase 1 (TAK1) (Alemán et al., 2016b). These results emphasize the recent recognized fact that NETs formation is induced by different signaling pathways depending on diverse stimuli (Kenny et al., 2017). In the case of parasitic pathogens, such as *E. histolytica*, no receptor has been clearly identified as an inducer of NETs, and nothing is known about the signaling pathway activated by amoebas in neutrophils to induce NETs formation. Therefore, in this report we investigated whether *E. histolytica* leads to NETs formation via a signaling pathway that involves ERK activation. Neutrophils were stimulated by *E. histolytica* trophozoites and the effect of various pharmacological inhibitors on amoeba-induced NETs formation was assessed. Selective inhibitors of Raf, MEK, and NF-κB prevented *E. histolytica*-induced NET formation. In contrast, inhibitors of PKC and NADPH-oxidase, as previously reported, blocked PMA-induced (Hakkim et al., 2011), but not *E. histolytica*-induced NET formation. *E. histolytica* induced phosphorylation of ERK in a Raf and MEK dependent manner. Also, NF-κB phosphorylation was dependent on MEK. Our results indicate for the first time that *E. histolytica* triggers a signaling pathway to induce NETs formation, that involves Raf/MEK/ERK, but it is independent of PKC, ROS, Syk, and TAK1. Thus, amoebas activate neutrophils via a different pathway from the pathways activated by PMA or the IgG receptor FcγRIIIb.

MATERIALS AND METHODS

Neutrophils

Neutrophils (PMN) were purified from blood exactly as previously described (García-García et al., 2013). Adult healthy volunteers provided a written informed consent before donating blood. The Bioethics Committee at Instituto de Investigaciones Biomédicas—Universidad Nacional Autónoma de México (UNAM), approved the informed consent form, and all experimental procedures.

Entamoeba histolytica

Entamoeba histolytica trophozoites (strain HM1:IMSS) were cultured axenically at 37°C in TYIS-33 medium supplemented with 15% heat-inactivated adult bovine serum and Diamond vitamin Tween® 80 solution (Sigma-Aldrich; St. Louis, MO)

(Diamond et al., 1978). The cultures were incubated for 72 h and trophozoites were collected after cooling on ice for 5 min and then centrifuging at 300 × g for 5 min at 4°C. The pelleted trophozoites (amoebas) were resuspended in PBS.

Reagents

Bovine serum albumin (BSA) was from F. Hoffmann-La Roche Ltd. (Mannheim, Germany). UO126, a specific MEK (ERK kinase) inhibitor was obtained from Promega (Madison, WI, USA). The antibiotic LLZ 1640-2 (also known as (5Z)-7-Oxozeaenol; cas 66018-38-0) (catalog no. sc-202055), a specific TAK1 inhibitor, was from Santa Cruz Biotechnology (Santa Cruz, CA). Wortmannin, a phosphatidylinositol 3-kinase (PI3K) inhibitor; Gö6976, a protein kinase C (PKC) inhibitor; Gö6983, another PKC inhibitor; SB 203580, a p38 MAP kinase inhibitor (catalog number 559389); 4′,6-diamino-2-fenilindol (DAPI), a cell-permeable DNA-binding dye (catalog no. 268298); and 3-(1-methyl-1H-indol-3-yl-methylene)-2-oxo-2,3-dihydro-1H-indole-5-sulfonamide (iSyk), a Syk inhibitor (catalog no. 574711) were from Calbiochem/EMD Millipore (Billerica, MA). The cOmplete™ protease inhibitor cocktail (catalog no. 11697498001) and *PhosSTOP*™ phosphatase inhibitor cocktail (catalog no. 04906845001) were from Roche Diagnostics (Basel, Switzerland). Dihydrorhodamine 123 (catalog no. AS-85711) was from AnaSpec, Inc. (Fremont, CA, USA), and Dihydroethidium (catalog no. 12013) was from Cayman Chemical (Ann Arbor, MI, USA). Diphenyleneiodonium chloride (DPI), an NADPH-oxidase inhibitor (catalog no. D2926); (E)-3-[4-methylphenylsulfonyl]-2-propenenitrile (BAY 117082), an NF-κB inhibitor (catalog no. B5556); 3-(3,5-dibromo-4-hydroxybenzyliden)-5-iodo-1,3-dihydroindol-2-one (GW5074), a cRaf1 kinase inhibitor (catalog no. G6416); phorbol 12-myristate 13-acetate (PMA) (catalog no. P8139), and all other chemicals were from Sigma-Aldrich (St. Louis, MO). The following antibodies were used: rabbit polyclonal anti-histone H4 (acetyl K12) antibody (catalog No. ab61238), and rabbit polyclonal anti-citrulline antibody (catalog No. ab100932) from Abcam, Inc. (Cambridge, MA). Monoclonal antibody IgG2a (IB4) anti-integrin β2 (catalog no. sc-65254), mouse monoclonal IgG2a anti-phospho-ERK 1/2 (pTyr204) (catalog no. sc-7383), mouse monoclonal IgG1 anti-NF-κB p50 subunit (catalog no. sc-8414), and rabbit polyclonal anti phospho-NF-κB p50 subunit (pSer337) (catalog no. sc-33022) from Santa Cruz Biotechnology (Santa Cruz, CA). Monoclonal antibody IgG1 (3G8) anti-human CD16 (catalog no. 556617), and R-phycoerythrin (PE)-conjugated monoclonal antibody IgG2a (clone CLB-gran1 1.5) anti-human CD16b (catalog No. 550868) were from BD Pharmingen™ (San Diego, CA). Tetramethylrhodamine (TRITC) conjugate ZyMax™ goat anti-rabbit IgG (catalog No. 81-6114) was from Thermo Fisher Scientific (Carlsbad, CA). Rabbit monoclonal IgG anti-ERK 1/2 (catalog no. 4695) was from Cell Signaling Technology, Inc. (Beverly, MA). HRP-conjugated $F(ab')_2$ goat anti-mouse IgG (catalog No. 0855572), and HRP-conjugated $F(ab')_2$ goat anti-rabbit IgG (catalog No. 0855686) were from MP Biomedicals (Santa Ana, CA).

NET Formation Assay

Neutrophils (2.5×10^5) in 500 μl RPMI-1640 medium (Gibco®; Grand Island, NY) were added to each well of a 24-well plate (Costar® 3524; Corning Inc., Corning, NY), and incubated in a humidified incubator with 5% CO_2 at 37°C for 30 min. Then 100 μl of 120 nM PMA in PBS, or 100 μl an *E. histolytica* suspension (1.25×10^5 cell/ml) were added to each well. The amoeba to neutrophil ratio was 1:20, as determined previously (Ávila et al., 2016). Plates were incubated in 5% CO_2 at 37°C for 4 h. Next, 600 μl of 2% paraformaldehyde in PBS were gently added to each well, and the plates were incubated overnight in 5% CO_2 at 37°C. The fixative was removed by very gentle aspiration at the side of the well, and then the cells were stained with 150 nM DAPI in PBS for 30 min at room temperature. Finally, the plates were observed with a fluorescence inverted microscope model IX-70 from Olympus (Center Valley, PA). Images were captured with an Evolution-VF Cooled Color camera from Media Cybernetics (Rockville, MD), and the computer program Q Capture pro 6.0 from QIMAGING Surrey (British Columbia, Canada). Images were processed with the computer program ImageJ 1.47v from The National Institutes of Health (Bethesda, MD).

In selected experiments, PMN were incubated on ice for 30 min before stimulation, with the inhibitors: Gö6983 (1 μM), Gö6976 (1 μM), GW5074 (100 μM), UO126 (75 μM), DPI (10 μM), BAY 117082 (5 μM), iSyk (1 μM), antibody IB4 (10 μg/ml), Wortmannin (50 nM), LLZ 1640-2 (10 nM), SB 203580 (200 nM), or the vehicle dimethyl sulfoxide (DMSO) alone.

Immunofluorescence

For NETs staining, neutrophils (2×10^5) were incubated with *E. histolytica* trophozoites (1×10^4) in 200 μl RPMI-1640 medium (Gibco®; Grand Island, NY) using Lab-Tek™ chamber slides from Thermo Fisher Scientific (Rockford, IL). After 1 h, cultures were fixed with 4% formaldehyde for 10 min, then fixed cells were permeabilized with 0.2% Triton X-100 in PBS for 5 min, and washed three times with PBS. Cells were next blocked with 1% BSA, 0.3 M glycine, 0.1% Tween 20 in PBS for 30 min at 37°C, and then incubated with anti-histone H4 or anti-citrulline antibodies diluted 1/100 in 1% BSA, 0.1% Tween 20 in PBS during 1 h at room temperature. Next, cells were gently washed with cold PBS and incubated in the dark with TRITC–conjugated goat anti-rabbit IgG antibody diluted 1/50 in the same solution for 1 h at room temperature. Cells were finally washed with PBS and stained with 150 nM DAPI. Coverslips were mounted with Fluoroshield before observation in a fluorescence Olympus BX51 microscope.

Live Cell Imaging Quantification of NETs

NETs formation was quantitated by live imaging and an offline analysis similarly to previous reports (Hoffmann et al., 2016; van der Linden et al., 2017). Neutrophils (2.5×10^5) were incubated in 250 μl RPMI-1640 medium containing 500 nM SYTOX® Green in each well of a 48-well tissue culture plate (Costar® 3548; Corning Inc., Corning, NY). The plate was incubated for 20 min at 37°C in the dark, and then *E. histolytica* trophozoites (1.25×10^4) were added in 50 μl to each well. The amoeba to neutrophil ratio was 1:20. NET release was monitored with an Olympus fluorescence inverted microscope during a period of 240 min. Images were captured every 5 min with an Evolution-VF Cooled Color camera from Media Cybernetics (Rockville, MD), and the computer program Q Capture pro 6.0 from QIMAGING Surrey (British Columbia, Canada). Image files were saved in tiff format and converted to 8-bit grayscale. Images were processed with the computer program Fiji (version 2.0.0-rc-65/1.52b) (Schindelin et al., 2012). This method for NET quantification is based on previously described protocols (Brinkmann et al., 2013; Hoffmann et al., 2016; van der Linden et al., 2017). Briefly, scale was set and threshold adjusted to define the area of fluorescent DNA. Then the area of NETs was measured using the tool "analyze particles." Total area of all fluorescent particles indicated the amount of NETs formation. Unstimulated neutrophils had an area of $62 \pm 6.1\ \mu m^2$. Thus only particles larger than $70\ \mu m^2$ were considered NETs.

Spectrophotometric Quantification of NETs

NET formation was also quantified by detecting DNA release spectrophotometrically with the DNA-binding dye SYTOX® Green as previously described (Behnen et al., 2014; Gonzalez et al., 2014; Alemán et al., 2016a,b). Briefly, neutrophils were resuspended at 1×10^6 cell/ml in RPMI-1640 medium (Gibco®; Grand Island, NY), containing 500 nM SYTOX® Green (Molecular Probes, Inc.; Eugene, OR). Then, 100 μl of this cell suspension (1×10^5 PMN) were added to each well of a 96-well plate (Costar® 3590; Corning Inc., Corning, NY). Next, the plate was incubated at 37°C in a 5% CO_2 incubator for 20 min. Neutrophils were then stimulated by adding 20 μl of 120 nM PMA (20 nM final concentration), or 20 μl of an *E. histolytica* suspension (2.5×10^5 amoeba/ml) to each corresponding well. The amoeba to neutrophil ratio was 1:20. The plate was then incubated in a 35°C pre-warmed microplate reader, model Synergy HT from BioTek Instruments (Winooski, VT), for up to 4 h. For this assay, cells were not fixed. The fluorescence from the bottom of the plate was read every 5 min, using the 485 nm excitation and 528 emission filters.

Fluorescent Calcium Measurements

Neutrophils at 1×10^7 cell/ml in PBS with 1.5 mM Ca^{2+} and 1.5 mM Mg^{2+}, were loaded with Fura-2/AM (Calbiochem; San Diego, CA) and cytosolic calcium concentration calculated as previously described (Rosales and Brown, 1991, 1992; García-García et al., 2002). Briefly, 3×10^6 neutrophils in 1 ml PBS were transferred to a cuvette and then 1.5×10^5 amoebas were added in 80 μl PBS. Fluorescence changes were monitored with a Perkin Elmer (Waltham, MA) LS55 spectrofluorimeter, and calcium concentration calculated with the Perkin Elmer FL WinLab software, version 4.00.02.

FACS

Fluoresce labeling of neutrophil surface receptors for flow cytometry analysis was completed exactly as described (García-García et al., 2007).

Neutrophil Stimulation With Trophozoites and Protein Extraction

Neutrophils (1×10^6) in 500 μl PBS were placed in a 1.5 ml Eppendorf tube. Next, *E. histolytica* trophozoites (5×10^4) in 100 μl PBS were added. Cells were gently mixed and immediately incubated at 37°C in a water bath for various periods of time as indicated. At the end of the corresponding time, 0.8 ml of cold PBS were added and cells centrifuged at 6,000 rpm in a microcentrifuge for 2 min. The supernatant was removed by aspiration and the cell pellets were then lysed in cold RIPA buffer (150 mM NaCl, 5 mM EDTA, 50 mM Hepes, 0.5% sodium deoxycholate, 1% Non-idet P-40, 2 mM Na_3VO_4, pH = 7.5), supplemented with 1X cOmplete™ protease inhibitor cocktail and 1X *PhosSTOP*™ phosphatase inhibitor cocktail, which were added just before lysing the cells. Cell lysates were incubated on ice for 20 min, and then cleared by centrifugation. Cell lysates were immediately used for Western blotting.

Western Blotting

Western blots were performed as previously described (Reyes-Reyes et al., 2001). Briefly, proteins in cell lysates were resolved on SDS 10% PAGE, and then electrotransfered onto polyvinylidine fluoride (PVDF) membranes (Immobilon-P; Millipore, Bedford, MA). Membranes were incubated in blocking buffer [1% BSA, 5% non-fat dry milk (Carnation; Nestle, Glendale, CA), and 0.1% Tween® 20 in Tris-buffered saline (TBS: 50 mM Tris-HCl, 150 mM NaCl, pH = 7.5)] for 2 h at room temperature. Membranes were subsequently probed with the corresponding antibody in blocking buffer, overnight at 4°C, anti-phospho-ERK 1 (1/2,500 dilution), or anti-phospho NF-κB (1/2,500 dilution). Membranes were washed with TBS-Tween (TBS containing 0.1% Tween® 20) six times and incubated with a 1/3,000 dilution of the corresponding HRP-conjugated $F(ab')_2$ goat anti-mouse IgG or goat anti-rabbit IgG for 1 h at room temperature. After washing six more times with TBS-Tween, the membrane was developed with Immobilon Western chemiluminescent HRP substrate (catalog no. WBKLS0100) from EMD Millipore (Billerica, MA) according to the manufacturer's instructions. Afterwards, membranes were stripped with 0.2 M NaOH, reprobed with anti-ERK antibody (1/4,000 dilution), or anti-NF-κB antibody (1/2,500 dilution), to assess protein loading in PAGE gels.

Reactive Oxygen Species (ROS)

ROS production was assessed with three independent methods (Wojtala et al., 2014). First, the cell-permeative reagent 2′,7′-dichlorofluorescin diacetate (DCFDA) was used in a fluorescence spectroscopy assay. Second, Dihydrorhodamine 123 was used in a flow cytometry (FACS) assay. Third, Dihydroethidium was used in a fluorescence microscopy assay.

For ROS detection with DCFDA, the DCFDA-cellular ROS detection assay kit (catalog no. ab113851) from Abcam, Inc. (Cambridge, MA) was used following the manufacturer's instructions. Briefly, neutrophils were washed with 1X buffer and then incubated with 15 μM DCFDA in 1X buffer for

30 min at 37°C in the dark. After one wash in 1X buffer, neutrophils were resuspended at 1×10^6 cell/ml in 2X buffer. Fifty microliters of this neutrophil suspension (5×10^4 PMN) were added into each well of a 96-well clear-bottom black plate (Costar® 3614; Corning Inc., Corning, NY) and incubated for 20 min at 36°C in a plate-reader, model Synergy HT from BioTek Instruments (Winooski, VT). Then, 50 μl of 40 nM PMA (20 nM final concentration), or 50 μl of an *E. histolytica* suspension (2,500 amoebas) were added. Fluorescence was read every 2 min for 2 h at excitation 485 nm and emission 535 nm.

For ROS detection with dihydrorhodamine 123, neutrophils (1×10^6) were resuspended in 100 μl of 15 μM dihydrorhodamine 123 in PBS inside a 1.5 ml Eppendorf tube, and incubated for 30 min at 37°C in the dark. Neutrophils were then centrifuged at 4,000 rpm for 1 min in a microcentrifuge model 5415C (Eppendorf; Mississauga, Ontario, Canada), and after removing the supernatant, they were washed in 500 μl PBS. Finally, neutrophils were resuspended in 500 μl PBS. In the same tube covered with aluminum foil, 100 μl of 120 nM PMA in PBS (final concentration 20 nM), or 100 μl of an *E. histolytica* suspension (5×10^5 amoebas/ml) were added for PMN stimulation. Cells were incubated for 60 min at 37°C in a 5% CO_2 incubator, and then fixed by adding 600 μl of 2% paraformaldehyde. Finally, cells were analyzed by flow cytometry using a FACScalibur apparatus (Becton Dickinson; Franklin Lakes, NJ), with the 485 nm (excitation) and 520 nm (emission) filters. PMN were gated by dot-plot analysis and 10,000 cells were acquired per sample. Data analysis was performed using the Cellquest software (Becton Dickinson; Franklin Lakes, NJ).

For ROS detection with dihydroethidium, neutrophils (1×10^6) were resuspended in 100 μl of 15 μM dihydroethidium in PBS, and were incubated for 30 min at 37°C in the dark. Neutrophils were then centrifuged at 4,000 rpm (1,375 × g) for 1 min in a microcentrifuge and washed in 500 μl PBS. Next, neutrophils were resuspended in 500 μl PBS, and 250 μl of this cell suspension (5×10^5 PMN) were added to each well of a 48-well tissue culture plate (Costar® 3548; Corning Inc., Corning, NY). The plate was incubated for 20 min at 37°C in the dark, and then 50 μl of 120 nM de PMA in PBS (20 nM final concentration), or 50 μl of a *E. histolytica* suspension (5×10^5 amoebas/ml) were added to each well. The plate was incubated for 60 min at 37°C in a 5% CO_2 incubator. Next, 300 μl of 2% paraformaldehyde were added to each well for fixing the cells. After 30 min, the plates were observed with a fluorescence inverted microscope model IX-70 from Olympus (Center Valley, PA).

Statistical Analysis

Quantitative data were expressed as mean ± standard error of mean (SEM). Single variable data were compared by paired-sample Student's *t*-tests using the computer program KaleidaGraph®version 3.6.2 for Mac (Synergy Software; Reading, PA). Differences were considered statistically different at a value $p < 0.05$.

RESULTS

Entamoeba histolytica Induce NET Formation

NETs formation has been mostly studied by using PMA, a potent activator of PKC as an inducer of NETosis (Brinkmann et al., 2004). The antibody receptor FcγRIIIb also induces a strong activation of NETs formation (Alemán et al., 2016a,b). In addition, we recently reported that *E. histolytica* also induce NETs formation (Ávila et al., 2016), but there are not reports on the mechanism of NETs induction by these parasites. When human neutrophils were stimulated by PMA, NETs are detected after 2.5 h of stimulation (Fuchs et al., 2007). Complete NETs were seen, as previously reported, by 4 h after stimulation (**Figure 1A**). Stimulation with *E. histolytica* trophozoites also induced NETosis (**Figure 1**). The extracellular DNA fibers co-localized with neutrophil elastase and myeloperoxidase (Díaz-Godínez et al., 2018), as well as with histone H4 and citrulline (**Figure 1B**), confirming that these fibers were bona fide NETs. Live cell imaging showed that by 30 min after incubation with amoebas, NETs were already visible (**Figure 2A**). By 2 h about half of the total amount of NETs had already been formed, and by 2.5 h NETs reached a maximum level (**Figure 2A**). NETs formation was induced only in neutrophils that were in direct contact with *E. histolytica* trophozoites (**Figure 2B**). The NETs were produced around the amoebas and progressively covered the parasites (**Figure 2B**). Neutrophils that were not in contact with amoebas did not release DNA fibers and never became SYTOX® Green-positive (**Figure 2B**), suggesting that the signaling for NETosis comes from a receptor that directly recognizes the parasite. Quantification of NETs from live cell imaging analysis showed that amoeba-induced NETs were formed with a much faster kinetics than PMA-induced NETs. After stimulation with amoebas, NETs could be easily detected by 30 min (**Figure 3A**). The amount of NETs progressively increased during the following 2 h, attaining a maximum level by 2.5 h, that was even higher than the one induced by PMA (**Figure 3A**). Since NETs were exclusively formed by neutrophils joining amoebas and the fluorescence staining of external DNA only reflected NETs, the formation of NETs was also quantitated spectrophotometrically as previously reported (Alemán et al., 2016a,b). In accordance with live cell imaging analysis, neutrophils treated with PMA showed NETs (extracellular DNA fibers) after 2 h of stimulation reaching a maximum level by 4 h (**Figure 3B**). Stimulation of neutrophils with *E. histolytica* trophozoites also induced NETosis that could be detected by 30 min and reached a maximum level around 2.5 h (**Figure 3B**). Neutrophils alone only presented background fluorescence that did not increase during the time of the experiment, thus confirming the imaging data showing that neutrophils did not lose membrane integrity. Therefore, both quantification methods are equivalent and allowed us to reach similar conclusions. The difference in kinetics for NETosis suggested that the signaling induced by *E. histolytica* was different from the one induced by PMA. Hence, we next explored whether the signaling molecules reported to be required for NETs formation after PMA or FcγRIIIb stimulation were also required for *E. histolytica*-induced NETosis.

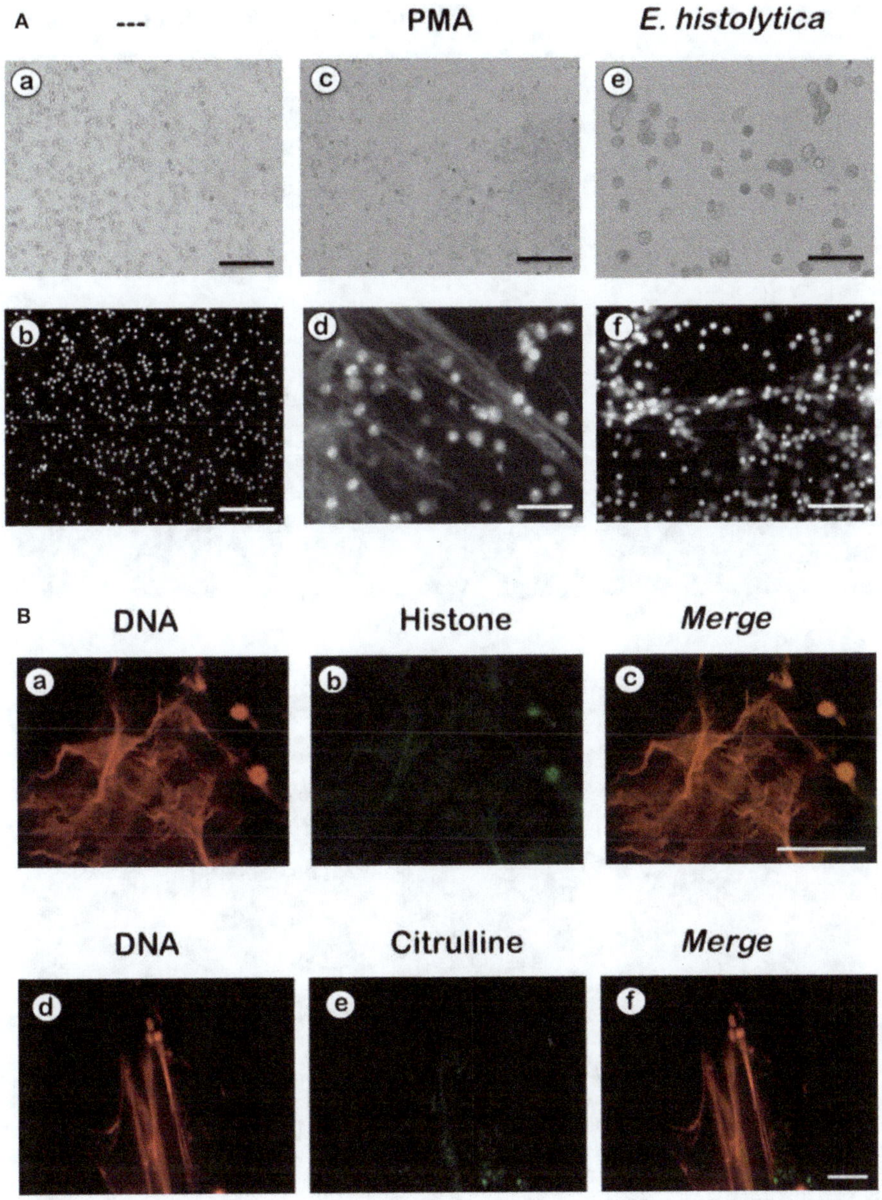

FIGURE 1 | *Entamoeba histolytica* induce NETs formation. **(A)** Human neutrophils (PMN) were left untreated (—), or were stimulated with 20 nM phorbol 12-myristate 13-acetate (PMA), or by *E. histolytica* trophozoites (amoeba to PMN ratio 1:20). After 4 h, cells were fixed and stained for DNA with DAPI. Microphotographs were taken with white light (a,c,e) or with fluorescent light (b,d,f) and are representative of more than 10 experiments. Scale bar is 100 μm. **(B)** Human neutrophils were stimulated with trophozoites during 4 h at 37°C. Cells were fixed and immunofluorescence was performed using anti-histone H4 or anti-citrulline antibodies followed by TRITC-conjugated anti-rabbit IgG antibody. DNA was stained with DAPI. Scale bar 50 is μm.

Entamoeba histolytica-Induced NETs Formation Is Dependent on Raf and MEK, but Not PKC

Because PMA is an activator of PKC, the involvement of this kinase in NET formation induced by *E. histolytica* was tested with two specific PKC inhibitors. PMN treated with PMA formed NETs as expected (**Figure 4**). However, when PMN were treated previously with Gö6983, an inhibitor of PKCα, PKCβ, and PKCγ isozymes (**Figure 4**), or with Gö6976, a conventional PKC inhibitor (**Figure 4**), NETs were not formed after PMA stimulation. In contrast, NETs formation after *E. histolytica* stimulation was not inhibited by these PKC inhibitors (**Figure 4**, Supplementary Figure 1). In addition, downstream of PKC, the Raf, MEK, ERK pathway has been reported to participate in NETs formation after PMA stimulation (Hakkim et al., 2011). When neutrophils were treated with GW5074, a specific Raf inhibitor, NETs were not formed after PMA stimulation (**Figure 4**), or after *E. histolytica* stimulation

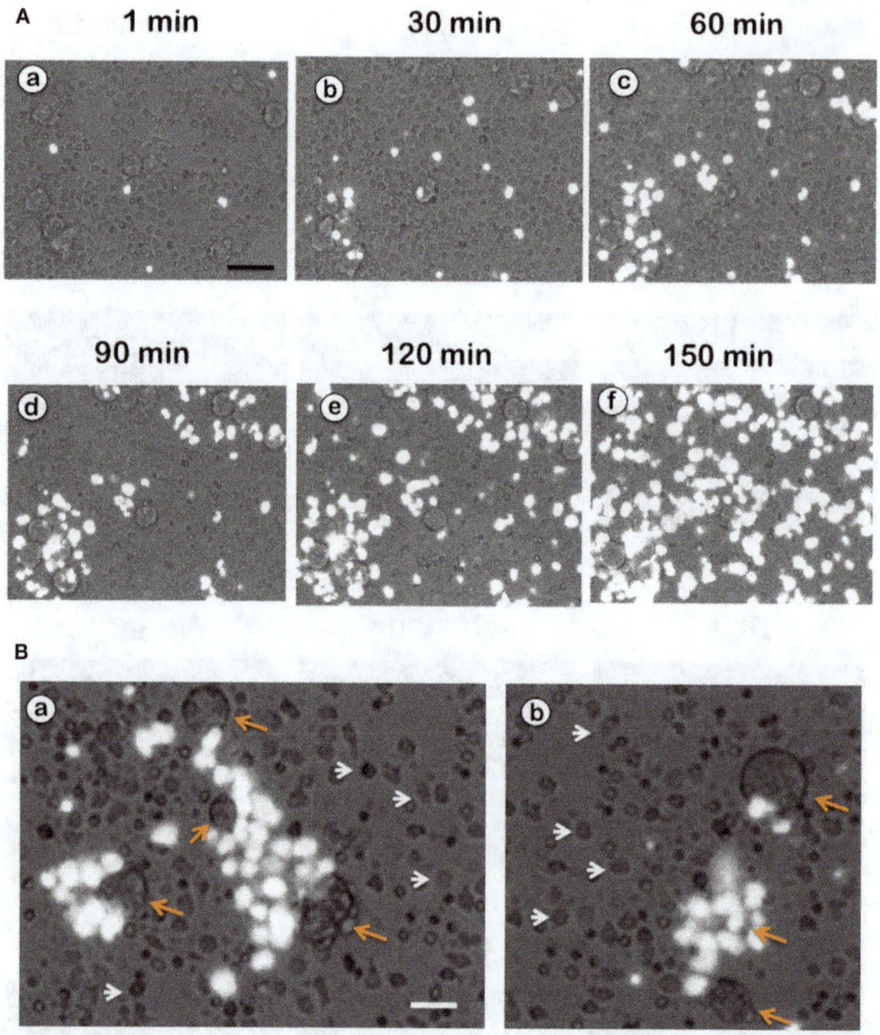

FIGURE 2 | Neutrophils in touch with *Entamoeba histolytica* release NETs. **(A)** Human neutrophils were stimulated with *E. histolytica* in the presence of SYTOX® Green. Live cell images were captured at different times with a fluorescence inverted microscope. External DNA fluorescence appears bright white in the pictures. Scale bar is 50 μm. **(B)** NETs formation was induced only in neutrophils that were in direct contact with *E. histolytica* trophozoites (orange arrows). The NETs were produced around the amoebas and progressively covered the parasites. Neutrophils that were not in contact with amoebas (white arrow heads) did not release DNA fibers and never became SYTOX® Green-positive. Scale bar is 25 μm.

(**Figure 4**, Supplementary Figure 2). In addition, when PMN were treated with UO126, a potent specific MEK inhibitor, NETs were not formed after PMA stimulation (**Figure 4**), or after *E. histolytica* stimulation (**Figure 4**, Supplementary Figure 3). These data suggested that *E. histolytica* stimulation led to NETs formation using Raf and MEK, but not through PKC activation.

Extracellular Calcium Is Required for *Entamoeba histolytica*-Induced NETs Formation

The involvement of MEK in amoeba-induced NETs formation suggested that also ERK would be involved. Since calcium plays a key role in ERK activation, and calcium mobilization is important for NETosis induced by other stimuli (Gupta et al., 2014), we explored the role of intracellular or extracellular calcium pools in *E. histolytica* induced NETosis. Neutrophils were placed in PBS with the calcium chelator EGTA, and then stimulated with the N-formylated chemotactic peptide formyl-methionyl-leucyl-phenylalanine (fMLF). As previously reported (Rosales and Brown, 1992), neutrophils showed an increase in cytosolic calcium concentration that comes from intracellular stores and is dependent on inositol 1,4,5-trisphosphate (IP_3) (**Figure 5A**). Then, after adding an excess of calcium outside the cells a second peak of cytosolic calcium was observed, indicating that an extracellular calcium flux is also activated by fMLF (Rosales and Brown, 1991, 1992) (**Figure 5A**). In contrast, when neutrophils were stimulated with E. *histolytica* trophozoites, no increase in cytosolic calcium concentration was detected. After, addition of an excess of calcium outside the cells, a robust calcium mobilization was observed (**Figure 5B**). This indicates that amoebas induce a calcium flux in neutrophils that comes

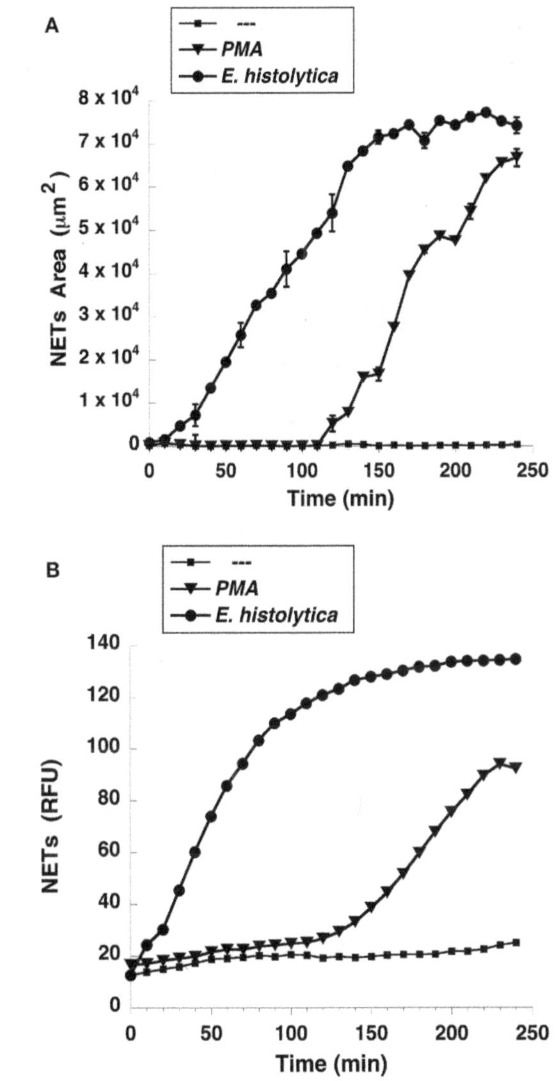

FIGURE 3 | *Entamoeba histolytica* induce NETs formation faster than PMA. Human neutrophils were left untreated (—), or were stimulated with 20 nM phorbol 12-myristate 13-acetate (PMA), or with *E. histolytica,* and then incubated for 4 h. The relative amount of NETs was estimated from **(A)** live cell images and reported as area of external DNA or **(B)** from SYTOX® Green fluorescence in relative fluorescent units (RFU) every 10 min. Data are mean ± SEM of three experiments done in triplicates.

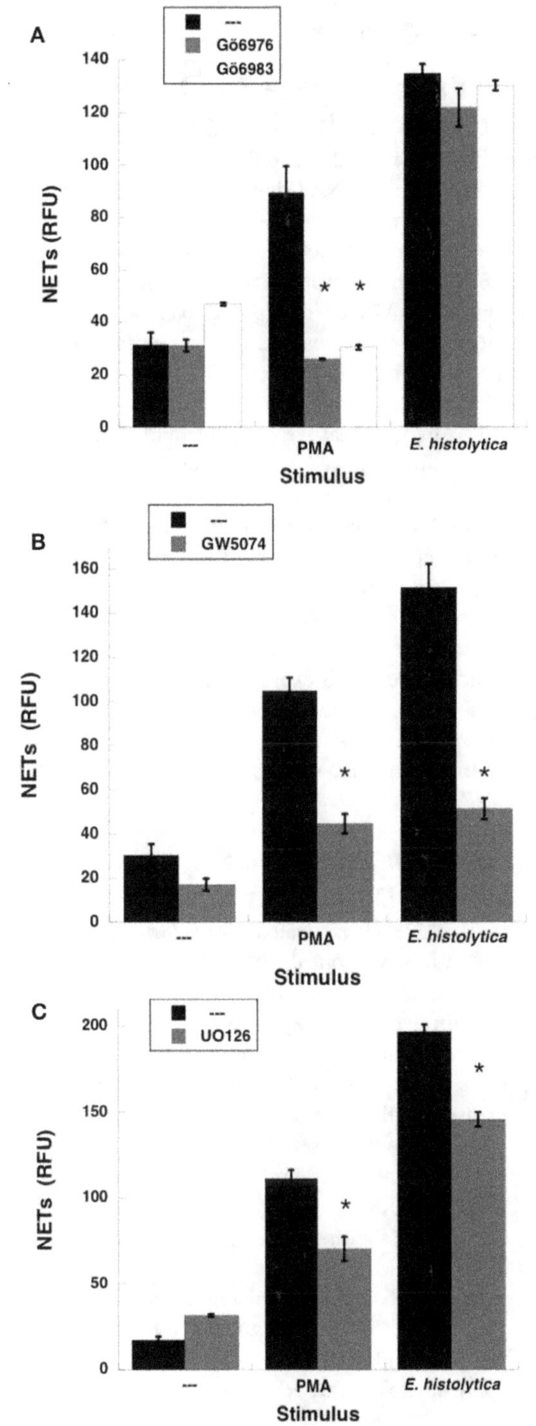

FIGURE 4 | *Entamoeba histolytica*-induced NETs formation is dependent on Raf and MEK, but not *PKC*. Human neutrophils were left untreated (—), stimulated with 20 nM phorbol 12-myristate 13-acetate (PMA), or with *E. histolytica* trophozoites. PMN were previously treated with solvent alone (—) or **(A)** with the PKC inhibitors Gö6976 (1 μM), or Gö6983 (1 μM); or **(B)** with the Raf inhibitor GW5074 (100 μM); or **(C)** with the MEK inhibitor UO126 (75 μM). The relative amount of NETs was estimated from SYTOX® Green fluorescence in relative fluorescent units (RFU) at 4 h after stimulation. Data are mean ± SEM of 3 experiments. Asterisks denote conditions that are statistically different from control ($p < 0.001$).

only from extracellular pools (**Figure 5C**). This extracellular calcium flux is important for NETs formation, because NETs were not formed when amoebas interacted with neutrophils in the presence of the calcium chelator EGTA (Díaz-Godínez et al., 2018). It has also been suggested that calcium mobilization required for NETosis involves the calcineurin pathway since cyclosporine A inhibited IL-8-induced NETosis (Gupta et al., 2014). However, in the case of amoebas, cyclosporine A did not prevent calcium mobilization nor NETs formation (data not shown). This suggests that *E. histolytica*-induced NETs formation requires extracellular calcium, but this calcium does not activate the calcineurin pathway.

Entamoeba histolytica Trophozoites Induced NETosis but Not Apoptosis

Live cell imaging revealed that only neutrophils in contact with amoebas released their DNA (**Figure 2**). In order to confirm that neutrophils were undergoing NETosis and no other forms of cell death in the presence of amoebas, the integrity of chromatin was analyzed. DNA from neutrophils treated with PMA, or with the calcium ionophore A23187, or exposed to amoebas did not show any fragmentation in agarose gels (Díaz-Godínez et al., 2018). In contrast, neutrophils exposed to 56°C for 1 h, a well-known inducer of apoptosis, showed fragmented DNA (Díaz-Godínez et al., 2018). Moreover, heat-treated neutrophils, and some PMA-treated neutrophils, showed an increase in surface expression of phosphatidylserine; while neutrophils exposed to A23187 or to amoebas did not show phosphatidylserine surface expression (Díaz-Godínez et al., 2018). In addition, it has been reported that neutrophils undergoing apoptosis lose the expression of the antibody receptor FcγRIIIb (CD16b) (Sim et al., 2005). However, neutrophils exposed to *E. histolytica* trophozoites, did not show any difference in FcγRIIIb expression, as indicated by binding of two different monoclonal antibodies specific for this receptor (**Figure 6**). Together these results confirm that amoebas induce NETs formation and not apoptosis when they are in contact with neutrophils.

Entamoeba histolytica-Induced NETs Formation Is Dependent on ERK

To confirm that ERK was activated after *E. histolytica* stimulation, neutrophils with or without the MEK inhibitor were incubated with amoebas and then ERK activation was detected by Western blotting. *E. histolytica* induced a rapid ERK phosphorylation, which reached a maximum at about 2 min after neutrophils and amoebas got in contact (**Figure 7A**). This phosphorylation then decreased with time and was barely detectable after 15 min. The antibodies used to detect ERK and phospho-ERK did not recognize any proteins from amoeba cell lysates (**Figure 7A**), thus ERK phosphorylation detected was only from neutrophils. *E. histolytica*-induced ERK phosphorylation was prevented by the MEK inhibitor UO126 (**Figure 7B**). Also, the Raf inhibitor GW5074 completely impeded *E. histolytica*-induced ERK phosphorylation (**Figure 7C**). These data suggested that *E. histolytica* induced, in neutrophils, the Raf, MEK, ERK signaling pathway to activate NETosis.

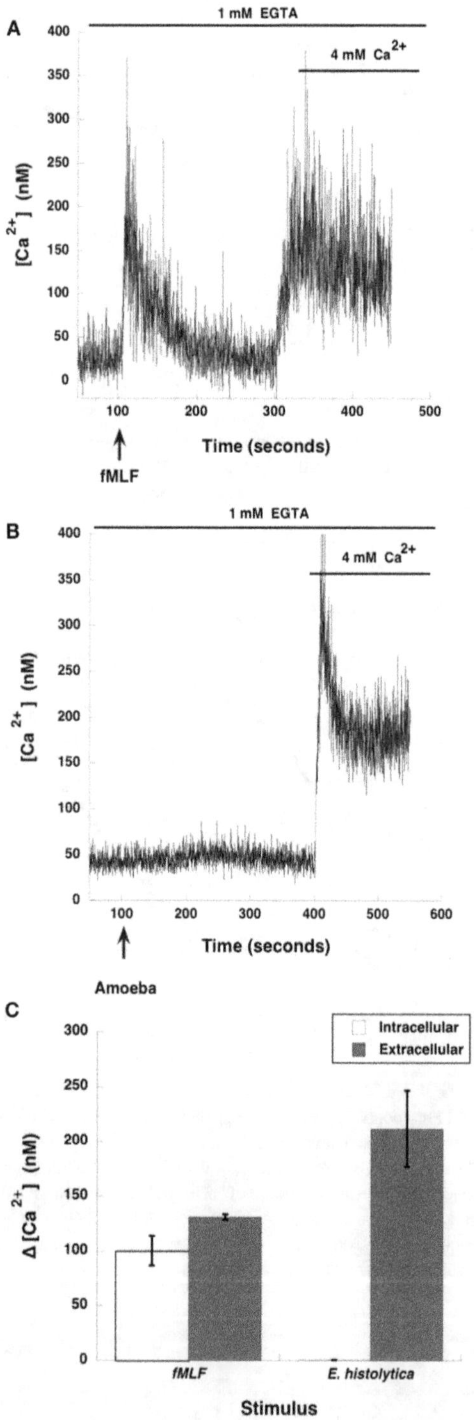

FIGURE 5 | *Entamoeba histolytica* trigger extracellular calcium mobilization in neutrophils. Human neutrophils were incubated with fura-2 for 30 min and then placed in PBS with EGTA. Neutrophils were stimulated (arrow) with **(A)** 10 nM formyl-methionyl-leucyl-phenylalanine (fMLF), or were stimulated with **(B)** *E. histolytica* trophozoites (amoeba). After about 250 s, an excess (4 mM) Ca^{2+} was added to the buffer. Changes in cytosolic calcium concentration were assessed by measuring the variations in fluorescence of fura-2-loaded cells. Tracings are representative of three experiments. **(C)** The increase of cytosolic calcium concentration (Δ [Ca^{2+}]) is shown from intracellular or extracellular calcium pools. Data are mean ± SEM of three experiments.

The NADPH-Oxidase Inhibitor DPI Reduced *Entamoeba histolytica*-Induced NETs Formation

NETs formed after PMA stimulation require activation of NADPH-oxidase and formation of ROS (Patel et al., 2010; Almyroudis et al., 2013; Björnsdottir et al., 2015). Thus, we explored the involvement of these molecules in *E. histolytica*-induced NETs formation. Neutrophils treated with diphenyleneiodonium (DPI), a NADPH-oxidase inhibitor,

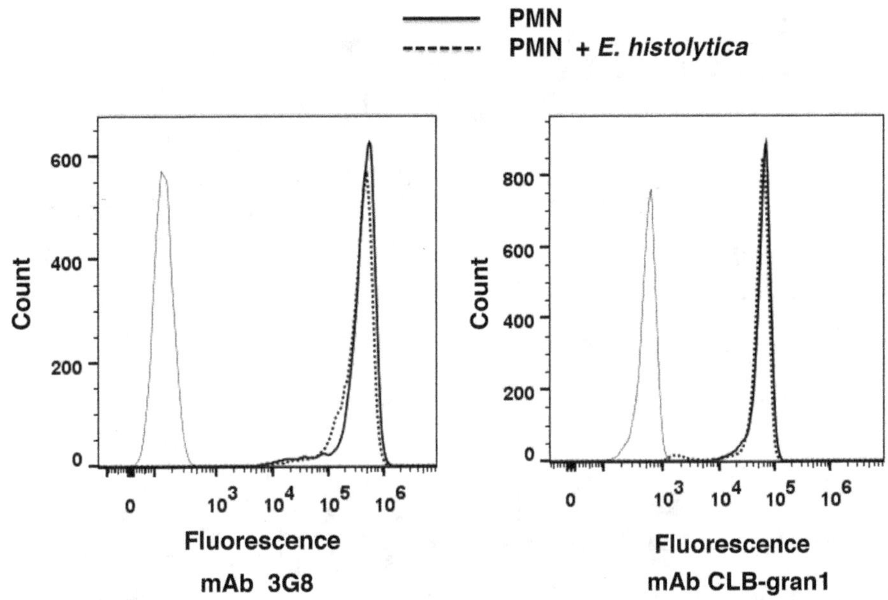

FIGURE 6 | *Entamoeba histolytica* trophozoites did not change surface expression of receptor FcγRIIIb (CD16b). Human neutrophils were not stimulated (solid line) or were stimulated with *E. histolytica* trophozoites (dashed line) for 30 min at 37°C. Then, cells were fluorescence-stained with secondary antibody only (thin line), or with monoclonal antibody (mAb) 3G8 or with mAb CLB-gran1, both specific against FcγRIIIb, as described in section Materials and Methods. Fluorescence intensity was then analyzed by flow cytometry. Histograms are representative of three independent determinations.

were not able to form NETs after PMA stimulation (**Figure 8**). Similarly, DPI-treated neutrophils did not efficiently form NETs after *E. histolytica* stimulation (**Figure 8**). However, because inhibition by DPI of *E. histolytica*-induced NETs formation was only to about half (**Figure 8**), we decided to use apocynin, a different inhibitor of NADPH-oxidase (Kim et al., 2012) and also a ROS scavenger (Heumüller et al., 2008). As expected, apocynin inhibited PMA-induced NETosis, indicating that this mechanism depends on ROS production (Díaz-Godínez et al., 2018). In contrast, apocynin did not decrease amoeba-induced NETs formation, suggesting that this type of NETosis is independent of ROS production by NADPH oxidases (Díaz-Godínez et al., 2018). In order to clarify the different effect of these two NADPH-oxidase inhibitors, we decided to directly assess ROS production after *E. histolytica* stimulation of neutrophils. When neutrophils were treated with PMA or with tert-butyl hydrogen peroxide (TBHP), a positive control for ROS production, ROS were generated in great amounts and could be easily detected with the 2′,7′-dichlorofluorescin diacetate (DCFDA) method (**Figure 9A**). To our surprise, however, *E. histolytica* stimulation of neutrophils did not induce any ROS production (**Figure 9A**). Consequently, the effect of DPI did not seem to be related to inhibition of ROS production. Cell viability was then tested in the presence of DPI. Neutrophils remained viable in the presence of DPI for more than 2 h (**Figure 9B**). In contrast, *E. histolytica* trophozoites began losing viability around 45 min after treatment with DPI. By 90 min, only about 20% amoebas were still viable. Finally, by 2 h most amoebas were not alive (**Figure 9B**). Therefore, the effect of DPI on NETs production was not due to inhibition of ROS production, but due to a toxic effect on *E. histolytica*.

Entamoeba histolytica Did Not Induce ROS Production

In order to confirm that *E. histolytica* did not induce ROS production, neutrophils were loaded with dihydrorhodamine 123 or with dihydroethidium, and ROS production assessed by flow cytometry and fluorescence microscopy respectively. When neutrophils were treated with PMA, a strong increase in dihydrorhodamine 123 fluorescence could be easily detected by flow cytometry (**Figure 10A**) indicating the presence of ROS. Similarly, PMA induced ROS could be easily detected by fluorescence microscopy (**Figure 10B**). In contrast, *E. histolytica* did not cause any rise in fluorescence from these ROS indicators (**Figure 10**). Thus, clearly *E. histolytica* did not induce any ROS production from neutrophils. These data suggest that amoebas can induce NETs production by a signaling pathway that is independent of ROS.

Entamoeba histolytica-Induced NETs Formation Is Dependent on NF-κB

NETs formation after PMA stimulation requires activation of NF-κB (Lapponi et al., 2013). Thus, we explored the involvement of this molecule in *E. histolytica*-induced NET formation. As previously reported (Alemán et al., 2016a), neutrophils treated with BAY117082, an NF-κB inhibitor, were not able to form NETs after PMA stimulation (**Figure 11**, Supplementary Figure 4). Similarly, neutrophils treated with BAY117082 did not

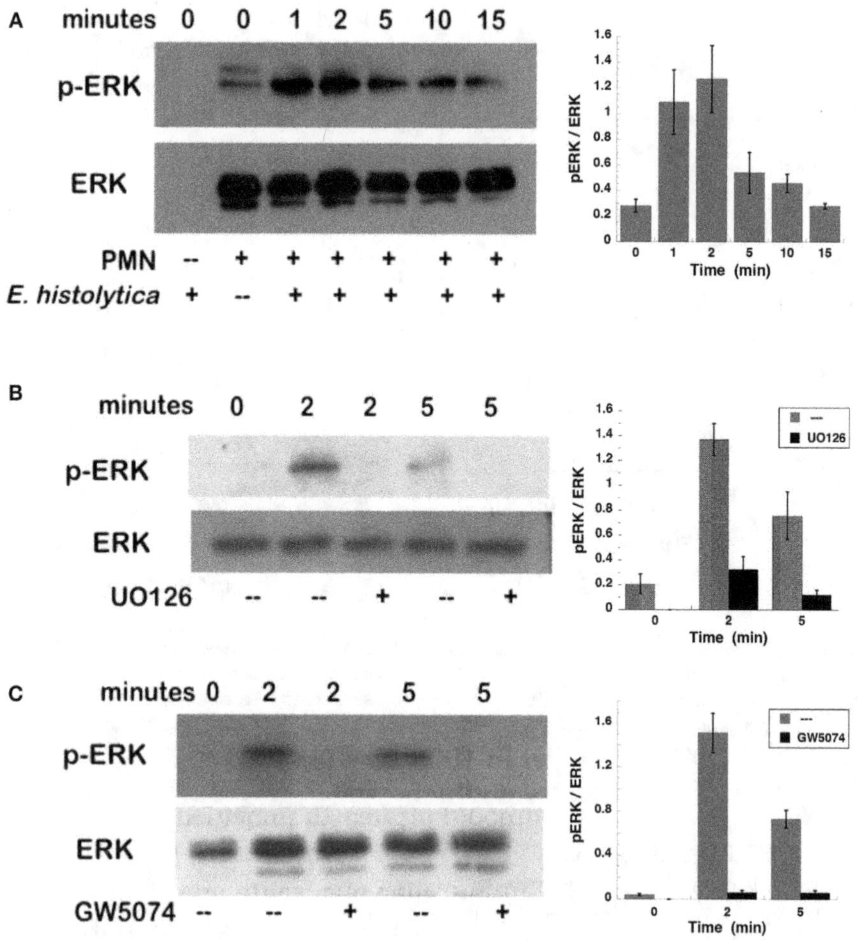

FIGURE 7 | *Entamoeba histolytica* induce activation of ERK. Human neutrophils were stimulated with *E. histolytica* trophozoites for various periods of time, and then cell lysates were prepared. Neutrophils were **(A)** left untreated, or previously treated with **(B)** the MEK inhibitor UO126 (75 μM), or with **(C)** the Raf inhibitor GW5074 (100 μM). Proteins were resolved by SDS-PAGE, and then Western blotted for phosphorylated-ERK (p-ERK) (upper panel) or for total ERK (lower panel) to show equal loading of proteins. Plots on the right show densitometric analysis for the ratio of pERK/ERK. Data are mean ± SEM of three experiments.

form NETs efficiently after *E. histolytica* stimulation (**Figure 11**, Supplementary Figure 4). To confirm that NF-κB was activated after *E. histolytica* stimulation, phosphorylation of NF-κB was detected by Western blotting. *E. histolytica* induced a rapid and transient NF-κB phosphorylation, which reached a maximum at about 1 min after neutrophils and amoebas got in contact (**Figure 12A**). This phosphorylation then decreased with time and was barely detectable after 10 min. The antibodies used to detect NF-κB and phospho- NF-κB did not recognize any proteins from amoeba cell lysates (**Figure 12A**). *E. histolytica*-induced NF-κB activation was completely blocked by the NF-κB inhibitor BAY117082 (**Figure 12B**). In addition, the MEK inhibitor UO126 also blocked *E. histolytica*-induced NF-κB phosphorylation (**Figure 12C**), indicating that activation of NF-κB is downstream from the ERK signaling pathway. Together these data suggested that amoebas could induce the formation of NETs independently of NADPH-oxidase activation, but with the involvement of NF-κB activation.

Entamoeba histolytica-Induced NETs Formation Is Independent on Syk, TAK1, PI3K, p38 MAPK, and β2 Integrins

When neutrophils are stimulated through the FcγRIIIb, the kinases Syk and TAK1 are involved in a signaling pathway that leads to NETs formation (Alemán et al., 2016a,b). Similarly some reports suggest that β2 integrins are required for NETs formation (Raftery et al., 2014; Rossaint et al., 2014). Thus, we explored whether these signaling molecules were also involved in *E. histolytica*-induced NETs formation. Neutrophils pretreated with iSyk, a specific Syk inhibitor formed NETs efficiently after both PMA and *E. histolytica* stimulation (**Figure 13**). Similarly, inhibition of TAK1 with the antibiotic LLZ 1640-2, or inhibition of β2 integrins with the blocking monoclonal antibody IB4 did not have any effect on NETs formation (**Figure 13**, Supplementary Figure 5). Also, inhibition of phosphatidylinositol 3-kinase (PI3K) with Wortmannin slightly

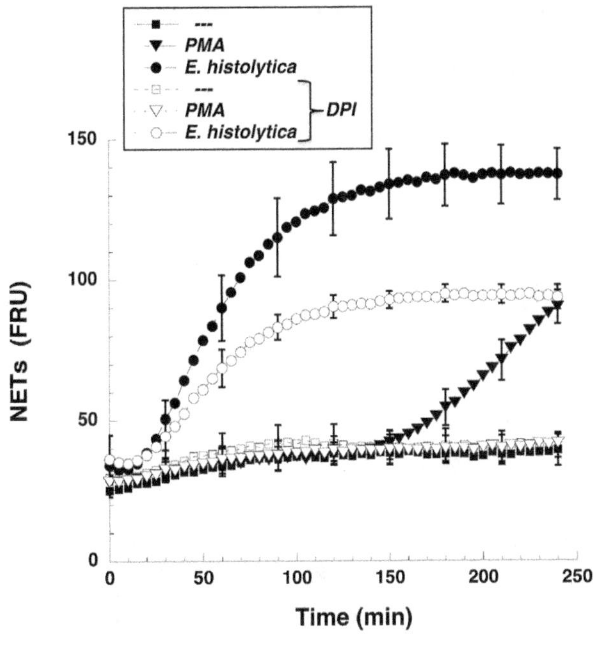

FIGURE 8 | The NADPH-oxidase inhibitor DPI reduced *Entamoeba histolytica*-induced NETs formation. Human neutrophils were not stimulated (−), or were stimulated with 20 nM phorbol 12-myristate 13-acetate (PMA), or with *E. histolytica trophozoites*. Some neutrophils were previously treated with 10 μM diphenyleneiodonium (DPI), a NADPH-oxidase inhibitor (open symbols). The relative amount of NETs was estimated from SYTOX® Green fluorescence in relative fluorescent units (RFU) during 4 h after stimulation. Data are mean ± SEM of three experiments.

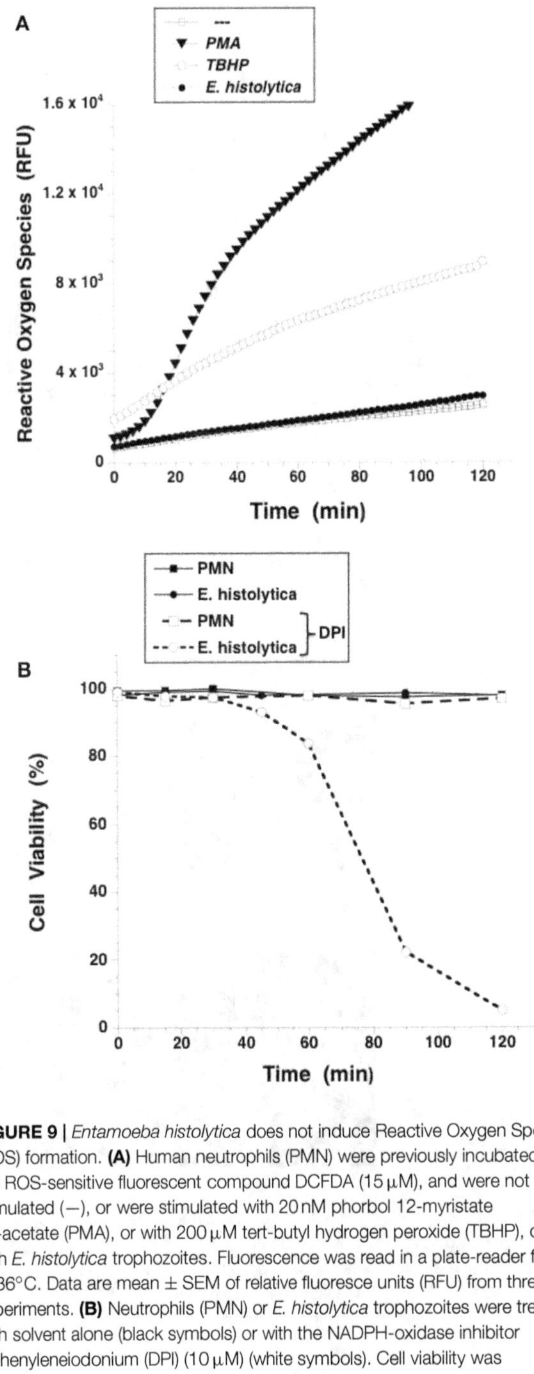

FIGURE 9 | *Entamoeba histolytica* does not induce Reactive Oxygen Species (ROS) formation. **(A)** Human neutrophils (PMN) were previously incubated with the ROS-sensitive fluorescent compound DCFDA (15 μM), and were not stimulated (−), or were stimulated with 20 nM phorbol 12-myristate 13-acetate (PMA), or with 200 μM tert-butyl hydrogen peroxide (TBHP), or with *E. histolytica* trophozoites. Fluorescence was read in a plate-reader for 2 h at 36°C. Data are mean ± SEM of relative fluoresce units (RFU) from three experiments. **(B)** Neutrophils (PMN) or *E. histolytica* trophozoites were treated with solvent alone (black symbols) or with the NADPH-oxidase inhibitor diphenyleneiodonium (DPI) (10 μM) (white symbols). Cell viability was estimated by Trypan Blue exclusion every 15 min.

reduced, as previously reported (Alemán et al., 2016a), PMA-induced NETosis, but had no effect on *E. histolytica*-induced NETs formation (**Figure 13**). Finally, inhibition of p38 MAP kinase with the specific inhibitor SB 203580 did not have any effect on NETs formation (**Figure 13**, Supplementary Figure 5). Together these data indicate that these signaling molecules are not involved in the signal pathway activated by amoebas to induce NETs formation.

DISCUSSION

Neutrophils present several antimicrobial defense mechanisms, including phagocytosis (Rosales and Uribe-Querol, 2017), respiratory burst, degranulation (Kolaczkowska and Kubes, 2013; Mayadas et al., 2014), and the formation of NETs (Yipp et al., 2012). Many pathogens, including virus, bacteria, fungi, and parasites are capable of inducing NETs formation (Papayannopoulos and Zychlinsky, 2009). Although the list of pathogens that induce NETs keeps growing every day, our knowledge about the molecular mechanisms that initiate this neutrophil function is very limited. Recently, we have reported that *E. histolytica* trophozoites were capable of inducing NETosis in human neutrophils (Ávila et al., 2016), but the role of this process in amoebiasis and the molecular mechanisms implicated in NETs formation were not clarified. In this report, we describe for the first time the *E. histolytica*-induced signaling to activate NETs formation. This signaling pathway involves Raf/MEK/ERK, but it is independent of PKC, ROS, Syk, and TAK1 (**Figure 14**).

Neutrophils, the most abundant leukocytes in blood, are rapidly recruited to sites of infection, where they act as the first line of defense against invading pathogens (Kolaczkowska and Kubes, 2013). Neutrophil activation, through various membrane receptors (Mócsai et al., 2015), is important for initiation of the

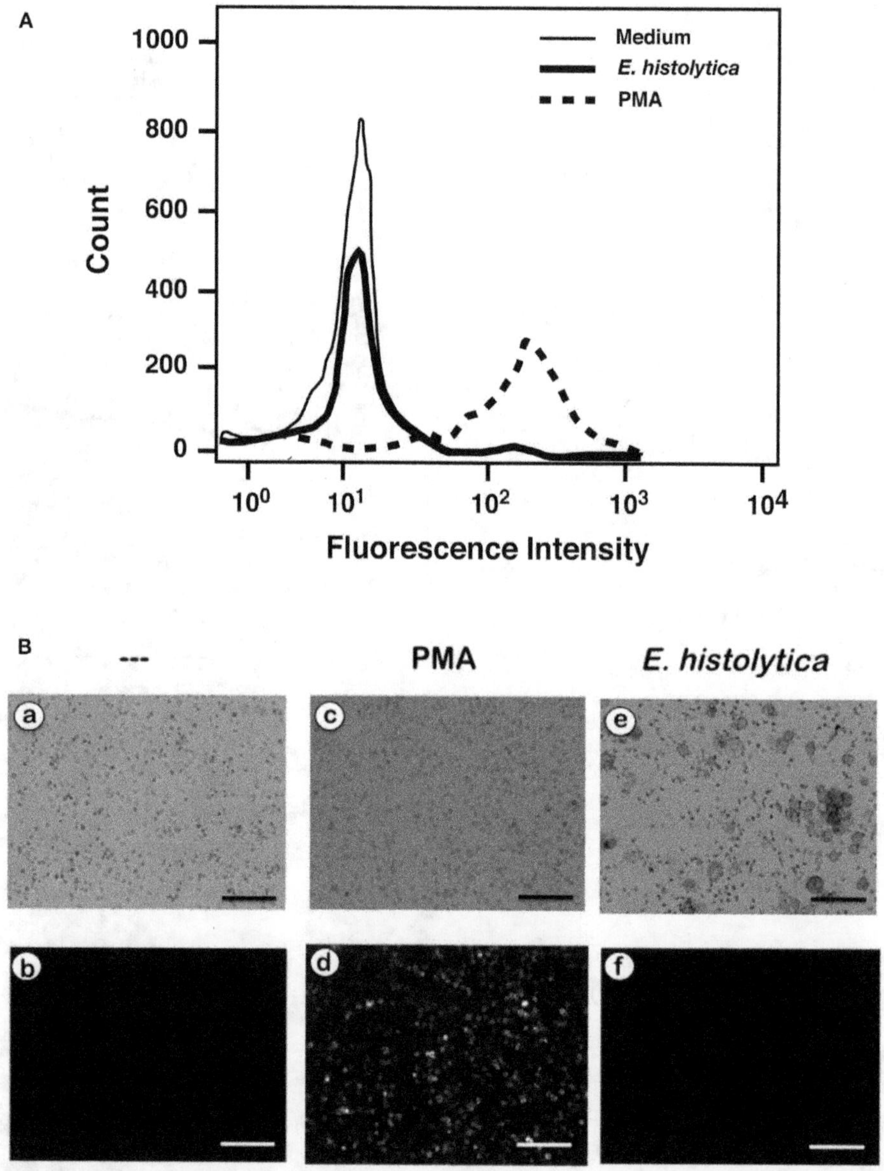

FIGURE 10 | *Entamoeba histolytica* does not induce Reactive Oxygen Species (ROS) formation. Human neutrophils were previously incubated with the ROS-sensitive fluorescent compounds **(A)** dihydrorhodamine 123 (15 μM), or **(B)** dihydroethidium (15 μM). Next, neutrophils were not stimulated (—), or were stimulated with 20 nM phorbol 12-myristate 13-acetate (PMA), or with *E. histolytica* trophozoites. After 1 h, cells were analyzed by flow cytometry **(A)** or by fluorescence microscopy **(B)**. Data are representative of three independent experiments. Bar is 100 μm.

various defense mechanisms of these cells. NETs are extracellular fibers formed by chromatin covered with histones (Neeli and Radic, 2012) and antimicrobial proteins derived from neutrophil granules (Brinkmann et al., 2004). NETs seem to act as a physical barrier for preventing pathogen disemination (Papayannopoulos and Zychlinsky, 2009). NETs also display antimicrobial activity that is independent of phagocytosis (Urban et al., 2006). Despite the fact that many pathogens, including virus, bacteria, fungi, and parasites (Papayannopoulos and Zychlinsky, 2009) have all been reported to induce NET formation, no particular receptor for PAMPs has been identified on the neutrophil membrane as responsible for inducing this neutrophil response. However, TLRs have been suggested to participate (Yipp et al., 2012). Only two receptors on the human neutrophil have been reported to be genuine activators of NETs release, the IgA receptor FcαR (Aleyd et al., 2014), and the IgG receptor FcγRIIIb (Behnen et al., 2014; Alemán et al., 2016a). In the case of human protozoan parasites, NETs formation has been described to occur in response to *L. amazonensis*, *L. major*, *L. chagasi*, *L. donovani* promastigotes (Guimarães-Costa et al., 2009; Gabriel et al., 2010; Hurrell et al., 2015), *T. gondii* (Abi Abdallah et al., 2012), *T. cruzi* (Sousa-Rocha et al., 2015), and

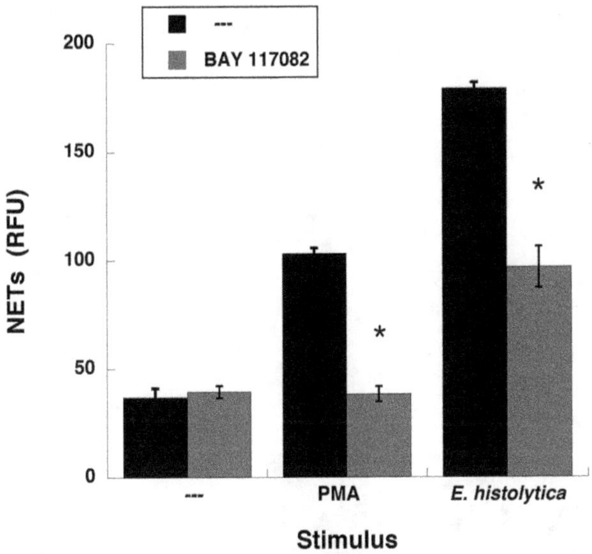

FIGURE 11 | *Entamoeba histolytica*-induced NET formation is dependent on NF-κB. Human neutrophils were not stimulated (—), or were stimulated with 20 nM phorbol 12-myristate 13-acetate (PMA), or with *E. histolytica* trophozoites. Neutrophils were previously treated with solvent alone (—) or with the NF-κB inhibitor BAY 117082 at 5 μM. The relative amount of NETs was estimated from SYTOX® Green fluorescence in relative fluorescent units (RFU) at 4 h after stimulation. Data are mean ± SEM of four experiments. Asterisks denote conditions that are statistically different from control ($p < 0.03$).

E. histolytica (Ávila et al., 2016; Ventura-Juarez et al., 2016). Yet, the mechanism of NETs induction by any of these parasites remains unknown.

Most studies on NETs formation have been conducted with phorbol 12-myristate 13-acetate (PMA) stimulation (Brinkmann et al., 2004; Fuchs et al., 2007). PMA is a direct activator of protein kinase C (PKC), and therefore inhibition of PKC has been shown to block NETs formation (Neeli and Radic, 2013). In agreement with those reports, we found that two different inhibitors of PKC indeed blocked NETs formation after PMA stimulation. In contrast, *E. histolytica*-induced NETs formation was not affected by PKC inhibition. Since PMA directly activates PKC, any possible receptor involved is bypassed. Thus, in the case of amoeba, it seems that the receptor(s) involved can connect with downstream signaling molecules required for NETosis without the need for PKC. This result indicates that PKC is not always necessary for NETs formation. In contrast, the ERK signaling pathway seems to be a common denominator for NETs formation. In the case of PMA-induced NETosis, it was found that PKC leads to activation of the Raf/MEK/ERK pathway (Hakkim et al., 2011). In the case of FcγRIIIb stimulation, we also found that the ERK pathway is important for NETs formation (Alemán et al., 2016a,b). Now, we describe that *E. histolytica* also induces activation of the Raf/MEK/ERK pathway for NETs formation, but independently of PKC (**Figure 14**). Nevertheless, we could not identify a particular receptor that would recognize amoeba and activate the Raf/MEK/ERK signaling cascade. Several possible receptors on the neutrophil are candidates for amoeba recognition, including some TLRs. Our group continues exploring this line of research.

Whatever the neutrophil receptor for amoeba is, it clearly connects to Raf kinase and activates ERK signaling. At present, there is no information of how Raf can be activated after *E. histolytica* recognition by neutrophils. Since Raf is primarily activated by the small GTPase Ras (Lavoie and Therrien, 2015), it is possible that amoebas trigger Ras activation and in turn Raf signaling. But, Raf can also be activated by several other means, including PKC (Takahashi et al., 1999), other small GTPases (Mishra et al., 2005), and even independently of GTPases (Rouquette-Jazdanian et al., 2012). Receptors for growth factors that are usually receptor tyrosine kinases (RTK) activate Raf via the small GTPases Ras (Lavoie and Therrien, 2015) or Rap1 (Mishra et al., 2005). Yet, some RTK, such as the vascular endothelial growth factor (VEGF) receptor can activate Raf independently of Ras using PKC instead (Takahashi et al., 1999). Similarly, in lymphocytes the T-cell receptor uses Pak1 kinase to activate Raf-1 and MEK independently of Ras or PKC (Rouquette-Jazdanian et al., 2012). Thus, in the case of amoebas, Raf activation could be achieved via either a small GTPase or Pak1 kinase. However, another possibility for Raf activation seems more likely to be involved in amoeba-induced Raf activation. In keratinocytes, stimulation with extracellular calcium resulted in activation of Raf and ERK pathway, without the involvement of Ras (Schmidt et al., 2000). In addition, this Raf activation did not connect to the JNK or p38 pathways. In *E. histolytica*-induced NETs formation, we also found strong calcium mobilization (**Figure 5**), and ERK but not p38 activation (**Figure 13**). Therefore, the extracellular calcium flux into neutrophils that are in contact with amoebas may also serve to activate the Raf/MEK/ERK pathway. This possibility is actually being explored in our laboratory.

An important difference between PMA-induced and amoeba-induced as well as FcγRIIIb-induced NETs formation was the time required for NETs release. As previously reported, release of NETs after PMA was detected 3–4 h after stimulation and was dependent on ROS, since the NADPH-oxidase inhibitor DPI abolished NETs release (Brinkmann et al., 2004; Fuchs et al., 2007). In contrast *E. histolytica*-induced NETs release was much rapid and stronger than the one induced by PMA (**Figure 3**). This response was similar to the rapid, oxidant-independent NETs release described after *Staphylococcus aureus* stimulation of neutrophils (Pilsczek et al., 2010). ROS are required for NETs formation in most cases (Brinkmann et al., 2004, 2010; Fuchs et al., 2007; Parker et al., 2012a), but ROS are not sufficient, since ROS production induced by phagocytosis cannot initiate NETs formation (Branzk and Papayannopoulos, 2013). ROS production was not detected when human neutrophils were mixed with *E. histolytica* trophozoites (Díaz-Godínez et al., 2018) and (**Figures 9, 10**). Therefore, NETs formed after amoeba recognition by neutrophils seem to be independent of ROS. Because, generation of ROS has been reported during the interaction of neutrophils with *E. histolytica* trophozoites (Sim et al., 2005), our data suggest that the mechanism of NETs formation induced by amoebas is independent of ROS.

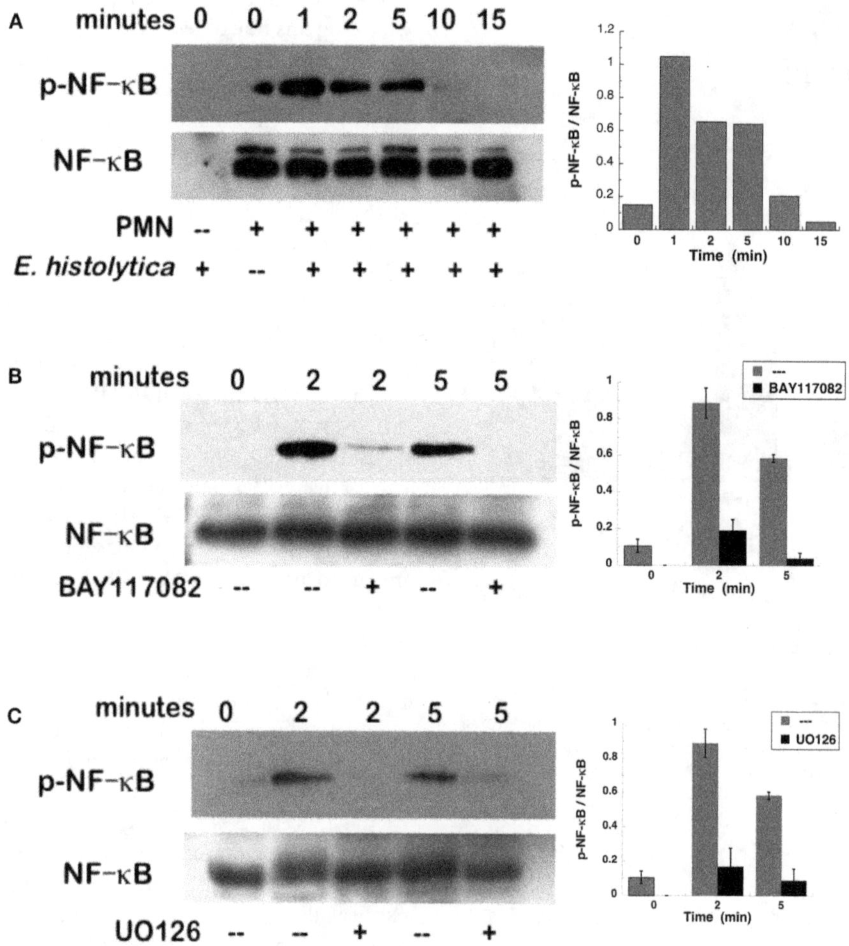

FIGURE 12 | *Entamoeba histolytica* induce activation of NF-κB. Human neutrophils were stimulated with *E. histolytica* trophozoites for various periods of time, and then cell lysates were prepared. Neutrophils were **(A)** left untreated, or previously treated with **(B)** the NF-κB inhibitor BAY117082 (5 μM), or with **(C)** the MEK inhibitor UO126 (75 μM). Proteins were resolved by SDS-PAGE, and then Western blotted for phosphorylated-NF-κB (p-NF-κB) (upper panel) or for total NF-κB (lower panels) to show equal loading of proteins. Plots on the right show densitometric analysis for the ratio of p-NF-κB/NF-κB. Data are mean ± SEM of three experiments.

Also, it has been previously suggested that interaction of amoebas with neutrophils results in apoptosis (Sim et al., 2005). We did not find evidence for apoptosis of neutrophils interacting with *E. histolytica* trophozoites (Díaz-Godínez et al., 2018). We do not know exactly the reasons for the different results between that initial report and our present results. Apoptosis was evaluated by surface expression of phosphatidylserine and FcγRIIIb (CD16b) by FACS, and by cleavage of caspases in Western blots (Sim et al., 2005). Under conditions similar to those presented in that report (Sim et al., 2005), we did not detect any increase in phosphatidylserine expression (Díaz-Godínez et al., 2018), or any decrease in CD16b expression using two different antibodies anti-CD16 (**Figure 6**). In addition, no DNA degradation typical of apoptosis could be detected in our cells (Díaz-Godínez et al., 2018). Thus, we think neutrophils do not really undergo apoptosis from interacting with amoebas. Careful reading of the initial report reveals that neutrophils alone kept in culture at 37°C for 1 h entered spontaneously into apoptosis, as suggested by having 27% of neutrophils positive for propidium iodide staining and 29% of neutrophils stained for annexin-V, a marker for phosphatidylserine (Sim et al., 2005). These percentages increased in the presence of *E. histolytica* trophozoites and were interpreted as amoebas inducing apoptosis of neutrophils (Sim et al., 2005). Also, the cleavage of caspases was very high in neutrophils alone (Sim et al., 2005), suggesting that neutrophils were already in apoptosis without interacting with amoebas. In addition, reduction of CD16 expression was used as a marker for apoptotic neutrophils. Although, apoptotic neutrophils show reduced expression of CD16 (Dransfield et al., 1994), the rapid loss of CD16 expression is better associated with the response of neutrophils to inflammatory signals (Moldovan et al., 1999). Moreover, neutrophils respond to inflammatory signals by producing ROS (Mayadas et al., 2014; El-Benna et al., 2016), and we did not find any evidence for ROS production in the presence of amoebas. Hence, it seems that, in the initial report, neutrophils were stimulated by other means,

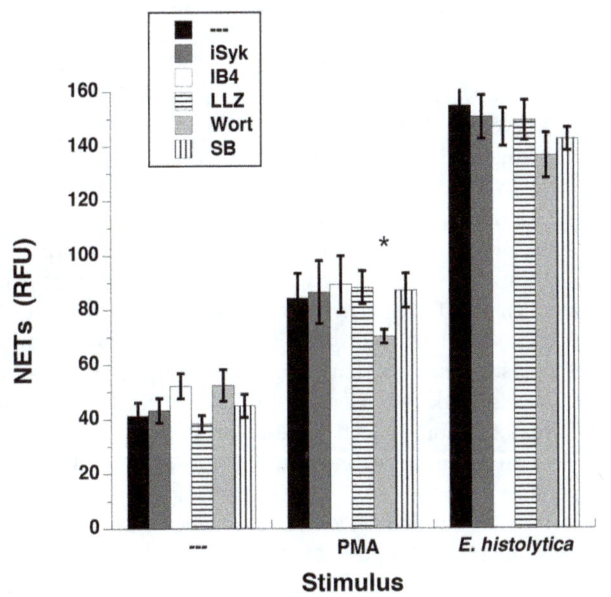

FIGURE 13 | *Entamoeba histolytica*-induced NET formation is independent on Syk, TAK1, β2 integrins, PI3K, and p38 MAPK. Human neutrophils were left untreated (—), stimulated with 20 nM phorbol 12-myristate 13-acetate (PMA), or with *E. histolytica* trophozoites. PMN were previously treated with solvent alone (—) or 1 μM iSyk, a Syk inhibitor, or 10 μg/ml of the blocking monoclonal antibody anti-β2 integrins (IB4), or 10 nM LLZ 1640-2 (LLZ), a TAK1 inhibitor, or 50 nM Wortmannin (Wort), a PI3K inhibitor, or 200 nM SB203580 (SB), a p38 MAPK inhibitor. The relative amount of NETs was estimated from SYTOX® Green fluorescence in relative fluorescent units (RFU) at 4 h after stimulation. Data are mean ± SEM of three experiments. Asterisk denotes a condition that was statistically different from control ($p < 0.05$).

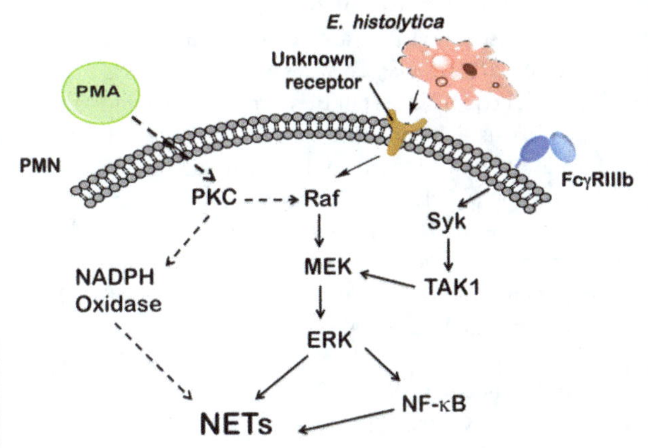

FIGURE 14 | Model for signaling in neutrophils to induce NETosis after *Entamoeba histolytica* engagement. In human neutrophils, phorbol 12-myristate 13-acetate (PMA) can directly activate (dashed arrows) protein kinase C (PKC), which in turn leads to activation of the Raf/MEK/ERK pathway. These kinases finally promote NETs formation. PKC is also required for NADPH-oxidase activation to form reactive oxygen species, which are required for NETs formation after PMA stimulation. In contrast, *E. histolytica* trophozoites are recognized by neutrophils via a, yet unknown, receptor, which connects to the Raf/MEK/ERK pathway. Also the nuclear factor kappa B (NF-κB) is activated to promote NETs formation. The antibody receptor FcγRIIIb also induces NETs formation via spleen tyrosine kinase (Syk) and transforming growth factor-β-activated kinase 1 (TAK1), which connects to MEK (Alemán et al., 2016b). Other signaling molecules (not shown), such as phosphatidylinositol 3-kinase (PI3K), and p38 MAP kinase are not involved in *E. histolytica* signaling to NETs formation.

and in consequence some of the cells underwent apoptosis, independently of amoebas.

We believe that a different scenario is taking place when *E. histolytica* trophozoites interact with neutrophils. Upon recognition of trophozoites, only the neutrophils in direct contact with the parasite release DNA fibers that can completely cover the amoeba (**Figure 2B**). Since, neutrophils cannot phagocytize large cells (Rosales and Uribe-Querol, 2017), they prefer to release NETs in those cases (Urban et al., 2006; Branzk et al., 2014) to prevent the pathogen from escaping. Thus, instead of the amoeba inducing neutrophil apoptosis, it is the neutrophil attacking the trophozoite by undergoing NETosis.

The exact role of NADPH oxidase-dependent ROS for NETs formation remains unclear. When neutrophils were stimulated by *Candida albicans* or by Group B *Streptococcus* (GBS), NETs were formed normally by healthy neutrophils when ROS were eliminated by the ROS scavenger pyrocatechol (Kenny et al., 2017), suggesting a ROS-independent via for NETosis. Yet, neutrophils from chronic granulomatous disease (CGD) patients were not able to form NETs in response to the same stimuli (Kenny et al., 2017), indicating a need for ROS in NETs formation. Possible explanations proposed by the authors are that in the case of GBS there was some residual ROS activity, and in the case of *C. albicans* the fungus itself produces low levels of ROS that the neutrophil can use to activate NETosis (Kenny et al., 2017). In addition, other pathogens, such as *L. amazonensis*, have also been reported to induce NETs in the absence of ROS production (Rochael et al., 2015; DeSouza-Vieira et al., 2016). Together, these studies suggest that PMA absolutely depends on NADPH oxidase derived ROS for NETs formation, while *C. albicans* and GBS can elude this need to some degree, and parasites such as *L. amazonensis* and *E. histolytica* can induce NETosis in complete absence of ROS. In addition to these parasites, various other stimuli can also induce NETosis independently of NADPH oxidase activity, including nicotine, calcium ionophores, uric acid, and immune complexes (Parker et al., 2012b; Arai et al., 2014; Hosseinzadeh et al., 2016; Kraaij et al., 2016). Yet, other sources of ROS such as the mitochondrial respiratory chain or exogenous hydrogen peroxide produced by microorganisms have been considered key for NETosis induced by calcium ionophores (Douda et al., 2015) and by *C. albicans* (Kenny et al., 2017). Therefore, we cannot abandon the possibility that another ROS source, producing amounts that might not be detected with the methodology we used here, play a role in the amoeba-induced NETosis.

Although, the Raf/MEK/ERK pathway has a central role for NETs formation induced by both PMA- and *E. histolytica*, as shown by MEK inhibition blocking NETosis, the role of ERK in NETs formation remains unclear. Previously, it was reported that ERK is required for NADPH-oxidase activation (Hakkim et al.,

2011), placing ERK upstream of ROS production. However, it has also been suggested that ROS are downstream of ERK activation (Keshari et al., 2013). Since, as discussed above, ROS are essential for PMA-induced NETosis, but they are not needed for amoeba-induced NETosis, it seems that NADPH-oxidase activation for NET formation, may proceed not only through an ERK pathway, but also independently of ERK activation, depending on the stimulus (Neeli et al., 2009; Kenny et al., 2017). The actual targets downstream of ERK required for NETosis are still unknown.

One possible molecule activated downstream of ERK that has been implicated in PMA-induced NETosis is the nuclear factor kappa B (NF-κB) (Lapponi et al., 2013). Similarly, *E. histolytica*-induced NETosis was blocked when NF-κB activation was prevented (**Figures 11, 12**). How NF-κB connects to NETs formation is a mystery. No clear function for this transcription factor has been reported. Originally, it was proposed that NF-κB would be required to increase the inflammatory response of neutrophils (Lapponi et al., 2013), but this idea has not been formally tested. In addition, it was reported that upon PMA stimulation, gene transcription does not have any role in NETs formation (Sollberger et al., 2016). Moreover, NF-κB is not always needed for NETosis. In the case of FcγRIIIb-induced NETs formation NF-κB was found not to be involved (Alemán et al., 2016b). Thus, the participation for this transcription factor in NETosis seems to depend on the type of stimuli used, and needs further exploration.

A possible explanation for the role of NF-κB, and other transcription factors, in NETosis has been provided recently. Through transcriptomics analyses of neutrophils, it was shown that the transcriptional activity reflects the degree of DNA decondensation occurring during NETs formation (Khan and Palaniyar, 2017). Interestingly, although both ROS-dependent and ROS-independent NETs formation require transcriptional activity, transcription starts at multiple loci in all chromosomes earlier in the rapid ROS-independent NETosis (induced by calcium ionophore A23187) than in the ROS-dependent NETosis (induced by PMA) (Khan and Palaniyar, 2017). Moreover, extensive citrullination of histones in multiple loci was found only during calcium-mediated NETosis, suggesting that citrullination of histone contributes to the rapid DNA decondensation seen in ROS-independent NETosis (Khan and Palaniyar, 2017). These data are in agreement with our findings that amoeba-induced NETs formation is rapid, requires calcium, is independent of ROS, and presents citrullination of histones. Therefore, the rapid activation of NF-κB (**Figure 12**) seems a reflection of the earlier transcriptional activity required for the rapid ROS-independent *E. histolytica*-induced NETs formation.

It is now generally recognized that there are several mechanisms of inducing NETs formation (Zawrotniak and Rapala-Kozik, 2013; Kenny et al., 2017; Papayannopoulos, 2018), but the particular signaling pathways involved remain confusing. Other signaling molecules that have been suggested to participate in NETosis initiated by the FcγRIIIb are Syk (Popa-Nita et al., 2009) and transforming growth factor-β-activated kinase 1 (TAK1) (Alemán et al., 2016b); in NETosis initiated by immune complexes is phosphatidylinositol 3-kinase (PI3K) (Behnen et al., 2014); in NETosis initiated by LPS (Neeli et al., 2009) and by yeast (Byrd et al., 2013) are p38 MAP kinase, and β2 integrins. Activation of Syk by PMA is dependent on PKC (Popa-Nita et al., 2009). However, inhibition of Syk with iSyk slightly reduced PMA-induced NETosis (Alemán et al., 2016a) and had no effect on *E. histolytica*-induced NETosis. In the case of FcγRIIIb, iSyk prevented TAK1 phosphorylation and NETs formation (Alemán et al., 2016a). This effect is interpreted as a result of Syk being activated by receptor engagement leading then to TAK1 activation (**Figure 14**). In the case of *E. histolytica*, the receptor used by neutrophils to recognize amoebas is still unknown. Thus, most likely this putative receptor does not use Syk to deliver a signal for NET formation. Similarly, inhibition of TAK1, PI3-K, or p38 MAP kinase had no effect on *E. histolytica*-induced NETosis (**Figure 14**). Thus, the putative receptor for *E. histolytica* recognition most likely connects to the Raf/MEK/ERK pathway independently of these signaling molecules (**Figure 14**). As discussed above, a possible connection for Raf activation might be the extracellular calcium flux.

Blocking β2 integrins with antibodies against both CD11b and CD18 chains prevented NET formation by LPS (Neeli et al., 2009), by β-glucan (Byrd et al., 2013), and by immobilized immune complexes (Behnen et al., 2014). However, integrin ligands are not sufficient to induce NETs formation in isolated neutrophils (Branzk and Papayannopoulos, 2013). Similarly, in our case selective crosslinking of β2 integrins with mAb IB4 also did not induce any NETs formation (Alemán et al., 2016a). Also, the mAb IB4 did not block FcγRIIIb-induced NETs formation (Alemán et al., 2016b). Similarly, blocking β2 integrins with mAb IB4 also did not inhibit *E. histolytica*-induced NETs formation (**Figure 13**). The involvement of β2 integrins in NET formation might be more related to the adhesion requirement of neutrophils to form NETs (Brinkmann et al., 2010) than to a signaling capacity of the integrin. Therefore, previous reports suggest that β2 integrins cooperate with other receptors to induce NETosis, but our data suggest that β2 integrins do not participate in NETs formation after *E. histolytica* engagement by neutrophils.

In conclusion, to our knowledge, we show for the first time that *E. histolytica* activates a signaling pathway for inducing NETs formation, that involves Raf/MEK/ERK, but it is independent of PKC, ROS, Syk, and TAK1. Hence, amoebas activate neutrophils to release NETs via a different pathway from the pathways activated by PMA or by the IgG receptor FcγRIIIb (**Figure 14**). Our results also support the idea that various stimuli promote NETs release via different signaling pathways.

AUTHOR CONTRIBUTIONS

ZF performed most of the experiments and analyzed data. CD-G performed experiments and discussed data. NM performed Western blots. OA performed calcium experiments and discussed data. EU-Q performed live cell imaging and statistical analysis, discussed data, and prepared figures. JC designed the research, analyzed data, and contributed reagents. CR designed the research, performed statistical analysis, prepared figures, organized the references, and wrote the paper.

FUNDING

Research in the authors' laboratories was supported in part by Grant 284830 (to JC) and Grant 254434 (to CR) from Consejo Nacional de Ciencia y Tecnología (CONACyT), Mexico (http://conacyt.mx), by Grant IN206316 (to JC) from Dirección General de Asuntos del Personal Académico, Universidad Nacional Autónoma de México (http://dgapa.unam.mx), and by a special Grant for encouragement of medical research (to JC) from the Miguel Alemán Valdés Foundation, Mexico (https://www.miguelaleman.org).

ACKNOWLEDGMENTS

Authors thank Mario Nézquiz Avendaño (Facultad de Medicina—UNAM) for culturing and providing *E. histolytica* trophozoites; José Pedraza Chaverri (Facultad de Química—UNAM) for providing dihydrorhodamine 123, dihydroethidium and for advice on ROS assays; and José Carlos Blanco-Camarillo (Instituto de Investigaciones Biomédicas—UNAM) for FACS assays.

REFERENCES

Abi Abdallah, D. S., Lin, C., Ball, C. J., King, M. R., Duhamel, G. E., and Denkers, E. Y. (2012). *Toxoplasma gondii* triggers release of human and mouse neutrophil extracellular traps. *Infect. Immun.* 80, 768–777. doi: 10.1128/IAI.05730-11

Alemán, O. R., Mora, N., Cortes-Vieyra, R., Uribe-Querol, E., and Rosales, C. (2016a). Differential use of human neutrophil Fcγ receptors for inducing neutrophil extracellular trap formation. *J. Immunol. Res.* 2016:142643. doi: 10.1155/2016/2908034

Alemán, O. R., Mora, N., Cortes-Vieyra, R., Uribe-Querol, E., and Rosales, C. (2016b). Transforming growth factor-β-activated kinase 1 is required for human FcγRIIIb-induced neutrophil extracellular trap formation. *Front. Immunol.* 7:277. doi: 10.3389/fimmu.2016.00277

Aleyd, E., van Hout, M. W., Ganzevles, S. H., Hoeben, K. A., Everts, V., Bakema, J. E., et al. (2014). IgA enhances NETosis and release of neutrophil extracellular traps by polymorphonuclear cells via Fcα receptor I. *J. Immunol.* 192, 2374–2383. doi: 10.4049/jimmunol.1300261

Almyroudis, N. G., Grimm, M. J., Davidson, B. A., Röhm, M., Urban, C. F., and Segal, B. H. (2013). NETosis and NADPH oxidase: at the intersection of host defense, inflammation, and injury. *Front. Immunol.* 4:45. doi: 10.3389/fimmu.2013.00045

Arai, Y., Nishinaka, Y., Arai, T., Morita, M., Mizugishi, K., Adachi, S., et al. (2014). Uric acid induces NADPH oxidase-independent neutrophil extracellular trap formation. *Biochem. Biophys. Res. Commun.* 443, 556–561. doi: 10.1016/j.bbrc.2013.12.007

Asgharpour, A., Gilchrist, C., Baba, D., Hamano, S., and Houpt, E. (2005). Resistance to intestinal *Entamoeba histolytica* infection is conferred by innate immunity and Gr-1$^+$ cells. *Infect. Immun.* 73, 4522–4529. doi: 10.1128/IAI.73.8.4522-4529.2005

Ávila, E. E., Salaiza, N., Pulido, J., Rodríguez, M. C., Díaz-Godínez, C., Laclette, J.P., et al. (2016). *Entamoeba histolytica* trophozoites and lipopeptidophosphoglycan trigger human neutrophil extracellular traps. *PLos ONE* 11:e0158979. doi: 10.1371/journal.pone.0158979

Behnen, M., Leschczyk, C., Möller, S., Batel, T., Klinger, M., Solbach, W., et al. (2014). Immobilized immune complexes induce neutrophil extracellular trap release by human neutrophil granulocytes via FcγRIIIB and Mac-1. *J. Immunol.* 193, 1954–1965. doi: 10.4049/jimmunol.1400478

Bianchi, M., Hakkim, A., Brinkmann, V., Siler, U., Seger, R. A., Zychlinsky, A., et al. (2009). Restoration of NET formation by gene therapy in CGD controls aspergillosis. *Blood* 114, 2619–2622. doi: 10.1182/blood-2009-05-221606

Björnsdottir, H., Welin, A., Michaëlsson, E., Osla, V., Berg, S., Christenson, K., et al. (2015). Neutrophil NET formation is regulated from the inside by myeloperoxidase-processed reactive oxygen species. *Free Radic. Biol. Med.* 89, 1024–1035. doi: 10.1016/j.freeradbiomed.2015.10.398

Branzk, N., and Papayannopoulos, V. (2013). Molecular mechanisms regulating NETosis in infection and disease. *Semin. Immunopathol.* 35, 513–530. doi: 10.1007/s00281-013-0384-6

Branzk, N., Lubojemska, A., Hardison, S. E., Wang, Q., Gutierrez, M. G., Brown, G. D., et al. (2014). Neutrophils sense microbe size and selectively release neutrophil extracellular traps in response to large pathogens. *Nat. Immunol.* 15, 1017–1025. doi: 10.1038/ni.2987

Brinkmann, V., Goosmann, C., Kühn, L. I., and Zychlinsky, A. (2013). Automatic quantification of *in vitro* NET formation. *Front. Immunol.* 3:413. doi: 10.3389/fimmu.2012.00413

Brinkmann, V., Laube, B., Abu Abed, U., Goosmann, C., and Zychlinsky, A. (2010). Neutrophil extracellular traps: how to generate and visualize them. *J. Vis. Exp.* 36:e1724. doi: 10.3791/1724

Brinkmann, V., Reichard, U., Goosmann, C., Fauler, B., Uhlemann, Y., Weiss, D. S., et al. (2004). Neutrophil extracellular traps kill bacteria. *Science* 303, 1532–1535. doi: 10.1126/science.1092385

Byrd, A. S., O'Brien, X. M., Johnson, C. M., Lavigne, L. M., and Reichner, J. S. (2013). An extracellular matrix-based mechanism of rapid neutrophil extracellular trap formation in response to *Candida albicans*. *J. Immunol.* 190, 4136–4148. doi: 10.4049/jimmunol.1202671

Cornick, S., and Chadee, K. (2017). *Entamoeba histolytica*: host parasite interactions at the colonic epithelium. *Tissue Barriers* 5:e1283386. doi: 10.1080/21688370.2017.1283386

Deniset, J. F., and Kubes, P. (2014). Recent advances in understanding neutrophils. *F1000Res.* 5:2912. doi: 10.12688/f1000research.9691.1

DeSouza-Vieira, T., Guimarães-Costa, A., Rochael, N. C., Lira, M. N., Nascimento, M. T., Lima-Gomez, P. S., et al. (2016). Neutrophil extracellular traps release induced by *Leishmania*: role of PI3Kγ, ERK, PI3Kσ, PKC, and [Ca^{2+}]. *J. Leukoc. Biol.* 100, 801–810. doi: 10.1189/jlb.4A0615-261RR

Diamond, L. S., Harlow, D. R., and Cunnick, C. C. (1978). A new medium for the axenic cultivation of *Entamoeba histolytica* and other *Entamoeba*. *Trans. R. Soc. Trop. Med. Hyg.* 72, 431–432.

Díaz-Godínez, C., Fonseca, Z., Néquiz, M., Laclette, J. P., Rosales, C., and Carrero, J. C. (2018). *Entamoeba histolytica* trophozoites induce a rapid non-classical NETosis mechanism independent of NOX2-derived reactive oxygen species and PAD4 activity. *Front. Cell. Infect. Microbiol.* 8:184. doi: 10.3389/fcimb.2018.00184

Dickson-Gonzalez, S. M., de Uribe, M. L., and Rodriguez-Morales, A. J. (2009). Polymorphonuclear neutrophil infiltration intensity as consequence of *Entamoeba histolytica* density in amebic colitis. *Surg. Infect.* 10, 91–97. doi: 10.1089/sur.2008.011

Douda, D. N., Khan, M. A., Grasemann, H., and Palaniyar, N. (2015). SK3 channel and mitochondrial ROS mediate NADPH oxidase-independent NETosis induced by calcium influx. *Proc. Natl. Acad. Sci. U.S.A.* 112, 2817–2822. doi: 10.1073/pnas.1414055112

Dransfield, I., Buckle, A. M., Savill, J. S., McDowall, A., Haslett, C., and Hogg, N. (1994). Neutrophil apoptosis is associated with a reduction in CD16 (Fc gamma RIII) expression. *J. Immunol.* 153, 1254–1263.

El-Benna, J., Hurtado-Nedelec, M., Marzaioli, V., Marie, J. C., Gougerot-Pocidalo, M. A., and Dang, P. M. (2016). Priming of the neutrophil respiratory burst: role in host defense and inflammation. *Immunol. Rev.* 273, 180–193. doi: 10.1111/imr.12447

Espinosa-Cantellano, M., and Martínez-Palomo, A. (2000). Pathogenesis of intestinal amebiasis: from molecules to disease.

Clin. Microbiol. Rev. 13, 318–331. doi: 10.1128/CMR.13.2.318-331.2000

Estrada-Figueroa, L. A., Ramírez-Jiménez, Y., Osorio-Trujillo, C., Shibayama, M., Navarro-García, F., García-Tovar, C., et al. (2011). Absence of CD38 delays arrival of neutrophils to the liver and innate immune response development during hepatic amoebiasis by *Entamoeba histolytica*. *Parasite Immunol.* 33, 661–668. doi: 10.1111/j.1365-3024.2011.01333.x

Fuchs, T. A., Abed, U., Goosmann, C., Hurwitz, R., Schulze, I., Wahn, V., et al. (2007). Novel cell death program leads to neutrophil extracellular traps. *J. Cell Biol.* 176, 231–241. doi: 10.1083/jcb.200606027

Gabriel, C., McMaster, W. R., Girard, D., and Descoteaux, A. (2010). *Leishmania donovani* promastigotes evade the antimicrobial activity of neutrophil extracellular traps. *J. Immunol.* 185, 4319–4327. doi: 10.4049/jimmunol.1000893

García-García, E., Brown, E. J., and Rosales, C. (2007). Transmembrane mutations to FcγRIIA alter its association with lipid rafts: implications for receptor signaling. *J. Immunol.* 178, 3048–3058. doi: 10.4049/jimmunol.178.5.3048

García-García, E., Rosales, R., and Rosales, C. (2002). Phosphatidylinositol 3-kinase and extracellular signal-regulated kinase are recruited for Fc receptor-mediated phagocytosis during monocyte to macrophage differentiation. *J. Leukoc. Biol.* 72, 107–114. doi: 10.1189/jlb.72.1.107

García-García, E., Uribe-Querol, E., and Rosales, C. (2013). A simple and efficient method to detect nuclear factor activation in human neutrophils by flow cytometry. *J. Vis. Exp.* 74:e50410. doi: 10.3791/50410

Ghenghesh, K. S., Ghanghish, K., BenDarif, E. T., Shembesh, K., and Franka, E. (2016). Prevalence of *Entamoeba histolytica*, *Giardia lamblia*, and *Cryptosporidium spp.* in Libya: 2000-2015. *Libyan J. Med.* 11:32088. doi: 10.3402/ljm.v11.32088

Gonzalez, A. S., Bardoel, B. W., Harbort, C. J., and Zychlinsky, A. (2014). Induction and quantification of neutrophil extracellular traps. *Methods Mol. Biol.* 1124, 307–318. doi: 10.1007/978-1-62703-845-4_20

Guimarães-Costa, A. B., Nascimento, M. T., Froment, G. S., Soares, R. P., Morgado, F. N., Conceição-Silva, F., et al. (2009). *Leishmania amazonensis* promastigotes induce and are killed by neutrophil extracellular traps. *Proc. Natl. Acad. Sci. U.S.A.* 106, 6748–6753. doi: 10.1073/pnas.0900226106

Gupta, A. K., Giaglis, S., Hasler, P., and Hahn, S. (2014). Efficient neutrophil extracellular trap induction requires mobilization of both intracellular and extracellular calcium pools and is modulated by cyclosporine A. *PLoS ONE* 9:e97088. doi: 10.1371/journal.pone.0097088

Hakkim, A., Fuchs, T. A., Martinez, N. E., Hess, S., Prinz, H., Zychlinsky, A., et al. (2011). Activation of the Raf-MEK-ERK pathway is required for neutrophil extracellular trap formation. *Nat. Chem. Biol.* 7, 75–77. doi: 10.1038/nchembio.496

Heumüller, S., Wind, S., Barbosa-Sicard, E., Schmidt, H. H., Busse, R., Schröder, K., et al. (2008). Apocynin is not an inhibitor of vascular NADPH oxidases but an antioxidant. *Hypertension* 51, 211–217. doi: 10.1161/HYPERTENSIONAHA.107.100214

Hoffmann, J. H., Schaekel, K., Gaiser, M. R., Enk, A. H., and Hadaschik, E. N. (2016). Interindividual variation of NETosis in healthy donors: introduction and application of a refined method for extracellular trap quantification. *Exp. Dermatol.* 25, 895–900. doi: 10.1111/exd.13125

Hosseinzadeh, A., Thompson, P. R., Segal, B. H., and Urban, C. F. (2016). Nicotine induces neutrophil extracellular traps. *J. Leukoc. Biol.* 100, 1105–1112. doi: 10.1189/jlb.3AB0815-379RR

Hurrell, B. P., Schuster, S., Grün, E., Coutaz, M., Williams, R. A., Held, W., et al. (2015). Rapid sequestration of *Leishmania mexicana* by neutrophils contributes to the development of chronic lesion. *PLoS Pathog.* 11:e1004929. doi: 10.1371/journal.ppat.1004929

Jarillo-Luna, R. A., Campos-Rodríguez, R., and Tsutsumi, V. (2002). *Entamoeba histolytica*: immunohistochemical study of hepatic amoebiasis in mouse. Neutrophils and nitric oxide as possible factors of resistance. *Exp. Parasitol.* 101, 40–56. doi: 10.1016/S0014-4894(02)00021-8

Kenny, E. F., Herzig, A., Krüger, R., Muth, A., Mondal, S., Thompson, P. R., et al. (2017). Diverse stimuli engage different neutrophil extracellular trap pathways. *Elife* 6:e24437. doi: 10.7554/eLife.24437

Keshari, R. S., Verma, A., Barthwal, M. K., and Dikshit, M. (2013). Reactive oxygen species-induced activation of ERK and p38 MAPK mediates PMA-induced NETs release from human neutrophils. *J. Cell. Biochem.* 114, 532–540. doi: 10.1002/jcb.24391

Khan, M. A., and Palaniyar, N. (2017). Transcriptional firing helps to drive NETosis. *Sci. Rep.* 7:41749. doi: 10.1038/srep41749

Kim, S. Y., Moon, K. A., Jo, H. Y., Jeong, S., Seon, S. H., Jung, E., et al. (2012). Anti-inflammatory effects of apocynin, an inhibitor of NADPH oxidase, in airway inflammation. *Immunol. Cell Biol.* 90, 441–448. doi: 10.1038/icb.2011.60

Kolaczkowska, E., and Kubes, P. (2013). Neutrophil recruitment and function in health and inflammation. *Nat. Rev. Immunol.* 13, 159–175. doi: 10.1038/nri3399

Kraaij, T., Tengström, F. C., Kamerling, S. W., Pusey, C. D., Scherer, H. U., Toes, R. E., et al. (2016). A novel method for high-throughput detection and quantification of neutrophil extracellular traps reveals ROS-independent NET release with immune complexes. *Autoimmun. Rev.* 15, 577–584. doi: 10.1016/j.autrev.2016.02.018

Lapponi, M. J., Carestia, A., Landoni, V. I., Rivadeneyra, L., Etulain, J., Negrotto, S., et al. (2013). Regulation of neutrophil extracellular trap formation by anti-inflammatory drugs. *J. Pharmacol. Exp. Ther.* 345, 430–437. doi: 10.1124/jpet.112.202879

Lavoie, H., and Therrien, M. (2015). Regulation of RAF protein kinases in ERK signalling. *Nat. Rev. Mol. Cell Biol.* 16, 281–298. doi: 10.1038/nrm3979

Lozano, R., Naghavi, M., Foreman, K., Lim, S., Shibuya, K., Aboyans, V., et al. (2012). Global and regional mortality from 235 causes of death for 20 age groups in 1990 and 2010: a systematic analysis for the global burden of disease study 2010. *Lancet* 380, 2095–2128. doi: 10.1016/S0140-6736(12)61728-0

Mayadas, T. N., Cullere, X., and Lowell, C. A. (2014). The multifaceted functions of neutrophils. *Annu. Rev. Pathol.* 9, 181–218. doi: 10.1146/annurev-pathol-020712-164023

Mishra, S., Smolik, S. M., Forte, M. A., and Stork, P. J. (2005). Ras-independent activation of ERK signaling via the torso receptor tyrosine kinase is mediated by Rap1. *Curr. Biol.* 15, 366–370. doi: 10.1016/j.cub.2005.02.022

Mócsai, A., Walzog, B., and Lowell, C. A. (2015). Intracellular signalling during neutrophil recruitment. *Cardiovasc. Res.* 107, 373–385. doi: 10.1093/cvr/cvv159

Moldovan, I., Galon, J., Maridonneau-Parini, I., Roman Roman, S., Mathiot, C., Fridman, W. H., et al. (1999). Regulation of production of soluble Fc gamma receptors type III in normal and pathological conditions. *Immunol. Lett.* 68, 125–134. doi: 10.1016/S0165-2478(99)00041-3

Moonah, S. N., Jiang, N. M., and Petri, W. A. Jr. (2013). Host immune response to intestinal amebiasis. *PLoS Pathog.* 9:e1003489. doi: 10.1371/journal.ppat.1003489

Mortimer, L., and Chadee, K. (2010). The immunopathogenesis of *Entamoeba histolytica*. *Exp. Parasitol.* 126, 366–380. doi: 10.1016/j.exppara.2010.03.005

Nakada-Tsukui, K., and Nozaki, T. (2016). Immune response of amebiasis and immune evasion by *Entamoeba histolytica*. *Front. Immunol.* 7:175. doi: 10.3389/fimmu.2016.00175

Neeli, I., and Radic, M. (2012). Knotting the NETs: analyzing histone modifications in neutrophil extracellular traps. *Arthritis Res. Ther.* 14:115. doi: 10.1186/ar3773

Neeli, I., and Radic, M. (2013). Opposition between PKC isoforms regulates histone deimination and neutrophil extracellular chromatin release. *Front. Immunol.* 4:38. doi: 10.3389/fimmu.2013.00038

Neeli, I., Dwivedi, N., Khan, S., and Radic, M. (2009). Regulation of extracellular chromatin release from neutrophils. *J. Innate Immun.* 1, 194–201. doi: 10.1159/000206974

Olivos-García, A., Carrero, J. C., Ramos, E., Nequiz, M., Tello, E., Montfort, I., et al. (2007). Late experimental amebic liver abscess in hamster is inhibited by cyclosporine and N-acetylcysteine. *Exp. Mol. Pathol.* 82, 310–315. doi: 10.1016/j.yexmp.2006.09.005

Papayannopoulos, V. (2018). Neutrophil extracellular traps in immunity and disease. *Nat. Rev. Immunol.* 18, 134–147. doi: 10.1038/nri.2017.105

Papayannopoulos, V., and Zychlinsky, A. (2009). NETs: a new strategy for using old weapons. *Trends. Immunol.* 30, 513–521. doi: 10.1016/j.it.2009.07.011.

Parker, H., Albrett, A. M., Kettle, A. J., and Winterbourn, C. C. (2012a). Myeloperoxidase associated with neutrophil extracellular traps is active and mediates bacterial killing in the presence of hydrogen peroxide. *J. Leukoc. Biol.* 91, 369–376. doi: 10.1189/jlb.0711387

Parker, H., Dragunow, M., Hampton, M. B., Kettle, A. J., and Winterbourn, C. C. (2012b). Requirements for NADPH oxidase and myeloperoxidase in neutrophil extracellular trap formation differ depending on the stimulus. *J. Leukoc. Biol.* 92, 841–849.doi: 10.1189/jlb.1211601

Patel, S., Kumar, S., Jyoti, A., Srinag, B. S., Keshari, R. S., Saluja, R., et al. (2010). Nitric oxide donors release extracellular traps from human neutrophils by augmenting free radical generation. *Nitric Oxide* 22, 226–234. doi: 10.1016/j.niox.2010.01.001

Pérez-Tamayo, R., Martínez, R. D., Montfort, I., Becker, I., Tello, E., and Pérez-Montfort, R. (1991). Pathogenesis of acute experimental amebic liver abscess in hamsters. *J. Parasitol.* 77, 982–988.

Pérez-Tamayo, R., Montfort, I., García, A. O., Ramos, E., and Ostria, C. B. (2006). Pathogenesis of acute experimental liver amebiasis. *Arch. Med. Res.* 37, 203–209. doi: 10.1016/j.arcmed.2005.10.007

Pilsczek, F. H., Salina, D., Poon, K. K., Fahey, C., Yipp, B. G., Sibley, C. D., et al. (2010). A novel mechanism of rapid nuclear neutrophil extracellular trap formation in response to *Staphylococcus aureus*. *J. Immunol.* 185, 7413–7425. doi: 10.4049/jimmunol.1000675

Popa-Nita, O., Proulx, S., Paré, G., Rollet-Labelle, E., and Naccache, P. H. (2009). Crystal-induced neutrophil activation: XI. Implication and novel roles of classical protein kinase C. *J. Immunol.* 183, 2104–2114. doi: 10.4049/jimmunol.0900906

Prathap, K., and Gilman, R. (1970). The histopathology of acute intestinal amebiasis. A rectal biopsy study. *Am. J. Pathol.* 60, 229–246

Raftery, M. J., Lalwani, P., Kräutkramer, E., Peters, T., Scharffetter-Kochanek, K., Krüger, R., et al. (2014). β2 integrin mediates hantavirus-induced release of neutrophil extracellular traps. *J. Exp. Med.* 211, 1485–1497. doi: 10.1084/jem.20131092

Remijsen, Q., Vanden Berghe, T., Wirawan, E., Asselbergh, B., Parthoens, E., De Rycke, R., et al. (2011). Neutrophil extracellular trap cell death requires both autophagy and superoxide generation. *Cell. Res.* 21, 290–304. doi: 10.1038/cr.2010.150

Reyes-Reyes, M., Mora, N., Zentella, A., and Rosales, C. (2001). Phosphatidylinositol 3-kinase mediates integrin-dependent NF-kB and MAPK activation through separate signaling pathways. *J. Cell Sci.* 114, 1579–1589. Available online at: http://jcs.biologists.org/content/114/8/1579.long

Rochael, N. C., Guimarães-Costa, A. B., Nascimento, M. T., DeSouza-Vieira, T. S., Oliveira, M. P., Garcia e Souza, L. F., et al. (2015). Classical ROS-dependent and early/rapid ROS-independent release of neutrophil extracellular traps triggered by *Leishmania* parasites. *Sci. Rep.* 5:18302. doi: 10.1038/srep18302

Rosales, C., and Brown, E. J. (1991). Two mechanisms for IgG Fc receptor-mediated phagocytosis by human neutrophils. *J. Immunol.* 146, 3937–3944.

Rosales, C., and Brown, E. J. (1992). Signal transduction by neutrophil IgG Fc receptors: dissociation of $[Ca^{+2}]$ rise from IP_3. *J. Biol. Chem.* 267, 5265–5271.

Rosales, C., and Uribe-Querol, E. (2017). Phagocytosis: a fundamental process in immunity. *BioMed Res. Int.* 2017:9042851. doi: 10.1155/2017/9042851

Rossaint, J., Herter, J. M., Van Aken, H., Napirei, M., Döring, Y., Weber, C., et al. (2014). Synchronized integrin engagement and chemokine activation is crucial in neutrophil extracellular trap-mediated sterile inflammation. *Blood* 123, 2573–2584. doi: 10.1182/blood-2013-07-516484

Rouquette-Jazdanian, A. K., Sommers, C. L., Kortum, R. L., Morrison, D. K., and Samelson, L. E. (2012). LAT-independent Erk activation via Bam32-PLC-γ1-Pak1 complexes: GTPase-independent Pak1 activation. *Mol. Cell* 48, 298–312. doi: 10.1016/j.molcel.2012.08.011

Salata, R. A., and Ravdin, J. I. (1986). The interaction of human neutrophils and *Entamoeba histolytica* increases cytopathogenicity for liver cell monolayers. *J. Infect. Dis.* 154, 19–26

Schindelin, J., Arganda-Carreras, I., Frise, E., Kaynig, V., Longair, M., Pietzsch, T., et al. (2012). Fiji: an open-source platform for biological-image analysis. *Nat. Methods* 9, 676–682. doi: 10.1038/nmeth.2019

Schmidt, M., Goebeler, M., Posern, G., Feller, S. M., Seitz, C. S., Brocker, E. B., et al. (2000). Ras-independent activation of the Raf/MEK/ERK pathway upon calcium-induced differentiation of keratinocytes. *J. Biol. Chem.* 275, 41011–41017. doi: 10.1074/jbc.M003716200

Seydel, K. B., Li, E., Zhang, Z., and Stanley, S. L. Jr. (1998). Epithelial cell-initiated inflammation plays a crucial role in early tissue damage in amebic infection of human intestine. *Gastroenterology* 115, 1446–1453. doi: 10.1016/S0016-5085(98)70023-X

Seydel, K. B., Zhang, T., and Stanley, S. L. Jr. (1997). Neutrophils play a critical role in early resistance to amebic liver abscesses in severe combined immunodeficient mice. *Infect. Immun.* 65, 3951–3953.

Sim, S., Yong, T. S., Park, S. J., Im, K. I., Kong, Y., Ryu, J. S., et al. (2005). NADPH oxidase-derived reactive oxygen species-mediated activation of ERK1/2 is required for apoptosis of human neutrophils induced by *Entamoeba histolytica*. *J. Immunol.* 174, 4279–4288. doi: 10.4049/jimmunol.174.7.4279

Sollberger, G., Amulic, B., and Zychlinsky, A. (2016). Neutrophil extracellular trap formation is independent of *de novo* gene expression. *PLoS ONE* 11:e0157454. doi: 10.1371/journal.pone.0157454

Sousa-Rocha, D., Thomaz-Tobias, M., Diniz, L. F., Souza, P. S., Pinge-Filho, P., and Toledo, K. A. (2015). *Trypanosoma cruzi* and its soluble antigens induce NET release by stimulating toll-like receptors. *PLoS ONE* 10:e0139569. doi: 10.1371/journal.pone.0139569

Takahashi, T., Ueno, H., and Shibuya, M. (1999). VEGF activates protein kinase C-dependent, but Ras-independent Raf-MEK-MAP kinase pathway for DNA synthesis in primary endothelial cells. *Oncogene* 18, 2221–2230. doi: 10.1038/sj.onc.1202527

Tellevik, M. G., Moyo, S. J., Blomberg, B., Hjøllo, T., Maselle, S. Y., Langeland, N., et al. (2015). Prevalence of *Cryptosporidium parvum/hominis*, *Entamoeba histolytica* and *Giardia lamblia* among young children with and without diarrhea in Dar es Salaam, Tanzania. *PLoS Negl. Trop. Dis.* 9:e0004125. doi: 10.1371/journal.pntd.0004125

Tsutsumi, V., and Martinez-Palomo, A. (1988). Inflammatory reaction in experimental hepatic amebiasis. An ultrastructural study. *Am. J. Pathol.* 130, 112–119.

Tsutsumi, V., Mena-López, R., Anaya-Velázquez, F., and Martínez-Palomo, A. (1984). Cellular bases of experimental amebic liver abscess formation. *Am. J. Pathol.* 117, 81–91.

Urban, C. F., Reichard, U., Brinkmann, V., and Zychlinsky, A. (2006). Neutrophil extracellular traps capture and kill Candida albicans yeast and hyphal forms. *Cell. Microbiol.* 8, 668–676. doi: 10.1111/j.1462-5822.2005.00659.x

van der Linden, M., Westerlaken, G. H. A., van der Vlist, M., van Montfrans, J., and Meyaard, L. (2017). Differential signalling and kinetics of neutrophil extracellular trap release revealed by quantitative live imaging. *Sci. Rep.* 7:6529. doi: 10.1038/s41598-017-06901-w

Velazquez, C., Shibayama-Salas, M., Aguirre-Garcia, J., Tsutsumi, V., and Calderon, J. (1998). Role of neutrophils in innate resistance to *Entamoeba histolytica* liver infection in mice. *Parasite Immunol.* 20, 255–262. doi: 10.1046/j.1365-3024.1998.00128.x

Ventura-Juarez, J., Campos-Esparza, M., Pacheco-Yepez, J., López-Blanco, J. A., Adabache-Ortíz, A., Silva-Briano, M., et al. (2016). *Entamoeba histolytica* induces human neutrophils to form NETs. *Parasite Immunol.* 38, 503–509. doi: 10.1111/pim.12332

Verkerke, H. P., Petri, W. A. Jr, and Marie, C. S. (2012). The dynamic interdependence of amebiasis, innate immunity, and undernutrition. *Semin. Immunopathol.* 34, 771–785. doi: 10.1007/s00281-012-0349-1

Walsh, J. A. (1986). Problems in recognition and diagnosis of amebiasis: estimation of the global magnitude of morbidity and mortality. *Rev. Infect. Dis.* 8, 228–238

Wojtala, A., Bonora, M., Malinska, D., Pinton, P., Duszynski, J., and Wieckowski, M. R. (2014). Methods to monitor ROS production by fluorescence microscopy and fluorometry. *Methods Enzymol.* 542, 243–262. doi: 10.1016/B978-0-12-416618-9.00013-3

Yipp, B. G., Petri, B., Salina, D., Jenne, C. N., Scott, B. N., Zbytnuik, L. D., et al. (2012). Infection-induced NETosis is a dynamic process involving neutrophil multitasking *in vivo*. *Nat. Med.* 18, 1386–1393. doi: 10.1038/nm.2847

Zawrotniak, M., and Rapala-Kozik, M. (2013). Neutrophil extracellular traps (NETs) - formation and implications. *Acta Biochim. Pol.* 60, 277–284. Available online at: http://www.actabp.pl/pdf/3_2013/277.pdf

15

A Novel Heat Shock Element (HSE) in *Entamoeba histolytica* that Regulates the Transcriptional Activation of the *EhPgp5* Gene in the Presence of Emetine Drug

*Alma Nieto [1], David G. Pérez Ishiwara [1], Esther Orozco [2], Virginia Sánchez Monroy [1] and Consuelo Gómez García [1]**

[1] Laboratorio de Biomedicina Molecular I, Escuela Nacional de Medicina y Homeopatía, Instituto Politécnico Nacional, Mexico City, Mexico, [2] Departamento de Infectómica y Patogénesis Molecular, Centro de Investigación y de Estudios Avanzados del Instituto Politécnico Nacional, Mexico City, Mexico

***Correspondence:**
Consuelo Gómez García
cgomezg@ipn.mx

Transcriptional regulation of the multidrug resistance *EhPgp5* gene in *Entamoeba histolytica* is induced by emetine stress. *EhPgp5* overexpression alters the chloride-dependent currents that cause trophozoite swelling, diminishing induced programmed cell death (PCD) susceptibility. In contrast, antisense inhibition of P-glycoprotein (PGP) expression produces synchronous death of trophozoites and the enhancement of the biochemical and morphological characteristics of PCD induced by G418. Transcriptional gene regulation analysis identified a 59 bp region at position −170 to −111 bp promoter as putative emetine response elements (EREs). However, insights into transcription factors controlling *EhPgp5* gene transcription are missing; to fill this knowledge gap, we used deletion studies and transient CAT activity assays. Our findings suggested an activating motif (−151 to −136 bp) that corresponds to a heat shock element (HSE). Gel-shift assays, UV-crosslinking, binding protein purification, and western blotting assays revealed proteins of 94, 66, 62, and 51 kDa binding to the *EhPgp5* HSE that could be heat shock-like transcription factors that regulate the transcriptional activation of the *EhPgp5* gene in the presence of emetine drug.

Keywords: multidrug resistance, HSE, *Entamoeba histolytica*, *EhPgp5*, emetine, stress

INTRODUCTION

The multidrug resistance phenotype (MDR) is a phenomenon in which the cell is able to survive in the presence of a drug and shows cross-resistance to a variety of structurally unrelated drugs across membranes in a wide range of organisms (Moons, 2003). The MDR phenotype has been identified in several organisms from mammals to prokaryotes provoking serious problems for the treatment and control of different illness, such as cancer, sepsis, and several parasitoses, such as malaria, leishmaniasis, and others (Juranka et al., 1989).

The P-glycoprotein (PGP) an ATP-dependent membrane-bound transporter is the major protein involved in the MDR phenotype (Mickley et al., 1989). In humans, the PGP is encoded by two *MDR* genes (*MDR1* and *MDR3*) (Chin et al., 1989); in mice, by *mdr1a* and *mdr1b* (Cui et al., 2009); in *Leishmania major*, by *lmmdr1* and *lmmdr2;* and in *Plasmodium falciparum*, by *pfmdr1* and the *pfmdr2* (Grogl et al., 1991). Interestingly, the largest *mdr* gene family described until now is present in *Entamoeba histolytica* (Orozco et al., 2001), the protozoan parasite responsible for human amoebiasis, which causes an estimated 50 million cases of invasive disease and 70,000 deaths per year (World Health Organization, 1998). The multigenic amoeba *mdr* family is composed of *EhPgp1*, *EhPgp2*, *EhPgp5*, and *EhPgp6* genes. A differential gene expression pattern has been documented in drug-sensitive (clone A) and drug-resistant (clone C2) trophozoites (Descoteaux et al., 1995). *EhPgp1* is constitutively expressed in trophozoites from clones A and C2 (Gómez et al., 1996). In contrast, the *EhPgp5* gene showed inducible expression due to the presence of emetine in culture medium (Descoteaux et al., 1995). The transcript of this gene was not detected in clones A and C2 growth without drug. However, when C2 trophozoites were cultured in the presence of emetine, expression of the *EhPgp5* gene increased in a drug concentration-dependent manner (Descoteaux et al., 1995). Although an increase in the *EhPgp5* mRNA half-life was reported (López-Camarillo et al., 2003), its expression was mainly dependent on transcriptional activation (Pérez et al., 1998). The *EhPgp5* promoter region, from −170 to +30 bp, was able to efficiently drive the expression of CAT reporter gene when trophozoites from clones A and C2 were cultured under drug pressure (Pérez et al., 1998), suggesting that specific emetine response elements (EREs) were present in this region. Additionally, functional assays suggested that the putative ERE could be localized between −170 and −111 bp of the *EhPgp5* gene promoter (Nieto et al., 2005).

To investigate the relevance of ERE to *EhPgp5* gene transcription, deletions, and transient CAT activity studies were performed here. Our findings suggested an activating motif (−151 to −136 bp) that corresponds to a heat shock element (HSE). Gel-shift assays, UV-crosslinking, binding protein purification, and western blotting assays revealed proteins binding to the *EhPgp5* HSE that could be heat shock-like transcription factors, which regulate transcriptional activation of the *EhPgp5* gene in the presence of emetine drug.

MATERIALS AND METHODS

E. histolytica Cultures

Trophozoites of clones A and C2 (strain HM1: IMSS) (Orozco et al., 1985) were axenically cultured in TY1-S-33 medium (Diamond et al., 1978). Emetine stress was exerted by the incubation of trophozoites from clones A or C2 in 8 or 20 μM emetine, respectively, for 24 h.

In Silico Search for Potential Transcription Binding Sites

The TRANSFACT database (MatInspector software) was used to identify potential transcription factor binding sites in the *EhPgp5* promoter (Matys et al., 2006).

Plasmid Constructions

To perform transfection experiments, several plasmids were constructed by inserting PCR-amplified *EhPgp5* gene core promoter fragments into multiple cloning sites of the pBSCAT-ACT plasmid (Gómez et al., 1998). The constructs performed are shown in **Figures 1A,B**. Constructs with specific mutations in the CdxA, YY1, and HSE regions were performed by PCR amplification using the primers shown in **Figure 1C**. Promoter-less (pBSCAT-ACT) and minimal p259Pgp5 promoter constructs (Pérez et al., 1998) were used as negative and positive controls, respectively. The pA5′A3′CAT plasmid (Nickel and Tannich, 1994), which contains a 480 bp fragment from the *actin* gene promoter, was used as an internal control of transfection efficiency. Correct sequence orientation of the cloned fragments was determined by sequencing analysis.

Transfection and Cat Assays

Transfection assays were performed by electroporation (Nickel and Tannich, 1994). Briefly, 10^6 trophozoites of clones A and C2 were transfected with 100 μg of the different plasmid constructs (ΔCdxA-Pgp5, ΔCdxA-YY1-Pgp5, Δ5HSE-Pgp5, pmuCdxAPgp5, pmuYY1cPgp5, pmuYY1gPgp5, pmuHSEPgp5, pmHSE-TTCPgp5, p-sinHSEPgp5, p259Pgp5, pBSCAT-ACT, and pA5′A3′CAT). Electroporated trophozoites were transferred into plastic flasks (Nalgene, NY, USA) containing 50 ml of TYI-S-33 medium and were incubated for 48 h at 37°C. Two hours after electroporation, we added 8 μM emetine to clone A or 20 μM emetine to clone C2. CAT activities were measured by two-phase diffusion assay using 5 μg of trophozoite extracts and 200 μl of chloramphenicol (1.25 mM), which were incubated with [^{14}C]-butyril-CoA (NEN Life Science Products, MA, USA) for 2 h. Protein concentrations were determined using Bradford's methods (Bradford, 1976). CAT activities were expressed as the cpm of the butyrylated derivatives. The background obtained from the trophozoites transfected with the pBSCAT-ACT plasmid was subtracted from the measurements given by the plasmids containing the different promoter constructions. CAT activities were determined in the linear range of assays, representing three independent experiments performed in triplicate. The efficiency of the transfection experiments was monitored by the activity of pA5′A3′CAT plasmid (Nickel and Tannich, 1994).

Nuclear Extracts (NEs)

NEs were prepared from trophozoites of clones A and C2 grown in the presence [clones $A_{(8)}$ and $C2_{(20)}$] or absence (clones A and C2) of emetine, following Schreiber et al.'s protocol (Schreiber et al., 1989), modified by Gómez et al. (1998). Protein concentrations were determined by Bradford's methods (Bradford, 1976).

Electrophoretic Mobility Gel-Shift Assays

Double-stranded oligonucleotides of the *EhPgp5* HSE sequence from −150 to −137 bp (HSE-S-16, 5′-ATAGAAATTTTTCATA-3′) were synthesized and labeled using T4 polynucleotide kinase (Invitrogen, CA, USA) in the presence of [γ-^{32} P]-ATP. Specific activity was determined by scintillation counting.

A

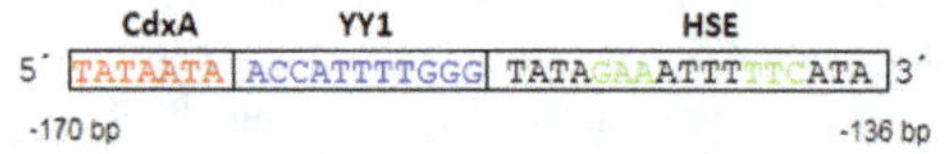

B

Element deleted	Consensus sequences deleted (bp)	Generate construction
CdxA	(-170 to -163)	pΔCdxA-Pgp5 (-163 to +30), AAAA**CGCAG**ACCATTTTGGGTATA
CdxA-YY1	(-170 to -150)	pΔCdxA-YY1-Pgp5 (-150 to +30) AAAA**CTGCAG**TAGAATTTCATA
5HSE	(-170 to -143)	pΔ 5 HSE-Pgp5 (-144 to + 30) AAAA**CTGCAG**TTTTTCATAATAGTA

C

Primers to generate mutations of different regions CdxA, YY1 and HSE	
Primer sequence 5′-3′	**Name construction**
AAAA**CTGCAG**TATA**CGC**ACCATT	pmuCdxA
AAAA**CTGCAG**TATAATAAC**AGC**TTTGGG	pmuYY1c
AAAA**CTGCAG**TATAATAACCATTTT**TAT**TATAGA	pmuYY1g
AAAA**CTGCAG**TATAATAACCATTTTGGGTATA**TCG**ATTTTT	pmuHSE
AAAA**CTGCAG**TATAATAACCATTTTGGGTATAGAAATT**AGATGA**AATAGTAAA	pmHSE-TTC
AAAA**CTGCAG**TATAATAACCATTTTGGGT**GACTGCTCGACGTGAC**ATAGTAAATA	sin-HSE
CCCAAGCTTGTATGCTGGTTCACTTGTCATGCGAAT	EhPgp5As36

FIGURE 1 | Plasmid constructions in the *EhPgp5* gene core promoter. **(A)** Schematic representation of three consensus sequences in the *EhPgp5* gene promoter (−170 to −136 bp). CdxA, YY1, and HSE motifs are marked in red, blue, and green in the rectangles, respectively. **(B)** Constructs generated by deletion of each consensus sequence of the *EhPgp5* gene core promoter (−170 to −136 bp). **(C)** Primers used to generate different mutations in CdxA, YY1, and HSE motifs. Mutations are underlined and bolded in black. Restriction sites for *Pst*I and *Hind* III are bolded in black. The last sequence is the antisense primer used for all constructs.

Gel-shift assays were performed in triplicate as described previously (Gómez et al., 1998). Briefly, we used 0.5–1 ng of labeled probes (10,000 cpm), 1 μg of poly [d (I-C)] (Amersham Pharmacia Biotech, NJ, USA), 20 μg of NE from trophozoites and 10% glycerol in DNA–protein binding buffer. For competition assays, 150-fold molar excess of unlabeled oligonucleotides was incubated with NE at 4°C for 10 min prior to adding the radiolabeled probes. As competitors, we used poly [d (I-C)] and the double-stranded oligonucleotides S-34 (5′-TATAATAACCATTTTGGGTATAGAAATTTTTCAT-3′) and HSEm (5′-ATATCGATTTTTCATA-3′).

UV-Crosslinking and Western Blot Experiments

UV-crosslinking assays were performed according to Ausubel et al. (1994) with some modifications. Standard gel-shift mixtures using NE from trophozoites of both clones grown in the absence or presence of emetine and the radiolabeled HSE probe were scaled up five-fold and were exposed to irradiation in a 312 nm UV-transilluminator (Bio-Rad, CA, USA) for 10 min at 4°C; then, the proteins were separated by 15 % SDS-PAGE (Laemmli, 1970). The gels were dried and analyzed by autoradiography. DNA cross-linked proteins were analyzed by western blot using the standard procedure (Ausubel et al., 1994). The membranes were incubated with 2 μg of human anti-HSF1 (H-311, Santa Cruz Biotechnology, TX, USA) in 5% non-fat dry milk and 0.05% Tween-20 in phosphate-buffered saline (PBS), with a pH of 7.4, overnight at 4°C. The proteins were revealed by peroxidase-conjugated anti-rabbit secondary antibodies (ZYMED Laboratories, CA, USA) (1:3000) and were immunodetected by a chemiluminescence system (ECL Plus ™, Amersham Pharmacia Biotech, NJ, USA). The assays were repeated at least three times for each studied condition.

Purification of *E. Histolytica* Proteins

E. histolytica proteins that bind to the HSE sites of the *EhPgp5* gene core promoter were partially purified three separate times under non-denaturing conditions using a DNA-binding protein purification kit (Roche, CA, USA) and NE from trophozoites of both clones $A_{[8]}$ and $C2_{[20]}$. Concatemeric polynucleotides were prepared by PCR amplification of the HSE probe. The oligomer was coupled to magnetic particles coated with streptavidin, as described by the manufacturer. Seventy-five micrograms of NE from trophozoites were mixed with the magnetic particles in protein buffer, poly [d (I-C)] and poly-L-lysine. Then, NE was incubated at 4°C for 60 min. After extensive washing, proteins bound to the particles were eluted with elution buffer containing 2 M KCl. All of the fractions were analyzed by 10% SDS-PAGE (Laemmli, 1970). The gels were silver stained or transferred to nitrocellulose membranes for western blotting assays. Purified fractions were added to DNA–protein binding reactions to perform EMSA, as described above.

Statistical Analysis

All of the data are expressed as the means ± SDs. IBM SPSS software, version 23, was used to compare all of the groups to each other. For all tests, $p < 0.05$ was considered significant.

RESULTS

Structural Characterization of the −170 to −111 bp of the *EhPgp5* Gene Core Promoter

Previously, a functional region of 59 bp (−170 to −111 bp) of the *EhPgp5* gene promoter was involved in the induction of *EhPgp5* gene expression (Nieto et al., 2005). To detect specific transcription elements within this region, we performed a bioinformatic search for the presence of consensus sequences of different transcription factors within the 59-bp *EhPgp5* gene promoter region, using the TransFact database. The structural analysis of this sequence revealed the presence of putative consensus sequences for CdxA (−170 to −164 bp) and YY1 (−163 to −153 bp) transcription factors and, interestingly, a HSE at −151 to −136 bp (**Figure 1A**).

Functional Identification of the ERE in the Region from −170 to −111 bp of the *EhPgp5* Gene Core Promoter

To identify whether these cis-regulatory elements direct specific *EhPgp5* gene expression in *E. histolytica* drug-sensitive [$A_{(8)}$] and drug-resistant [$C2_{(20)}$] clones grown in the presence of 8 and 20 μM emetine, respectively, we performed a series of mutations and deletions within the 59 bp region. Different constructs were generated, as described in the Materials and Methods section (**Figures 1B,C**). These plasmids contain internal deletions of CdxA, YY1, or HSE sequences.

Transfection assays of all constructs were performed in trophozoites from clones A and C2. In transfected trophozoites of both clones grown without emetine, no CAT activities were detected with any constructs, compared to the CAT activity developed by pA5′A3′CAT plasmid (**Figure 2**). However, when emetine was added to the culture medium after electroporation, we observed significantly higher CAT activities with all the constructs, similar to the activity shown by the *EhPgp5* gene core promoter (p259Pgp5 plasmid) (**Figure 2**), except with the pΔ5-HSEPgp5 plasmid. No significant differences were observed in the CAT activities shown by ΔCdxAPgp5, ΔCdxA-YY1Pgp5, pmuCdxAPgp5, pmuYY1cPgp5, and pmuYY1gPgp5, suggesting that CdxA and YY1 putative consensus sequences were not involved in *EhPgp5* gene transcriptional activation. In contrast, the construct pΔ5-HSEPgp5 that does not contain six of 16 bases that form the putative HSE element (ataGAAatttTTCata) displayed significant CAT activity reductions of 80 and 78% in trophozoites from clones $A_{[8]}$ and $C2_{[20]}$, respectively.

The HSE Element Is Indispensable to Activating *EhPgp5* Gene Transcription

To demonstrate that the putative HSE (−151 to −136 bp) is responsible for activating *EhPgp5* gene expression by emetine, we generated three new constructs introducing point mutations into the putative HSE. pmuHSEPgp5 contains three nucleotide replacements in the central inverted repeated GAA of HSE (ATA**GAA**ATTTT**TC**ATA→ ATA**TCG**ATTTTTCATA); pmHSE-TTCPgp5 had three base changes in the inverted repeated TTC and its flanking bases (ATA**GAA**ATTT**TTC**ATA→ ATAGAAATTA**GAT**GAA), and in p-sinHSEPgp5, the HSE sequence was completely replaced (GACTGCTCGACGTGAC). We transfected these constructs into trophozoites from clones A and C2 and then cultured them in the absence or presence of 8 or 20 μM emetine, respectively. The results showed that all of the constructs presented CAT activities in trophozoites from both clone cultures without emetine (**Figure 3**). However, a dramatic difference in expression was observed when emetine was added to the cultures, and the plasmid pmuHSEPgp5 presented higher CAT activity, similar to that shown by the p259Pgp5 minimal promoter (**Figure 3**). The activities observed were similar in both clones [$A_{(8)}$ and $C2_{(20)}$], suggesting that the changes introduced into the GAA sequence from the HSE did not affect the transcriptional activation. Interestingly, the plasmid pmHSE-TTCPgp5 presented a strong CAT activity reduction in trophozoites from both clones, suggesting that the second repeat of the HSE was indispensable to *EhPgp5* gene expression. Moreover, when the HSE was eliminated, CAT reporter gene activity was not detected, either in trophozoites of clone $A_{[8]}$ or in trophozoites of clone $C2_{[20]}$.

The *EhPgp5* HSE Is Recognized by Nuclear Proteins from *E. histolytica* Trophozoites from Sensitive and Resistant Clones

As a second approach to gaining insight into the role of HSEs in the promoter activity of the *EhPgp5* gene, we analyzed DNA–protein interactions using gel shift and competition assays. Gel electrophoretic mobility shift assays were performed to obtain evidence of nuclear protein binding to the putative HSE. Double-stranded synthetic oligonucleotides containing the *EhPgp5* HSE were incubated with NE from clones A, $A_{[8]}$, C2, and $C2_{[20]}$. Additionally, oligonucleotides containing the wild-type consensus HSE and the HSEm mutated at the repeated GAA and the region of 34 bp of the *EhPgp5* promoter from −170 to −136 bp, which contains the CdxA, YY1, and HSE sequences, were used as specific competitors. As demonstrated in **Figures 4A,B**, the HSE was specifically recognized by nuclear proteins from *E. histolytica* clones grown in the presence or absence of emetine, forming one DNA–protein complex that had identical electrophoretic mobility using NE from both clones. Interestingly, the intensity of the complex was enhanced when the DNA probe was incubated with NE from the trophozoites from clones $A_{[8]}$ and $C2_{[20]}$ (**Figures 4A–D**, lanes 2 and 7). Competition assays showed that formation of the complex with the HSE probe was efficiently blocked by the wild-type HSE and the S34 oligonucleotides when a 150-fold molar excess was used (**Figures 4A–E**, lanes 3, 5, 8, and 10) but not with the HSEm, for which the DNA–protein complexes only diminished (**Figures 4A–E**, lanes 4 and 9), suggesting that the DNA–protein interaction was partially affected by changing the GAA repeated

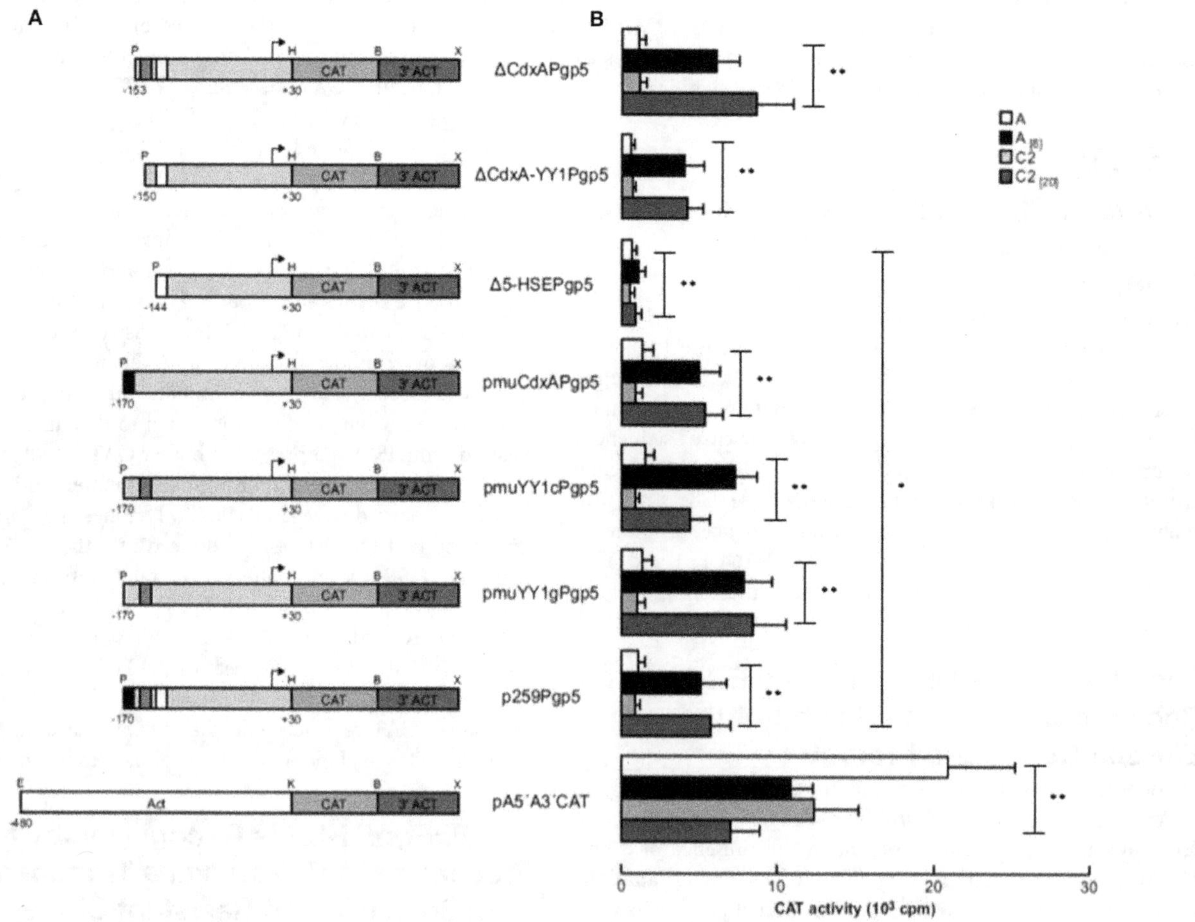

FIGURE 2 | Functional identification of the ERE in the region from −170 to −111 bp of the *EhPgp5* gene core promoter. **(A)** Schematic representation of the constructs used for the transfection assays. All of the plasmids contain the CAT reporter gene and the 3′-flanking actin region (3′ ACT). Arrows, transcription initiation sites. P, *Pst*I; H, *Hind*III; B, *Bam*HI; X, *Xho*I; E, *EcoR*I; K, *Kpn*I. CdxA, YY1, and HSE motifs are in black, gray and white boxes, respectively. **(B)** Bars show the average of CAT activity (cpm) of the transfected plasmids obtained by the two-phase diffusion assays ± SD, representative of three independent experiments performed in duplicate ($^*p < 0.05$; $^{**}p < 0.001$). The background given by the trophozoites transfected with pBSCAT-ACT plasmid was subtracted in all of the experiments. The efficiency of the transfection assays was monitored by the activities given by the pA5′A3′CAT plasmid.

sequence. However, this change did not interfere with the *EhPgp5* promoter activity (**Figures 4A,B**). In contrast, when poly [d(I-C)] was used as a non-specific competitor (350-fold molar excess), the DNA–protein complex formation was not affected (**Figures 4A–D**, lanes 6 and 11).

Molecular Weights of the Nuclear Proteins Binding to the *EhPgp5* HSE

To identify the nuclear proteins binding to the *EhPgp5* HSE, we performed UV-crosslinking assays after gel shift. Two main proteins of 51 and 34 kDa after correction for the bound probe (61 and 44 kDa) were found in both clones incubated with or without emetine (**Figure 5**). The HSE-protein interactions were specific due to complex formation being prevented by a 150-fold molar excess of cold oligonucleotide (lane 5), while binding proteins were not inhibited using the unspecific competitor poly [d (I-C)] (lane 6), indicating the specificity of the complexes. The bands obtained using the NE trophozoites from both clones grown in the presence of emetine (**Figures 5A,C,E,F**), were more intense than the bands obtained using the NE trophozoites from both clones grown in the absence of emetine (**Figures 5B,D–F**).

Putative Heat Shock Transcription Factor Binds to the *EhPgp5* HSE

To identify the proteins interacting with the *EhPgp5* HSE, we searched for putative heat shock transcription factors (HSTF) by western blot assays of the UV-crosslinked complexes from trophozoites of clones A, $A_{[8]}$, C2, and $C2_{[20]}$ using the human heterologous antibody anti-HSF1. As shown in **Figure 5G**, a band of 51 kDa was detected after correction for the bound probe from the DNA–protein complex formed with the HSE element. The band was stronger (20%) in $C2_{[20]}$, trophozoites (**Figure 5H**). In trophozoites from both clones grown without emetine, a very slight signal was detected (data not show).

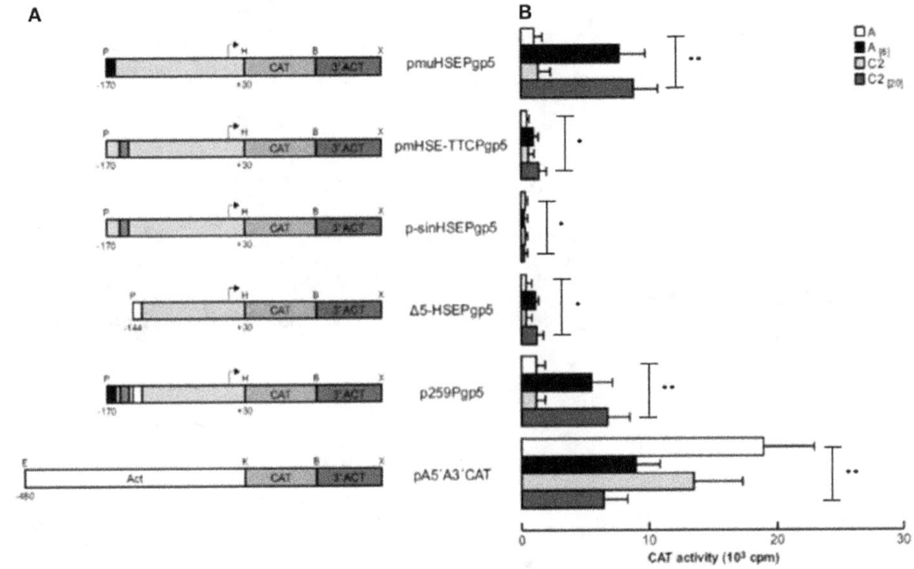

FIGURE 3 | Functional identification of the putative HSE element in the region from −170 to −111 bp of the *EhPgp5* gene core promoter. **(A)** Schematic representation of the constructs used for the transfection assays. All of the plasmids contain the CAT reporter gene and the 3′-flanking actin region (3′ ACT). Arrows, transcription initiation sites. P, *Pst*I; H, *Hind*III; B, *Bam*HI; X, *Xho*I; E, *Eco*RI; K, *Kpn*I. CdxA, YY1, and HSE motifs are in black, gray and white boxes, respectively. **(B)** Bars show the average CAT activity (cpm) of the transfected plasmids obtained by the two-phase diffusion assays ± SD, representative of three independent experiments performed in duplicate. The background given by the trophozoites transfected with pBSCAT-ACT plasmid was subtracted in all of the experiments. The efficiency of transfection assays was monitored by the activities given by the pA5′A3′CAT plasmid. Vertical bars and asterisks indicate significant differences (*$p < 0.05$; **$p < 0.001$).

Partial Purification of the Proteins Binding to the *EhPgp5* HSE

We performed partial purification of proteins that bind to the HSE using the DNA-binding protein purification kit from Roche Molecular Biochemical (Roche, CA, USA), NE from trophozoites of clones $A_{[8]}$ and $C2_{[20]}$ and a concatamerized oligonucleotide containing the HSE. Two main and defined enrichment purified proteins of ~94 and 66 kDa, respectively, were detected on a silver-stained SDS-polyacrylamide gel in NE from trophozoites of clone $A_{[8]}$, (**Figure 6A**, lane 3), while two proteins of 62 and 51 kDa were purified from the NE from the trophozoites of clone $C2_{[20]}$ (**Figure 6D**, lane 3). To determine whether purified proteins were also detected by the HSTF1 heterologous antibody, we performed western blot assays. The results showed that both pairs of proteins, 94 and 66 kDa and 62 and 51 kDa from $A_{[8]}$ and $C2_{[20]}$ trophozoites, respectively, were recognized by the human anti-HSTF1 (**Figures 6B,E**). These results supported the idea that the proteins that binding to the *EhPgp5* HSE could be putative heat shock like transcription factors.

Furthermore, the semipurified proteins from both clones were used to determine whether these proteins could bind to the HSE sequence. As shown in **Figures 6C,F,G,H** (lane 2), two specific DNA–protein complexes were observed with the semipurified proteins of clones $A_{[8]}$ and $C2_{[20]}$. The complexes were highly specific due to being completely inhibited by a 150-fold molar excess of the same unlabeled wild-type HSE and S34 oligonucleotides (lanes 3 and 5), and 350-fold molar excess of poly [d(I-C)] did not affect complex formation (lane 6). Interestingly, the HSEm did not affect complex formation (**Figures 6C,F–H** lane 4).

DISCUSSION

The *EhPgp5* gene and its encoded P-glycoprotein (EhPGP5) have functional relevance in different mechanisms of *E. histolytica* parasites. On the one hand, the antisense inhibition of gene expression enhances the PCD of trophozoites in the presence of G418; on the other hand, gene overexpression alters the chloride-dependent currents and confers drug resistance to emetine (Pérez et al., 1998; Bañuelos et al., 2002; Delgadillo et al., 2002; Medel Flores et al., 2013).

Therefore, due to the relevance of EhPGP5 for different cellular processes, its transcription must be finely regulated. To determine the molecular effectors up-regulating *EhPgp5* gene expression, our group performed the structural and functional characterization of *EhPgp5* gene promoter (Pérez et al., 1998) in trophozoites growth in the absence and presence of emetine, delimiting a 59 bp region at the position from −170 to −111 bp, in which putative EREs were found (Nieto et al., 2005).

Here, we investigated for the first time the functional roles of motifs found in promoter activity. Consensus DNA-binding sequences for different transcription factors are well conserved throughout evolution, and different databases of transcription factors and promoters have been established to develop algorithms, as well as computer methods to predict sequence target sites for specific DNA-binding proteins (Boeva,

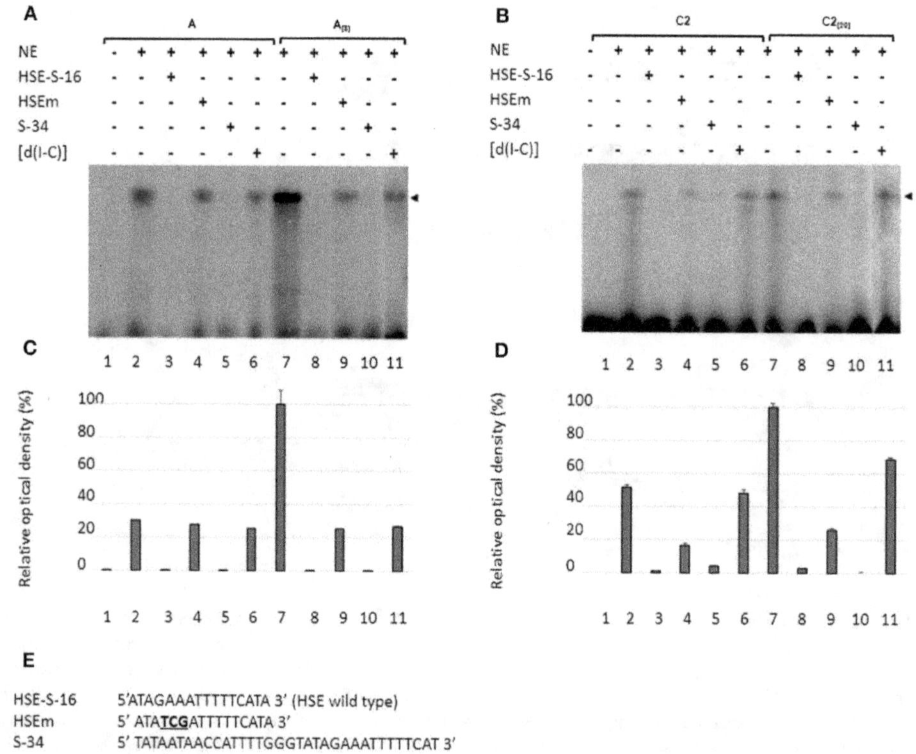

FIGURE 4 | Nuclear protein binding with the putative HSE element of the *EhPgp5* gene core promoter. Gel shift assays were performed with 20 μg of NE from clones: **(A)** A and $A_{[8]}$, **(B)** C2 and $C2_{[20]}$, 1 ng of [γ-^{32}P]-radiolabeled double-stranded fragment of different unlabeled oligonucleotides (150-fold molar excess). Lane 1, free probe; lanes 2 and 7, no competitor; lanes 3 and 8 specific competitor unlabeled straight (150-fold molar excess); lanes 4 and 9, specific competitor with the HSE mutated at the repeated GAA; lanes 5 and 10, specific competitor containing the CdxA, YY1, and HSE consensus sequences; lanes 6 and 11 unspecific competitor (350-fold molar excess of poly [d(I–C)]). Arrowheads indicate the specific complexes formed. **(C,D)** Densitometric analysis of DNA-binding interaction with NE from clones A and $A_{[8]}$ and C2 and $C2_{[20]}$, respectively. **(E)** Sequence of the *EhPgp5* HSE used as a probe (HSE-S-16) and the competitors (HSEm and S-34). Mutations are underlined and bolded in black. Data presented in this figure are representative of three independent experiments.

2016). The bioinformatic screening revealed three consensus sequences for CdxA, YY1, and HSE, recognized by the CdxA, Ying Yang 1 (YY1), and HSTF proteins, respectively (Perisic et al., 1989; Shi et al., 1991; Margalit et al., 1993).

In *E. histolytica,* seven putative HSEs located in *EhrabB*, three in *Ehhsp100* and four in *Ehmlbp* gene promoter have been reported (Bernes et al., 2005; Romero-Díaz et al., 2007; Katz et al., 2012). Functional CAT assays driven by *EhrabB* promoter demonstrated that CAT activity increased by two times when trophozoites were exposed to heat shock stress (42°C) (Romero-Díaz et al., 2007). Deletion of HSEs from *Ehmlbp* gene promoter down-regulated CAT reporter gene expression in trophozoites exposed to heat shock (Katz et al., 2012), while the activity of the HSEs present in *Ehhsp100* gene promoter has not yet been studied. Comparison of the HSE from the *EhPgp5* gene promoter with those reported in *E. histolytica* showed greater similarity with the HSEs of the *Ehhsp100* gene promoter. Both sequences were formed by two motifs; however, the orientation of the *EhPgp5* HSE (ATA**GAA**ATTTT**TTC**ATA) is head-tail (GAA and TTC), while that of the *Ehhsp100* is head-head (AAG**GAA**CTT**GAA**GAA), containing a gap of four and three bases between them, respectively (Bernes et al., 2005). In contrast, Tchénio et al. (2006) that osteosarcoma cells became doxorubicin resistant by overexpression of the MDR1 gene, induced by the HSE. These results together supported the idea that HSE within the *EhPgp5* gene promoter is relevant for its expression in trophozoite culture under emetine drug pressure, which is a stress situation. Functional analyses of the HSE (nGAAnnTTCn) in other organisms have demonstrated that the GAA and TTC motifs contain indispensable bases for DNA–protein interactions and consequently for promoter activation (Enoki and Sakurai, 2011). Mutations or deletions of these motifs decreased or abolished the promoter activity of the *RPN4* and *PDR3* genes in *Saccharomyces cerevisiae* and *BnGolS1* in plant cells in a similar manner to that we observed for the *EhPgp5* HSE (Hahn et al., 2006; Lang et al., 2017). We demonstrated here that CAT activity was abolished by complete HSE substitution or by TTC (GAT) mutation, strongly supporting that emetine increases the activity of the *EhPgp5* gene promoter via HSE.

Using DNA–protein interactions, western blots from crosslinked and semipurified proteins employing heterologous HSTF antibodies indicated that HSE interacts with an HSTF-like factor present in both sensitive and resistant trophozoites;

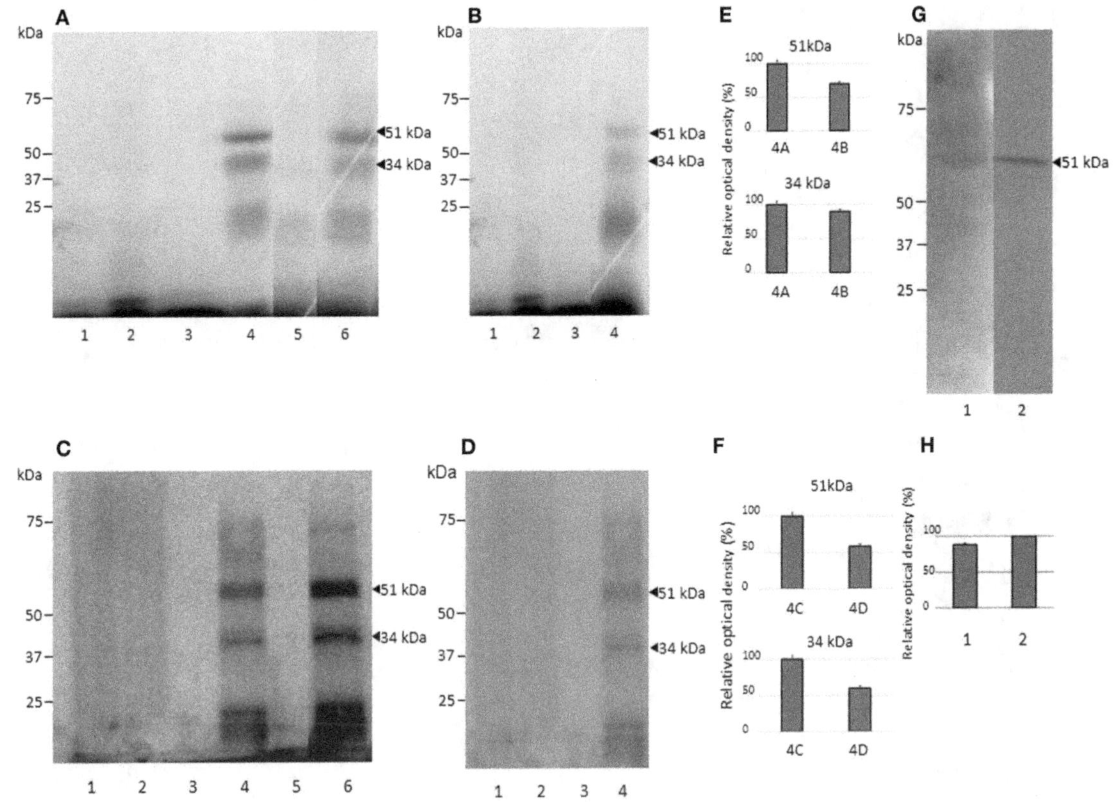

FIGURE 5 | Molecular weight of the nuclear proteins binding to the *EhPgp5* HSE and their immunorelation to human HSF. UV-crosslinking analyses after EMSA in A and C2 clone grown in the presence **(A,C)** or in the absence **(B,D)** of emetine. One hundred micrograms of NE from clones A **(A,B)** and C2 **(C,D)** trophozoites were UV cross-linked to 5 ng of the γ^{32}P-ATP radiolabeled HSE probe for 10 min at 4°C, and DNA–protein complexes were electrophoresed through 15% SDS-PAGE, followed by exposure to X-ray film. Lane 1, UV untreated HSE probe; lane 2, UV irradiation of HSE probe; lane 3, UV untreated complete binding reaction; lane 4, UV treatment of complete binding reaction; lane 5, probe (150-fold molar excess); lane 6, unspecific competitor poly [d(I-C)]. Arrowheads, DNA–protein complexes after correction for the bound probe. Relative densitometry of each protein in clones $A_{[8]}$ and A **(E)** and $C2_{[20]}$ and C2 **(F)**. **(G)** Western blot assay of UV cross-linked DNA–protein complexes of clones $A_{[8]}$ and $C2_{[20]}$ using heterologous antibodies to anti-HSF1 from humans with their corresponding densitometric values. **(H)** Lane 1, clone $A_{[8]}$; and lane 2, clone $C2_{[20]}$. All assays were performed on three different occasions.

however, functional CAT assays demonstrated that the promoter was active only in the presence of emetine, suggesting that binding of HSTF-like factor is not sufficient to drive promoter activity. Several pieces of evidence from other systems have shown that HSTF factors present a multistep activation mechanism (trimerization, phosphorylation, and translocation to nucleus) to activate gene expression (Sorger and Pelham, 1988; Høj and Jakobsen, 1994; Sandqvist et al., 2009). These factors are activated in the presence of stress induced by heat, oxidative stress, heavy metals, bacterial toxins, and drugs between others (Høj and Jakobsen, 1994; Akerfelt et al., 2007). In amoebas, it was reported that the HSE from *Ehhsp100* promoter was recognized by a 37 kDa protein when the trophozoites were exposed to heat shock (Bernes et al., 2005), while a 25 kDa protein bound to the HSE in *Ehmlbp* promoter also under heat shock (Katz et al., 2012).

Different experimental procedures performed here showed that HSE interacts with 94, 66, and 51 kDa proteins in sensitive trophozoites, while in resistant ones, HSE interacts with 62 and 51 kDa, both recognized by HSTF antibodies.

Differences found in the molecular weights of EhHSTF-like proteins interacting with the HSE in sensitive and resistant clones could be due to: (i) translational modifications; (ii) formation of homodimers or homotrimers; or (iii) interactions with other proteins, for example, molecular weight changes in human HSFs by different posttranslational modifications, mainly phosphorylation (Sorger et al., 1987; Larson et al., 1988; Baler et al., 1993; Sarge et al., 1993). These factors are able to trimerize or interact with different proteins, such as CHIP (C-terminus of HSP70-interacting protein) (Murata et al., 2003), DDL-1 and DDL-2, forming a complex that stabilizes HSF1 monomers (Chiang et al., 2012), or with HSP70 and HSP90 to keep HSTF1 in an inactive state preventing trimerization (Zou et al., 1998) or even more perhaps interacting with other human HSFs (HSF1, HSF2, HSF3, and HSF4) (Rabdiran et al., 1991; Schuetz et al., 1991; Nakai et al., 1997). In this parasite, eight Hsps (101, 100, 90, 70, 60, 40, 20, and 10) have been identified, and some of them have been characterized, showing their participation in heat shock stress (Bernes et al., 2005; Ximénez et al., 2017). These results suggest that amoebas

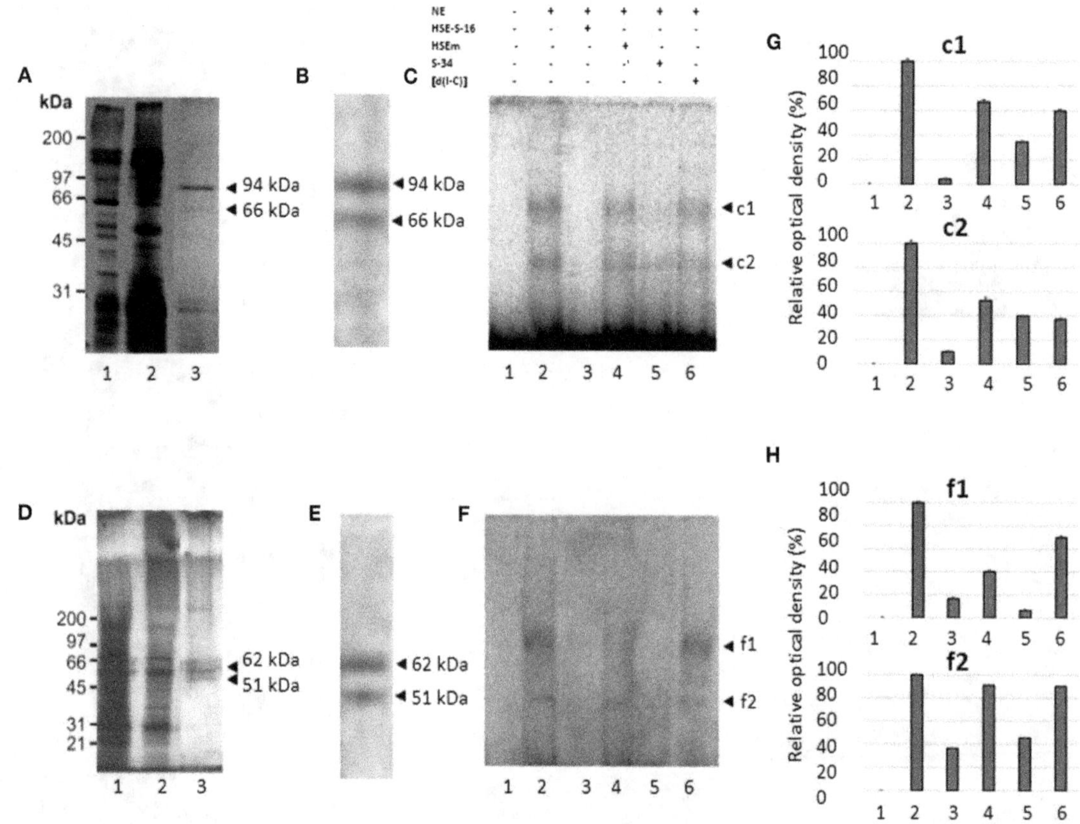

FIGURE 6 | Purification, immunodetection, and DNA-interaction of the nuclear proteins that bind to the HSE element **(A,D)**. 10% SDS-PAGE of protein fractions obtained from the purification protocol of NE from clones $A_{[8]}$ and $C2_{[20]}$, respectively. Lane 1, NE (5 μg); lane 2, non-retained fraction; and lane 3, partially purified fraction. **(B,E)** Western blot analysis of fractions obtained from the purification protocol of NE of clones $A_{[8]}$ and $C2_{[20]}$, respectively. Arrowheads, silver stained polypeptides detected by antibodies against HSF1 from humans. **(C,F)** EMSA using [γ-^{32}P]-ATP radiolabeled HSE probe and partially purified fraction from clones $A_{[8]}$ and $C2_{[20]}$, respectively. Lane 1, free probe; lane 2, no competitor; lane 3, specific competitor unlabeled straight (150-fold molar excess); lane 4, specific competitor with the HSE mutated; lane 5, specific competitor containing the CdxA, YY1, and HSE consensus sequences; lane 6, unspecific competitor (350-fold molar excess of poly[d(I–C)]). Arrowheads, specific complexes formed. **(G,H)** Relative amounts of DNA binding protein complexes with partial purification proteins of clones A[8] and C2[20], respectively. Each bar indicates the mean ± SE. Data presented in this figure are representative of three independent experiments.

might contain an HSTF demonstrated in other organisms, which is responsible for controlling the expression of the *hsp* genes (Driedonks et al., 2015). In the literature, it has been described that HSF is a master regulator of stress-responsive genes among organisms as distantly related as bacteria and humans (Guertin et al., 2010). Moreover, in the *E. histolytica* genome, seven putative HSTFs are present that could interact with the HSE of the *EhPgp5* gene promoter in trophozoites grown in the presence of emetine (Bernes et al., 2005; Loftus et al., 2005; Macías-Arguelles, in preparation). However, we do not know which of the seven factors is being expressed and is regulating *EhPgp5* gene expression. HSFs are characterized by their ability to bind to the HSE; but, in organisms containing different HSFs, such as humans, mice, and chickens, it has been described that each is able to regulate different genes (Driedonks et al., 2015).

The findings presented here provide evidence of the participation of a novel HSE that requires a putative HSTF-like factor(s) to regulate the transcriptional activation of the multidrug-resistant *EhPgp5* gene in trophozoites exposed to emetine, as has been reported in human MDR1 multidrug-resistance gene. However, the underlying mechanisms explaining how a putative EhHSTF recognizes and binds to the HSE, how emetine activates the *EhPgp5* promoter via EhHSTF, and which of the seven EhHSTFs binds to the HSE remain to be discovered.

AUTHOR CONTRIBUTIONS

AN: Data acquisition and analysis or for the work. DP: interpretation of data and revision of intellectual content. EO: Revision of intellectual content. VS: Draft the work and revision of intellectual content. CG: Design of the work and revision of intellectual content.

ACKNOWLEDGMENTS

This work was supported by the Consejo Nacional de Ciencia y Tecnología (CONACyT-39986) and Instituto Politécnico Nacional (Secretaría de Investigación y Posgrado). We would like to thank Alfredo Padilla for his help with the artwork.

REFERENCES

Akerfelt, M., Trouillet, D., Mezger, V., and Sistonen, L. (2007). Heat shock factors at a crossroad between stress and development. *Ann. N. Y. Acad. Sci.* 1113, 15–27. doi: 10.1196/annals.1391.005

Ausubel, F. M., Brent, R., Kingston, R. E., Moore, D. D., Seidman, J. G., Smith, J. A., et al. (1994). *Current Protocols in Molecular Biology*. New York, NY: John Wiley and Sons.

Baler, R., Dahl, G., and Voellmy, R. (1993). Activation of human heat shock genes is accompanied by oligomerization, modification, and rapid translocation of heat shock transcription factor HSF1. *Mol. Cell. Biol.* 13, 2486–2496 doi: 10.1128/MCB.13.4.2486

Bañuelos, C., Orozco, E., Gómez, C., González, A., Medel, O., Mendoza, L., et al. (2002). "Cellular location and function of the P-glycoproteins (EhPgps)" in *Entamoeba histolytica* Multidrug-Resistant Trophozoites. *Microb. Drug Resist.* 8, 291–300. doi: 10.1089/10766290260469552

Bernes, S., Siman-Tov, R., and Ankri, S. (2005). Epigenetic and classical activation o *Entamoeba histolytica* heat shock protein 100 (EHsp100) expression. *FEBS Lett.* 579, 6395–6402. doi: 10.1016/j.febslet.2005.09.101

Boeva, V. (2016). Analysis of genomic sequence motifs for deciphering transcription factor binding and transcriptional regulation in eukaryotic cells. *Front. Genet.* 7:24. doi: 10.3389/fgene.2016.00024

Bradford, M. M. (1976). A rapid and sensitive method for the quantitation of microgram quantities of protein utilizing the principle of protein-dye binding. *Anal. Biochem.* 72, 248–254. doi: 10.1016/0003-2697(76)90527-3

Chiang, W. C., Ching, T. T., Lee, H. C., Mousigian, C., and Hsu, A. L. (2012). HSF-1 regulators DDL-1/2 link insulin-like signaling to heat-shock responses and modulation of longevity. *Cell* 148, 322–334. doi: 10.1016/j.cell.2011.12.019

Chin, J. E., Soffir, R., Noonan, K. E., Choi, K., and Roninson, I. B. (1989). Structure and expression of the human MDR (P-glycoprotein) gene family. *Mol. Cell. Biol.* 9, 3808–3820 doi: 10.1128/MCB.9.9.3808

Cui, Y. J., Cheng, X., Weaver, Y. M., and Klaassen, C. D. (2009). Tissue distribution, gender-divergent expression, ontogeny, and chemical induction of multidrug resistance transporter genes (Mdr1a, Mdr1b, Mdr2) in mice. *Drug Metab. Dispos.* 37, 203–210. doi: 10.1124/dmd.108.023721

Delgadillo, D. M., Pérez, D. G., Gómez, C., Ponce, A., Paz, F., Bañuelos, C., et al. (2002). The *Entamoeba histolytica* EhPgp5 (MDR-like) protein induces swelling of the trophozoites and alters chloride-dependent currents in *Xenopus laevis* oocytes. *Microb. Drug Resist.* 8, 15–26. doi: 10.1089/10766290252913719

Descoteaux, S., Ayala, P., Samuelson, J., and Orozco, E. (1995). Increase in mRNA of multiple Eh pgp genes encoding P-glycoprotein homologues in emetine-resistant *Entamoeba histolytica* parasites. *Gene* 164, 179–184 doi: 10.1016/0378-1119(95)00533-C

Diamond, L. S., Harlow, D. R., and Cunnick, C. C. (1978). A new medium for the axenic cultivation of *Entamoeba histolytica* and other Entamoeba. *Trans. R. Soc. Trop. Med. Hyg.* 72, 431–432 doi: 10.1016/0035-9203(78)90144-X

Driedonks, N., Xu, J., Peters, J. L., Park, S., and Rieu, I. (2015). Multi-level interactions between heat shock factors, heat shock proteins, and the redox system regulate acclimation to heat. *Front. Plant Sci.* 6:999. doi: 10.3389/fpls.2015.00999

Enoki, Y., and Sakurai, H. (2011). Diversity in DNA recognition by heat shock transcription factors (HSFs) from model organisms. *FEBS Lett.* 585, 1293–1298. doi: 10.1016/j.febslet.2011.04.014

Gómez, C., Pérez, D. G., López-Bayghen, E., and Orozco, E. (1998). Transcriptional analysis of the EhPgp1 promoter of *Entamoeba histolytica* multidrug-resistant mutant. *J. Biol. Chem..* 273, 7277–7284. doi: 10.1074/jbc.273.13.7277

Gómez, M. D., Pérez, D. G., Ayala, P., Samuelson, J., and Orozco, E. (1996). Physiology and molecular biology of multidrug resistance in *Entamoeba histolytica. Arch. Med. Res.* 27, 421–425

Grogl, M., Martin, R. K., Oduola, A. M., Milhous, W. K., and Kyle, D. E. (1991). Characteristics of multidrug resistance in Plasmodium and Leishmania: detection of P-glycoprotein-like components. *Am. J. Trop. Med. Hyg.* 45, 98–111 doi: 10.4269/ajtmh.1991.45.98

Guertin, M. J., Petesch, S. J., Zobeck, K. L., Min, I. M., and Lis, J. T. (2010). Drosophila heat shock system as a general model to investigate transcriptional regulation. *Cold Spring Harb. Symp. Quant. Biol.* 75, 1–9. doi: 10.1101/sqb.2010.75.039

Hahn, J. S., Neef, D. W., and Thiele, D. J. (2006). A stress regulatory network for co-ordinated activation of proteasome expression mediated by yeast heat shock transcription factor. *Mol. Microbiol.* 60, 240–251. doi: 10.1111/j.1365-2958.2006.05097.x

Høj, A., and Jakobsen, B. K. (1994). A short element required for turning off heat shock transcription factor: evidence that phosphorylation enhances deactivation. *EMBO J.* 13, 2617–2624.

Juranka, P. F., Zastawny, R. L., and Ling, V. (1989). P-glycoprotein: multidrug-resistance and a superfamily of membrane-associated transport proteins. *FASEB J.* 14, 2583–2592.

Katz, S., Kushnir, O., Tovy, A., Siman Tov, R., and Ankri, S. (2012). The *Entamoeba histolytica* methylated LINE-binding protein EhMLBP provides protection against protein heat shock. *Cell. Microbiol.* 14, 58–70. doi: 10.1111/j.1462-5822.2011.01697.x

Laemmli, U. K. (1970). Cleavage of structural proteins during the assembly of the head of bacteriophage T4. *Nature* 227, 680–685 doi: 10.1038/227680a0

Lang, S., Lui, X., Xue, H., Li, X., and Wang, X. (2017). Functional characterization of BnHSFA4a as a heat shock transcription factor in controlling the re-establishment of desiccation tolerance in seeds. *J. Exp. Bot.* 68, 2361–2375. doi: 10.1093/jxb/erx097

Larson, J. S., Schuetz, T. J., and Kingston, R. E. (1988). Activation *in vitro* of sequence-specific DNA binding by a human regulatory factor. *Nature* 335, 372–375. doi: 10.1038/335372a0

Loftus, B., Anderson, I., Davies, R., Alsmark, U. C., Samuelson, J., Amedeo, P., et al. (2005). The genome of the protist parasite *Entamoeba histolytica. Nature* 433, 865–868. doi: 10.1038/nature03291

López-Camarillo, C., Luna-Arias, J. P., Marchat, L. A., and Orozco, E. (2003). EhPgp5 MRNA stability is a regulatory event in the *Entamoeba histolytica* multidrug resistance phenotype. *J. Biol. Chem.* 278, 11273–11280. doi: 10.1074/jbc.M211757200

Margalit, Y., Yarus, S., Shapira, E., Gruenbaum, Y., and Fainsod, A. (1993). Isolation and characterization of target sequences of the chicken CdxA homeobox gene. *Nucleic Acids Res.* 21, 4915–4922. doi: 10.1093/nar/21.21.4915

Matys, V., Kel-Margoulis, O. V., Fricke, E., Liebich, I., Land, S., Barre-Dirrie, A., et al. (2006). TRANSFAC and its module TRANSCompel: transcriptional gene regulation in eukaryotes. *Nucleic Acids Res.* 34, D108–D110. doi: 10.1093/nar/gkj143

Medel Flores, O., Gómez García, C., Sánchez Monroy, V., Villalba Magadaleno, J. D., Nader García, E., and Pérez Ishiwara, D. G. (2013). *Entamoeba histolytica* P-glycoprotein (EhPgp) inhibition, induce trophozoite acidification and enhance programmed cell death. *Exp. Parasitol.* 135, 532–540. doi: 10.1016/j.exppara.2013.08.017

Mickley, L. A., Bates, S. E., Richert, N. D., Currier, S., Tanaka, S., Foss, F., et al. (1989). Modulation of the expression of a multidrug resistance gene (mdr-1/P-glycoprotein) by differentiating agents. *J. Biol. Chem.* 264, 18031–18040.

Moons, A. (2003). Ospdr9, which encodes a PDR-type ABC transporter, is induced by heavy metals, hypoxic stress and redox perturbations in rice roots. *FEBS Lett.* 553, 370–376. doi: 10.1016/S0014-5793(03)01060-3

Murata, S., Chiba, T., and Tanaka, K. (2003). CHIP: a quality-control E3 ligase collaborating with molecular chaperones. *Int. J. Biochem. Cell Biol.* 35, 572–578. doi: 10.1016/S1357-2725(02)00394-1

Nakai, A., Tanabe, M., Kawazoe, Y., Inazawa, J., Morimoto, R. I., and Nagata, K. (1997). HSF4, a new member of the human heat shock factor family which lacks properties of a transcriptional activator. *Mol. Cell. Biol.* 17, 469–481. doi: 10.1128/MCB.17.1.469

Nickel, R., and Tannich, E. (1994). Transfection and transient expression of chloramphenicol acetyltransferase gene in the protozoan parasite *Entamoeba histolytica. Proc. Natl. Acad. Sci. U.S.A.* 91, 7095–7098. doi: 10.1073/pnas.91.15.7095

Nieto, A., Pérez, D. G., Orozco, E., Paz, F., and Gómez, C. (2005). *Entamoeba histolytica* EhPgp5 transcriptional activation depends on putative emetine response elements. *Exp. Parasitol.* 110, 233–237. doi: 10.1016/j.exppara.2005.03.016

Orozco, E., López, C., Gómez, C., Pérez, D. G., Marchat, L., Ba-uelos, C., et al. (2001). Multidrug resistance in the protozoan parasite *Entamoeba histolytica. Parasitol. Int.* 51, 353–359. doi: 10.1016/S1383-5769(02)00041-7

Orozco, E., Suárez, M. E., and Sánchez, T. (1985). Differences in adhesion, phagocytosis and virulence of clones from *Entamoeba histolytica*, strain HM1:IMSS. *Int. J. Parasitol.* 15, 655–660. doi: 10.1016/0020-7519(85)90012-8

Pérez, D. G., Gómez, C., López-Bayghen, E., Tannich, E., and Orozco, E. (1998). Transcriptional analysis of the EhPgp5 promoter of *Entamoeba histolytica* multidrug-resistant mutant. *J. Biol. Chem.* 273, 7285–7292. doi: 10.1074/jbc.273.13.7285

Perisic, O., Xiao, H., and Lis, J. T. (1989). Stable binding of Drosophila heat shock factor to head-to-head and tail-to-tail repeats of a conserved 5 bp recognition unit. *Cell* 59, 797–806. doi: 10.1016/0092-8674(89)90603-X

Rabdiran, S. K., Giorgi, G., Clos, J., and Wu, C. (1991). Molecular cloning and expression of a human heat shock factor, HSF1. *Proc. Natl. Acad. Sci. U.S.A.* 88, 6906–6910. doi: 10.1073/pnas.88.16.6906

Romero-Díaz, M., Gómez, C., López-Reyes, I., Martínez, M. B., Orozco, E., and Rodríguez, M. A. (2007). Structural and functional analysis of the *Entamoeba histolytica* EhrabB gene promoter. *BMC Mol. Biol.* 8:82. doi: 10.1186/1471-2199-8-82

Sandqvist, A., Björk, J. K., Akerfelt, M., Chitikova, Z., Grichine, A., Vourc'h, C., et al. (2009). Heterotrimerization of heat-shock factors 1 and 2 provides a transcriptional switch in response to distinct stimuli. *Mol. Biol. Cell* 20, 1340–1347. doi: 10.1091/mbc.E08-08-0864

Sarge, K. D., Murphy, S. P., and Morimoto, R. I. (1993). Activation of heat shock gene transcription by heat shock factor 1 involves oligomerization, acquisition of DNA-binding activity, and nuclear localization and can occur in the absence of stress. *Mol. Cell. Biol.* 13, 1392–1407. doi: 10.1128/MCB.13.3.1392

Schreiber, E., Matthias, P., Müeller, M. M., and Schaffner, W. (1989). Rapid detection of octamer binding proteins with 'mini-extracts', prepared from a small number of cells. *Nucleic Acid Res.* 17:6419. doi: 10.1093/nar/17.15.6419

Schuetz, T. J., Gallo, G. J., Sheldon, L., Tempst, P., and Kingston, R. E. (1991). Isolation of a cDNA for HSF2: evidence for two heat shock factor genes in human. *Proc. Natl. Acad. Sci. U.S.A.* 88, 6911–6915. doi: 10.1073/pnas.88.16.6911

Shi, Y., Seto, E., Chang, L. S., and Shenk, T. (1991). Transcriptional repression by YY1, a human GLI-Krüppel-related protein, and relief of repression by adenovirus E1A protein. *Cell* 67, 377–388. doi: 10.1016/0092-8674(91)90189-6

Sorger, P. K., and Pelham, H. R. (1988). Yeast heat shock factor is an essential DNA-binding protein that exhibits temperature-dependent phosphorylation. *Cell* 54, 855–864. doi: 10.1016/S0092-8674(88)91219-6

Sorger, P. K., Lewis, M. J., and Pelham, H. R. (1987). Heat shock factor is regulated differently in yeast and HeLa cells. *Nature* 239, 81–84. doi: 10.1038/329081a0

Tchénio, T., Havard, M., Martinez, L. A., and Dautry, F. (2006). Heat Shock-independent induction of multidrug resistance by heat shock factor 1. *Mol. Cell. Biol.* 26, 580–591. doi: 10.1128/MCB.26.2.580-591.2006

World Health Organization (1998). *The World Health Report 1998: Life in the 21st Century: a Vision for All.* Geneva: World Health Organization.

Ximénez, C., González, E., Nieves, M., Maga-a, U., Morán, P., Gudiño-Zayas, M., et al. (2017). Differential expression of pathogenic genes of *Entamoeba histolytica* vs E. dispar in a model of infection using human liver tissue explants. *PLoS ONE* 12:e0181962. doi: 10.1371/journal.pone.0181962

Zou, J., Guo, Y., Guettouche, T., Smith, D. F., and Voellmy, R. (1998). Repression of heat shock transcription factor HSF1 activation by HSP90 (HSP90 complex) that forms a stress-sensitive complex with HSF1. *Cell* 94, 471–480 doi: 10.1016/S0092-8674(00)81588-3

16

Immune Response of Amebiasis and Immune Evasion by *Entamoeba histolytica*

*Kumiko Nakada-Tsukui[1] and Tomoyoshi Nozaki[1,2]**

[1] Department of Parasitology, National Institute of Infectious Diseases, Tokyo, Japan, [2] Graduate School of Life and Environmental Sciences, University of Tsukuba, Tsukuba, Japan

Correspondence:
Tomoyoshi Nozaki
nozaki@nih.go.jp

Entamoeba histolytica is a protozoan parasite and the causative agent of amebiasis. It is estimated approximately 1% of humans are infected with *E. histolytica*, resulting in an estimate of 100,000 deaths annually. Clinical manifestations of amebic infection range widely from asymptomatic to severe symptoms, including dysentery and extra-intestinal abscesses. Like other infectious diseases, it is assumed that only ~20% of infected individuals develop symptoms, and genetic factors of both the parasite and humans as well as the environmental factors, e.g., microbiota, determine outcome of infection. There are multiple essential steps in amebic infection: degradation of and invasion into the mucosal layer, adherence to the intestinal epithelium, invasion into the tissues, and dissemination to other organs. While the mechanisms of invasion and destruction of the host tissues by the amebae during infection have been elucidated at the molecular levels, it remains largely uncharacterized how the parasite survive in the host by evading and attacking host immune system. Recently, the strategies for immune evasion by the parasite have been unraveled, including immunomodulation to suppress IFN-γ production, elimination of immune cells and soluble immune mediators, and metabolic alterations against reactive oxygen and nitrogen species to fend off the attack from immune system. In this review, we summarized the latest knowledge on immune reaction and immune evasion during amebiasis.

Keywords: *Entamoeba histolytica*, cysteine protease, glycosidase, mucin, phagocytosis, oxidative stress, metabolism

INTRODUCTION

Entamoeba histolytica is an enteric protozoan parasite that infects humans, and is the etiological agent of amebiasis. Amebiasis remains a worldwide health problem accounting for up to 100,000 deaths annually (1, 2). Transmission occurs via ingestion of food and water contaminated with amebic cysts (1, 3, 4). In endemic areas, exposure can be extremely high: an annual incidence of 40% was estimated among children in an urban slum in Bangladesh (5). In some parts of Asia and Australia, amebiasis is endemic among men who have sex with men (MSM) and can be transmitted sexually (6–9). Majority of infections with *E. histolytica* remain asymptomatic, while ~20% of the cases develop clinical manifestations, such as dysentery, which is characterized by colonic mucosal invasion and tissue destruction (10). Invasive disease includes dysentery and extra-intestinal amebiasis, most commonly amebic liver abscesses (ALAs), which occur in approximately 1% of symptomatic cases in developing countries and around 17% in Japan (11, 12).

When amebic trophozoites invade the colonic epithelium, they activate immune response in the human host. In order to survive in the host, the repression of host immune systems and the control of the environment of parasitism are crucial. For instance, during extraintestinal dissemination, the amebae must transiently survive in the blood vessels and the spleen, in which a network of immune cells and humoral factors are present, and the amebae are exposed to high concentrations of oxygen (*E. histolytica* are anaerobic or microaerophilic). To persist in such environment, amebae must subvert detection by antibody and complement, and resist oxidative and nitrosative attack. In this review, we summarize our current knowledge on immune response during amebic infection (**Figure 1**) and the parasite's strategies to evade from host immune system (**Figure 2**).

IMMUNE RESPONSE DURING AMEBIC INFECTION

Course of Amebic Infection

Entamoeba histolytica infection is initiated by parasite adherence to the colonic mucin layer. Trophozoites express a galactose

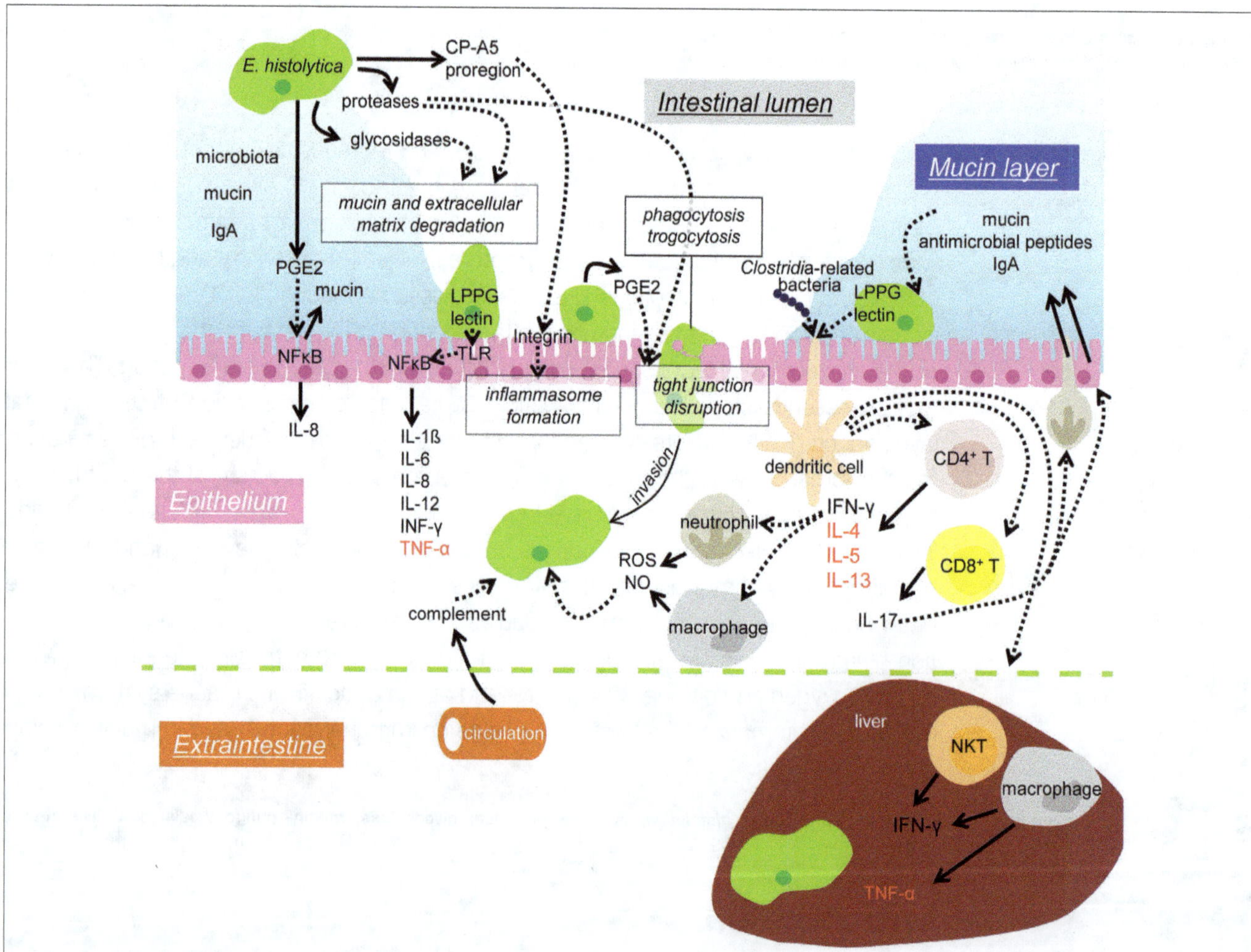

FIGURE 1 | Mechanisms of colonization and invasion by *E. histolytica* trophozoites and host immune responses to suppress and control amebic infection. In the lumen of the large intestine, the IEC layer is covered by the mucus layer (blue), which contains secreted mucin and IgA from the host and commensal microbiota. Proteases and glycosidases secreted from the amebae are involved in the degradation of mucin and extracellular matrix. The pro-domain of EhCP-A5 binds to and activate integrin and enhances the inflammasome formation of leading to pro-inflammatory responses. PGE2 also secreted from the amebae causes mucin hypersecretion and depletion of mucin from the IECs. PGE2 also elicits signaling in a cascade leading to NFκB activation in the IECs and induces IL-8 secretion. The Gal/GalNAc lectin (lectin) and LPPG on the ameba's surface binds to TLR2 and leads to NFκB activation and pro-inflammatory cytokine release for IEC. PGE2 also helps to disrupt tight junction function of the epithelium and enhances the amebic infiltration. Phagocytosis and trogocytosis are also involved in removal of host cells and invasion into the host tissue. Infiltrating trophozoites are attacked by complement from the circulation, ROS and NO from neutrophils and macrophages. The Gal/GalNAc lectin and LPPG activate CD4, CD8 T cells, and NKT cells, and, thus, enhances protective cellular immunity. CD4 T cells produce IFN-γ, IL-4, IL-5, and IL-13, and CD8 T cells produce IL-17. IL-17 induces neutrophil infiltration and enhances secretion of mucin, antimicrobial peptides, and IgA into the colonic lumen. When disseminated to the liver, the amebae are attached and removed by the dense mediated by IFN-γ secreted by NKT cells. TNF-α secreted from hepatic macrophages leads to abscess formation. Solid arrows depict secretion of soluble proteins and dotted arrows indicate interaction or signal transduction. Cytokines mainly beneficial for an elimination of the amebae are shown in black, while those involved in disease manifestations are shown in red.

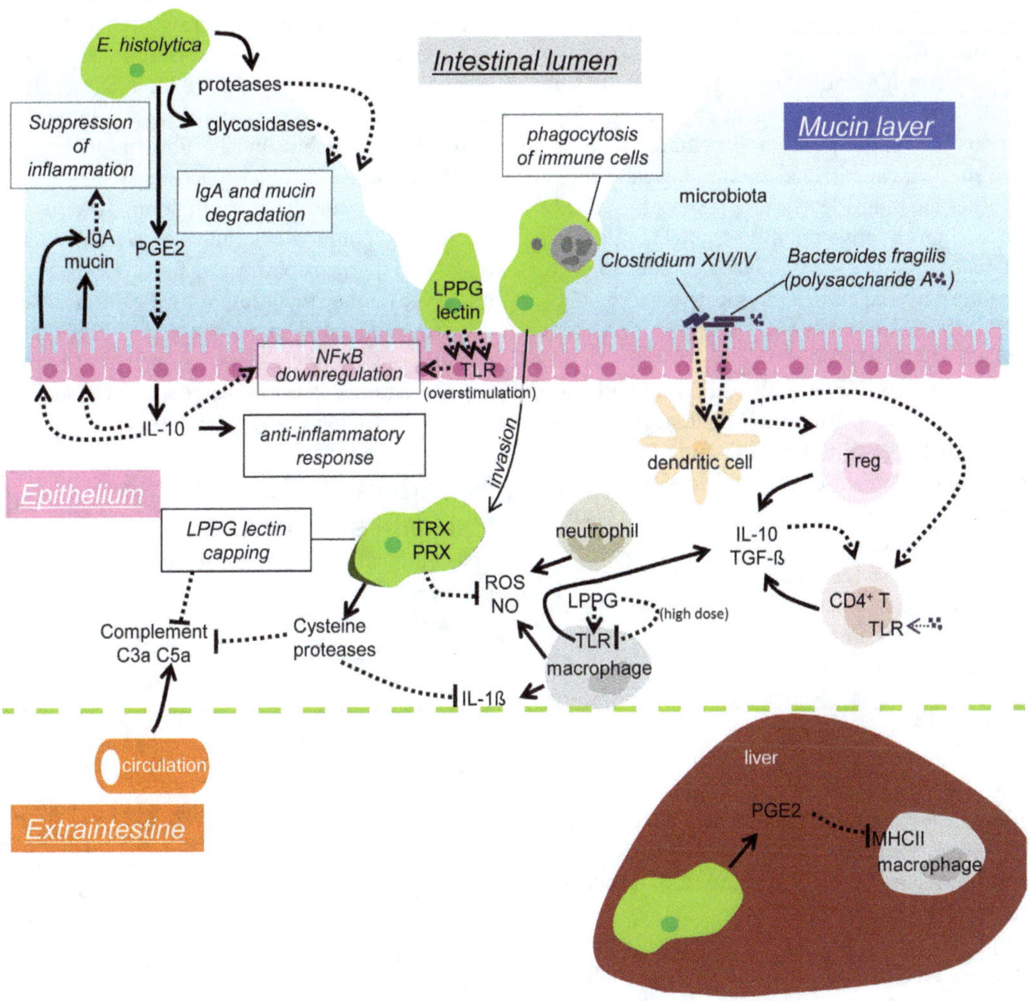

FIGURE 2 | Possible mechanisms of immune evasion during amebiasis. Secreted or surface proteases of the amebae degrade IgA in the mucosal layer. PGE2 from the amebae induces IL-10 secretion from the IECs, and in turn stimulates mucin and IgA secretion, which likely prevents unnecessary inflammation. Overstimulation of TLR causes downregulation of NFκB activation. Removal of infiltrating immune cells by phagocytosis/trogocytosis helps to reduce immune responses. Some commensal microbiota, namely *Clostridium* XIV and IV groups and *Bacteroides fragilis,* induce Treg cells to downregulate immune responses. Polysaccharide A from *B. fragilis* binds to TLR2 on CD4 T cells and induces IL-10 production. The amebae in the tissues and the blood stream evade from complement by surface receptor capping (LPPG, lectin) and degradation of C3a and C5a by cysteine proteases. Cysteine proteases also degrade IL-1β, antioxidative stress defense by the TRX and PRX systems fends off the attack from ROS and NO from activated neutrophils and macrophages. LPPG binds to TLR2 on monocytes and macrophages, which leads to secretion of cytokines, including IL-10 and TGF-β. High doses of LPPG downregulate TLR2 gene expression in monocyte and cause negative feedback of protective immune responses. PGE2 from the amebae and the host causes downregulation of MHC class II expression on macrophages in the liver, which results in anti-inflammation.

and *N*-acetyl-D-galactosamine specific lectin (Gal/GalNAc lectin) on the cell surface and attach to host mucin and colonic epithelial cells (13). The colonized parasites are capable of extensive tissue destruction. Beside the pore-forming proteins, amoebapores (14, 15), hydrolytic enzymes, particularly cysteine proteases (CP), are considered to be essential weapons of the parasite to penetrate the epithelium and destroy components of the host's extracellular matrix (ECM) (16–20). During and after penetration into the submucosal region, amebic trophozoites interact directly and indirectly with host immune and non-immune cells.

Humoral Immunity

While the mucosal layer in the gastrointestinal tract generally serves as a primary physical barrier against intestinal pathogens, the intestinal immune response is the secondary defense to *E. histolytica* infection. Mucosal immunoglobulins (Ig) are the major component of the human intestinal defense mechanism (21). Among them, secretory IgA is one of the most abundant Ig produced by plasma cells and functions by preventing pathogens from adhering and removing the mucosal barrier (21). Haque and colleagues showed that the presence of Gal/GalNAc lectin-specific IgA antibodies in the stool correlated with reduced re-infection rates with *E. histolytica* in a study on susceptible children from Bangladesh (5, 22, 23). This implication was also confirmed with patients who had recovered from ALA. Increases in anti-Gal/GalNAc lectin IgA antibodies in post-ALA patients were associated with clearance of subsequent amebic infections, demonstrating that post-ALA patients developed a higher immune responsiveness and maintained immunological memory (24, 25). On the other hand, IgG levels have either protective or non-protective effects on the susceptibility to amebic infections depending upon major IgG subclasses induced by infection (i.e., IgG1 and IgG2 induced by Th2 and Th1, respectively) (26, 27).

Cell-Mediated Immunity

Cell-mediated immune responses are also important for host defense against *E. histolytica*. During the initial stage of infection, intestinal epithelial cells (IECs) bind to and recognize the carbohydrate recognition domain of the Gal/GalNAc lectin via toll-like receptor (TLR)-2/4, which activates NFκB and leads to the production of inflammatory cytokines, including IL-1β, IL-6, IL-8, IL-12, IFN-γ, and TNF-α (28–30). IECs are the second line of barriers against pathogens after the mucosal layer and the first line of host cells to encounter microbial/parasite antigens, they express an array of pathogen recognition receptors (PRRs), including TLRs (31). IFN-γ is involved in clearance of infection, whereas IL-4 and TNF-α are associated with disease (32–35). In fact, IFN-γ production by peripheral mononuclear cells was shown to be correlated with protection from future *E. histolytica* infection in children (36) and the serum level of IL-4 was high in patients with invasive amebiasis (27, 37). It has been also shown that IFN-γ-producing CD4+ T cells and IL-17-producing CD8+ T cells are involved protection in vaccinated mice (38, 39). IL-17 plays multiple roles in protection against amebic infection, including induction of secretion of mucin and antimicrobial peptides, increase in IgA transport across the intestinal epithelium, and promotion of neutrophil infiltration (40–43).

IFN-γ-activated neutrophils and macrophages have amebicidal activity *in vitro* (44, 45). *In vivo*, neutrophils predominated in amebic lesions where the macrophages were infrequent, suggesting importance of neutrophils for clearance of amebae (46). Production of reactive oxygen species (ROS) and nitric oxide (NO) via NAD(P)H oxidase complex and iNOS, respectively, play critical roles in killing trophozoites (45, 47). In experimental ALA, protection was mediated by IFN-γ from natural killer T cells (NKTs), while TNF-α-producing macrophages increased tissue damage (32, 33). Taken together, both humoral and cell-mediated immune responses play important roles against amebic infection.

MICROBIOTA-MEDIATED MODIFICATIONS OF PARASITE VIRULENCE AND HOST IMMUNE RESPONSE

Microbiota Affects Energy Metabolism and Growth of the Amebae

The adult human intestine has trillions of bacteria composed of more than hundreds of species. Recent studies have suggested that the intestinal bacterial microbiota may influence the outcome of protozoan infections (48, 49). The growth and survival of *E. histolytica* trophozoites depends on nutrients from the host and the microbiota. The bacterial microbiota produces glycosidases that degrade complex polysaccharides into forms available for the absorption by the amebae and the host (50). Microbial glycosidase activity determines the levels of free colonic carbohydrates (the glycobiome). Thus, microbiota potentially influences central energy metabolism of *E. histolytica* trophozoites. Since *E. histolytica* has numerous glycosidases, including amylases, β-hexosaminidases, and lysozymes encoded in its genome (51–55), and can degrade a panel of polysaccharides to yield monocarbohydrates, the activity and regulation of amebic glycosidases also influence available carbohydrate concentrations.

Microbiota Influences the Parasite's Virulence

The commensal bacteria are generally protective against enteric pathogens. However, *E. histolytica* infection requires the presence of enteric bacteria. Germ-free animals were resistant to *E. histolytica* infection, but the introduction of a single bacterial species restored amebic pathogenesis (56, 57).

It has been shown that axenization (i.e., removal of associating bacteria) of xenically cultivated trophozoites decreases virulence, and incubation of axenic trophozoites with live bacteria restored virulence in a contact-dependent manner (58, 59). Incubation of *E. histolytica* trophozoites with the enteropathogenic *Escherichia coli* (EHEC) or *Shigella dysenteriae* increased amebic adherence to and cytotoxicity against MDCK cell monolayer (60). These observations indicate the enteric microbiota influence *E. histolytica* virulence during human infection (also see Perturbation of the Enteric Microbiota by *E. histolytica*).

The microbiota-dependent glycobiome has an emerging role in regulating the virulence of enteric pathogenic bacteria, such as EHEC, *Clostridium difficile,* and *Salmonella enterica* serovar Typhimurium (*S. typhimurium*) (61–63). EHEC has a fucose-responsive regulator of virulence genes, while *C. difficile* growth is promoted with high concentrations of free sialic acid reproduced by sialidase from associating bacteria (*Bacteroides thetaiotaomicron*). Similarly, the *in vivo* virulence of *S. typhimurium* was shown to be dependent on both fucose and sialic acid (63). It has been shown that glucose starvation enhances *E. histolytica* virulence, motility, and lectin expression via URE-3BP (64, 65). This finding suggests that the ameba has an ability to sense glucose (and possibly other monosugars) to modulate its virulence. The amebae and the bacterial microbiota influence each other by providing energy source and degrading available carbohydrates.

Microbiota Affects Host Immune Response

Gut microbiota plays a number of physiological roles involving digestion, metabolism, extraction of nutrients, synthesis of vitamins, prevention against colonization by pathogens, and immunomodulation (66–68). It has been demonstrated that *Bacteroides fragilis* and cluster XIV and IV of *Clostridium* species induce the development of regulatory T (Treg) cells in the colon (69, 70). Treg cells have the ability to suppress inflammatory responses through the production of anti-inflammatory cytokines, including IL-10 and TGF-β, and are considered to be involved in self-tolerance (71, 72). The beneficial effect of *B. fragilis* depends on the expression of polysaccharide A, which is a unique surface polysaccharide that binds to TLR2 on CD4+ T cells (72). Microbiota-mediated immunomodulation is evident in several diseases, e. g., Rheumatoid arthritis, diabetes, obesity, and cancer (73–78). It seems that *E. histolytica* requires the intestinal microbiota for pathogenesis, and, conversely, the parasite also needs to disrupt the homeostasis of the microbiota during infection.

STRATEGIES FOR IMMUNE EVASION OF *E. histolytica*

Disruption of Host Physical Barriers and Soluble Immune Mediators by Hydrolases

Glycosidases

Hydrolases secreted by *E. histolytica* trophozoites are involved in the elimination of immune cells and degradation and/or activation of soluble immune mediators, as well as disruption of the host gut and liver epithelia (29, 55, 79–84). The mucosal layer between the lumen and the epithelia forms a physical barrier. Degradation of carbohydrates in the barrier is crucial for the initiation of colonization by the amebae. Human intestinal mucus is mainly composed of highly glycosylated mucins (85). Among >20 human mucins, MUC2 is the major gel-forming mucin secreted by goblet cells of the small and large intestines (86, 87). When the amebae colonize the colonic epithelia, they binds to secreted mucin oligosaccharides with the Gal/GalNAc lectin and penetrate through the mucosal layer. In this process, the amebae decompose the mucin barrier to finally reach and subsequently attach on IEC (13).

Secreted proteins by *E. histolytica* trophozoites displayed glycosidase activities, including β-*N*-acetyl-D-glucosaminidase, α-D-glucosidase, β-D-galactosidase, β-L-fucosidase, and α-*N*-acetyl-D-galactosaminidase (88). Among these glycosidases, β-*N*-acetyl-D-glucosaminidase showed the highest activity (88, 89). Thus, β-*N*-acetyl-D-glucosaminidase activity likely have a central role in degrading carbohydrates on mucin and exposing its protein backbone (88). It was previously demonstrated that the amount of intracellular and secreted β-*N*-acetyl-D-glucosaminidase activity increased by complement in the serum (90, 91). Huldt et al. also suggested that hexosaminidase activity plays a role in the amebic virulence (90).

Recently, it has been shown that knock down of a β-amylase gene by siRNA caused reduction in the degradation of the mucosal layer and the invasion into the human colon in an *ex vivo* experiment (55). Furthermore, the β-amylase gene was found upregulated after contact with colon tissues (55). Mucin degradation by amebic glycosidases may also affect the central metabolism of the amebae *per se* and also the microbiota equilibrium in the colon since highly glycosylated mucin is a carbon source for the amebae and the colonic microbiota (92, 93).

Cysteine Proteases

The *E. histolytica* genome has ~50 genes encoding CPs (20), which likely reflects robust biological importance of CPs. Of these, however, only four proteins, EhCP-A1, EhCP-A2, EhCP-A5, and EhCP-A7, are highly expressed under culture conditions and altogether account for more than 90% of the proteolytic activity in trophozoite extracts (94). After mucin was digested by amebic glycosidases, the protein backbone of mucin is degraded by robust CPs. Altogether, these mucin-digesting glycosidases and proteases are the ameba's first line strategy to overcome the innate defense of the mucus barrier.

As suggested by various studies, among the four major CPs, EhCP-A5 appears to play a pivotal role in virulence, including immunomodulation (80, 95–102). EhCP-A5 has a capacity to bind integrin via the RGD motif in the pro region, and elicits pro-inflammatory response in Caco-2 cells *in vitro* and the murine colon via NLRP3 inflammasome activation independent of the CP activity (100, 102, 103). CPs are also known to modulate cell-mediated immunity by activating pro-inflammatory cytokines and also modulate humoral immunity (see below).

Involvement of Glycosidases and Proteases for Extraintestinal Propagation

When *E. histolytica* trophozoites propagate extraintestinally, they take a route similar to that of cancer metastasis (104), which requires both glycosidases and proteases for the disintegration of the basement membrane and entry into circulation (105–107). In case of ALA, amebic glycosidases and proteases are also needed to survive in the blood vessels (see Degradation of Immunoglobulins and Complements), and to destroy Kupffer cells, the epithelial cells, ECM, and hepatocytes in the liver. Thibeaux and colleagues have recently demonstrated that EhCP-A5 secreted from the amebae activates host matrix metalloproteases (MMP), a well-known mediator of ECM degradation (84). Recombinant EhCP-A5 restored the invasiveness of the *EhCP-A5* gene-silenced trophozoites, suggesting that proteases from both the ameba and the host contribute to the tissue invasion process. In contrast to proteases, the roles of glycosidases in pathophysiology of amebiasis are not well demonstrated. It is evident in cancer metastasis that the level of serum β-hexosaminidase correlates with the likeliness of liver metastasis in variety of cancers, including colon, breast, stomach, pancreas, small bowel, kidney, testis, melanoma, lymphoma, and myeloma (108). Increased levels of tissue β-hexosaminidase were also reported for breast, kidney, pancreas, thyroid, colon, ovary, brain, salivary gland, stomach, and larynx cancers (109–112). Thus, it is conceivable by analogy that amebic glycosidases are involved in tissue invasion and extraintestinal dissemination.

Degradation of Immunoglobulins and Complements

As described above, the major component responsible for the intestinal immune response against amebic infection is secreted

Igs. It was demonstrated that anti-Gal/GalNAc lectin IgA reduces trophozoite colonization in the colon (5, 23, 25, 113–117). Intriguingly, *E. histolytica* surface-associated CP [most likely EhCP-A5, (118)] cleaves human IgA (16, 119). Amebic CPs are capable of cleaving both isotypes, i.e., IgA1 and IgA2 (119, 120). Furthermore, amebic CPs can also inactivate circulating IgG and, thus, believed to be involved in the survival during tissue invasion and extraintestinal propagation (18). Degradation of IgG in the blood could prevent activation of the classical pathway of the complement system and immune cells that harbor Fc receptors (19).

When the trophozoites are exposed to the intravascular immune system, complements are the major component that mediates trophozoite destruction. *E. histolytica* trophozoites evade from a complement attack by cleaving and inactivating anaphylatoxins C5a and C3a with CPs (79). C5a and C3a are potent activators of inflammation and enhance the release of histamine from mast cells, lysosomal enzymes from leukocytes, and pro-inflammatory cytokines, including IL-6 and TNF-α, from macrophages (121–123). C5a and C3a also increase vascular permeability and attract immune cells (122, 123). Reduction of these anaphylatoxins detracts from immune detection of the amebae in the blood and reduces inflammation in amebic lesions. It also partially explains the lack of severe inflammation in advanced colitis and ALA region.

Degradation of Cytokines

Cysteine proteases are also known to modulate cell-mediated immunity by activating pro-inflammatory cytokine IL-1β and inactivation of pro- and mature IL-18 (82, 124). It is not concluded, however, if these changes are protective against or deleterious for amebic infection.

Cell Surface Decorations to Evade Host Immunity

Glycosylphosphatidylinositol-Anchored Proteins

Entamoeba histolytica is also capable of evading from complement attach by decorating their surface with glycosylphosphatidylinositol (GPI)-anchored proteins. GPI is a glycolipid required for anchoring many proteins and glycoconjugates to the cell surface in most of eukaryotes (125–127). *E. histolytica* trophozoites expose on their cell surface a complex GPI-anchored glycoconjugate, designated lipopeptidophosphoglycan (LPPG) (128, 129). LPPG on the cell surface is a component of glycocalyx that is composed of oligosaccharides of glycoproteins and glycolipids and afford trophozoites protection by creating an impervious layer to complement (130, 131). It was demonstrated that complement-susceptible *Entamoeba dispar* trophozoites possess a much thinner structure of LPPG-containing glycocalyx, which is consistent with the premise that LPPG is important for the evasion from complement (130). It is also known that antibody against human CD59, a cell surface protein that prevents auto-lysis by inhibiting the formation of the membrane attack complex (MAC) antibody cross-reacts with Gal/GalNAc lectin and a 21 kDa surface protein (132, 133). Later, it was shown that the Gal/GalNAc lectin contains a CD59-like region on the cell surfaces that prevents MAC formation (132). These data suggest that the Gal/GalNAc lectin is a cross-reactive CD59 homolog of the ameba and have a similar function as CD59. In agreement with these results, global inhibition of GPI-anchor formation leaves *E. histolytica* trophozoites susceptible to complement-mediated lysis (131). However, functionality of 21 kDa protein as an inhibitor of MAC formation and its molecular identity has yet to be elucidated.

Surface Receptor Capping

Surface receptor capping is another strategy to hide from the immune system by disposing of the surface molecules that have been recognized by Igs or complements (134, 135). During cell movement, surface-bound immune complexes are translocated toward the uroid, where capped ligands accumulate (136). This polar re-distribution can be induced by concanavalin A (Con A) or anti-amebic polyclonal antibodies (137). It has been reported that serine protease, *E. histolytica* rhomboid protease (ROM1), is involved in the translocation of the complex to the base of the caps and subsequent release of the materials in the cap (135, 138). It is of note that ROM1 also cleaves the transmembrane domain of the heavy subunit of the Gal/GalNAc lectin (138). As the lectin heavy subunit is highly immunogenic, its release from the plasma membrane by ROM1 may interfere with host immune response directed to amebae.

Killing and Phago/Togocytosis of Immune Cells

Contact-Dependent Cell Killing

Immobilization and killing of immune cells also serves as an ameba's strategy for evasion from immune surveillance. Amebic trophozoites are able to kill a variety of cells, including neutrophils, T lymphocytes, macrophages, and a variety of tissue culture lines (116, 139–141). Adherence of the ameba triggers multiple intracellular events leading to cytotoxic effects to the mammalian cells. Such events include increased intracellular Ca^{2+}, production of ROS, loss of membrane integrity, DNA fragmentation, phosphatidylserine exposure on the cell surface, and caspase-3 activation (116, 117, 139–144). It was reported that after host cell killing, *E. histolytica* preferentially ingest the dead cells (117, 140, 143). This observation is consistent with the theory that clearance of dead cells and debris by phagocytosis helps to minimize pro-inflammatory responses (145, 146). A phagocytosis-defective line of *E. histolytica* apparently showed decreased virulence *in vitro* and *in vivo*, suggesting a potential causal link between phagocytosis and virulence (147, 148).

Huston and colleagues demonstrated that *E. histolytica* preferentially ingests apoptotic Jurkat cells via recognition of phosphatidylserine and collectins (140, 149). Amebic calreticulin was found to be the surface receptor for host C1q, and required for phagocytosis of apoptotic cells, but it did not directly mediate cell killing (150). A few recent studies have started to unveil the detailed molecular mechanisms involved in the ameba phagocytosis (151, 152). However, the molecular events that take place in host immune cells in particular to suppress (or augment) immune response, together with a missing link between the surface receptor to the internalization machinery, remains totally unknown.

Trogocytosis

Ralston and colleagues have recently reported *E. histolytica* trophozoites ingested pieces of intact living cells via trogocytosis (*"trogo"* = nibbling) (153). When trophozoites were incubated with a combination of live and pre-killed host cells (Jurkat T cells), the live cells were ingested by trogocytosis, while the pre-killed host cells were ingested as a whole by canonical phagocytosis. Trogocytosis is an active process that resembles phagocytosis in some ways, i.e., it requires physiological temperature, actin rearrangements, Gal/GalNAc lectin, C2 domain-containing protein kinase, and phosphatidylinositol 3-phosphate kinase signaling, and it is accompanied with a rapid rise in intracellular Ca^{2+} concentrations. Trogocytosed host cells finally were killed. Trogocytosis of murine IEC was also evident in the *in vivo* animal model, suggesting that both trogocytosis of live host cells and phagocytosis of dead cells are important for pathogenesis and sustained parasitism of *E. histolytica*. Since amebic contact can potentially results in multiple outcomes: apoptosis and necrosis, followed by phagocytosis, or trogocytosis, it remains to be elucidated what factors and conditions differentiate these distinct manners of killing and ingestion of target host cells.

IFN-γ

Entamoeba histolytica regulates IFN-γ for survival in the host. In CBA mice, which are susceptible to *E. histolytica* cecal infection, the amebic infection led to upregulation of Th2 (IL-4, IL-5, and IL-13) and Th17 (IL-17) cytokine responses, while Th1 cytokines, IL-12p35 and IFN-γ, were suppressed (154). This indicates that suppression of INF-γ causes susceptibility of amebiasis. From cohort studies in Bangladesh, susceptible children with malnutrition showed lower IFN-γ levels (36, 155). Analysis of asymptomatic carriers of *E. histolytica* showed that carriers had higher levels of IFN-γ, while patients with invasive amebiasis displayed higher levels of IL-4 (35). The significance of IFN-γ in susceptibility is also implicated for ALA. It is known that more than 80% of all ALA cases occur in adult males (156–158), and the male predominance is attributable to testosterone (159). Lotter and colleagues showed that testosterone inhibits IFN-γ secretion from invariant natural killer T (iNKT) cells stimulated by LPPG, a physiological ligand for CD1d (159). iNKT cells are a subset of NKT cells that recognize lipid antigens in the context of CD1d and produce IFN-γ and IL-4. *E. histolytica* LPPG is presented on CD1d to invariant TCR and activates iNKT cells in combination with TLR signaling. αGalCer, a CD1d agonist, stimulates production of both IFN-γ and IL-4, whereas LPPG induces IFN-γ but not IL-4 production (33). These data suggest that iNKT cells provide a link between innate and adaptive immunity due to their capacity to produce large amounts of IFN-γ and IL-4 that can bias the immune response into either a Th1 or Th2 direction. Production of IFN-γ helps clearance of *E. histolytica* infection and controls abscess formation, whereas an adequate level of IFN-γ reduces the trophozoite number and pro-inflammatory response at a low level, and may balance for trophozoites to survive.

IL-10

It is known that anti-inflammatory cytokine, IL-10, plays a critical role to maintain the mucosal barrier. IL-10-deficient mice have compromised and highly permeable mucosal barriers and develop spontaneous intestinal inflammation in response to normal microflora (160). A murine amebic colitis model demonstrated that IL-10 from hematopoietic cells (CD4+ T cells) acting upon the non-hematopoietic compartment (IEC) is required for innate resistance to parasite invasion (161). Furthermore, it has been shown that IL-10 enhances MUC2 production, suppresses activation of antigen-presenting cells, induces B cell class-switching to IgA, has anti-apoptotic effects on IECs, reduces pro-inflammatory NFκB signaling in IECs, and promotes induction of CD4+ Treg cells (162–165). Interestingly, in asymptomatic carriers, no elevation of IL-10 level was observed. On the other hand, the IL-10 level was increased in dysenteric and ALA patients (27, 37). These studies indicate that invasion of the colon and liver by *E. histolytica* elicits an anti-inflammatory immune response and may successfully suppress immune reaction to the amebae. Altogether, the ameba needs to balance IL-10 and inflammatory cytokine levels to establish infection. It was shown that peritoneal monocytes and macrophages exposed to LPPG secreted TNF-α, IL-6, IL-8, IL-12, and IL-10 via TLR2 (166). It has been also shown that high doses of LPPG down-regulated TLR2 gene expression (166, 167). Thus, LPPG-driven signaling may activate a negative feedback loop that attenuates inflammatory responses. The mechanisms of the suppression of IL-10 production by the ameba remain to be elucidated (see below).

Suppression of NFκB in IECs

Entamoeba histolytica trophozoites secrete materials that induce a protective response in human IECs (168, 169), the first line of host cells to encounter microbial antigens, via PRRs, including TLRs. Upon binding to their ligand, PRRs trigger activation of a transcription factor NFκB. Gut homeostasis requires continuous activation of NFκB by TLR signaling in response to intestinal bacteria (170), commensal microbes can also disrupt NFκB signaling to attenuate pro-inflammatory IEC responses (171). It has been shown that secreted components from *E. histolytica* trophozoites induce a protective response in human IECs that primed by macrophage secretions through suppression of NFκB via heat shock protein response and increase resistance of IECs to apoptosis (168). Thus, it appears that *E. histolytica* elicits a stress response to IECs and promotes a hyporesponsive state toward trophozoites. The amebic factors that induce NFκB suppression have not yet determined. The factors that activate TLR2, i.e., LPPG and Gal/GalNAc lectin, are candidates involved in this pathway (172).

Prostaglandin PGE2

Entamoeba histolytica trophozoites produce and secrete prostaglandin 2 (PGE2), which have contact-independent effects on tight junction integrity and ion absorption. Secreted amebic PGE2 binds to prostaglandin E receptor 4 (EP4) on IECs, disrupts tight junctions, and increases luminal Cl^- secretion (173, 174). PGE2 secreted from the amebae elicits inflammatory response in IECs by increasing IL-8 production by IECs (173). PGE2 is a potent mucin secretagogue (175) that can overcome luminal barrier function by causing hypersecretion and, thus, depletion of the protective mucus barrier (176). On the contrary, it has been also reported that during invasive amebiasis, local PGE2 has anti-inflammatory effect. In animal model of chronic ALA, hepatic granuloma macrophages do not respond to IFN-γ and LPS and do not produce inflammatory cytokines, show decrease in MHC class II expression, and are unable to kill trophozoites (47, 177, 178). This suppression is local during chronic ALA and is directly caused by the parasite (47, 177). A culture supernatant and an unknown soluble protein component of *E. histolytica* trophozoites decrease class II major histocompatibility complex (MHC II) immune-associated (Ia) antigen expression through a PGE2-dependent manner (178). Inhibition of macrophage PGE2 synthesis can partially recover MHC II Ia expression and TNF-α expression (177, 178). However, inhibition of PGE2 synthesis does not recover iNOS expression or amebicidal activity in the deactivated macrophage (177). A continuous supply of parasite-derived PGE2 likely prevents iNOS expression and full recovery of MHC II and TNF-α, possibly through a concentration-dependent effect of PGE2. In short, ameba-secreted PGE2 represses inflammation in ALA, which is beneficial for survival, whereas it likely enhances destruction of the colon.

PERTURBATION OF THE ENTERIC MICROBIOTA BY *E. histolytica*

It has been reported that *E. histolytica* infection alters the microbiota composition. *E. histolytica*-induced dysbiosis was characterized by fewer *Bacteroides*, *Clostridia*, *Lactobacillus*, *Campylobacter*, and *Eubacterium* species, and increased *Bifidobacterium* species (179). *In vitro* experiments have shown that *E. histolytica* preferentially ingest some bacterial species (59, 180). It is known that amoebapores, a family of the major pore-forming peptides, have differential activity against bacteria and eukaryotes (15). Furthermore, *E. histolytica* infection induces production of colonic antimicrobial peptides, while the trophozoites degrade them (181). A recent study has shown that dendritic cells from the mouse intestine where *Clostridia*-related bacteria colonized provide IL-17A-dependent protection against amebic colitis (182). Detailed molecular events remain to be elucidated, however, by examining how alternations of the microbiota modulate host immune responses against amebic intestinal infection. Altogether, microbiota can be modulated by amebic infection, and in turn concentrations of carbohydrates (and other compounds) that affect growth and virulence of the amebae can strongly influence outcome of infection. It remains to be elucidated whether and how the amebae modulate the intestinal microbiota for their survival and parasitism.

STRATEGY FOR OXIDATIVE STRESS MANAGEMENT AND METABOLIC CONTROL

Lack of Respiration and Antioxidative Stress Management in *E. histolytica*

Entamoeba histolytica trophozoites are microaerophilic and consume oxygen. They tolerate low levels of oxygen tension. *E. histolytica* lacks a conventional respiratory electron transport chain that terminates in the reduction of O_2 to H_2O. However, it does respire and tolerates up to 5% oxygen in the gas phase (183–185). The parasite lacks most of the components of antioxidant defense mechanisms that are widely present in other prokaryotic and eukaryotic organisms, such as catalase, peroxidase, glutathione, and the glutathione-recycling enzymes glutathione peroxidase and glutathione reductase (184, 185). However, during tissue invasion, trophozoites must fend off reactive oxygen and nitrogen species produced by activated immune cells through the respiratory burst. Thus, trophozoites must use antioxidative stress defense to survive immune surveillance.

Anti-Oxidative Stress Response Contributes to Immune Evasion in *E. histolytica*

Entamoeba histolytica trophozoites contain high levels of cysteine, instead of glutathione, as the major thiol in the cell. They possess several enzymes to defend from oxidative stress, such as peroxiredoxin (Prx), superoxide dismutase, flavoprotein A, ferredoxin, thioredoxin (Trx), and Trx reductase (186, 187). The Trx/Trx reductase system is crucial for buffering sensitive proteins under oxidative stress (188). The amebicidal drugs, metronidazole and auranofin, are known to disrupt Trx (189, 190). Interestingly, the oxidative stress increases *E. histolytica* virulence. It has been shown that oxidative stress causes upregulation of a stress-induced adhesion factor and a phospholipid transporting P-type ATPase/flippase (187). Both genes are involved in adhesion and phagocytosis. Oxidative stress also alters metabolic flux, including glycerol and chitin biosynthesis, potentially triggering encystation (191). Furthermore, it has been shown that *E. histolytica* (HM-1:IMSS) responds more strongly to oxidative stress than *E. dispar* and *E. histolytica* non-virulent Rahman strain, and surface localization of Prx in HM-1:IMSS is associated with virulence (186). Altogether, antioxidative defense mechanisms in *E. histolytica* are associated with pathogenesis. For more details on the anti-oxidative management in *E. histolytica,* a recent review should be consulted (192).

CONCLUSION

Our understanding of molecular mechanisms of the parasite's pathogenesis, such as adherence to host cells, induction of apoptosis, degradation of mucin and ECM, tissue invasion, and phago/trogocytosis of host cells, has greatly advanced in recent years. So have mechanisms of immune evasion, such as induction of IL-10 and suppression of INF-γ, degradation of Igs, complement, and pro-inflammatory cytokines. In addition, defense against ROS and NO and evasion from antibody and complement-dependent killing also plays important roles in survival in the host. Furthermore, mutual signaling among the three domains in the complex network of the parasite, the human, and the microbiota with polymorphic genetic backgrounds affect outcome of amebic infection. Further research is needed to elucidate the molecular basis of the complex interaction in the intestinal ecosystem.

AUTHOR CONTRIBUTIONS

KN-T and TN have made substantial, direct, and intellectual contribution to the work and approved it for publication.

ACKNOWLEDGMENTS

This work was supported by a Grant-in-Aid for Scientific Research from the Ministry of Education, Culture, Sports, Science, and Technology (MEXT) of Japan (23117001, 23117005, 26293093, 26111524), a grant for research on emerging and re-emerging infectious diseases from Japan Agency for Medical Research and Development (AMED), a grant for Science and Technology Research Partnership for Sustainable Development (SATREPS) from AMED and Japan International Cooperation Agency (JICA) to TN.

REFERENCES

Ackers J, Clark CG, Diamond LS, Duchêne M, Cantellano ME, Jackson TF, et al. WHO/PAHO/UNESCO report. A consultation with experts on amoebiasis. Mexico City, Mexico 28-29 January, 1997. *Epidemiol Bull* (1997) **18**:13–4.

Lozano R, Naghavi M, Foreman K, Lim S, Shibuya K, Aboyans V, et al. Global and regional mortality from 235 causes of death for 20 age groups in 1990 and 2010: a systematic analysis for the global burden of disease study 2010. *Lancet* (2012) **380**:2095–128. doi:10.1016/S0140-6736(12)61728-0

Ali IK, Clark CG, Petri WA Jr. Molecular epidemiology of amebiasis. *Infect Genet Evol* (2008) **8**:698–707. doi:10.1016/j.meegid.2008.05.004

Ximénez C, Morán P, Rojas L, Valadez A, Gómez A. Reassessment of the epidemiology of amebiasis: state of the art. *Infect Genet Evol* (2009) **9**:1023–32. doi:10.1016/j.meegid.2009.06.008

Haque R, Ali IM, Sack RB, Farr BM, Ramakrishnan G, Petri WA Jr. Amebiasis and mucosal IgA antibody against the *Entamoeba histolytica* adherence lectin in Bangladeshi children. *J Infect Dis* (2001) **183**:1787–93. doi:10.1086/320740

Hung CC, Chang SY, Ji DD. *Entamoeba histolytica* infection in men who have sex with men. *Lancet Infect Dis* (2012) **12**:729–36. doi:10.1016/ S1473-3099(12)70147-0

Watanabe K, Gatanaga H, Escueta-de Cadiz A, Tanuma J, Nozaki T, Oka S. Amebiasis in HIV-1-infected Japanese men: clinical features and response to therapy. *PLoS Negl Trop Dis* (2011) **5**:e1318. doi:10.1371/journal.pntd.0001318

Haghighi A, Kobayashi S, Takeuchi T, Masuda G, Nozaki T. Remarkable genetic polymorphism among *Entamoeba histolytica* isolates from a limited geographic area. *J Clin Microbiol* (2002) **40**:4081–90. doi:10.1128/JCM.40.11.4081-4090.2002

Haghighi A, Kobayashi S, Takeuchi T, Thammapalerd N, Nozaki T. Geographic diversity among genotypes of *Entamoeba histolytica* field isolates. *J Clin Microbiol* (2003) **41**:3748–56. doi:10.1128/JCM.41.8.3748-3756.2003

Haque R, Mondal D, Karim A, Molla IH, Rahim A, Faruque AS, et al. Prospective case-control study of the association between common enteric protozoal parasites and diarrhea in Bangladesh. *Clin Infect Dis* (2009) **48**:1191–7. doi:10.1086/597580

Haque R, Huston CD, Hughes M, Houpt E, Petri WA Jr. Amebiasis. *N Engl J Med* (2003) **348**:1565–73. doi:10.1056/NEJMra022710

Infectious Disease Surveillance Center, National Institute of Infectious Diseases of Japan. *HIV/AIDS in Japan in the Year of 2013. IASR*. Vol. **35**. (2014). p. 223–4. Available from: http://www.nih.go.jp/niid/ja/id/969-dis- ease-based/a/entamoeba-histolytica/idsc/iasr-in/4978-kj4151.html

Petri WA Jr, Haque R, Mann BJ. The bittersweet interface of parasite and host: lectin-carbohydrate interactions during human invasion by the parasite *Entamoeba histolytica. Annu Rev Microbiol* (2002) **56**:39–64. doi:10.1146/annurev.micro.56.012302.160959

Leippe M. Amoebapores. *Parasitol Today* (1997) **13**:178–83. doi:10.1016/S0169-4758(97)01038-7

Bruhn H, Riekens B, Berninghausen O, Leippe M. Amoebapores and NK-lysin, members of a class of structurally distinct antimicrobial and cytolytic peptides from protozoa and mammals: a comparative functional analysis. *Biochem J* (2003) **375**:737–44. doi:10.1042/BJ20030250

Kelsall BL, Ravdin JI. Degradation of human IgA by *Entamoeba histolytica. J Infect Dis* (1993) **168**:1319–22. doi:10.1093/infdis/168.5.1319

Schulte W, Scholze H. Action of the major protease from *Entamoeba histolytica* on proteins of the extracellular matrix. *J Protozool* (1989) **36**:538–43. doi:10.1111/j.1550-7408.1989.tb01092.x

Tran VQ, Herdman S, Torian BE, Reed SL. The neutral cysteine proteinase of *Entamoeba histolytica* degrades IgG and prevents its binding. *J Infect Dis* (1998) **177**:508–11. doi:10.1086/517388

Que X, Reed SL. Cysteine proteinases and the pathogenesis of amebiasis. *Clin Microbiol Rev* (2000) **13**:196–206. doi:10.1128/CMR.13.2.196-206.2000

Tillack M, Biller L, Irmer H, Freitas M, Gomes MA, Tannich E, et al. The *Entamoeba histolytica* genome: primary structure and expression of proteolytic enzymes. *BMC Genomics* (2007) **8**:170. doi:10.1186/1471-2164-8-170

Lamm ME. Current concepts in mucosal immunity. IV. How epithelial transport of IgA antibodies relates to host defense. *Am J Physiol* (1998) **274**:G614–7.

Haque R, Duggal P, Ali IM, Hossain MB, Mondal D, Sack RB, et al. Innate and acquired resistance to amebiasis in bangladeshi children. *J Infect Dis* (2002) **186**:547–52. doi:10.1086/341566

Haque R, Mondal D, Duggal P, Kabir M, Roy S, Farr BM, et al. *Entamoeba histolytica* infection in children and protection from subsequent amebiasis. *Infect Immun* (2006) **74**:904–9. doi:10.1128/IAI.74.2.904-909.2006

Abd-Alla MD, Jackson TF, Rogers T, Reddy S, Ravdin JI. Mucosal immunity to asymptomatic *Entamoeba histolytica* and *Entamoeba dispar* infection is associated with a peak intestinal antilectin immunoglobulin A antibody response. *Infect Immun* (2006) **74**:3897–903. doi:10.1128/ IAI.02018-05

Ravdin JI, Abd-Alla MD, Welles SL, Reddy S, Jackson TF. Intestinal anti- lectin immunoglobulin A antibody response and immunity to *Entamoeba dispar* infection following cure of amebic liver abscess. *Infect Immun* (2003) **71**:6899–905. doi:10.1128/IAI.71.12.6899-6905.2003

Kaur U, Sharma AK, Sharma M, Vohra H. Distribution of *Entamoeba histolytica* Gal/GalNAc lectin-specific antibody response in an endemic area. *Scand J Immunol* (2004) **60**:524–8. doi:10.1111/j.0300-9475.2004.01512.x

Bernin H, Marggraff C, Jacobs T, Brattig N, Le VA, Blessmann J, et al. Immune markers characteristic for asymptomatically infected and diseased *Entamoeba histolytica* individuals and their relation to sex. *BMC Infect Dis* (2014) **14**:621. doi:10.1186/s12879-014-0621-1

Gay NJ, Gangloff M. Structure and function of toll receptors and their ligands. *Annu Rev Biochem* (2007) **76**:141–65. doi:10.1146/annurev.biochem.76.060305.151318

Bansal D, Ave P, Kerneis S, Frileux P, Boché O, Baglin AC, et al. An ex-vivo human intestinal model to study *Entamoeba histolytica* pathogenesis. *PLoS Negl Trop Dis* (2009) **3**:e551. doi:10.1371/journal.pntd.0000551

Galván-Moroyoqui JM, Del CarmenDomínguez-Robles M, Meza I. Pathogenic bacteria prime the induction of toll-like receptor signalling in human colonic cells by the Gal/GalNAc lectin carbohydrate recognition domain of *Entamoeba histolytica. Int J Parasitol* (2011) **41**:1101–12. doi:10.1016/j.ijpara.2011.06.003

Kumar H, Kawai T, Akira S. Pathogen recognition by the innate immune system. *Int Rev Immunol* (2011) **30**:16–34. doi:10.3109/08830185.2010.529976

Helk E, Bernin H, Ernst T, Ittrich H, Jacobs T, Heeren J, et al. TNFα-mediated liver destruction by Kupffer cells and Ly6Chi monocytes during *Entamoeba histolytica* infection. *PLoS Pathog* (2013) **9**:e1003096. doi:10.1371/journal.ppat.1003096

Lotter H, González-Roldán N, Lindner B, Winau F, Isibasi A, Moreno-Lafont M, et al. Natural killer T cells activated by a lipopeptido- phosphoglycan from *Entamoeba histolytica* are critically important to control amebic liver abscess. *PLoS Pathog* (2009) **5**(5):e1000434. doi:10.1371/journal. ppat.1000434

Peterson KM, Shu J, Duggal P, Haque R, Mondal D, Petri WA Jr. Association between TNF-α and *Entamoeba histolytica* diarrhea. *Am J Trop Med Hyg* (2010) **82**:620–5. doi:10.4269/ajtmh.2010.09-0493

Sánchez-Guillén Mdel C, Pérez-Fuentes R, Salgado-Rosas H, Ruiz-Argüelles A, Ackers J, Shire A, et al. Differentiation of *Entamoeba histolytica/Entamoeba dispar* by PCR and their correlation with humoral and cellular immunity in individuals with clinical variants of amoebiasis. *Am J Trop Med Hyg* (2002) **66**:731–7.

Haque R, Mondal D, Shu J, Roy S, Kabir M, Davis AN, et al. Correlation of interferon-γ production by peripheral blood mononuclear cells with childhood malnutrition and susceptibility to amebiasis. *Am J Trop Med Hyg* (2007) **76**:340–4.

Bansal D, Sehgal R, Chawla Y, Malla N, Mahajan RC. Cytokine mRNA expressions in symptomatic vs. asymptomatic amoebiasis patients. *Parasite Immunol* (2005) **27**:37–43. doi:10.1111/j.1365-3024.2005.00739.x

Guo X, Barrosom L, Becker SM, Lyerly DM, Vedvick TS, Reed SG, et al. Protection against intestinal amebiasis by a recombinant vaccine is transferable by T cells and mediated by gamma interferon. *Infect Immun* (2009) **77**:3909–18. doi:10.1128/IAI.00487-09

Guo X, Barroso L, Lyerly DM, Petri WA Jr, Houpt ER. CD4+ and CD8+ T cell- and IL-17-mediated protection against *Entamoeba histolytica* induced by a recombinant vaccine. *Vaccine* (2011) **29**:772–7. doi:10.1016/j. vaccine.2010.11.013

Liang SC, Tan XY, Luxenberg DP, Karim R, Dunussi-Joannopoulos K, Collins M, et al. Interleukin (IL)-22 and IL-17 are coexpressed by Th17 cells and cooperatively enhance expression of antimicrobial peptides. *J Exp Med* (2006) **203**(10):2271–9. doi:10.1084/jem.20061308

Nishida A, Lau CW, Zhang M, Andoh A, Shi HN, Mizoguchi E, et al. The membrane-bound mucin Muc1 regulates T helper 17-cell responses and colitis in mice. *Gastroenterology* (2012) **142**:865–74.e2. doi:10.1053/j. gastro.2011.12.036

Cao AT, Yao S, Gong B, Elson CO, Cong Y. Th17 cells upregulate polymeric Ig receptor and intestinal IgA and contribute to intestinal homeostasis. *J Immunol* (2012) **189**:4666–73. doi:10.4049/jimmunol.1200955

Blaschitz C, Raffatellu M. Th17 cytokines and the gut mucosal barrier. *J Clin Immunol* (2010) **30**:196–203. doi:10.1007/s10875-010-9368-7

Ghadirian E, Denis M. In vivo activation of macrophages by IFN-γ to kill *Entamoeba histolytica* trophozoites in vitro. *Parasite Immunol* (1992) **14**:397–404. doi:10.1111/j.1365-3024.1992.tb00014.x

Lin JY, Chadee K. Macrophage cytotoxicity against *Entamoeba histolytica* trophozoites is mediated by nitric oxide from L-arginine. *J Immunol* (1992) **148**:3999–4005.

Espinosa-Cantellano M, Martínez-Palomo A. Pathogenesis of intestinal amebiasis: from molecules to disease. *Clin Microbiol Rev* (2000) **13**:318–31. doi:10.1128/CMR.13.2.318-331.2000

Denis M, Chadee K. Cytokine activation of murine macrophages for in vitro killing of *Entamoeba histolytica* trophozoites. *Infect Immun* (1989) **57**:1750–6.

Berrilli F, Di Cave D, Cavallero S, D'Amelio S. Interactions between parasites and microbial communities in the human gut. *Front Cell Infect Microbiol* (2012) **2**:141. doi:10.3389/fcimb.2012.00141

Gilchrist CA, Petri SE, Schneider BN, Reichman DJ, Jiang N, Begum S, et al. Role of the gut microbiota of children in diarrhea due to the protozoan parasite *Entamoeba histolytica*. *J Infect Dis* (2015). doi:10.1093/infdis/jiv772

Ouwerkerk JP, de Vos WM, Belzer C. Glycobiome: bacteria and mucus at the epithelial interface. *Best Pract Res Clin Gastroenterol* (2013) **27**:25–38. doi:10.1016/j.bpg.2013.03.001

Nakada-Tsukui K, Tsuboi K, Furukawa A, Yamada Y, Nozaki T. A novel class of cysteine protease receptors that mediate lysosomal transport. *Cell Microbiol* (2012) **14**:1299–317. doi:10.1111/j.1462-5822.2012.01800.x

Furukawa A, Nakada-Tsukui K, Nozaki T. Novel transmembrane receptor involved in phagosome transport of lysozymes and β-hexosaminidase in the enteric protozoan *Entamoeba histolytica*. *PLoS Pathog* (2012) **8**:e1002539. doi:10.1371/journal.ppat.1002539

Furukawa A, Nakada-Tsukui K, Nozaki T. Cysteine protease-binding protein family 6 mediates the trafficking of amylases to phagosomes in the enteric protozoan *Entamoeba histolytica*. *Infect Immun* (2013) **81**:1820–9. doi:10.1128/IAI.00915-12

Marumo K, Nakada-Tsukui K, Tomii K, Nozaki T. Ligand heterogeneity of the cysteine protease binding protein family in the parasitic protist *Entamoeba histolytica*. *Int J Parasitol* (2014) **44**:625–35. doi:10.1016/j.ijpara. 2014.04.008

Thibeaux R, Weber C, Hon CC, Dillies MA, Avé P, Coppée JY, et al. Identification of the virulence landscape essential for *Entamoeba histolytica* invasion of the human colon. *PLoS Pathog* (2013) **9**:e1003824. doi:10.1371/ journal. ppat.1003824

Phillips BP, Wolfe PA, Rees CW, Gordon HA, Wright WH, Reyniers JA. Studies on the amebabacteria relationship in amebiasis: comparative results of the intracecal inoculation of germfree, monocontaminated, and conven- tional guinea pigswith *Entamoeba histolytica*. *Am J Trop Med Hyg* (1955) **4**:675–92.

Phillips BP, Gorstein F. Effects of different species of bacteria on the pathol- ogy of enteric amebiasis in monocontaminated guinea pigs. *Am J Trop Med Hyg* (1966) **15**:863–8.

Wittner M, Rosenbaum RM. Role of bacteria in modifying virulence of *Entamoeba histolytica*: studies of amebae from axenic cultures. *Am J Trop Med Hyg* (1970) **19**:755–61.

Mirelman D, Feingold C, Wexler A, Bracha R. Interactions between *Entamoeba histolytica*, bacteria and intestinal cells. *Ciba Found Symp* (1983) **99**:2–30.

Galván-Moroyoqui JM, Del Carmen Domínguez-Robles M, Franco E, Meza I. The interplay between *Entamoeba* and enteropathogenic bacteria modulates epithelial cell damage. *PLoS Negl Trop Dis* (2008) **2**:e266. doi:10.1371/ journal. pntd.0000266

Flint HJ, Scott KP, Duncan SH, Louis P, Forano E. Microbial degradation of complex carbohydrates in the gut. *Gut Microbes* (2012) **3**:289–306. doi:10.4161/gmic.19897

Pacheco AR, Curtis MM, Ritchie JM, Munera D, Waldor MK, Moreira CG, et al. Fucose sensing regulates bacterial intestinal colonization. *Nature* (2012) **492**:113–7. doi:10.1038/nature11623

Ng KM, Ferreyra JA, Higginbottom SK, Lynch JB, Kashyap PC, Gopinath S, et al. Microbiota-liberated host sugars facilitate post-antibiotic expansion of enteric pathogens. *Nature* (2013) **502**:96–9. doi:10.1038/nature12503

Tovy A, Hertz R, Siman-Tov R, Syan S, Faust DM, Guillen N, et al. Glucose starvation boosts *Entamoeba histolytica* virulence. *PLoS Negl Trop Dis* (2011) **5**:e1247. doi:10.1371/journal.pntd.0001247

Gilchrist CA, Baba DJ, Zhang Y, Crasta O, Evans C, Caler E, et al. Targets of the *Entamoeba histolytica* transcription factor URE3-BP. *PLoS Negl Trop Dis* (2008) **2**:e282. doi:10.1371/journal.pntd.0000282

Jumpertz R, Le DS, Turnbaugh PJ, Trinidad C, Bogardus C, Gordon JI, et al. Energy-balance studies reveal associations between gut microbes, caloric-load, and nutrient absorption in humans. *Am J Clin Nutr* (2011) **94**:58–65. doi:10.3945/ajcn.110.010132

Purchiaroni F, Tortora A, Gabrielli M, Bertucci F, Gigante G, Ianiro G, et al. The role of intestinal microbiota and the immune system. *Eur Rev Med Pharmacol Sci* (2013) **17**:323–33.

Donia MS, Fischbach MA. HUMAN MICROBIOTA. Small molecules from the human microbiota. *Science* (2015) **349**:1254766. doi:10.1126/ science.1254766

Mazmanian SK, Round JL, Kasper DL. A microbial symbiosis factor prevents intestinal inflammatory disease. *Nature* (2008) **453**:620–5. doi:10.1038/ nature07008

Atarashi K, Tanoue T, Shima T, Imaoka A, Kuwahara T, Momose Y, et al. Induction of colonic regulatory T cells by indigenous *Clostridium* species. *Science* (2011) **331**:337–41. doi:10.1126/science.1198469

Sakaguchi S. The origin of FOXP3-expressing CD4+ regulatory T cells: thy- mus or periphery. *J Clin Invest* (2003) **112**:1310–2. doi:10.1172/JCI200320274

Round JL, Lee SM, Li J, Tran G, Jabri B, Chatila TA, et al. The toll-like receptor 2 pathway establishes colonization by a commensal of the human microbiota. *Science* (2011) **332**:974–7. doi:10.1126/science.1206095

Hot A, Miossec P. Effects of interleukin (IL)-17A and IL-17F in human rheumatoid arthritis synoviocytes. *Ann Rheum Dis* (2011) **70**:727–32. doi:10.1136/ard.2010.143768

Scher JU, Abramson SB. The microbiome and rheumatoid arthritis. *Nat Rev Rheumatol* (2011) 7:569–78. doi:10.1038/nrrheum.2011.121

Romano-Keeler J, Weitkamp JH, Moore DJ. Regulatory properties of the intestinal microbiome effecting the development and treatment of diabetes. *Curr Opin Endocrinol Diabetes Obes* (2012) **19**:73–80. doi:10.1097/MED.0b013e3283514d43

Wu HJ, Wu E. The role of gut microbiota in immune homeostasis and autoimmunity. *Gut Microbes* (2012) **3**:4–14. doi:10.4161/gmic.19320

Jin C, Henao-Mejia J, Flavell RA. Innate immune receptors: key regulators of metabolic disease progression. *Cell Metab* (2013) **17**:873–82. doi:10.1016/j.cmet.2013.05.011

Erdman SE, Poutahidis T. Gut bacteria and cancer. *Biochim Biophys Acta* (2015) **1856**:86–90. doi:10.1016/j.bbcan.2015.05.007

Reed SL, Ember JA, Herdman DS, DiScipio RG, Hugli TE, Gigli I. The extracellular neutral cysteine proteinase of *Entamoeba histolytica* degrades anaphylatoxins C3a and C5a. *J Immunol* (1995) **155**:266–74.

Ankri S, Stolarsky T, Bracha R, Padilla-Vaca F, Mirelman D. Antisense inhibition of expression of cysteine proteinases affects *Entamoeba histolytica*-induced formation of liver abscess in hamsters. *Infect Immun* (1999) **67**:421–2.

Stanley SL Jr. Amoebiasis. *Lancet* (2003) **361**:1025–34. doi:10.1016/ S0140-6736(03)12830-9

Que X, Kim SH, Sajid M, Eckmann L, Dinarello CA, McKerrow JH, et al. A surface amebic cysteine proteinase inactivates interleukin-18. *Infect Immun* (2003) **71**:1274–80. doi:10.1128/IAI.71.3.1274-1280.2003

Kissoon-Singh V, Mortimer L, Chadee K. *Entamoeba histolytica* cathep- sin-like enzymes: interactions with the host gut. *Adv Exp Med Biol* (2011) **712**:62–83. doi:10.1007/978-1-4419-8414-2_5

Thibeaux R, Avé P, Bernier M, Morcelet M, Frileux P, Guillén N, et al. The parasite *Entamoeba histolytica* exploits the activities of human matrix metalloproteinases to invade colonic tissue. *Nat Commun* (2014) **5**:5142. doi:10.1038/ncomms6142

Corfield AP. Mucins: a biologically relevant glycan barrier in mucosal protection. *Biochim Biophys Acta* (2015) **1850**:236–52. doi:10.1016/j.bbagen.2014.05.003

Carlstedt I, Herrmann A, Karlsson H, Sheehan J, Fransson L, Hansson G. Characterization of two different glycosylated domains from the insoluble mucin complex of rat small intestine. *J Biol Chem* (1993) **268**:18771–81.

Herrmann A, Davies JR, Lindell G, Martensson S, Packer NH, Swallow DM, et al. Studies on the "insoluble" glycoprotein complex from human colon. Identification of reduction-insensitive MUC2 oligomers and C-terminal cleavage. *J Biol Chem* (1999) **274**:15828–36. doi:10.1074/jbc.274.22.15828

Moncada D, Keller K, Chadee K. *Entamoeba histolytica*-secreted products degrade colonic mucin oligosaccharides. *Infect Immun* (2005) 73:3790–3. doi:10.1128/IAI.73.6.3790-3793.2005

Connaris S, Greenwell P. Glycosidases in mucin-dwelling protozoans. *Glycoconj J* (1997) **14**:879–82. doi:10.1023/A:1018554408558

Huldt G, Davies P, Allison AC, Schorlemmer HU. Interactions between *Entamoeba histolytica* and complement. *Nature* (1979) **18**:214–6. doi:10.1038/277214a0

Arias-Negrete S, Sabanero-López M, Villagómez-Castro JC. Biochemical analysis of *Entamoeba histolytica* HM1 strain resistant to complement lysis. *Arch Med Res* (1992) **23**:135–7.

Sonnenburg JL, Xu J, Leip DD, Chen CH, Westover BP, Weatherford J, et al. Glycan foraging in vivo by an intestine-adapted bacterial symbiont. *Science* (2005) **307**:1955–9. doi:10.1126/science.1109051

Qin J, Li R, Raes J, Arumugam M, Burgdorf KS, Manichanh C, et al. A human gut microbial gene catalogue established by metagenomic sequencing. *Nature* (2010) **464**:59–65. doi:10.1038/nature08821

Irmer H, Tillack M, Biller L, Handal G, Leippe M, Roeder T, et al. Major cysteine peptidases of *Entamoeba histolytica* are required for aggregation and digestion of erythrocytes but are dispensable for phagocytosisand cytopathogenicity. *Mol Microbiol* (2009) **72**:658–67. doi:10.1111/j.1365-2958.2009.06672.x

Bruchhaus I, Jacobs T, Leippe M, Tannich E. *Entamoeba histolytica* and *Entamoebadispar*: differences in numbers and expression of cysteineproteinase genes. *Mol Microbiol* (1996) **22**:255–63. doi:10.1046/j.1365-2958.1996.00111.x

Willhoeft U, Hamann L, Tannich E. A DNA sequence corresponding to the gene encoding cysteine proteinase 5 in *Entamoeba histolytica* is present and positionally conserved but highly degenerated in *Entamoeba dispar*. *Infect Immun* (1999) **67**:5925–9.

Hellberg A, Nickel R, Lotter H, Tannich E, Bruchhaus I. Overexpression of cysteine proteinase 2 in *Entamoeba histolytica* or *Entamoeba dispar* increases amoeba-induced monolayer destruction in vitro but does not augment amoebic liver abscess formation in gerbils. *Cell Microbiol* (2001) **3**:13–20. doi:10.1046/j.1462-5822.2001.00086.x

Tillack M, Nowak N, Lotter H, Bracha R, Mirelman D, Tannich E, et al. Increased expression of the major cysteine proteinases by stable episomal transfection underlines the important role of EhCP5 for the pathogenicity of *Entamoeba histolytica*. *Mol Biochem Parasitol* (2006) **149**:58–64. doi:10.1016/j.molbiopara.2006.04.009

Freitas MA, Fernandes HC, Calixto VC, Martins AS, Silva EF, Pesquero JL, et al. *Entamoeba histolytica*: cysteine proteinase activity and virulence. Focus on cysteine proteinase 5 expression levels. *Exp Parasitol* (2009) **122**:306–9. doi:10.1016/j.exppara.2009.04.005

Hou Y, Mortimer L, Chadee K. *Entamoeba histolytica* cysteine proteinase 5 binds integrin on colonic cells and stimulates NFkappaB-mediated pro-inflammatory responses. *J Biol Chem* (2010) **285**:35497–504. doi:10.1074/jbc.M109.066035

Thibeaux R, Dufour A, Roux P, Bernier M, Baglin AC, Frileux P, et al. Newly visualized fibrillar collagen scaffolds dictate *Entamoeba histolytica* invasion route in the human colon. *Cell Microbiol* (2012) **14**:609–21. doi:10.1111/j.1462-5822.2012.01752.x

Mortimer L, Moreaum F, Cornick S, Chadee K. The NLRP3 Inflammasome is a pathogen sensor for invasive *Entamoeba histolytica* via activation of $\alpha 5\beta 1$ integrin at the macrophage-amebae intercellular junction. *PLoS Pathog* (2015) **11**:e1004887. doi:10.1371/journal.ppat.1004887

Mortimer L, Moreau F, Cornick S, Chadee K. Gal-lectindependent contact activates the inflammasome by invasive *Entamoeba histolytica*. *Mucosal Immunol* (2014) **7**:829–41. doi:10.1038/mi.2013.100

Leroy A, Mareel M, De Bruyne G, Bailey G, Nelis H. Metastasis of *Entamoeba histolytica* compared to colon cancer: one more step in invasion. *Invasion Metastasis* (1995) **14**:177–91.

Bernacki RJ, Niedbala MJ, Korytnyk W. Glycosidases in cancer and invasion. *Cancer Metastasis Rev* (1985) **4**:81–101. doi:10.1007/BF00047738

Liotta LA. Tumor invasion and metastases: role of the basement membrane. *Am J Pathol* (1984) **117**:339–48.

Coghlin C, Murray GI. Current and emerging concepts in tumour metastasis. *J Pathol* (2010) **222**:1–15. doi:10.1002/path.2727

Plucinsky MC, Prorok JJ, Alhadeff JA. Variant serum beta-hexosaminidase as a biochemical marker of malignancy. *Cancer* (1986) **58**:1484–7. doi:10.1002/1097-0142(19861001)58:7<1484:AID-CNCR2820580718>3.0.CO;2-R

Bosmann HB, Hall TC. Enzyme activity in invasive tumors of human breast and colon. *Proc Natl Acad Sci USA* (1974) **71**:1833–7. doi:10.1073/ pnas.71.5.1833

Gil-Martín E, Rodríguez-Berrocal J, Páez de la Cadena M, Fernández-Briera

Alterations of glycosidases in human colonic adenocarcinoma. *Clin Biochem* (1997) **30**:17–25. doi:10.1016/S0009-9120(96)00123-3

Ramessur KT, Greenwell P, Nash R, Dwek MV. Breast cancer invasion is mediated by beta-N-acetylglucosaminidase (beta-NAG) and associated with a dysregulation in the secretory pathway of cancer cells. *Br J Biomed Sci* (2010) **67**:189–96.

Choromańska B, Luto M, Szajda SD, Waszkiewicz N, Kępka A, Janica J, et al. Activity of N-acetyl-β-hexosaminidase and its isoenzymes A and B in cancer. *Postepy Hig Med Dosw (Online)* (2011) **65**:752–8. doi:10.5604/17322693.966833

Chadee K, Petri WA Jr, Innes DJ, Ravdin JI. Rat and human colonic mucins bind to and inhibit adherence lectin of *Entamoeba histolytica*. *J Clin Invest* (1987) **80**:1245–54. doi:10.1172/JCI113199

Saffer LD, Petri WA Jr. Role of the galactose lectin of *Entamoeba histolytica* in adherence-dependent killing of mammalian cells. *Infect Immun* (1991) **59**:4681–3.

Guerrant RL, Brush J, Ravdin JI, Sullivan JA, Mandell GL. Interaction between *Entamoeba histolytica* and human polymorphonuclear neutrophils. *J Infect Dis* (1981) **143**:83–93. doi:10.1093/infdis/143.1.83

Ravdin JI, Moreau F, Sullivan JA, Petri WA Jr, Mandell GL. Relationship of free intracellular calcium to the cytolytic activity of *Entamoeba histolytica*. *Infect Immun* (1988) **56**:505–12.

Huston CD, Boettner DR, Miller-Sims V, Petri WA Jr. Apoptotic killing and phagocytosis of host cells by the parasite *Entamoeba histolytica*. *Infect Immun* (2003) **71**:964–72. doi:10.1128/IAI.71.2.964-972.2003

Jacobs T, Bruchhaus I, Dandekar T, Tannich E, Leippe M. Isolation and molecular characterization of a surface-bound proteinase of *Entamoeba histolytica*. *Mol Microbiol* (1998) **27**:269–76. doi:10.1046/j.1365-2958.1998.00662.x

Garcia-Nieto RM, Rico-Mata R, Arias-Negrete S, Avila EE. Degradation of human secretory IgA1 and IgA2 by *Entamoeba histolytica* surface-associated proteolytic activity. *Parasitol Int* (2008) **57**:417–23. doi:10.1016/j.parint.2008.04.013

Macpherson AJ, McCoy KD, Johansen F, Brandtzaeg P. The immune geography of IgA induction and function. *Mucosal Immunol* (2008) **1**:11–22. doi:10.1038/mi.2007.6

Walport MJ. Complement: second of two parts. *N Engl J Med* (2001) **344**:1140–4. doi:10.1056/NEJM200104123441506

Köhl J. Anaphylatoxins and infectious and non-infectious inflammatory diseases. *Mol Immunol* (2001) **38**:175–87. doi:10.1016/S0161-5890(01)00041-4

Gasque P. Complement: a unique innate immune sensor for danger signals. *Mol Immunol* (2004) **41**:1089–98. doi:10.1016/j.molimm.2004.06.011

Zhang Z, Wang L, Seydel KB, Li E, Ankri S, Mirelman D, et al. *Entamoeba histolytica* cysteine proteinases with interleukin-1 beta converting enzyme (ICE) activity cause intestinal inflammation and tissue damage in amoebiasis. *Mol Microbiol* (2000) **37**:542–8. doi:10.1046/j.1365-2958.2000.02037.x

Mayor S, Riezman H. Sorting GPI-anchored proteins. *Nat Rev Mol Cell Biol* (2004) **5**:110–20. doi:10.1038/nrm1309

Fujita M, Kinoshita T. GPI-anchor remodeling: potential functions of GPI-anchors in intracellular trafficking and membrane dynamics. *Biochim Biophys Acta* (2012) **1821**:1050–8. doi:10.1016/j.bbalip.2012.01.004

Saha S, Anilkumar AA, Mayor S. GPI-anchored protein organization and dynamics at the cell surface. *J Lipid Res* (2015). doi:10.1194/jlr.R062885

Isibasi A, Santa Cruz M, Soto Montano X, Ramirez A, Kumate J. Localization of a lipopeptidophosphoglycan extracted by phenol-water from trophozoites of the HK-9 strain of *Entamoeba histolytica*. *Arch Invest Med (Mex)* (1982) **13**:57–62.

Guha-Niyogi A, Sullivan DR, Turco SJ. Glycoconjugate structures of parasitic protozoa. *Glycobiology* (2001) **11**:45R–59R. doi:10.1093/glycob/11.4.45R

Bhattacharya A, Arya R, Clark CG, Ackers JP. Absence of lipophosphogly- can-like glycoconjugates in *Entamoeba dispar*. *Parasitology* (2000) **120**:31–5. doi:10.1017/S0031182099005259

Weber C, Blazquez S, Marion S, Ausseur C, Vats D, Krzeminski M, et al. Bioinformatics and functional analysis of an *Entamoeba histolytica* mannosyltransferase necessary for parasite complement resistance and hepatical infection. *PLoS Negl Trop Dis* (2008) **2**:e165. doi:10.1371/journal.pntd.0000165

Braga L, Ninomiya H, McCoy JJ, Eacker S, Wiedmer T, Pham C, etal. Inhibition of the complement membrane attack complex by the galactose-specific adhesion of *Entamoeba histolytica*. *J Clin Invest* (1992) **90**:1131–7. doi:10.1172/JCI115931

Ventura-Juárez J, Campos-Rodríguez R, Jarillo-Luna RA, Muñoz-Fernández L, Escario-G-Trevijano JA, Pérez-Serrano J, et al. Trophozoites of Entamoeba histolytica express a CD59-like molecule in human colon. *Parasitol Res* (2009) **104**:821–6. doi:10.1007/s00436-008-1262-3

Calderón J, de Lourdes Muñoz M, Acosta HM. Surface redistribution and release of antibody-induced caps in entamoebae. *J Exp Med* (1980) **151**:184–93. doi:10.1084/jem.151.1.184

Baxt LA, Baker RP, Singh U, Urban S. An *Entamoeba histolytica* rhomboid protease with atypical specificity cleaves a surface lectin involved in phagocytosis and immune evasion. *Genes Dev* (2008) **22**:1636–46. doi:10.1101/gad.1667708

Bailey GB, Day DB, McCoomer NE. Entamoeba motility: dynamics of cytoplasmic streaming, locomotion and translocation of surface bound particles, and organization of the actin cytoskeleton in *Entamoeba invadens*. *J Protozool* (1992) **39**:267–72. doi:10.1111/j.1550-7408.1992.tb01313.x

Espinosa-Cantellano M, Martínez-Palomo A. *Entamoeba histolytica*: mechanism of surface receptor capping. *Exp Parasitol* (1994) **79**:424–35. doi:10.1006/expr.1994.1104

Baker RP, Wijetilaka R, Urban S. Two *Plasmodium* rhomboid proteases preferentially cleave different adhesins implicated in all invasive stages of malaria. *PLoS Pathog* (2006) **2**:e113. doi:10.1371/journal.ppat.0020113

Ragland BD, Ashley LS, Vaux DL, Petri WA Jr. *Entamoeba histolytica*: target cells killed by trophozoites undergo DNA fragmentation which is not blocked by Bcl-2. *Exp Parasitol* (1994) **79**:460–7. doi:10.1006/expr.1994.1107

Huston CD, Houpt ER, Mann BJ, Hahn CS, Petri WA Jr. Caspase 3-dependent killing of host cells by the parasite *Entamoeba histolytica*. *Cell Microbiol* (2000) **2**:617–25. doi:10.1046/j.1462-5822.2000.00085.x

Sim S, Yong TS, Park SJ, Im KI, Kong Y, Ryu JS, et al. NADPH oxidase-derived reactive oxygen species-mediated activation of ERK1/2 is required for apoptosis of human neutrophils induced by *Entamoeba histolytica*. *J Immunol* (2005) **174**:4279–88. doi:10.4049/jimmunol.174.7.4279

Berninghausen O, Leippe M. Necrosis versus apoptosis as the mechanism of target cell death induced by *Entamoeba histolytica*. *Infect Immun* (1997) **65**:3615–21.

Boettner DR, Huston CD, Linford AS, Buss SN, Houpt E, Sherman NE, et al. *Entamoeba histolytica* phagocytosis of human erythrocytes involves PATMK, a member of the transmembrane kinase family. *PLoS Pathog* (2008) **4**:e8. doi:10.1371/journal.ppat.0040008

Ralston KS, Petri WA Jr. Tissue destruction and invasion by *Entamoeba histolytica*. *Trends Parasitol* (2011) **27**:254–63. doi:10.1016/j.pt.2011. 02.006

Fadok VA, Bratton DL, Konowal A, Freed PW, Westcott JY, Henson PM. Macrophages that have ingested apoptotic cells in vitro inhibit proinflammatory cytokine production through autocrine/paracrine mechanisms involving TGF-beta, PGE2, and PAF. *J Clin Invest* (1998) **101**:890–8. doi:10.1172/JCI1112

Poon IK, Lucas CD, Rossi AG, Ravichandran KS. Apoptotic cell clearance: basic biology and therapeutic potential. *Nat Rev Immunol* (2014) **14**:166–80. doi:10.1038/nri3607

Orozco E, Guarneros G, Martinez-Palomo A, Sánchez T. *Entamoeba histolytica*: phagocytosis as a virulence factor. *J Exp Med* (1983) **158**:1511–21. doi:10.1084/jem.158.5.1511

Rodríguez MA, Orozco E. Isolation and characterization of phagocytosis- and virulence-deficient mutants of *Entamoeba histolytica*. *J Infect Dis* (1986) **154**:27–32. doi:10.1093/infdis/154.1.27

Teixeira JE, Heron BT, Huston CD. C1q- and collectin-dependent phagocy- tosis of apoptotic host cells by the intestinal protozoan *Entamoeba histolytica*. *J Infect Dis* (2008) **198**:1062–70. doi:10.1086/591628

Vaithilingam A, Teixeira JE, Miller PJ, Heron BT, Huston CD. *Entamoeba histolytica* cell surface calreticulin binds human C1q and functions in amebic phagocytosis of host cells. *Infect Immun* (2012) **80**:2008–18. doi:10.1128/IAI.06287-11

Somlata, Bhattacharya S, Bhattacharya A. A C2 domain protein kinase initiates phagocytosis in the protozoan parasite *Entamoeba histolytica*. *Nat Commun* (2011) **2**:230. doi:10.1038/ncomms1199

Mansuri MS, Bhattacharya S, Bhattacharya A. A novel alpha kinase EhAK1 phosphorylates actin and regulates phagocytosis in *Entamoeba histolytica*. *PLoS Pathog* (2014) **10**:e1004411. doi:10.1371/journal.ppat.1004411

Ralston KS, Solga MD, Mackey-Lawrence NM, Somlata, Bhattacharya A, Petri WA Jr. Trogocytosis by *Entamoeba histolytica* contributes to cell killing and tissue invasion. *Nature* (2014) **508**:526–30. doi:10.1038/nature13242

Guo X, Stroup SE, Houpt E. Persistence of *Entamoeba histolytica* infection in CBA mice owes to intestinal IL-4 production and inhibition of protective IFN-γ. *Mucosal Immunol* (2008) **1**:139–46. doi:10.1038/mi.2007.18

Petri WA Jr, Mondal D, Peterson KM, Duggal P, Haque R. Association of malnutrition with amebiasis. *Nutr Rev* (2009) **67**:S207–15. doi:10.1111/j.1753-4887.2009.00242.x

Acuna-Soto R, Maguire JH, Wirth DF. Gender distribution in asymp- tomatic and invasive amebiasis. *Am J Gastroenterol* (2000) **95**:1277–83. doi:10.1111/j.1572-0241.2000.01525.x

Blessmann J, Van Linh P, Nu PA, Thi HD, Muller-Myhsok B, Buss H, et al. Epidemiology of amebiasis in a region of high incidence of amebic liver abscess in central Vietnam. *Am J Trop Med Hyg* (2002) **66**:578–83.

Blessmann J, Ali IK, Nu PA, Dinh BT, Viet TQ, Van AL, et al. Longitudinal study of intestinal *Entamoeba histolytica* infections in asymptomatic adult carriers. *J Clin Microbiol* (2003) **41**:4745–50. doi:10.1128/JCM.41.10.4745- 4750.2003

Lotter H, Helk E, Bernin H, Jacobs T, Prehn C, Adamski J, et al. Testosterone increases susceptibility to amebic liver abscess in mice and mediates inhibition of IFNγ secretion in natural killer T cells. *PLoS One* (2013) **8**:e55694. doi:10.1371/journal.pone.0055694

Madsen KL, Malfair D, Gray D, Doyle JS, Jewell LD, Fedorak RN. Interleukin-10 gene-deficient mice develop a primary intestinal permeability defect in response to enteric microflora. *Inflamm Bowel Dis* (1999) **5**:262–70. doi:10.1097/00054725-199911000-00004

Hamano S, Asgharpour A, Stroup SE, Wynn TA, Leiter EH, Houpt E. Resistance of C57BL/6 mice to amoebiasis is mediated by nonhemopoi- etic cells but requires hemopoietic IL-10 production. *J Immunol* (2006) **177**:1208–13. doi:10.4049/jimmunol.177.2.1208

Ruiz PA, Shkoda A, Kim SC, Sartor RB, Haller D. IL-10 gene-deficient mice lack TGF-beta/Smad signaling and fail to inhibit proinflammatory gene expression in intestinal epithelial cells after the colonization with colitogenic *Enterococcus faecalis*. *J Immunol* (2005) **174**:2990–9. doi:10.4049/jimmunol.174.5.2990

Schwerbrock NM, Makkink MK, van der Sluis M, Buller HA, Einerhand AW, Sartor RB, et al. Interleukin 10-deficient mice exhibit defective colonic Muc2 synthesis before and after induction of colitis by commensal bacteria. *Inflamm Bowel Dis* (2004) **10**:811–23. doi:10.1097/00054725-200411000-00016

Grazia Roncarolo M, Bacchetta R, Bordignon C, Narula S, Levings MK. Type 1 T regulatory cells. *Immunol Rev* (2001) **182**:68–79. doi:10.1034/j.1600-065X.2001.1820105.x

Zhou P, Streutker C, Borojevic R, Wang Y, Croitoru K. IL-10 modulates intestinal damage and epithelial cell apoptosis in T cell-mediated enteropathy. *Am J Physiol* (2004) **287**:G599–604. doi:10.1152/ajpgi.00063.2004

Maldonaldo-Bernal C, Kirschning CJ, Rosenstein Y, Rocha LM, Rios-Sarabia N, Espinosa-Cantellano M, et al. The innate immune response to *Entamoeba histolytica* lipopeptidophosphoglycan is medi- ated by toll-like receptors 2 and 4. *Parasite Immunol* (2005) **2**:127–37. doi:10.1111/j.1365-3024.2005.00754.x

Maldonado C, Trejo W, Ramirez A, Carrera M, Sánchez J, López-Macías C, et al. Lipophosphopeptidoglycan of *Entamoeba histolytica* induces an anti-inflammatory innate immune response and downregulation of toll-like receptor 2 (TLR-2) gene expression in human monocytes. *Arch Med Res* (2000) **31**:S71–3. doi:10.1016/S0188-4409(00)00199-5

Kammanadiminti SJ, Chadeem K. Suppression of NF-kappaB activation by *Entamoeba histolytica* in intestinal epithelial cells is mediated by heat shock protein 27. *J Biol Chem* (2006) **281**:26112–20. doi:10.1074/jbc. M601988200

Cho KN, Becker SM, Houpt ER. The NF-kappaB p50 subunit is protective during intestinal *Entamoeba histolytica* infection of 129 and C57BL/6 mice. *Infect Immun* (2010) **78**:1475–81. doi:10.1128/IAI.00669-09

Nenci A, Becker C, Wullaert A, Gareus R, van Loo G, Danese S, et al. Epithelial NEMO links innate immunity to chronic intestinal inflammation. *Nature* (2007) **446**:557–61. doi:10.1038/nature05698

Artis D. Epithelial-cell recognition of commensal bacteria and maintenance of immune homeostasis in the gut. *Nat Rev Immunol* (2008) **8**:411–20. doi:10.1038/nri2316

Ivory C, Kammanadiminti S, Chadee K. Innate resistance to *Entamoeba histolytica* in murine models. *Trends Parasitol* (2007) **23**:46–8. doi:10.1016/j.pt.2006.12.006

Dey I, Chadee K. Prostaglandin E2 produced by *Entamoeba histolytica* binds to EP4 receptors and stimulates interleukin-8 production in human colonic cells. *Infect Immun* (2008) **6**:5158–63. doi:10.1128/IAI.00645-08

Lejeune M, Moreau F, Chadee K. Prostaglandin E2 produced by *Entamoeba histolytica* signals via EP4 receptor and alters claudin-4 to increase ion permeability of tight junctions. *Am J Pathol* (2011) **179**:807–18. doi:10.1016/j.ajpath.2011.05.001

Belley A, Chadee K. Prostaglandin E(2) stimulates rat and human colonic mucin exocytosis via the EP(4) receptor. *Gastroenterology* (1999) **117**:1352–62. doi:10.1016/S0016-5085(99)70285-4

Moncada D, Keller K, Chadee K. *Entamoeba histolytica* cysteine proteinases disrupt the polymeric structure of colonic mucin and alter its protective func- tion. *Infect Immun* (2003) **71**:838–44. doi:10.1128/IAI.71.2.838-844.2003

Wang W, Keller K, Chadee K. *Entamoeba histolytica* modulates the nitric oxide synthase gene and nitric oxide production by macrophages for cyto- toxicity against amoebae and tumour cells. *Immunology* (1994) **83**:601–10.

Wang W, Chadee K. *Entamoeba histolytica* suppresses gamma interferon-induced macrophage class II major histocompatibility complex Ia molecule and I-Aβ mRNA expression by a prostaglandin E2-dependent mechanism. *Infect Immun* (1995) **63**:1089–94.

Verma AK, Verma R, Ahuja V, Paul J. Real-time analysis of gut flora in *Entamoeba histolytica* infected patients of northern India. *BMC Microbiol* (2012) **12**:183. doi:10.1186/1471-2180-12-183

Bracha R, Kobiler D, Mirelman D. Attachment and ingestion of bacteria by trophozoites of *Entamoeba histolytica*. *Infect Immun* (1982) **36**:396–406.

Cobo ER, He C, Hirata K, Hwang G, Tran U, Eckmann L, et al. *Entamoeba histolytica* induces intestinal cathelicidins but is resistant to cathelicidin-mediated killing. *Infect Immun* (2012) **80**:143–9. doi:10.1128/IAI.05029-11

Burgess SL, Buonomo E, Carey M, Cowardin C, Naylor C, Noor Z, et al. Bone marrow dendritic cells from mice with an altered microbiota provide interleukin 17A-dependent protection against *Entamoeba histolytica* colitis. *MBio* (2014) **5**:e01817. doi:10.1128/mBio.01817-14

Band RN, Cirrito H. Growth response of axenic *Entamoeba histolytica* to hydrogen, carbon dioxide, and oxygen. *J Protozool* (1979) **26**:282–6. doi:10.1111/j.1550-7408.1979.tb02781.x

Mehlotra RK. Antioxidant defense mechanisms in parasitic protozoa. *Crit Rev Microbiol* (1996) **22**:295–314. doi:10.3109/10408419609105484

Weinbach EC, Diamond LS. *Entamoeba histolytica*. I. Aerobic metabolism. *Exp Parasitol* (1974) **35**:232–43. doi:10.1016/0014-4894(74)90027-7

Vicente JB, Ehrenkaufer GM, Saraiva LM, Teixeira M, Singh U. *Entamoeba histolytica* modulates a complex repertoire of novel genes in response to oxidative and nitrosative stresses: implications for amebic pathogenesis. *Cell Microbiol* (2009) **11**:51–69. doi:10.1111/j.1462-5822.2008.01236.x

Rastew E, Vicente JB, Singh U. Oxidative stress resistance genes contribute to the pathogenic potential of the anaerobic protozoan parasite, *Entamoeba histolytica*. *Int J Parasitol* (2012) **42**:1007–15. doi:10.1016/j.ijpara.2012.08.006

Schlosser S, Leitschm D, Duchêne M. *Entamoeba histolytica*: identification of thioredoxin-targeted proteins and analysis of serine acetyltransferase-1 as a prototype example. *Biochem J* (2013) **451**:277–88. doi:10.1042/BJ20121798

Debnath A, Parsonage D, Andrade RM, He C, Cobo ER, Hirata K, et al. A high-throughput drug screen for *Entamoeba histolytica* identifies a new lead and target. *Nat Med* (2012) **18**:956–60. doi:10.1038/nm.2758

Leitsch D, Kolarich D, Wilson IB, Altmann F, Duchêne M. Nitroimidazole action in *Entamoeba histolytica*: a central role for thioredoxin reductase. *PLoS Biol* (2007) **5**:e211. doi:10.1371/journal.pbio.0050211

Husain A, Sato D, Jeelani G, Soga T, Nozaki T. Dramatic increase in glycerol biosynthesis upon oxidative stress in the anaerobic protozoan parasite *Entamoeba histolytica*. *PLoS Negl Trop Dis* (2012) **6**:e1831. doi:10.1371/journal.pntd.0001831

Jeelani G, Nozaki T. Entamoeba thiol-based redox metabolism: a potential target for drug development. *Mol Biochem Parasitol* (2016). doi:10.1016/j.molbiopara.2016.01.004

Permissions

All chapters in this book were first published by Frontiers; hereby published with permission under the Creative Commons Attribution License or equivalent. Every chapter published in this book has been scrutinized by our experts. Their significance has been extensively debated. The topics covered herein carry significant findings which will fuel the growth of the discipline. They may even be implemented as practical applications or may be referred to as a beginning point for another development.

The contributors of this book come from diverse backgrounds, making this book a truly international effort. This book will bring forth new frontiers with its revolutionizing research information and detailed analysis of the nascent developments around the world.

We would like to thank all the contributing authors for lending their expertise to make the book truly unique. They have played a crucial role in the development of this book. Without their invaluable contributions this book wouldn't have been possible. They have made vital efforts to compile up to date information on the varied aspects of this subject to make this book a valuable addition to the collection of many professionals and students.

This book was conceptualized with the vision of imparting up-to-date information and advanced data in this field. To ensure the same, a matchless editorial board was set up. Every individual on the board went through rigorous rounds of assessment to prove their worth. After which they invested a large part of their time researching and compiling the most relevant data for our readers.

The editorial board has been involved in producing this book since its inception. They have spent rigorous hours researching and exploring the diverse topics which have resulted in the successful publishing of this book. They have passed on their knowledge of decades through this book. To expedite this challenging task, the publisher supported the team at every step. A small team of assistant editors was also appointed to further simplify the editing procedure and attain best results for the readers.

Apart from the editorial board, the designing team has also invested a significant amount of their time in understanding the subject and creating the most relevant covers. They scrutinized every image to scout for the most suitable representation of the subject and create an appropriate cover for the book.

The publishing team has been an ardent support to the editorial, designing and production team. Their endless efforts to recruit the best for this project, has resulted in the accomplishment of this book. They are a veteran in the field of academics and their pool of knowledge is as vast as their experience in printing. Their expertise and guidance has proved useful at every step. Their uncompromising quality standards have made this book an exceptional effort. Their encouragement from time to time has been an inspiration for everyone.

The publisher and the editorial board hope that this book will prove to be a valuable piece of knowledge for researchers, students, practitioners and scholars across the globe.

List of Contributors

Koushik Das
Graduate School of Medicine, The University of Tokyo, Bunkyō, Japan

Francisco Javier Rendón-Gandarilla, Víctor Álvarez-Hernández, Elizabeth J. Castañeda-Ortiz, Helios Cárdenas-Hernández, Rosa Elena Cárdenas-Guerra, Lilia López-Canovas and Elisa Azuara-Liceaga
Posgrado en Ciencias Genómicas, Universidad Autónoma de la Ciudad de Mexico, Mexico City, Mexico

Bibiana Chávez-Munguía and Anel Lagunes-Guillen and Dxinegueela Zanatta
Departamento de Infectómica y Patogénesis Molecular, Centro de Investigación y de Estudios Avanzados del Instituto Politécnico Nacional, Mexico City, Mexico

Esther Orozco
Departamento de Infectómica y Patogénesis Molecular, Centro de Investigación y de Estudios Avanzados del Instituto Politécnico Nacional, Mexico City, Mexico

Enrique Gonzalez Rivas, Cecilia Ximenez, Miriam Enriqueta Nieves-Ramirez, Patricia Moran Silva, Oswaldo Partida-Rodríguez, Eric Hernandez Hernandez, Liliana Rojas Velázquez, Angelica Serrano Vázquez and Ulises Magaña Nuñez
Laboratorio de Inmunología, Unidad de Investigación de Medicina Experimental, Facultad de Medicina, Universidad Nacional Autónoma de México (UNAM), Ciudad de Mexico, Mexico

Mark Bonner
International Institute of Periodontology, Victoriaville, QC, Canada

Manuel Fresno and Núria Gironès
Centro de Biología Molecular Severo Ochoa, Consejo Superior de Investigaciones Científicas, Universidad Autónoma de Madrid, Madrid, Spain
Instituto de Investigación Sanitaria del Hospital Universitario de La Princesa, Madrid, Spain

Nancy Guillén
Institut Pasteur, Paris, France Centre National de la Recherche Scientifique, CNRSERL9195, Paris, France

Julien Santi-Rocca
Science and Healthcare for Oral Welfare, Toulouse, France

Natsuki Watanabe
Department of Parasitology, National Institute of Infectious Diseases, Tokyo, Japan
Graduate School of Life and Environmental Sciences, University of Tsukuba, Tsukuba, Japan

Tomohiko Maehama
Division of Molecular and Cellular Biology, Graduate School of Medicine, Kobe University, Kobe, Japan

Preeti Shahi, France Moreau and Kris Chadee
Department of Microbiology, Immunology and Infectious Diseases, Snyder Institute for Chronic Diseases, University of Calgary, Calgary, AB, Canada

Diana Torres-Cifuentes and José M. Galindo-Rosales
RNA Laboratory, Department of Biochemistry, Centro de Investigación y de Estudios Avanzados del Instituto Politécnico Nacional, Mexico City, Mexico

Odila Saucedo-Cárdenas
Departamento de Histología, Facultad de Medicina, Universidad Autónoma de Nuevo León, Monterrey, Mexico
División de Genética, Centro de Investigación Biomédica del Noreste, Instituto Mexicano del Seguro Social, Monterrey, Mexico

Jesús Valdés
Departamento de Bioquímica, Centro de Investigación y de Estudios Avanzados del Instituto Politécnico Nacional, Mexico City, Mexico
RNA Laboratory, Department of Biochemistry, Centro de Investigación y de Estudios Avanzados del Instituto Politécnico Nacional, Mexico City, Mexico

María S. Mendoza-Figueroa
Departamento de Bioquímica, Centro de Investigación y de Estudios Avanzados del Instituto Politécnico Nacional, Mexico City, Mexico
Departamento de Atención a la Salud, Universidad Autónoma Metropolitana-Xochimilco, Mexico City, Mexico

Eddy E. Alfonso-Maqueira
Departamento de Bioquímica, Centro de Investigación y de Estudios Avanzados del Instituto Politécnico Nacional, Mexico City, Mexico

Cristina Vélez
Departamento de Biología Celular, Centro de Investigación y de Estudios Avanzados del Instituto Politécnico Nacional, Mexico City, Mexico

Elisa I. Azuara-Liceaga and Selene Zárate
Posgrado en Ciencias Genómicas, Universidad Autónoma de la Ciudad de Mexico, Mexico City, Mexico

Nicolás Villegas-Sepúlveda
Departamento de Biomedicina Molecular, Centro de Investigación y de Estudios Avanzados del Instituto Politécnico Nacional, Mexico City, Mexico

César Díaz-Godínez, Zayda Fonseca, Juan P. Laclette, Carlos Rosales and Julio C. Carrero
Laboratory of Immunology, Department of Immunology, Instituto de Investigaciones Biomédicas, Universidad Nacional Autónoma de México, Mexico City, Mexico
Departamento de Inmunología, Instituto de Investigaciones Biomédicas, Universidad Nacional Autónoma de México, Mexico City, Mexico

Mario Néquiz
Laboratory of Immunopathology, Department of Experimental Medicine, Hospital General de México, Facultad de Medicina, Universidad Nacional Autónoma de México, Mexico City, Mexico

Itzel López-Rosas
Catedrática CONACYT, Laboratorio de Genómica Funcional y Biología Molecular, Colegio de Postgraduados Campus Campeche, Campeche, Mexico
CONACyT Research Fellow - Colegio de Postgraduados Campus Campeche, Campeche, Mexico

César López-Camarillo, Yarely M. Salinas-Vera, Olga N. Hernández-de la Cruz, María Elizbeth Álvarez Sánchez
Posgrado en Ciencias Genómicas, Universidad Autónoma de la Ciudad de Mexico, Mexico City, Mexico

Carlos Palma-Flores
Catedrático CONACYT, Instituto Politécnico Nacional, Mexico City, Mexico

Osbaldo Resendis-Antonio
Instituto Nacional de Medicina Genómica y Coordinación de la Investigación Científica, Red de Apoyo a la Investigación, Universidad Nacional Autónoma de Mexico, Mexico City, Mexico

Carlos Pérez-Plasencia
Unidad de Biomedicina, Facultad de Estudios Superiores-Iztacala, Universidad Nacional Autónoma de México, Mexico City, Mexico
Instituto Nacional de Cancerología, Mexico City, Mexico

Esther Ramírez-Moreno and Laurence A. Marchat
Programa en Biomedicina Molecular y Red de Biotecnología, Escuela Nacional de Medicina y Homeopatía, Instituto Politécnico Nacional, Mexico City, Mexico
Escuela Nacional de Medicina y Homeopatía, Instituto Politécnico Nacional, Ciudad de Mexico, Mexico City, Mexico

Jesús Valdés-Flores
Departamento de Bioquímica, CINVESTAV, Ciudad de Mexico, Mexico City, Mexico

Juan D. Ospina-Villa
Escuela Nacional de Medicina y Homeopatía, Instituto Politécnico Nacional, Ciudad de Mexico, Mexico City, Mexico

Abigail Betanzos
Consejo Nacional de Ciencia y Tecnología, Mexico City, Mexico
Departamento de Infectómica y Patogénesis Molecular, Centro de Investigación y de Estudios Avanzados del Instituto Politécnico Nacional, Mexico City, Mexico

Cecilia Bañuelos
Coordinación General de Programas de Posgrado Multidisciplinarios, Programa de Doctorado Transdisciplinario en Desarrollo Científico y Tecnológico para la Sociedad, Centro de Investigación y de Estudios Avanzados del Instituto Politécnico Nacional, Mexico City, Mexico

Elizabeth Hernández-Nava
Programa de Cáncer de Ovario, Instituto Nacional de Cancerología, Mexico City, Mexico

Patricia Cuellar
Centro Regional de Educación Superior, Universidad Autónoma de Guerrero, Chilpancingo, Mexico

Carlos Ortuño-Pineda
Unidad Académica de Ciencias Químico Biológicas, Universidad Autónoma de Guerrero, Chilpancingo, Mexico

Nancy Mora and Omar R. Alemán
Departamento de Inmunología, Instituto de Investigaciones Biomédicas, Universidad Nacional Autónoma de México, Mexico City, Mexico

Eileen Uribe-Querol
División de Estudios de Posgrado e Investigación, Facultad de Odontología, Universidad Nacional Autónoma de México, Mexico City, Mexico

Alma Nieto, David G. Pérez Ishiwara, Virginia Sánchez Monroy and Consuelo Gómez García
Laboratorio de Biomedicina Molecular I, Escuela Nacional de Medicina y Homeopatía, Instituto Politécnico Nacional, Mexico City, Mexico

Kumiko Nakada-Tsukui
Department of Parasitology, National Institute of Infectious Diseases, Tokyo, Japan

Tomoyoshi Nozaki
Department of Parasitology, National Institute of Infectious Diseases, Tokyo, Japan
Graduate School of Life and Environmental Sciences, University of Tsukuba, Tsukuba, Japan
Department of Biomedical Chemistry, Graduate School of Medicine, The University of Tokyo, Tokyo, Japan
Graduate School of Medicine, The University of Tokyo, Bunkyō, Japan

Index

O

P

R

S

T

U

V

www.ingramcontent.com/pod-product-compliance
Lightning Source LLC
LaVergne TN
LVHW081023210926
848485LV00004B/938

* 9 7 8 1 6 3 9 2 7 8 6 7 1 *